weightwatchers

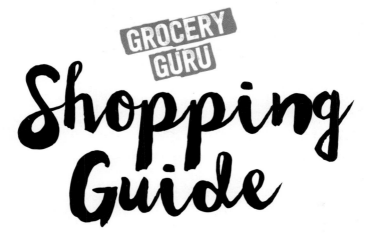

GROCERY GURU

Shopping Guide

WEIGHT WATCHERS is the registered trademark of Weight Watchers International, Inc. The SmartPoints Weight Loss System, trademark, and formula are proprietary to Weight Watchers International, Inc. U.S. patent pending.

©2015 Weight Watchers International, Inc. All rights reserved.

Printed in U.S. A.

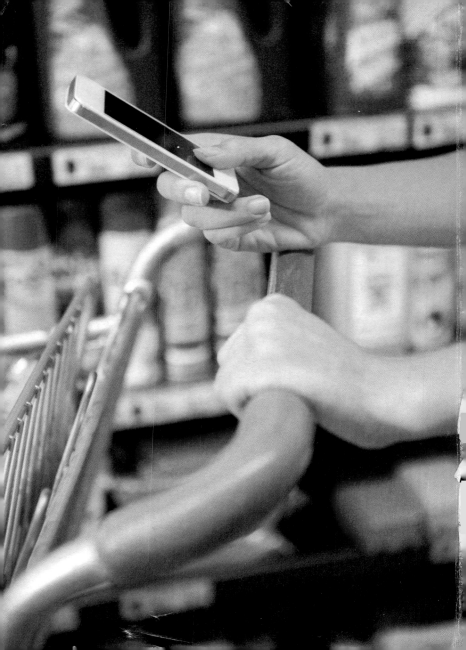

Table of *contents*

welcome to Grocery Guru

2016 is going to be a great year! We've updated the Program, and in your hands are some of the results. With SmartPoints™ values for all the foods members love, you'll be on your way to reaching your weight-loss goals.

In this **book** you will find:

- SmartPoints™ values for each and every food item listed.

- Our indispensable **Complete A-Z Food List,** streamlined to focus on the items members track most. And for those following the **Simply Filling** technique, no-count foods are marked with an icon (**O**) to make finding them easy.

- The latest **Brand Name Food List,** filled with thousands and thousands of items members track most. Each section begins with a shopping guide to help you find what you're looking for fast.

- The latest list of **Weight Watchers Food Products** available in grocery stores, and at participating meeting room locations.

- A user-friendly **Index,** with all the categories of our brand-name listings alphabetized, along with their page numbers, to make finding what you're looking for a cinch.

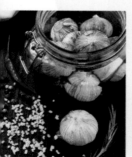
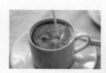
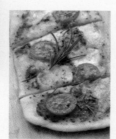
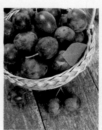

A note about branded foods:

In order to help make finding what you're looking for and comparison shopping easier, products in the **Brand Name Food List** are grouped by category. However, for many products there are numerous categories into which a product could be placed. Therefore, if you can't find the product you're looking for in a specific category, try another category. The **Index** at the end of the book is a great resource for finding categories, and the pages where they begin.

Inclusion of the products in this book does not imply endorsement or sponsorship of such products by Weight Watchers International, Inc. Endorsed products are specifically marked as such on the products' labels.

A note about the SmartPoints™ value for each listing:

The SmartPoints™ values for the foods in this book were calculated by Weight Watchers International, Inc. using the most current nutrition information supplied by manufacturers and available from the USDA at the time of the book's publication. However, since product formulations may change during the year, it's a good idea to continue to use the nutrition labels on products to confirm SmartPoints™ values.

One more thing to keep in mind:

Note that the alcohol content of certain foods, especially alcoholic beverages, can impact their total SmartPoints™ values. Because alcohol is not typically included on nutrition labels, you might notice discrepancies with the values of alcoholic beverages you see in these lists and that you calculate with nutrition information. For beverages that contain alcohol, as with all the products in this book, you can feel confident using the SmartPoints™ values listed here.

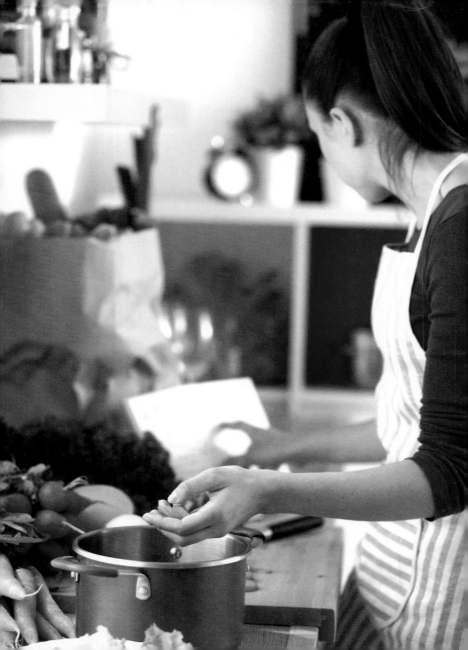

Complete A-Z
food list

Complete A-Z Food List

A

Alcoholic beverages

bourbon, 1 ½ fl oz	4
brandy, 1 ½ fl oz	3
cognac, 1 ½ fl oz	4
crème de menthe, 1 ½ fl oz	8
gin, 1 ½ fl oz	3
Irish cream, 1 ½ fl oz	6
kahlua, 1 ½ fl oz	8
liqueur, any type other than those listed here, 1 ½ fl oz	9
liqueur, coffee with cream, 34 proof, 1 ½ fl oz	7
liqueur, coffee, 63 proof, 1 ½ fl oz	11
liqueur, orange-flavored, 1 ½ fl oz	7
mirin, 1 fl oz	1
rum, 1 ½ fl oz	3
sake, 1 fl oz	1
schnapps, any flavor, 1 ½ fl oz	13
scotch, 1 ½ fl oz	3
tequila, 1 ½ fl oz	3
vodka, 1 ½ fl oz	3
vodka, raspberry-flavored, 1 ½ fl oz	3
whiskey, 1 ½ fl oz	3

Alcoholic mixed drinks

bay breeze, 5 ½ fl oz	7
bellini, 6 fl oz	6
black Russian, 3 fl oz	11
bloody Mary, 5 fl oz	5
brandy Alexander, 3 fl oz	13
chocolate mudslide, frozen, 12 fl oz	42
cosmopolitan, 3 ½ fl oz	7
daiquiri, 3 fl oz	7
daiquiri, strawberry, frozen, 7 fl oz	11
gin and diet tonic, 5 fl oz	4
gin and tonic, 5 fl oz	6
gin gimlet, 2 ½ fl oz	5
highball, 5 fl oz	6
Jack and cola, 5 fl oz	6
Jack and diet cola, 5 fl oz	4
kamikazi, 4 ½ fl oz	15
Long Island iced tea, 8 fl oz	18
mai tai, 3 ½ fl oz	11
Manhattan, 4 fl oz	10
Manhattan, dry, 4 fl oz	10
Manhattan, perfect, 4 fl oz	10
Manhattan, scotch, 4 fl oz	10
Margarita, 6 fl oz	11
martini, 2 fl oz	6
martini, chocolate, 2 ½ fl oz	7
martini, sour apple, 3 fl oz	10
mimosa, 6 fl oz	4
mojito, 12 fl oz	8
old-fashioned, 4 fl oz	12
piña colada, 6 fl oz	16
piña colada, canned, 3 fl oz	9
Rob Roy, 4 fl oz	10
rum and cola, 5 fl oz	6
rum and diet cola, 5 fl oz	4
sakatini, 3 fl oz	6
screwdriver, 6 fl oz	7
sex on the beach, 6 fl oz	8
Singapore sling, 6 fl oz	8
tequila sunrise, canned, 3 fl oz	3
Tom Collins, 6 fl oz	4
vodka and cranberry juice, 5 fl oz	7
vodka and diet soda, 5 fl oz	4
vodka gimlet, 3 fl oz	5
vodka tonic, 5 fl oz	6
vodka, flavored, and soda, any type, 5 fl oz	4
whiskey sour, 4 fl oz	7
whiskey sour (prepared from mix), 1 ½ fl oz	2

● No Count	SmartPoints™ value
whiskey sour (prepared with water, whiskey, and powder mix), 3 ½ fl oz	8
white Russian, 3 fl oz	10
All-fruit spread	
1 Tbsp	2
Almond milk	
plain, unsweetened, 8 fl oz	1
Almond paste	
firmly packed, 1 Tbsp	3
Almonds	
¼ cup	4
blanched, ¼ cup	6
chopped, ¼ cup	5
dry-roasted, ¼ cup	6
honey-roasted, ¼ cup	6
marcona, 1 cup	26
oil-roasted, ¼ cup	7
sliced, ¼ cup	4
slivered, ¼ cup	5
smoked, 23 pieces	5
Aloo gobi	
1 cup	4
Aloo palak	
1 cup	4
Amaranth	
● cooked, 1 cup	7
Ambrosia	
½ cup	4
Anchovy paste	
1 Tbsp	1
Apple	
baked, with nuts, butter, and sugar, 1 medium	12
candied, 1 medium	16
canned, sliced, sweetened with sugar, drained, ½ cup	4
caramel, 1 medium	16
dried, ¼ cup	3
dried, stewed, sweetened with sugar, ¼ cup	2

● No Count	SmartPoints™ value
● dried, stewed, without sugar, ¼ cup	0
● fresh, frozen, cooked, or canned, without added sugar	0
Apple brown Betty	
1 cup	12
Apple crisp	
8 oz	17
Applesauce	
● fresh, frozen, cooked, or canned, without added sugar	0
Apricots	
canned, in extra light syrup, 1 cup	4
canned, in heavy syrup, drained, 1 cup	9
● fresh, frozen, cooked, or canned, without added sugar	0
frozen, sweetened with sugar, ½ cup	7
halves, canned, in heavy syrup, with skin, 1	1
halves, canned, in juice, with skin, 1	1
halves, canned, in light syrup, with skin, 1	1
halves, dried, ¼ cup	4
halves, dried, stewed, with sugar, ½ cup	4
● halves, dried, stewed, without sugar, ¼ cup	3
Arroz con gandules (rice with pigeon peas)	
1 cup	11
Arroz con pollo	
11 oz	16
Artichoke	
● fresh, frozen, cooked, or canned, without added sugar or oil	0
Artichoke hearts	
● fresh, frozen, cooked, or canned, without added sugar or oil	0
marinated, 1 cup	6

Complete A-Z Food List

O No Count	SmartPoints™ value
Artichoke, stuffed	
7 ¾ oz	18
Arugula	
O fresh, frozen, cooked, or canned, without added sugar or oil	0
Asparagus	
O fresh, frozen, cooked, or canned, without added sugar or oil	0
Avocado	
Hass, fresh, ¼	2
pureed or mashed, ¼ cup	3

B

	SmartPoints™ value
Baba ghanoush	
¼ cup	4
Bacon	
cooked, crisp, 3 slices (1 oz)	5
imitation, cooked, 3 slices (½ oz)	1
reduced/low-sodium, uncooked, 3 slices (2 ¾ oz)	9
reduced-fat, cooked, crisp, 3 slices (1 oz)	3
reduced-fat, uncooked, 3 slices (1 ¾ oz)	3
turkey, cooked, crisp, 3 slices (1 ½ oz)	3
turkey, uncooked, 3 slices (1 ½ oz)	3
uncooked, 3 slices (4 oz)	15
vegetarian, uncooked, ½ oz	2
Bacon bits	
imitation, 1 Tbsp	1
Bacon fat	
1 Tbsp	5
Bacon grease	
1 tsp	2
Bacon, Canadian	
cooked, 3 slices (2 ½ oz)	3
pan-fried, 3 slices (1 ½ oz)	1
O uncooked, 2 slices (2 oz)	1

O No Count	SmartPoints™ value
Bagel	
any type, 1 small or ½ large (2 oz)	5
asiago cheese, restaurant-type, 1 (4 ½ oz)	10
blueberry, restaurant-type, 1 (4 oz)	10
cinnamon-raisin, small, 1 (2 ½ oz)	6
everything, restaurant-type, 1 (4 oz)	9
multigrain, restaurant-type, 1 (4 oz)	9
onion, restaurant-type, 1 (4 oz)	9
plain, restaurant-type, 1 (4 oz)	9
poppy seed, restaurant-type, 1 (4 oz)	9
pumpernickel, restaurant-type, 1 (4 oz)	8
salt, restaurant-type, 1 (4 oz)	8
sesame, restaurant-type, 1 (4 oz)	12
wheat, restaurant-type, 1 (4 oz)	9
Bagel chips	
1 oz	4
fat-free, 1 oz	4
Baked Alaska	
1 piece (3 ½ oz)	10
Baking mix	
buttermilk, ⅓ cup	5
Baking powder	
1 tsp	0
Baking soda	
1 tsp	0
Baklava	
1 piece (2 ½ oz)	14
store-bought, 1 piece (2 oz)	11
Balsamic glaze	
1 Tbsp	1
Bamboo shoots	
O fresh, frozen, cooked, or canned, without added sugar or oil	0

12

Banana

dehydrated or freeze-dried, ¼ cup	4
○ fresh, frozen, cooked, or canned, without added sugar	0

Banana bread

with nuts, 1 piece (2 ½ oz)	10
without nuts, 1 piece (2 ¼ oz)	9

Banana chips

banana chips, ¼ cup	16

Barley

○ cooked, 1 cup	6
○ quick-cooking, cooked, 1 cup	6
○ uncooked, 2 oz	6

Bean curd skin

○ 2 oz	1

Beans

○ black, canned, ½ cup	3
○ black, canned, low-sodium, ½ cup	3
○ black, cooked, ½ cup	3
○ black, dry, ¼ cup	4
○ broadbeans (fava), canned, ½ cup	2
○ broadbeans (fava), cooked, ½ cup	2
○ broadbeans (fava), uncooked, ¼ cup	3
○ butter, canned, ½ cup	2
○ cannellini, canned, ½ cup	4
○ cranberry (Roman), canned, ½ cup	3
○ cranberry (Roman), cooked, ½ cup	3
○ French, cooked, ½ cup	3
○ garbanzo beans (chickpeas), cooked, ½ cup	3
○ garbanzo beans (chickpeas), dry, ¼ cup	5
○ great northern, canned, ½ cup	4

○ great northern, cooked, ½ cup	2
○ great northern, dry, ¼ cup	4
○ green snap, canned	0
○ green snap, cooked	0
○ green snap, fresh, frozen, cooked, or canned, without added sugar or oil	0
○ green, cooked	0
○ green, fresh, frozen, cooked, or canned, without added sugar or oil	0
○ kidney, cooked, ½ cup	3
○ kidney, dry, ¼ cup	4
○ lima, canned, ½ cup	2
○ lima, cooked, ½ cup	3
○ lima, dry, ¼ cup	4
○ mung, cooked, ½ cup	2
○ mung, dry, ¼ cup	5
○ navy, canned, ½ cup	4
○ navy, cooked, ½ cup	3
○ navy, dry, ¼ cup	4
○ pink, cooked, ½ cup	3
○ pinto, canned, ½ cup	3
○ pinto, cooked, ½ cup	3
○ pinto, dry, 1 cup	17
○ small white, cooked, ½ cup	3
○ small white, dry, ¼ cup	4
○ wax, cooked	0
○ wax, fresh, frozen, cooked, or canned, without added sugar or oil	0
○ white, canned, ½ cup	4
○ white, cooked, ½ cup	3
○ white, dry, ¼ cup	4
○ yellow snap, canned	0
○ yellow snap, cooked	0
○ yellow snap, fresh, frozen, cooked, or canned, without added sugar or oil	0

Complete A-Z Food List

○ No Count	SmartPoints™ value
Beans and franks	
1 cup	18
Beans, baked	
½ cup	7
canned, ½ cup	5
deli, ½ cup	7
fast food, 6 ¼ oz	9
vegetarian, canned, ½ cup	4
with beef, canned, ½ cup	5
with franks, canned, ½ cup	7
with pork and sweet sauce, canned, ½ cup	5
with pork, canned, ½ cup	4
Beans, black, and rice	
1 cup	6
Beans, red, and rice	
1 cup	7
Beans, refried	
½ cup	6
black, canned, ½ cup	3
canned, ½ cup	3
○ fat-free, canned, ½ cup	2
red, canned, ¼ cup	2
○ reduced-sodium, canned, ½ cup	3
with sausage, canned, ½ cup	7
Beef	
back ribs, lean and fat, cooked, 3 oz	10
back ribs, lean and fat, uncooked, 3 oz	10
back ribs, lean, trimmed, cooked, 3 oz	7
blade roast, lean, trimmed, cooked, 3 oz	5
bottom round, trimmed, uncooked, 4 oz	6
○ brains, cooked, 3 oz	3
brisket, cooked, 3 oz	11
brisket, lean, trimmed, cooked, 3 oz	4

○ No Count	SmartPoints™ value
brisket, lean, trimmed, uncooked, 4 oz	4
brisket, trimmed, uncooked, 4 oz	9
chuck, arm pot roast, cooked, 3 oz	7
chuck, arm pot roast, lean, trimmed, cooked, 3 oz	3
chuck, blade roast, cooked, 3 oz	9
chuck, blade roast, trimmed, cooked, 3 oz	5
chuck, boneless, lean, trimmed, uncooked, 4 oz	3
cube steak, cooked, 3 oz	3
○ cube steak, trimmed, cooked, 3 oz	2
○ eye round, lean, trimmed, uncooked, 4 oz	2
○ eye round, steak or roast, trimmed, cooked, 3 oz	2
fillet mignon, cooked, 3 oz	9
○ fillet mignon, lean, trimmed, cooked, 3 oz	3
○ fillet mignon, trimmed, uncooked, 4 oz	3
○ flank, lean, trimmed, cooked, 3 oz	3
○ flank, lean, uncooked, 4 oz	3
○ flank, uncooked, 4 oz	3
KC strip, cooked, 3 oz	5
○ KC strip, lean, trimmed, cooked, 3 oz	3
○ KC strip, lean, trimmed, uncooked, 4 oz	3
New York steak, cooked, 3 oz	5
○ New York steak, lean, trimmed, cooked, 3 oz	3
New York steak, uncooked, 4 oz	7
porterhouse steak, cooked, 3 oz	9
porterhouse steak, trimmed, cooked, 3 oz	7
rib eye, lean, trimmed, cooked, 3 oz	5

● No Count	SmartPoints™ value
rib, large end, cooked, 3 oz	9
rib, large end, trimmed, cooked, 3 oz	9
rib, small end, trimmed, cooked, 3 oz	5
rib, whole (ribs 6-12), lean and fat, cooked, 3 oz	10
rib, whole (ribs 6-12), lean and fat, uncooked, 4 oz	12
rib, whole (ribs 6-12), lean, cooked, 3 oz	5
rib, whole (ribs 6-12), lean, uncooked, 4 oz	4
round, lean and fat, uncooked, 4 oz	6
● round, lean, trimmed, cooked, 3 oz	3
● round, lean, uncooked, 4 oz	3
round, steak or roast, cooked, 3 oz	5
● rump roast, lean, trimmed, cooked, 3 oz	3
● shank, lean, trimmed, uncooked, 4 oz	2
shortribs, lean and fat, cooked, 3 oz	14
shortribs, lean and fat, uncooked, 4 oz	17
shortribs, trimmed, cooked, 3 oz	8
shortribs, trimmed, uncooked, 4 oz	9
sirloin, cooked, 3 oz	5
● sirloin, lean, trimmed, cooked, 3 oz	3
● sirloin, lean, trimmed, uncooked, 4 oz	2
sirloin, trimmed, cooked, 3 oz	4
skirt steak, cooked, 3 oz	5
skirt steak, lean, trimmed, cooked, 3 oz	5
● steak (round or loin cuts), lean, trimmed, cooked, 3 oz	3

● No Count	SmartPoints™ value
steak, flat-iron, cooked, 3 oz	5
steak, flat-iron, uncooked, 4 oz	5
steak, regular, cooked, 3 oz	8
strip sirloin, cooked, 3 oz	6
● strip sirloin, lean, trimmed, cooked, 3 oz	3
● strip sirloin, lean, trimmed, uncooked, 4 oz	3
t-bone steak, cooked, 3 oz	8
t-bone steak, lean, trimmed, cooked, 3 oz	6
t-bone steak, lean, trimmed, uncooked, 4 oz	7
tenderloin roast, cooked, 3 oz	6
● tenderloin roast, lean, trimmed, cooked, 3 oz	3
● tenderloin roast, lean, trimmed, uncooked, 4 oz	3
tenderloin roast, lean, uncooked, 4 oz	3
tongue, cooked, 3 oz	8
top round, trimmed, uncooked, 4 oz	4
● tripe, cooked, 3 oz	2
Beef au poivre	
3 oz	7
Beef Bourguignon	
1 cup	17
Beef gordita	
4 oz	14
Beef jerky or stick	
1 oz	3
Beef macaroni, with tomato sauce	
frozen, reduced-fat, 9 ½ oz	9
Beef masala	
1 cup	6
Beef sandwich steak	
processed, uncooked, 3 oz	9
sliced, frozen, prepared, 3 oz	10

Complete A-Z Food List

● No Count	SmartPoints™ value
Beef stroganoff with noodles	
1 cup Stroganoff with 1 cup noodles	21
Beef Wellington	
5 oz	15
Beef with barbecue sauce	
frozen, 2 oz	6
Beef, barbecued	
back ribs, 3 oz	7
brisket, 3 oz	9
shortribs, 3 oz	16
Beef, corned	
canned, 3 oz	6
cooked, 3 oz	6
lean, cooked, 3 oz	6
uncooked, 4 oz	7
Beef, country-fried	
patty, 3 oz	8
patty, store-bought, 3 oz	8
Beef, cured	
breakfast strips, cooked, 3 oz	12
thin-sliced, 3 oz	3
Beef, dried	
3 oz	2
Beef, ground	
75% lean/25% fat, cooked, 3 oz	6
75% lean/25% fat, uncooked, 4 oz	11
80% lean/20% fat, cooked, 3 oz	6
80% lean/20% fat, uncooked, 4 oz	9
85% lean/15% fat, cooked, 3 oz	6
85% lean/15% fat, uncooked, 4 oz	7
90% lean/10% fat, cooked, 3 oz	4
90% lean/10% fat, uncooked, 4 oz	5
● 93% lean/ 7% fat, cooked, 3 oz	3
● 93% lean/7% fat, uncooked, 4 oz	3

● No Count	SmartPoints™ value
● 95% lean/5% fat, cooked, 3 oz	3
● 95% lean/5% fat, uncooked, 4 oz	3
patties, frozen, cooked, 3 oz	8
sirloin, cooked, 3 oz	4
sirloin, uncooked, 4 oz	5
Beef, smoked	
● chopped, 3 oz	2
Beefalo	
● cooked, 3 oz	3
● uncooked, 4 oz	3
Beer	
ginger, 12 fl oz	11
light, 12 fl oz	3
malt, 8 fl oz	5
non-alcoholic, 12 fl oz	2
regular, 12 fl oz	5
Beets	
● fresh, frozen, cooked, or canned, without added sugar or oil	0
pickled, ½ cup	4
Beignet	
beignet, 1 (¾ oz)	3
prepared from dry mix, 1 (¾ oz)	4
Berries, mixed	
● fresh, frozen, cooked, or canned, without added sugar	0
Bhuna gosht	
bhuna gosht, 1 cup	8
Bialy	
1 (3 oz)	8
Biryani	
chicken, 1 cup	12
lamb, 1 cup	19
Biscuit	
2 ½" diameter, 1 (1 ½ oz)	4
cheese, 1 (1 ¾ oz)	8
prepared from dry mix, 1 (2 oz)	6
prepared from refrigerated dough, 1 (1 oz)	3

○ No Count	SmartPoints™ value
prepared from refrigerated dough, lower fat, 1 (¾ oz)	2
store-bought, 1 (1 ¼ oz)	4
Biscuit breakfast	
biscuit, with egg and bacon, fast food, 1 (5 ⅓ oz)	15
with egg and ham, fast food, 1 (6 ¾ oz)	14
with egg and sausage, fast food, 1 (6 ⅓ oz)	19
with egg and steak, fast food, 1 (5 ¼ oz)	13
with egg, cheese, and bacon, fast food, 1 (5 oz)	14
with egg, fast food, 1 (4 ¾ oz)	11
Biscuit dough, refrigerated	
2 ½" diameter, 1 ½ oz	4
lower fat, 1 (¾ oz)	2
mixed grain, 1 ½ oz	3
Biscuit mix	
⅓ cup	6
buttermilk, reduced-fat, ⅓ cup	6
Bistec de palomilla (Cuban fried steak)	
3 oz	5
Blackberries	
canned, in heavy syrup, ½ cup	6
○ fresh, frozen, cooked, or canned, without added sugar	0
Blackened chicken	
3 oz	10
Blackened fish	
6 oz	14
Blackened steak	
3 oz	9
Blanquette of veal	
1 cup	5
Blintz	
cheese, 3 (14 ½ oz)	24
cheese, frozen, 3 (6 ¾ oz)	9
fruit, frozen, 3 (6 ¾ oz)	10
potato, frozen, 3 (6 ¾ oz)	9

○ No Count	SmartPoints™ value
Blueberries	
canned, in heavy syrup, ½ cup	7
canned, in heavy syrup, drained, ½ cup	9
dried, sweetened with sugar, ¼ cup	7
○ fresh, frozen, cooked, or canned, without added sugar	0
frozen, sweetened with sugar, 1 cup	11
Bok choy	
○ fresh, frozen, cooked, or canned, without added sugar or oil	0
Bologna	
beef, 2 oz	6
beef and pork, low-fat, 2 oz	4
beef, low-fat, 2 oz	4
beef, reduced-sodium, 2 oz	6
chicken and pork, 2 oz	7
chicken, pork, and beef, 2 oz	5
chicken, turkey, and pork, 2 oz	6
Lebanon, beef, 2 oz	2
pork, 2 oz	6
pork and turkey, light, 2 oz	4
turkey, 2 oz	4
Bouillon	
any type, low-sodium, dehydrated, 1 Tbsp	1
beef, canned, 1 cup	0
beef, cube, 1	0
beef, cube, prepared with water, 1 cup	0
beef, granules, ¼ cup	4
chicken, cube, 1	0
chicken, dehydrated, prepared with water, 1 cup	0
vegetable, cube, 1	0
Boysenberries	
canned, in heavy syrup, ½ cup	7
○ fresh, frozen, cooked, or canned, without added sugar	0

● No Count	SmartPoints™ value
Bran	
corn, uncooked, 2 oz	3
oat, uncooked, ¼ cup	1
wheat, uncooked, 2 Tbsp	0
Brazil nuts	
¼ cup	7
Bread	
7-grain, 1 slice (1 oz)	2
any type (white, wheat, rye, Italian, French, pumpernickel), 1 slice (1 oz)	2
challah, 1 slice (1 ½ oz)	3
cheese, 1 slice (1 ¾ oz)	6
cinnamon-raisin swirl, 1 slice (1 ¼ oz)	4
cracked-wheat, 1 slice (1 oz)	2
egg, 1 slice (1 ½ oz)	3
French baguette, 1 piece (2 ¼ oz)	5
French, whole-wheat, 1 loaf (10 oz)	19
high-fiber (3 g or more dietary fiber per slice), 1 slice (1 oz)	2
Italian, 1 slice (1 oz)	2
jalapeño, 1 slice (1 ½ oz)	4
mixed-grain, 1 slice (1 oz)	2
oat bran, 1 slice (1 oz)	2
oatmeal, 1 slice (1 oz)	2
peasant, 1 slice (1 oz)	2
potato, 1 slice (1 oz)	3
protein-enriched (includes gluten), 1 slice (⅔ oz)	1
pumpernickel, 1 slice (1 oz)	2
raisin, 1 slice (1 oz)	2
● reduced-calorie, any type, 1 slice (¾ oz)	1
rice bran, 1 slice (1 oz)	2
rye, 1 slice (1 oz)	2
● sandwich, thin, 1 (1 ½ oz)	3
sourdough, 1 slice (1 ¼ oz)	3
wheat, 1 slice	2

● No Count	SmartPoints™ value
wheat bran, 1 slice (1 ¼ oz)	3
wheat germ, 1 slice (1 oz)	2
white, 1 slice (1 oz)	2
white wheat, 1 slice (1 oz)	2
white, low-sodium, 1 slice (1 oz)	2
white, prepared from recipe, 1 slice (1 ½ oz)	3
white, prepared from recipe, made with fat-free milk, 1 slice (1 ½ oz)	3
white, prepared from recipe, made with reduced-fat (2%) milk, 1 slice (1 ½ oz)	3
whole-wheat, 1 slice (1 oz)	2
whole-wheat, prepared from recipe, 1 slice (1 oz)	3
● whole-wheat, sandwich, thin, 1 (1 ½ oz)	3
Bread, Boston brown	
1 slice (1 ½ oz)	3
canned, 1 slice (1 ½ oz)	3
Bread, date-nut	
1 slice (2 ½ oz)	11
Bread, focaccia	
1 slice (2 oz)	4
any type, store-bought, 1 slice (2 oz)	4
Bread, garlic	
1 slice (1 ½ oz)	8
frozen, 1 slice (1 ½ oz)	5
Bread, Irish soda	
1 slice (3 ½ oz)	12
Bread, pan Cubano	
6 ½" x 3", 1 (4 ¾ oz)	12
Bread, Portuguese sweet	
1 slice (3 oz)	10
Bread, pumpkin	
1 slice (3 oz)	13
Bread, zucchini	
1 (2 oz)	9

Breadcrumbs

dried, plain, ¼ cup	3
dried, seasoned, ¼ cup	3
fresh, ¼ cup	1
panko, ¼ cup	3
panko, whole-wheat, ¼ cup	3
whole-wheat, ¼ cup	2

Breadstick

cheese, 1 (¼ oz)	1
hard, any type, 1 (⅓ oz)	1
soft, 1 (1 ¼ oz)	3

Breadstick dough

refrigerated, 1 oz	2

Breakfast, frozen

scrambled eggs and sausage with hashed brown potatoes, 6 oz	12

Brioche

1 (1 oz)	5

Broccoli

○ broccoli, frozen, chopped, cooked, ½ cup	0
○ fresh, frozen, cooked, or canned, without added sugar or oil	0

Broccoli rabe

○ fresh, frozen, cooked, or canned, without added sugar or oil	0

Broccoli slaw

○ fresh	0

Broccolini

○ fresh, frozen, cooked, or canned, without added sugar or oil	0

Broccoli-rice casserole

5 oz	7

Broth

beef, any type, 1 cup	0
beef, canned, 1 cup	0
beef, canned, condensed, ½ cup	0
beef, canned, condensed, prepared with equal volume water, 1 cup	0

beef, dehydrated, prepared with water, 1 cup	0
beef, fat-free, 1 cup	0
○ beef, reduced-sodium, 1 cup	0
○ beef, with tomato juice, 1 cup	3
chicken, canned, 1 cup	1
chicken, canned, condensed, ½ cup	1
chicken, fat-free, 1 cup	0
○ chicken, fat-free, reduced-sodium, 1 cup	0
○ chicken, low-sodium, canned, 1 cup	1
chicken, ready-to-serve, 1 cup	0
fish, 1 cup	1
scotch, 1 cup	7
scotch, canned, condensed, ½ cup	2
scotch, canned, condensed, prepared with equal volume water, 1 cup	2
vegetable, 1 cup	1
○ vegetable, reduced-sodium, 1 cup	1

Brownie

2" square, fast food, 1 (2 oz)	11
fat-free, store-bought, 1 (1 ½ oz)	6
low-fat, store-bought, 1 (1 ½ oz)	8
prepared, 1 (2 ½ oz)	15
prepared from dry mix, special dietary, 1 (¾ oz)	3
walnut, restaurant-type, 4 ⅔ oz	26

Brownie mix

regular, ¼ package (5 ⅓ oz)	24
special dietary, ¼ package (2 oz)	8

Bruschetta

3 oz	4

Brussels sprouts

○ fresh, frozen, cooked, or canned, without added sugar or oil	0

● No Count	SmartPoints™ value
Bubble and squeak	
bubble and squeak, 7 ¾ oz	6
Bubble tea (milk tea)	
8 fl oz	4
Buckwheat	
● uncooked, 2 oz	5
Buffalo wings	
cooked, 1 (1 ½ oz)	4
frozen, prepared without fat, 1 (1 oz)	2
Buffalo, water	
● cooked, 3 oz	1
● uncooked, 4 oz	1
Buffalo/bison	
● free range, top round steak, cooked, 3 oz	1
● free range, top round steak, uncooked, 4 oz	1
ground, cooked, 3 oz	4
ground, uncooked, 4 oz	6
● lean, all visible fat trimmed, cooked, 3 oz	2
● lean, all visible fat trimmed, uncooked, 4 oz	2
● top sirloin steak, cooked, 3 oz	3
● top sirloin steak, uncooked, 4 oz	2
Bulgogi (beef stir fry)	
4 ⅓ oz	4
Bulgur	
● cooked, 1 cup	4
● uncooked, 2 oz	5
Burrito	
bean, 1 small (6")	8
bean and cheese, reduced-fat, store-bought, 1 (5 ½ oz)	7
bean and cheese, store-bought, 1 (5 oz)	10
bean, fast food, 2 pieces (7 ⅔ oz)	14

● No Count	SmartPoints™ value
beef and bean, store-bought, 1 (5 oz)	12
beef and cheese, 1 large (5 ¾ oz)	11
beef and cheese, 1 small (3 ½ oz)	7
beef or chicken and cheese, reduced-fat, store-bought, 1 small (4 oz)	7
breakfast (egg, cheese and bacon, ham, or sausage), store-bought, 1 (3 ½ oz)	8
breakfast, ham and cheese, frozen, 1 package (3 ½ oz)	6
chicken and cheese, 1 large (8")	9
chicken and cheese, 1 small (6")	6
chicken, store-bought, 1 (5 oz)	8
vegetable, 1 large (11 oz)	15
vegetable, 1 small (5 ½ oz)	7
with beans and cheese, fast food, 1 (6 ½ oz)	12
with beans and chili peppers, fast food, 7 oz	14
with beans and meat, fast food, 8 oz	13
with beans, cheese, and beef, fast food, 1 piece (8 ½ oz)	14
with beans, cheese, and chili peppers, fast food, 12 oz	20
with beef and chili peppers, fast food, 7 oz	13
with beef, cheese, and chili peppers, fast food, 2 pieces (10 ¾ oz)	18
with beef, fast food, 2 pieces (8 oz)	16
with fruit, fast food, 1 (2 ½ oz)	10
Butter	
ghee, 1 tsp	2
light, 1 Tbsp	3
regular, 1 Tbsp	5
whipped, 1 Tbsp	3

Butter chicken

1 cup	10

Butter substitute

without fat, powder, 1 Tbsp	1

C

Cabbage

○ all varieties, fresh, frozen, cooked, or canned, without added sugar or oil	0

Cabbage, pickled

Japanese-style, fresh, pickled, ¼ cup	0

Café au lait

made with reduced-fat (2%) milk, 6 fl oz	3

Café mocha

made with fat-free milk, without whipped cream, 8 fl oz	7
made with reduced-fat (2%) milk, with whipped cream, 8 fl oz	10

Cake

angel food, 1 piece (2 oz)	4
angel food, store-bought, 1 piece (1 ¾ oz)	5
apple, 1 slice (3 oz)	10
baba au rhum, 3 ¼ oz	15
Boston cream pie, store-bought, 1 piece (3 ¼ oz)	11
carrot, restaurant-type, 1 piece (6 oz)	29
carrot, with cream cheese icing, 6 ½ oz	29
cherry fudge, with chocolate frosting, 1 piece (2 ½ oz)	9
chocolate, with chocolate frosting, store-bought, 5 oz	25
chocolate, without frosting, prepared from recipe, 1/12 cake (3 ⅓ oz)	12
coffee cake, 1 piece (3 ¼ oz)	14

coffee cake, cheese, 1 piece (2 ⅔ oz)	11
coffee cake, cinnamon, store-bought, 1 piece (2 oz)	10
coffee cake, cinnamon, with crumb topping, prepared from mix, 1 piece (2 oz)	7
coffee cake, crème filled, with chocolate frosting, 1 (3 ¼ oz)	12
coffee cake, fat-free, store-bought, 1 piece (2 oz)	6
coffee cake, fruit, 1 piece (1 ¾ oz)	7
corn, sweet, 4 oz	16
double chocolate, restaurant-type, 1 piece (5 ⅓ oz)	27
fat-free, store-bought, 1 piece (3 ½ oz)	9
fruitcake, 1 piece (2 oz)	9
fruitcake, store-bought, 1 piece (1 ½ oz)	6
gingerbread, prepared from recipe, 1 piece (2 ½ oz)	12
honey, 1 piece (4 oz)	14
panettone, 1 piece (1 ½ oz)	10
petit four, 1 (1 oz)	5
pineapple upside-down, ⅑ of 8" square (4 oz)	12
pound, 1 piece (5" x 3" x 1")	15
pound, butter, store-bought, 1 piece (1 ¾ oz)	8
pound, fat-free, 1 cake (12 oz)	42
pound, store-bought, 1 piece (2 ½ oz)	13
sachertorte, 1 piece (2 ¾ oz)	15
shortcake, store-bought, 1 piece (1 oz)	4
shortcake, biscuit type, prepared from recipe, 1 piece (2 ¼ oz)	10
shortcake, strawberry, 1 piece (4 ⅓ oz)	12
sponge, 1 piece (1 ½ oz)	5
sponge, Passover, 1 piece (2 ½ oz)	6

○ No Count	SmartPoints™ value
sponge, store-bought, 1 piece (1 ⅓ oz)	5
sugar-free, store-bought, 1 piece (2 ½ oz)	7
white, with coconut frosting, prepared from recipe, ¹⁄₁₂ cake (4 oz)	21
white, without frosting, prepared from recipe, 1 piece (2 ½ oz)	11
with icing, ¹⁄₁₂ of 9" layer cake or 3" square	23
with icing, store-bought, 1 piece (3 oz)	13
yellow, with chocolate frosting, store-bought, 5 oz	25
yellow, with vanilla frosting, store-bought, 1 piece (2 ⅓ oz)	12
yellow, without frosting, prepared from recipe, ¹⁄₁₂ cake (2 ⅓ oz)	8

Cake mix

○ No Count	SmartPoints™ value
angel food, 1 oz	5
banana, ⅛ package (2 ⅓ oz)	12
carrot, pudding-type, ⅛ package (2 oz)	8
chocolate, pudding-type, ⅛ package (2 ¼ oz)	11
chocolate, regular, 1 oz	5
coffee cake, cinnamon, with crumb topping, 1 oz	5
devil's food, 1 oz	5
German chocolate, ¼ package (4 ½ oz)	20
gingerbread, 1 oz	5
marble, pudding-type, ⅛ package (2 ¼ oz)	13
vanilla, ⅛ package (2 ¼ oz)	13
white, ⅛ package (2 ¼ oz)	13
white, pudding-type, enriched, 1 oz	5
white, regular, 1 oz	5
yellow, ⅛ package (2 ¼ oz)	12
yellow, regular, enriched, 1 oz	5

Cake, snack

○ No Count	SmartPoints™ value
crème filled, sponge, 1 (1 ½ oz)	7
crème-filled, chocolate, with frosting, 1 (1 ¾ oz)	9
crème-filled, store-bought, 1 (1 oz)	5

Calamari

fried, 3 ½ oz	13
○ grilled, 3 oz	2

Calzone

ham and cheese, 7 oz	18

Candy, chocolate

any type other than those listed here, 1 ½ oz	12
candy bar, chocolate toffee, 1 (1 ⅓ oz)	10
candy bar, fun-size, 1 (⅔ oz)	4
caramels, chocolate-flavor roll, 6 (1 ½ oz)	7
coffee beans, milk chocolate-covered, 1 oz	8
dark, 60-69% cacao solids, 1 oz	8
dark, 70-85% cacao solids, 1 oz	8
fondant, sweet chocolate-coated, 1 (1 ½ oz)	9
milk chocolate, with almonds, 1 ½ oz	11
milk chocolate, with rice cereal, 1 ½ oz	11
mints, chocolate-covered, 1 (1 ¼ oz)	8
peanuts, chocolate-covered, 1	1
raisins, chocolate-covered, ¼ cup	10

Candy, non-chocolate

butterscotch, 3 (½ oz)	4
candy bits, yogurt-covered, 1 oz	6
candy cane, any type, 1 (½ oz)	3
candy corn, 1 oz	6
candy rolls, yogurt-covered, fruit-flavored, 1 (¾ oz)	4
caramels, 1 oz	6

cotton candy, 1 oz	6
fondant, prepared from recipe, 1 oz	6
gum drops, 1	1
gum drops, low-calorie, 1	1
hard, 1 piece	1
hard, low-calorie, 1	1
jelly beans, 10	2
licorice, 1 oz	4
licorice rope, 1 (⅔ oz)	3
lollipop, 1 (1 oz)	6
nougat, with almonds, 1 piece (½ oz)	3
peanut bar, 1 (1 ½ oz)	9
peanut brittle, 1 ¼ oz	6
peanut brittle, store-bought, 1 oz	6
praline, 1 (1 ⅓ oz)	8
sesame, ¾ oz	5
sesame crunch, 20 (1 ¼ oz)	7
taffy, 1 piece (1 oz)	6
Cannelloni	
cheese, with meat sauce, 2 shells with ½ cup sauce (12 oz)	21
cheese, with tomato sauce, 2 shells with ½ cup sauce (12 oz)	17
cheese, with tomato sauce, frozen, 7 oz	9
meat, with cream sauce, 2 shells with ½ cup sauce (12 oz)	25
meat, with tomato sauce, 2 shells with ½ cup sauce (12 oz)	18
spinach and cheese, with cream sauce, 2 shells with ½ cup sauce (12 oz)	22
spinach and cheese, with tomato sauce, 2 shells with ½ cup sauce (12 oz)	14
Cannoli	
1 (3 oz)	12

Cantaloupe	
○ fresh, frozen, cooked, or canned, without added sugar	0
Capers	
1 Tbsp	0
Caponata (eggplant appetizer)	
6 ½ oz	5
store-bought, ½ cup	5
Cappuccino	
○ made with fat-free milk, 8 fl oz	2
made with reduced-fat (2%) milk, 8 fl oz	3
made with whole milk, 8 fl oz	3
powder, any flavor, 1 Tbsp	3
ready-made, from machine, any flavor, 8 fl oz	3
Caramel macchiato	
made with fat-free milk, 8 fl oz	6
made with reduced-fat (2%) milk, 8 fl oz	7
Carne asada	
5 oz	12
Carnitas	
5 ½ oz	8
Carob	
sweetened with sugar, 3 oz	24
unsweetened, ¼ cup	4
Carrots	
○ baby	0
○ fresh, frozen, cooked, or canned, without added sugar or oil	0
Casaba melon	
○ fresh, frozen, cooked, or canned, without added sugar	0
Cashew chicken	
3 oz chicken with ⅓ cup sauce	7
Cashews	
¼ cup	6
dry-roasted, ¼ cup	7
oil-roasted, ¼ cup	6

● No Count	SmartPoints™ value
Cassava	
½ cup	5
Cassoulet	
1 cup	13
Cauliflower	
● fresh, frozen, cooked, or canned, without added sugar or oil	0
Cavatelli with sausage and broccoli	
1 cup	8
Caviar	
any type, 1 Tbsp	1
spread, store-bought, 1 Tbsp	1
Celeriac	
● fresh, frozen, cooked, or canned, without added sugar or oil	0
Celery	
● fresh, frozen, cooked, or canned, without added sugar or oil	0
Cereal bars/snack bars	
cereal bar, fat-free, 1 (1 ½ oz)	6
cereal bar, regular, 1 (1 ¼ oz)	4
cereal bar, rice and wheat, 1 (¾ oz)	3
granola bar, chocolate-covered, 1 (1 oz)	6
granola bar, hard, chocolate chip, 1 (¾ oz)	4
granola bar, hard, peanut butter, 1 (¾ oz)	3
granola bar, hard, with almonds, 1 (¾ oz)	4
granola bar, nut and raisin, soft, uncoated, 1 (1 oz)	4
granola bar, peanut butter, soft, milk chocolate-coated, 1 (1 oz)	6
granola bar, peanut butter, soft, uncoated, 1 (1 oz)	4
granola bar, plain, hard, 1 (1 oz)	4
granola bar, raisin, soft, uncoated, 1 (1 ½ oz)	7
granola bar, reduced-calorie, 1 (1 oz)	4

● No Count	SmartPoints™ value
granola bar, soft, chocolate chip, 1 (1 ½ oz)	7
granola bar, soft, chocolate chip, graham, and marshmallow, 1 (1 oz)	4
granola bar, soft, uncoated, 1 (1 oz)	4
granola bar, with coconut, chocolate-coated, 1 (1 oz)	7
granola bars, uncoated, 1 (1 oz)	4
snack bar, crisped rice, chocolate chip, 1 (1 oz)	4
snack bar, mixed berry, 1 (1 ⅓ oz)	6
snack bar, rice (crisp) and marshmallow treat, store-bought, 1 (¾ oz)	4
Cereal, hot	
● cream of rice, cooked, 1 cup	4
● cream of wheat, cooked, 1 cup	3
● farina, cooked, 1 cup	4
farina, uncooked, ¼ cup	4
● grits, corn, cooked, 1 cup	5
grits, corn, uncooked, ¼ cup	4
● grits, corn, white, quick, cooked, 1 cup	4
● grits, corn, yellow, quick, cooked, 1 cup	4
● oat bran, cooked, 1 cup	2
● oatmeal, cooked, 1 cup	5
oatmeal, flavored, cooked, 1 cup	8
● oatmeal, instant, plain, cooked, 1 cup	5
oatmeal, instant, unflavored, uncooked, 1 packet (1 oz)	3
oatmeal, instant, with cinnamon and spice, uncooked, 1 packet (1 ½ oz)	7
oatmeal, instant, with raisins and spice, uncooked, 1 packet (1 ½ oz)	6
oatmeal, uncooked, ¼ cup	2
● oats, old-fashioned, cooked, 1 cup	5

oats, old-fashioned, uncooked, ¼ cup | 2

oats, quick, uncooked, ¼ cup | 2

oats, rolled, uncooked, ¼ cup | 2

○ oats, steel-cut, cooked, 1 cup | 4

oats, steel-cut, uncooked, ¼ cup | 4

○ whole-wheat, natural, cooked, 1 cup | 4

whole-wheat, natural, uncooked, ¼ cup | 2

Cereal, ready-to-eat

amaranth flakes, 1 cup | 4

any type, with sugar substitute, 1 cup | 3

bran flakes, 1 cup | 4

corn flakes, 1 cup | 3

crispy rice, 1 cup | 3

frosted, 1 cup | 7

granola, homemade, 1 cup | 20

granola, low-fat, 1 cup | 13

granola, store-bought, 1 cup | 19

museli, with dried fruit and nuts, 1 cup | 11

nuggets, 1 cup | 12

oat bran, 1 cup | 6

oat, corn, and wheat squares, sweetened with sugar, maple flavor, 1 cup | 5

puffed rice, 1 cup | 2

puffed wheat, 1 cup | 1

raisin bran, 1 cup | 8

○ shredded wheat, bite size, 1 oz | 3

whole-grain, fortified, 1 cup | 4

Ceviche

½ cup | 2

Chalupa (pork and bean dish)

1 cup | 8

Champagne

5 fl oz | 4

Chana dal

1 cup | 6

Chana masala

1 cup | 10

Char shiu bao (Chinese roast pork bun)

1 (2 ½ oz) | 6

Cheese ball

store-bought, 1 oz | 3

Cheese fries, restaurant-type

9 oz | 22

Cheese snacks

cheese puffs, hot, 1 oz | 3

cheese straws, 1 oz | 1

cheese twists or balls, 1 oz | 5

snack pack, cheese and breadstick, 1 oz | 4

snack pack, cheese and pretzel, 1 oz | 3

Cheese spread

garlic and herb, reduced-fat, 2 Tbsp | 3

pasteurized process, American, 1 oz | 3

pimiento, reduced-fat, store-bought, 1 oz | 2

pimiento, regular, store-bought, 1 oz | 3

Cheese sticks

breaded, prepared without fat, store-bought, 1 (½ oz) | 2

Cheese, American

1 slice (1 oz) | 4

cheese product, yellow loaf, 1 oz | 5

cold pack cheese food, 1 oz | 3

○ fat-free, 1 oz | 1

low-fat, singles, 1 slice (¾ oz) | 1

spread, 1 oz | 3

Cheese, asiago

1 oz | 5

Cheese, blue

1 oz | 4

crumbled, reduced-fat, ¼ cup | 3

○ No Count	SmartPoints™ value
Cheese, brick	
1 oz	4
Cheese, brie	
1 oz	4
Cheese, camembert	
1 oz	3
Cheese, caraway	
1 oz	4
Cheese, cheddar or colby	
1 oz	4
○ fat-free, 1 oz	0
○ fat-free, shredded, ¼ cup	1
low-fat, 1 oz	1
low-sodium, 1 oz	4
reduced-fat, 1 oz	3
shredded, ¼ cup	4
shredded, low-fat, ¼ cup	1
Cheese, Cheshire	
1 oz	4
Cheese, cottage	
○ fat-free, 1 cup	2
fat-free, with fruit, 1 cup	8
low-fat (1%), 1 cup	3
low-fat (1%), with vegetables, 1 cup	3
reduced-fat (2%), 1 cup	5
regular (4%), 1 cup	6
regular (4%), with fruit, 1 cup	6
with vegetables, 1 cup	6
Cheese, cream	
⅓ less-fat, 1 Tbsp	2
○ fat-free, 1 Tbsp	0
○ fat-free, 2 Tbsp	1
light, 1 Tbsp	1
regular, 1 Tbsp	2
whipped, 1 Tbsp	2
Cheese, edam	
1 oz	4
Cheese, farmer	
1 oz	3

○ No Count	SmartPoints™ value
Cheese, feta	
1 oz	3
crumbled, 1 oz	3
○ fat-free, 1 oz	0
reduced-fat, 1 oz	2
Cheese, fontina	
1 oz	4
Cheese, fromage frais (soft cheese with fruit)	
1 oz	1
Cheese, gjetost	
1 oz	5
Cheese, goat	
hard-type, 1 oz	5
reduced-fat, 1 oz	2
semisoft-type, 1 oz	4
soft-type, 1 oz	3
Cheese, gorgonzola	
1 oz	4
Cheese, gouda	
1 oz	4
Cheese, gruyère	
1 oz	4
Cheese, hard or semisoft	
○ fat-free, 1 oz	1
○ fat-free, 1 slice (¾ oz)	1
low-fat, 1 oz	2
low-fat, 1 slice (¾ oz)	2
regular, 1 oz	4
regular, 1 slice (¾ oz)	3
Cheese, havarti	
1 oz	4
Cheese, limburger	
1 oz	4
Cheese, manchego	
1 oz	4
shredded, 1 cup	16
Cheese, mascarpone	
1 oz	6

Cheese, Mexican

queso anejo, 1 oz	4
queso asadero, 1 oz	4
queso chihuahua, 1 oz	4
reduced-fat, shredded, ¼ cup	3

Cheese, Monterey Jack

1 oz	4
shredded, reduced-fat, 1 oz	3

Cheese, mozzarella

cheese substitute, 1 oz	3
○ fat-free, shredded, ¼ cup	0
fresh, 1 oz	3
low-sodium, 1" cubes, 1 oz	2
low-sodium, diced, 1 oz	2
low-sodium, shredded, 1 oz	2
low-sodium, sliced, 1 oz	2
part-skim, 1 oz	2
part-skim, shredded, 1 oz	2
sticks, breaded, frozen, prepared without fat, 1 oz	3
sticks, fried, family-style, restaurant-type, 8 ⅔ oz	26
whole milk, 1 oz	3
whole milk, low-moisture, 1 oz	3

Cheese, mozzarella, fried

1 piece (1 ¾ oz)	6

Cheese, muenster

1 oz	4
low-fat, 1" cubes, 1 oz	3
low-fat, shredded, 1 oz	3
low-fat, sliced, 1 oz	3

Cheese, Neufchâtel

1 oz	3

Cheese, non-dairy

imitation, American or cheddar, 1 oz	3

Cheese, non-dairy

imitation, American or cheddar, low-cholesterol, 1" cubed, 1 oz	3
imitation, American or cheddar, low-cholesterol, shredded, 1 oz	3

Cheese, paneer

1 oz	4
fried, 1 oz	3

Cheese, Parmesan

1 oz	4
fat-free, 1 Tbsp	0
grated, 1 oz	4
low-sodium, grated, 1 oz	4
Parmigiano Reggiano, shredded, ¼ cup	3
reduced-fat, 1 oz	3
shredded, ¼ cup	3

Cheese, pepper jack

1 oz	4

Cheese, port de salut

1 oz	4

Cheese, pot

1 cup	2

Cheese, provolone

1 oz	4
reduced-fat, 1 oz	3

Cheese, queso blanco

crumbled, 1 oz	3

Cheese, queso cotija

1 oz	4

Cheese, queso fresco

fresh, crumbled, 1 oz	3

Cheese, queso seco

dry white, grated, 1 oz	3

Cheese, ricotta

○ fat-free, ½ cup	2
part-skim, ½ cup	5
ricotta salata, 1 oz	3
whole milk, ½ cup	8

Cheese, Romano

1 oz	4
Pecorino Romano, grated, ¼ cup	3

● No Count	SmartPoints™ value
Cheese, Roquefort	
1 oz	4
crumbled, ¼ cup	4
Cheese, soy	
cream cheese, 1 oz	3
curd soybean, 1 oz	1
● fat-free, 2 oz	1
● Parmesan-flavored, 1 oz	3
● regular, 1 oz	1
Cheese, Swiss	
1 oz	4
● fat-free, 1 oz	0
● fat-free, shredded, ¼ cup	1
low-fat, 1 oz	1
low-fat, shredded, 1 tsp	0
pasteurized process, 1 oz	3
pasteurized process cheese food, 1 oz	3
Cheese, tilsit	
1 oz	4
Cheeseburger on bun	
double, double decker bun, with condiments and special sauce, fast food, 1 (7 ¾ oz)	19
double, fast food, 1 (5 ¼ oz)	15
double, large patty, with condiments and vegetables, fast food, 1 (9 oz)	22
double, large patty, with condiments, fast food, 1 (10 oz)	25
double, large patty, with condiments, vegetables and mayonnaise, fast food, 1 (12 ½ oz)	30
double, regular patty and bun, with condiments, fast food, 1 (5 ½ oz)	15
double, regular patty, with condiments and vegetables, fast food, 1 (5 ¾ oz)	13
double, with bacon, fast food, 1 (10 oz)	26
large, fast food, 1 (6 ½ oz)	18

● No Count	SmartPoints™ value
large, with bacon and condiments, fast food, 1 (7 ½ oz)	20
large, with condiments and vegetables, fast food, 1 (8 ¼ oz)	16
microwave, 1 (4 ¾ oz)	14
plain, without mayonnaise, lettuce, and tomato, 1 (6 ⅔ oz)	14
single, large patty, with condiments, fast food, 1 (7 ¼ oz)	18
single, large patty, with condiments, vegetables and mayo, fast food, 1 (7 ½ oz)	19
single, regular patty, with condiments, fast food, 1 (4 ½ oz)	12
small, fast food, 1 (3 ½ oz)	10
small, with condiments and vegetables, fast food, 4 oz	10
triple, plain, fast food, 1 (8 ¾ oz)	25
with bacon, microwave, 1 (5 oz)	15
Cheesecake	
any type, fast food, 1 piece (2 ¾ oz)	12
frozen, 1 piece (4 oz)	17
prepared from mix, no-bake type, 1 piece (3 ½ oz)	12
with fruit topping, 1 piece (5 ⅔ oz)	19
without fruit topping, 1 piece (4 ½ oz)	18
Cherries	
chocolate-covered, 1 (½ oz)	3
dried, ¼ cup	8
● fresh, frozen, cooked, or canned, sweet or sour, without added sugar	0
maraschino, 1	0
sour, red, canned, in heavy syrup, ½ cup	7
sour, red, canned, in light syrup, ½ cup	5

● No Count	SmartPoints™ value
sweet, canned, in heavy syrup, ½ cup	6
sweet, canned, in juice, ½ cup	4
sweet, canned, in light syrup, ½ cup	5
sweet, frozen, sweetened with sugar, 1 cup	13
Chestnuts	
Chinese, boiled and steamed, ¼ cup	1
Chinese, roasted, ¼ cup	3
European, boiled and steamed, 1 oz	1
European, roasted, ¼ cup	3
Chicken	
barbecued, with skin, without bone, 3 oz	4
broilers or fryers, dark meat, with skin, without bone, cooked, 3 oz	5
broilers or fryers, dark meat, without skin and bone, cooked, 3 oz	4
broilers or fryers, dark meat, without skin and bone, uncooked, 4 oz	2
chicken skin only, rotisserie, barbecue, 3 oz	11
dark meat, cooked, 2 oz	2
light meat, cooked, 2 oz	2
roaster, with skin, with bone, uncooked, 4 oz	7
without skin and bone, roasted, 5 oz	5
Chicken a la king	
1 cup	15
Chicken adobo	
4 oz	6
Chicken and dumplings	
canned, 8 ½ oz	6
cooked, with skin, 5 oz	9
cooked, without skin, 5 oz	8
frozen, 8 ½ oz	6

● No Count	SmartPoints™ value
Chicken and meatball fricassee	
2 cups	9
Chicken and rice	
restaurant-type, 5 oz	6
Chicken asopao	
10 ½ oz	10
Chicken breast	
barbecued, with skin and bone, 4 ½ oz	8
cooked, with skin, without bone, 3 oz	3
● cooked, without skin and bone, 3 oz	2
fillet (without skin and bone), breaded, frozen, prepared without fat, 3 oz	4
● fillet (without skin and bone), grilled, 3 oz	2
● roasted, without skin and bone, 1 oz	1
rotisserie, barbecue, with skin, without bone, 3 oz	3
rotisserie, barbecue, without skin and bone, 3 oz	2
● rotisserie, without skin and bone, 3 oz	1
● uncooked, without skin and bone, 4 oz	2
Chicken cacciatore	
6 ½ oz	12
Chicken cordon bleu	
frozen, 4 ⅓ oz	12
Chicken creole	
without rice, 1 cup	6
Chicken crêpes	
10 ½ oz	18
Chicken cutlet	
pan-fried, 3 oz	4
Chicken drumstick	
barbecued, with skin and bone, 1 ½ oz	3
cooked, with skin, with bone, 3 oz	3

Complete A-Z Food List

○ No Count	SmartPoints™ value
cooked, with skin, without bone, 1 (3 ½ oz)	4
cooked, without skin and bone, 1 (3 ½ oz)	4
cooked, without skin, with bone, 3 oz	3
rotisserie, barbecue, with skin, without bone, 1 (2 ½ oz)	3
rotisserie, barbecue, without skin and bone, 1 (2 ½ oz)	2
uncooked, with skin, with bone, 4 oz	3
uncooked, without skin and bone, 4 oz	4
Chicken feet	
boiled, 1 oz	2
Chicken fingers	
family-style, restaurant-type, 4 oz	10
Chicken giblets	
cooked, ½ cup	2
Chicken gizzard	
● cooked, 3 oz	2
Chicken jalfrezi	
6 oz	7
Chicken Kiev	
6 ½ oz	21
frozen, 6 oz	11
Chicken leg (drumstick and thigh)	
roasted, with skin and bone, 1 (11 ¾ oz)	13
Chicken long rice	
1 cup	4
Chicken marsala	
10 ¾ oz	20
Chicken mole	
6 ¾ oz	7
Chicken nuggets	
fried, 2 ½ oz	8
fried, fast food, 6 (3 ¾ oz)	9
frozen, 3 oz	7
frozen, fat-free, 3 oz	2

○ No Count	SmartPoints™ value
Chicken paprika	
10 oz	9
Chicken paprikash	
1 ½ cups chicken mixture with ½ cup sauce	11
Chicken parmigiana	
patty, store-bought, 5 oz	8
with sauce, 5 oz with ½ cup sauce	13
without sauce, 5 ½ oz	10
Chicken patty	
breast, breaded, fat-free, prepared without fat, 3 oz	2
cooked, frozen, 3 oz	7
fried, frozen, 3 oz	6
uncooked, frozen, 4 oz	10
Chicken pilaf (kotta pilafi)	
13 ½ oz	12
Chicken shawarma	
2 oz	5
Chicken tenders	
breaded, frozen, prepared, 3 oz	6
cooked, breaded, 3 oz	6
family-style, restaurant-type, 7 oz	16
fast food, 3 oz	7
restaurant-type, 3 oz	4
Chicken thigh	
barbecued, with skin and bone, 3 oz	6
cooked, with skin, with bone, 3 oz	4
cooked, with skin, without bone, 5 oz	8
cooked, without skin and bone, 3 oz	5
cooked, without skin, with bone, 3 oz	4
roasted, with skin, without bone, 4 oz	4
roasted, without skin and bone, 4 oz	4

rotisserie, barbecue, with skin, without bone, 1 (3 ⅓ oz)	5
rotisserie, barbecue, without skin and bone, 1 (3 ⅓ oz)	4
uncooked, without skin and bone, 3 oz	2
uncooked, without skin, with bone, 1 oz	1
Chicken tikka	
4 oz	5
Chicken wing	
cooked, with skin and bone, 1 (3 oz)	6
glazed, barbecue flavor, frozen, 1 oz	2
rotisserie, barbecue, with skin, without bone, 1 (1 ¾ oz)	3
rotisserie, barbecue, without skin and bone, 1 (1 ¾ oz)	2
uncooked, with skin, with bone, 4 oz	6
uncooked, without skin, with bone, 4 oz	2
Chicken with cashews	
7 oz	12
Chicken, canned	
with broth, 3 oz	3
without broth, 3 oz	3
Chicken, fried	
breast, with skin and bone, 4 ½ oz	11
breast, with skin, with bone, breaded, fast food, 3 oz	5
breast, with skin, without bone, 3 oz	5
breast, without skin, with bone, without breading, fast food, 3 oz	2
drumstick, with skin and bone, 1 (1 ½ oz)	6
drumstick, with skin, with bone, breaded, fast food, 3 oz	6
drumstick, without skin and bone, 1 (1 ½ oz)	2

drumstick, without skin, with bone, without breading, fast food, 3 oz	3
light meat (from breast or wing), with skin, with bone, breaded, fast food, 3 oz	7
thigh, fried, with skin and bone, 3 oz	8
thigh, with skin, with bone, breaded, fast food, 3 oz	7
thigh, without skin, with bone, without breading, fast food, 3 oz	3
wing, with skin, with bone, with breading, fast food, 3 oz	7
wing, without skin, with bone, without breading, fast food, 3 oz	4
Chicken, ground	
○ breast, uncooked, 4 oz	1
cooked, 12 oz	15
cooked, 93% lean/7% fat, 3 oz	3
uncooked, 4 oz	4
Chicken, stewed	
with skin and bone, 11 ¾ oz	17
without skin and bone, 5 oz	5
Chicken-fried steak	
with cream gravy, 8 ¼ oz	22
without gravy, 6 oz	16
Chicory (curly endive)	
○ fresh, frozen, cooked, or canned, without added sugar or oil	0
Chile rellenos, beef and cheese	
without sauce, 7 ½ oz	24
Chili	
bean, in a cup, unprepared, 1 container (2 oz)	5
low-fat, canned, 1 cup	7
meat and beans, family-style, restaurant-type, 6 ½ oz	9
turkey, with beans, canned, 1 cup	6
turkey, without beans, canned, 1 cup	4
vegetarian, 1 cup	7

Complete A-Z Food List

Complete A-Z Food List

No Count	SmartPoints™ value
vegetarian, low-fat or fat-free, canned, 1 cup	5
with beans, canned, 1 cup	9
with beans, in a microwavable bowl, 1 cup	7
without beans, canned, 1 cup	8
without beans, frozen, 1 cup	16
Chili con carne	
fast food, 1 cup	7
with beans, 1 cup	6
without beans, 1 cup	8
Chili con queso	
¼ cup	8
store-bought, ¼ cup	4
Chili mac	
canned, 1 cup	8
Chimichanga	
beef, 1 (8 ¼ oz)	14
beef or chicken, with beans, frozen, 1 (6 ½ oz)	10
chicken, 1 (8 ¼ oz)	12
with beef and cheese, fast food, 1 (6 ½ oz)	15
with beef and red chili peppers, fast food, 6 ¾ oz	13
with beef, cheese, and red chili peppers, fast food, 1 (6 ½ oz)	12
with beef, fast food, 6 oz	13
Chinese beef and broccoli	
1 cup	4
frozen, 1 cup	9
Chinese chicken and broccoli	
1 cup	3
Chinese lemon chicken	
restaurant-type, 2 ½ oz	6
Chinese orange chicken	
restaurant-type, 2 oz	6
Chinese pepper steak	
3 oz	3

No Count	SmartPoints™ value
Chinese pork and broccoli	
6 ½ oz	4
Chinese roast pork	
1 cup	5
Chinese shrimp and broccoli	
6 ½ oz	2
Chinese vegetables	
prepared without oil, 1 cup	3
with beef, 1 cup	6
with chicken, 1 cup	5
with pork, 1 cup	8
with shrimp, 1 cup	5
with tofu, 1 cup	4
Chitterlings	
cooked, 3 oz	7
uncooked, 4 oz	8
Chocolate and candy, baking	
chocolate chips, mini, 1 Tbsp	3
chocolate chips, semisweet, 1 Tbsp	3
chocolate, baking, Mexican, squares, 1 piece (⅔ oz)	5
chocolate, baking, unsweetened, liquid, 1 Tbsp	3
chocolate, baking, unsweetened, squares, 1 piece (1 oz)	8
chocolate, bittersweet, 1 piece (½ oz)	3
chocolate, bittersweet, shavings, 1 Tbsp	2
chocolate, milk, shavings, 1 Tbsp	2
chocolate, unsweetened, grated, 1 Tbsp	2
chocolate, white, shavings, 1 Tbsp	2
cocoa powder, unsweetened, 1 Tbsp	0
cocoa powder, unsweetened, ¼ cup	2

milk chocolate chips, 1 Tbsp	3
peanut butter chips, 1 Tbsp	4
toffee baking bits, 1 Tbsp	3
white chocolate chips, 1 Tbsp	3
Chocolate drink	
8 fl oz	7
chocolate-flavor powdered beverage mix, ¼ cup	17
chocolate-flavor powdered beverage mix, prepared with whole milk, 8 fl oz	11
Cholent	
1 cup	5
Chop suey	
beef, 1 cup	6
chicken, 1 cup	4
pork, 1 cup	5
vegetable, 1 cup	3
Chorizo	
chicken, 1 oz	1
pork, 3 oz	13
Chow fun	
beef, 5 oz	10
chicken, 5 oz	10
pork, 5 oz	10
shrimp, 5 oz	10
Chow mein	
beef, 1 cup	4
beef, chicken, or pork, canned, 1 cup	2
chicken, 1 cup	4
pork, 1 cup	5
subgum chicken, 1 cup	4
Chutney	
2 Tbsp	3
mango, 2 Tbsp	3
tamarind, 2 Tbsp	3
Cilantro	
fresh, 1 Tbsp	0

Cinnamon bun	
frosted, 2 ¼ oz	12
homemade, 1 (4 oz)	11
mini, fast food, 1 (1 oz)	4
Clam juice	
2 Tbsp	0
Clams, baked	
6 (2 ½ oz)	11
Clams, breaded and fried	
3 oz	5
fast food, 4 oz	14
Clams, fried	
6 ½ oz	12
frozen, prepared without fat, 3 oz	9
Clams, stuffed	
frozen, prepared without fat, 3 oz	3
Clementine	
fresh	0
Cobbler	
fruit, 1 cup	22
fruit, frozen, 4 ½ oz	12
Cocktail mix	
daiquiri, bottled, 3 fl oz	4
margarita, bottled, 3 fl oz	6
piña colada, bottled, 3 fl oz	5
whiskey sour, bottled, 3 fl oz	5
Coconut	
dried, flaked, sweetened with sugar, 2 Tbsp	4
dried, without sugar, 2 Tbsp	10
flakes, unsweetened, 1 Tbsp	1
flakes, unsweetened, 1 tsp	0
fresh, ¼ cup	4
shredded, sweetened with sugar, 2 Tbsp	3
Coconut cream	
canned, 2 Tbsp	8

⬤ No Count	SmartPoints™ value
Coconut milk	
fresh, 8 fl oz	31
fresh, canned, 8 fl oz	25
light, store-bought, 8 fl oz	7
vanilla, 8 fl oz	5
Coconut rice	
Indian, 1 cup	8
Thai, 1 cup	16
Coconut shrimp	
4 jumbo (7 ½ oz)	22
Coconut water	
8 fl oz	2
Coffee	
brewed, black, decaffeinated, hot or iced, without sugar, 8 fl oz	0
brewed, black, hot or iced, without sugar, 8 fl oz	0
Coffee drink	
Jamaican, store-bought, 8 fl oz	5
with milk, canned, 8 fl oz	8
Coffee mix	
flavored, sugar-free, prepared, 8 fl oz	1
flavored, sugar-free, unprepared, 1 Tbsp	1
flavored, sweetened with sugar, prepared, 8 fl oz	3
Coffee substitute	
cereal beverage powder, instant, 1 Tbsp	1
cereal beverage powder, prepared with water, 8 fl oz	0
Coffee, instant	
powder or granules, decaffeinated, 1 Tbsp	0
powder or granules, regular, 1 Tbsp	0
powder, decaffeinated, with low-calorie sweetener, coffee and cocoa flavor, 1 Tbsp	4
powder, sweetened with sugar, French flavor, 1 Tbsp	2

⬤ No Count	SmartPoints™ value
powder, sweetened with sugar, mocha flavor, 1 Tbsp	1
powder, with low-calorie sweetener, mocha flavor, 1 Tbsp	5
Coffee, Irish	
7 fl oz	7
Coffee, Mexican	
6 fl oz	6
Colcannon	
1 cup	12
Coleslaw	
½ cup	5
family-style, restaurant-type, 3 ¾ oz	7
fast food, 6 ¾ oz	12
store-bought, 4 oz	6
Coleslaw mix	
⬤ shredded cabbage and carrots, packaged	0
Collards	
⬤ fresh, frozen, cooked, or canned, without added sugar or oil	0
Cookie	
amaretti, 1 (1 oz)	4
animal crackers, 13 (1 oz)	4
animal crackers, fast food, 1 oz	4
bar, 1 (1 ¼ oz)	5
biscotti, chocolate, 1 (1 oz)	6
biscotti, fat-free, 1 (1 oz)	5
biscotti, plain, 1 (1 oz)	6
butter, store-bought, 1 small (⅛ oz)	1
buttercrunch toffee, 1 (2 oz)	12
Chinese almond, 1 (½ oz)	3
chocolate chip, fast food, 2 oz	8
chocolate chip, oatmeal, sugar, or similar type, homemade, 1 (½ oz)	3
chocolate chip, oatmeal, sugar, or similar type, packaged, 1 (½ oz)	3

O No Count	SmartPoints™ value
chocolate chip, special dietary, 1 (¼ oz)	1
chocolate chip, store-bought, higher fat, 1 (⅓ oz)	2
chocolate chip, store-bought, soft-type, 1 (½ oz)	2
chocolate sandwich, with crème filling, 1 (⅓ oz)	2
chocolate sandwich, with crème filling, chocolate-coated, 1 (⅔ oz)	4
chocolate sandwich, with crème filling, special dietary, 1 (⅓ oz)	2
chocolate sandwich, with extra crème filling, 1 (½ oz)	3
chocolate wafers, 2 (½ oz)	2
coconut macaroons, prepared from recipe, 1 (¾ oz)	6
fig bar, 1 (½ oz)	3
fortune, 1 (¼ oz)	1
from refrigerated dough, baked, 2 (1 oz)	6
fruit bar, 1 (½ oz)	3
fudge, cake-type, 1 (¾ oz)	3
gingerbread, 1 (¾ oz)	4
gingersnaps, 1 (¼ oz)	1
hamantaschen, 1 (1 ⅓ oz)	4
kolache, fruit filled, 1 piece (2 oz)	7
kolache, without filling, 1 (2 oz)	6
kringla, 1 (¾ oz)	3
lace, 1 (¼ oz)	2
ladyfinger, 1 (⅓ oz)	2
ladyfingers, store-bought, 1 (½ oz)	2
macaroons, 1 (½ oz)	3
mandelbrot, 1 (2 oz)	8
marshmallow, chocolate-coated, 1 (½ oz)	2
Mexican wedding, 2 (½ oz)	3
molasses, 1 (½ oz)	2

O No Count	SmartPoints™ value
oatmeal, special dietary, 1 (¼ oz)	1
oatmeal, store-bought, 1 (⅔ oz)	3
oatmeal, store-bought, fat-free, 1 oz	4
peanut butter sandwich, regular, 1 (½ oz)	3
peanut butter sandwich, special dietary, 1 (⅓ oz)	2
peanut butter, store-bought, 1 (½ oz)	3
pecan shortbread, store-bought, 1 (½ oz)	3
rainbow, 1 (⅔ oz)	3
raisin, soft, 1 (½ oz)	3
reduced-calorie, store-bought, 1 (½ oz)	2
rosettes, 1 (⅛ oz)	1
rugalach, 1 (1 oz)	6
sesame seed, 2 (1 oz)	5
shortbread, store-bought, 1 (¼ oz)	1
social tea biscuit, 1	1
sugar wafers, with crème filling, 1 (⅓ oz)	2
sugar wafers, with crème filling, special dietary, 2 (¼ oz)	1
sugar, refrigerated dough, 1 (½ oz)	3
sugar, special dietary, 1 (¼ oz)	1
sugar, store-bought, 1 (½ oz)	3
sugar-free, store-bought, 1 (½ oz)	2
vanilla sandwich, with crème filling, 1 (½ oz)	3
vanilla wafers, 1 (⅕ oz)	1
vanilla wafers, reduced-fat, 1 (⅕ oz)	1
viennese wafers, with chocolate crème filling, 1 (1 oz)	6
white macadamia, restaurant-type, 1 (1 ¾ oz)	11

Cookie dough, refrigerated

chocolate chip, ¼ cup	11
oatmeal, 1 (½ oz)	3
peanut butter, 1 (½ oz)	3

Cookie mix

chocolate chip, 1 oz	6
oatmeal, 1 oz	6

Cooking spray

5 sprays	0
butter-flavored, 1 spray	0
olive oil, 1 spray	0

Coq au vin

7 oz	14

Coquilles St. Jacques

13 ⅔ oz	10

Corn cakes

1 (⅓ oz)	1

Corn casserole

6 oz	14

Corn chips

30 small or 10 large (1 oz)	5
barbecue-flavor, 1 oz	5

Corn dog

1 (2 ¾ oz)	6
fast food, 1 (6 oz)	15
frozen, prepared, 1 (2 ¾ oz)	7
mini, frozen, prepared, 1 (⅔ oz)	2

Corn flake crumbs

¼ cup	2

Corn nuts

1 oz	4
barbecue-flavor, 1 oz	4
chile picante, ⅓ cup	4
nacho-flavor, 1 oz	4

Corn on the cob

○	1 medium (7" long)	4
	cooked on the grill, with butter, 1 (4 oz)	8
○	frozen, cooked, ½ cup	2
	with butter, fast food, 1 (5 oz)	5

Corn, baby

○	ears, ½ cup	0

Corn, cream-style

½ cup	3
white, canned, ½ cup	3
yellow, canned, ½ cup	3

Corn, kernels

○	canned, with red and green peppers, ½ cup	2
○	cooked, ½ cup	2
○	dried, 1 oz	3
○	frozen, ½ cup	2
○	frozen, cooked, ½ cup	2
○	white, canned, ½ cup	2
○	white, uncooked, ½ cup	2
○	yellow, canned, vacuum packed, ½ cup	3
○	yellow, cooked, ½ cup	2
○	yellow, frozen, cooked, ½ cup	2
○	yellow, uncooked, ½ cup	2

Cornbread

2" square, 1 ¾ oz	4
Mexican, 1 piece (3 ⅔ oz)	12
prepared from dry mix, 1 (2 oz)	7
prepared from recipe, made with reduced-fat (2%) milk, 1 slice (2 ¼ oz)	5

Cornbread dressing

1 cup	11

Cornbread mix

¼ package (2 oz)	9

Cornish hen

	with skin, cooked, 3 oz	6
	with skin, uncooked, 4 oz	6
○	without skin, cooked, 3 oz	2
○	without skin, uncooked, 4 oz	2

Cornmeal

○	cooked, ¼ cup	1
○	uncooked, ¼ cup	3

Cornmeal mix

self-rising, ¼ cup	4

Cornstarch

1 Tbsp	1

Couscous

in a cup, unprepared, 1 container (2 oz)	6
semolina, cooked, 1 cup	5
uncooked, 2 oz	6
○ whole-wheat, cooked, 1 cup	6
○ whole-wheat, uncooked, 2 oz	6

Crab cake

4 ¾ oz	4
blue, 2 oz	2
fast food, 2 oz	5

Crab puff

2 oz	6

Crab rangoon

1 large (2 oz)	7
frozen, 5 ¼ oz	12

Crab, stuffed

frozen, 3 oz	3

Cracker meal

¼ cup	3

Crackers

arare, 1 oz	3
cheese squares, mini, reduced-fat, 1 oz	4
cheese squares, mini, regular, 1 oz	5
cheese, whole-grain, 1 oz	3
fat-free, 1 oz	3
graham, 2 (2 ½" each) or ½ oz	2
graham, chocolate-coated, 1 (½ oz)	3
graham, mini, any variety, 1 oz	5
graham, reduced-fat, 2 (2 ½" each) or ½ oz	2
graham, reduced-fat, cinnamon, 2 (2 ½" each) or ½ oz	2
graham, reduced-fat, cinnamon-honey, 2 (2 ½" each) or ½ oz	2
Italian toast snacks, store-bought, 1 oz	4
milk, 1 oz	4
multigrain, 1 oz	5
oyster, 1 oz	4
rice, 1 oz	3
rusk toast, 1 oz	3
rye, wafers, plain, 1 oz	3
rye, wafers, seasoned, 1 oz	3
saltines, 1 oz	4
saltines, fat-free, low-sodium, 1 oz	3
saltines, whole-wheat, 1 oz	3
snack, 1 oz	4
snack, sandwich-type, with filling (cheese, wheat, rye, toast, or wafer crackers with cheese, peanut butter, or cream cheese filling), 1 oz	4
wheat, regular, 1 oz	5
whole-wheat, 1 oz	4
whole-wheat, reduced-fat, 1 oz	3

Cranberries

dried, ¼ cup	5
○ fresh, frozen, cooked, or canned, without added sugar	0

Cranberry sauce

canned, 1 Tbsp	2

Crawfish pie

10 oz	19

Cream

clotted, 2 Tbsp	7
half and half, 2 Tbsp	2
half and half, fat-free, 2 Tbsp	1
light, 2 Tbsp	3
whipped, aerosol, 2 Tbsp	1
whipped, chocolate, aerosol, 2 Tbsp	1

Cream (cont'd)

○ No Count	SmartPoints™ value
whipped, unsweetened, homemade, 2 Tbsp	5
whipping, heavy, 2 Tbsp	5
whipping, light, 2 Tbsp	4
Cream puff	
1 (2 oz)	13
Cream substitute	
flavored, liquid, 1 Tbsp	2
flavored, powder, 1 tsp	1
light, powder, 1 tsp	0
liquid, light, 1 Tbsp	1
Cream, sour	
○ fat-free, 2 Tbsp	1
imitation, cultured, 2 Tbsp	3
light, 2 Tbsp	2
reduced-fat, 2 Tbsp	2
regular, 2 Tbsp	3
soy, 2 Tbsp	1
Creamed chipped beef	
1 cup	15
Creamed chipped chicken	
1 cup	16
Creamer	
fat-free, liquid, flavored, dairy, 2 Tbsp	2
fat-free, liquid, unflavored, dairy, 2 Tbsp	1
liquid, unflavored, non-dairy, 2 Tbsp	2
powder, non-dairy, 2 Tbsp	4
Crème brûlée	
½ cup	13
Crème fraiche	
2 Tbsp	5
Crêpes	
1 (6" diameter)	3
Crêpes Suzette	
2 (5 oz)	19
Crispbread	
1 oz	3

○ No Count	SmartPoints™ value
Croissant	
apple, 1 (2 oz)	6
butter, 1 (2 oz)	9
cheese, 1 (2 oz)	9
chocolate-filled, 1 (3 ¾ oz)	10
plain, 1 (1 ¾ oz)	9
Croissant breakfast	
with egg and cheese, fast food, 1 (4 ½ oz)	14
with egg, cheese, and bacon, fast food, 1 (4 ½ oz)	16
with egg, cheese, and ham, fast food, 1 (5 ½ oz)	17
with egg, cheese, and sausage, fast food, 1 (6 oz)	19
Croquette	
beef, 5 oz	11
chicken, 5 oz	10
turkey, breaded, frozen, 3 ½ oz	7
Croutons	
homemade, 7 (1 oz)	4
packaged, fat-free, 7 (¼ oz)	1
packaged, regular, 7 (1 oz)	4
plain, 7 (1 oz)	3
seasoned, 7 (1 ½ oz)	6
Cruller	
French, glazed, 1 (1 ½ oz)	7
glazed, 2 ¼ oz	10
Crumpet	
1 (2 oz)	5
Cuban rice	
1 cup	7
Cucumber	
○ fresh, frozen, cooked, or canned, without added sugar or oil	0
Cupcake	
any type, extra-large, with frosting, store-bought, 1 (4 ½ oz)	23
any type, large, with frosting, store-bought, 1 (3 oz)	15

any type, medium, with frosting, store-bought, 1 (2 oz)	9
any type, mini, with frosting, store-bought, 1 (1 oz)	5
any type, standard size, with 2 Tbsp frosting, prepared from mix, 1	14
chocolate, with frosting, low-fat, 1 (1 ½ oz)	6
crème-filled, store-bought, 1 (1 ¾ oz)	8

Currants
dried, ¼ cup	6
○ fresh, frozen, cooked, or canned, without added sugar	0

Curry
African fish, 4 oz	9
African shrimp, 4 oz	10
beef, 7 ½ oz	14
Bengali fish, 4 ½ oz fillet with 1 cup vegetables	12
chicken, 7 ½ oz	14
egg, 7 ½ oz	4
goat, 9 oz	5
lamb, 7 ½ oz	14
Massaman beef, 1 cup	33
panang, with beef, 1 cup	19
panang, with chicken, 1 cup	18
panang, with pork, 1 cup	21

Curry paste
green, 1 Tbsp	0
panang, 1 Tbsp	1
Thai, 1 Tbsp	2

Custard
½ cup	7

Custard, egg
baked, prepared from recipe, 5 oz	6
dry mix, ½ cup	3
prepared from dry mix, with reduced-fat (2%) milk, ½ cup	6
prepared from dry mix, with whole milk, ½ cup	6

D

Daikon (Chinese radish)
○ fresh, frozen, cooked, or canned, without added sugar or oil	0

Danish pastry
bear claw, restaurant-type, 1 (4 oz)	17
cheese, 1 (2 ½ oz)	9
cinnamon, 2 ¼ oz	10
cinnamon, fast food, 1 (3 oz)	14
fast food, 1 (3 ¼ oz)	15
fruit, 1 (2 ½ oz)	11
fruit, fast food, 1 (3 ⅓ oz)	13
nut, 2 ¼ oz	11
store-bought, 2 ¼ oz	10

Dates
dried, ¼ cup	6
○ fresh	0

Dessert topping
butterscotch or caramel, 2 Tbsp	6
caramel, fat-free, 2 Tbsp	6
fruit, 2 Tbsp	5
fudge, fat-free, 2 Tbsp	5
fudge, regular, 2 Tbsp	7
hot fudge, fat-free, 2 Tbsp	5
marshmallow crème, store-bought, 1 Tbsp	1
nuts in syrup, 2 Tbsp	7
powdered, 2 Tbsp	1
powdered, prepared with milk, 2 Tbsp	1
sprinkles, any type, 1 Tbsp	1
strawberry glaze, 2 Tbsp	3
whipped, dairy or non-dairy, frozen, 2 Tbsp	1
whipped, dairy or non-dairy, light or fat-free, aerosol or frozen, 2 Tbsp	1

Complete A-Z Food List

Deviled crab

½ cup	6

Deviled egg

2 stuffed halves (2 oz)	5

Dim sum

bean curd roll with shrimp and vegetables, 1 (3 ½ oz)	3
bean curd roll with vegetables, 1 (2 ½ oz)	3
sesame seed balls, 1 (2 oz)	9

Dip

artichoke, baked, 2 Tbsp	4
bean, fat-free, ½ cup	2
bean, fat-free, 2 Tbsp	0
black bean, fat-free, 2 Tbsp	1
guacamole, homemade or restaurant-type, 2 Tbsp	1
guacamole, store-bought, 2 Tbsp	2
Mexican 7-layer, 2 Tbsp	1
spinach, 2 Tbsp	4
spinach-artichoke, restaurant-type, 2 oz	5
strawberry-yogurt, 2 Tbsp	3

Dirty rice

1 cup	12
prepared from dry mix without fat, 1 cup	4

Dolma

4 (3 ¼ oz)	6
store-bought, 3 ½ oz	5

Donair

4 oz meat with onion, tomato, and 2 Tbsp sauce	21

Doro wat

1 cup	8

Doughnut

any type, store-bought, 1 (2 oz)	8
cake type, with icing, 1 (2 oz)	11
cake type, without icing, 1 (2 oz)	9
cake-type, sugared or glazed, 1 (2 oz)	9

cake-type, wheat, sugared or glazed, 1 (2 oz)	8
malasadas (Portuguese doughnuts), 1 ¼ oz	4
mini, chocolate-covered, store-bought, 1 (2 oz)	12
mini, powdered sugar-covered, store-bought, 1 (2 oz)	10
with crème filling, 1 (3 oz)	12
yeast, glazed, 1 (2 oz)	10
yeast, with jelly filling, 1 (3 oz)	12

Doughnut holes

yeast, glazed, 1 (½ oz)	2

Dried fruit, candied

¼ cup	8

Dried fruit, mixed

¼ cup	6

Drink mix, dairy

reduced-calorie, powder, 1 packet (¾ oz)	2

Drunken noodles

1 cup	7

Duck

domestic, cooked, with skin, ¼ (5 oz)	15
domestic, cooked, without skin and bone, 3 oz	4
uncooked, with skin, without bone, 4 oz	17
uncooked, without skin and bone, 4 oz	4

Duck a l'orange

duck a l'orange, ¼ duck with 2 Tbsp sauce	17

Dumpling

beef or pork, fried, 1 (1 ½ oz)	2
beef or pork, steamed, 1 (1 ½ oz)	2
chicken, fried, 1 (1 ½ oz)	1
chicken, steamed, 1 (1 ½ oz)	1
kroppkakor (potato dumpling), boiled, 1 (2 oz)	5

kroppkakor (potato dumpling), fried, 1 (2 oz)	5
palak vada (vegetable dumpling), fried, 1 (2 ½ oz)	6
palak vada (vegetable dumpling), steamed, 1 (2 oz)	3
potato, 5 ⅔ oz	4
shrimp, fried, 1 (1 ½ oz)	1
shrimp, steamed, 1 (1 ½ oz)	1
vegetarian, fried, 1 (¾ oz)	1
vegetarian, steamed, 1 (¾ oz)	1

E

Éclair

1 (5 ¼ oz)	16

Edamame

○	in pods, 1 cup	3
○	shelled, ½ cup	3

Egg foo yung

beef, 1 (3 oz)	5
chicken, 1 (2 ¾ oz)	5
pork, 1 (3 oz)	5
shrimp, 1 (2 ¾ oz)	4

Egg roll

beef, 1 (4 ½" long) or 2 ½ oz	7
chicken, 1 (4 ½" long) or 2 ½ oz	5
chicken, store-bought, 1 (3 oz)	5
pork, 1 (4 ½" long) or 2 ½ oz	6
pork, store-bought, 1 (3 oz)	5
restaurant-type, 1 (3 oz)	7
shrimp, 1 (4 ½" long) or 2 ½ oz	5
shrimp, store-bought, 1 (3 oz)	6
vegetable, store-bought, 1 (3 oz)	5

Egg roll snacks

pork or shrimp, store-bought, 3 oz	5
vegetable, store-bought, 3 oz	5

Egg roll wrapper

egg roll wrapper, 1 (½ oz)	1

Egg substitute

○	fat-free, ½ cup	1
○	regular, ½ cup	1

Eggnog

homemade, with liquor, 4 fl oz	16
homemade, without liquor, 8 fl oz	15
reduced-calorie, without liquor, store-bought, 8 fl oz	14
without liquor, store-bought, 8 fl oz	17

Eggplant

○	fresh, frozen, cooked, or canned, without added sugar or oil	0

Eggplant parmesan

frozen, 5 oz	6

Eggplant parmigiana

with sauce, 3" x 4" with ½ cup sauce	16
without sauce, 6 ½ oz	12

Eggplant, breaded and baked

without oil, 1 ½ oz	1

Eggplant, breaded and fried

2 slices (3" diameter) or 1 ½ oz	2

Eggs

○	1	2
	fried, 1	3
○	hard-boiled, 1	2
	scrambled, fast food, 2 eggs	7
	scrambled, with milk and butter, 2 eggs (½ cup)	6
○	whites only, 1	0
○	whites only, 3	1
○	whites only, 1 cup	1
○	whole, cooked or uncooked, 1	2
	yolks only, 1	2

Eggs benedict

8 ⅓ oz	24

Eggs, duck

1	4

● No Count	SmartPoints™ value
Elk	
● cooked, 3 oz	1
ground, cooked, 3 oz	4
ground, uncooked, 4 oz	5
● raw, 4 oz	1
Empanadas	
2 (1 ¾ oz)	7
beef, restaurant-type, 3 oz	10
Enchilada	
beef, 2 (10 ½ oz)	16
cheese, 2 (9 oz)	14
chicken, 2 (10 ½ oz)	12
pork, 2 (10 ½ oz)	16
sour cream, 1 (5 ½ oz)	12
with cheese and beef, fast food, 1 (6 ¾ oz)	11
with cheese, fast food, 1 (5 ⅔ oz)	12
Enchilada de camarones	
6 ¾ oz	5
Enchilada meal	
beef (2 enchiladas, beans, and rice), 11 ½ oz	12
cheese (2 enchiladas, beans and rice), 11 ½ oz	12
chicken (2 enchiladas, beans, and rice), 11 ½ oz	12
Enchirito	
with cheese, beef, and beans, fast food, 6 ¾ oz	11
Endive	
● fresh, frozen, cooked, or canned, without added sugar or oil	0
Energy drink	
regular, 8 fl oz	8
sugar-free, 8 fl oz	0
English muffin	
any type other than those listed here, 1 (2 oz)	4
● light, 1 (2 oz)	2

● No Count	SmartPoints™ value
● light, whole-wheat, 1 (2 oz)	3
raisin-cinnamon, 1 (2 oz)	5
white, 1 (2 oz)	4
with butter, fast food, 1 (2 oz)	6
English muffin breakfast	
egg and cheese with meat, frozen, 1 (4 ½ oz)	9
with cheese and sausage, fast food, 1 (4 oz)	13
with egg, cheese, and Canadian bacon, fast food, 1 (4 ½ oz)	9
with egg, cheese, and sausage, fast food, 1 (5 ¾ oz)	15
Escargots	
3 oz	14
Escarole	
● fresh, frozen, cooked, or canned, without added sugar or oil	0
Espresso	
brewed, 8 fl oz	0
instant, powder or granules, 1 oz	0
Étouffée	
crawfish, 1 cup	13
crawfish or shrimp, store-bought, 1 cup	8
shrimp, 1 cup	14
Extract	
almond, 1 Tbsp	2
lemon, 1 Tbsp	2
mint, 1 Tbsp	1
orange, 1 Tbsp	2
rum, 1 Tbsp	1
vanilla, 1 Tbsp	1
vanilla, imitation, 1 Tbsp	1
vanilla, imitation, without alcohol, 1 Tbsp	0

F

Fadge (Irish potato bread)
1 slice (3 ¼ oz)   3
Fajita
beef, 2 (9 oz)   15
chicken, 2 (8 ½ oz)   9
pork, 2 (10 ½ oz)   16
shrimp, 2 (9 oz)   9
vegetarian, 2 (11 oz)   14
Falafel in pita
1 large pita with 4 falafel patties   15
Falafel patty
4 (4 ½ oz)   10
prepared from mix, 2 ¼ oz   6
Farro
○ cooked, 1 cup   6
○ uncooked, ¼ cup   4
Fennel bulb
○ uncooked   0
Fettucine Alfredo
1 cup   25
with broccoli and chicken, frozen, 1 cup   13
Figs
canned, in heavy syrup, ½ cup   7
canned, in light syrup, ½ cup   5
dried, ¼ cup   5
dried, stewed, ¼ cup   4
○ fresh, frozen, cooked, or canned, without added sugar   0
Fish
anchovies, canned in oil, drained, 5   1
○ arctic char, cooked, 3 oz   2
○ arctic char, uncooked, 4 oz   4
○ bass, striped, cooked, 3 oz   1
○ bass, striped, uncooked, 4 oz   2
○ bluefish, cooked, 3 oz   2
○ bluefish, uncooked, 4 oz   2

○ carp, cooked, 3 oz   3
○ catfish, farm-raised, cooked, 3 oz   3
catfish, farm-raised, uncooked, 4 oz   3
○ catfish, wild, cooked, 3 oz   1
○ cod, Atlantic, canned, solids and liquid, 3 oz   1
○ cod, Atlantic, cooked, 3 oz   1
cod, Atlantic, dried, salted, 3 oz   2
○ cod, Atlantic, uncooked, 4 oz   1
○ cod, Pacific, cooked, 3 oz   1
○ cod, Pacific, uncooked, 4 oz   1
dried, 3 oz   2
eel, cooked, 3 oz   5
eel, uncooked, 4 oz   5
○ flounder, cooked, 3 oz   1
○ flounder, uncooked, 4 oz   1
○ grouper, cooked, 3 oz   1
○ grouper, uncooked, 4 oz   1
○ haddock, cooked, 3 oz   1
○ haddock, uncooked, 4 oz   1
○ halibut, cooked, 3 oz   1
○ halibut, uncooked, 4 oz   1
herring, cooked, 3 oz   4
lox, 3 oz   2
○ mackerel, canned, 3 oz   2
mackerel, cooked, 3 oz   4
mackerel, uncooked, 4 oz   4
○ mahi-mahi (dolphinfish), cooked, 3 oz   1
○ mahi-mahi (dolphinfish), uncooked, 4 oz   1
○ monkfish, cooked, 3 oz   1
○ monkfish, uncooked, 4 oz   1
○ orange roughy, cooked, 3 oz   1
○ orange roughy, uncooked, 4 oz   1
○ perch, cooked, 3 oz   1
○ perch, uncooked, 4 oz   1

Complete A-Z Food List

Complete A-Z Food List

○ No Count	SmartPoints™ value
● pike, cooked, 3 oz	1
● pollack, cooked, 3 oz	1
● pollack, uncooked, 4 oz	1
pompano, cooked, 3 oz	4
● rockfish, cooked, 3 oz	1
● rockfish, uncooked, 4 oz	1
sable, cooked, 3 oz	6
sable, smoked, 3 oz	6
sable, uncooked, 4 oz	6
salmon, Atlantic, farmed, cooked, 3 oz	4
● salmon, Atlantic, wild, cooked, 3 oz	3
● salmon, Atlantic, wild, uncooked, 4 oz	3
● salmon, canned, drained, 3 oz	2
salmon, chinook, cooked, 3 oz	5
salmon, chinook, uncooked, 4 oz	5
salmon, coho, farmed, raw, 4 oz	4
● salmon, coho, wild, cooked, 3 oz	3
● salmon, coho, wild, uncooked, 4 oz	3
salmon, cooked, 3 oz	4
● salmon, pink, canned, 3 oz	2
● salmon, pink, cooked, 3 oz	2
● salmon, pink, wild, canned, 2 oz	2
● salmon, pink, wild, uncooked, 4 oz	2
salmon, skinless fillet, uncooked, 4 oz	5
salmon, smoked, 3 oz	2
● salmon, sockeye, canned, 3 oz	3
● salmon, sockeye, cooked, 3 oz	3
● salmon, sockeye, uncooked, 4 oz	3
salmon, uncooked, 4 oz	5
sardines, canned in oil, drained, 2 oz	3
sardines, canned in tomato sauce, 3 oz	4

○ No Count	SmartPoints™ value
● sea bass, cooked, 3 oz	1
● sea bass, uncooked, 4 oz	1
● snapper, cooked, 3 oz	1
● snapper, uncooked, 4 oz	1
● sole, cooked, 3 oz	1
● sole, uncooked, 4 oz	1
● swordfish, cooked, 3 oz	3
swordfish, uncooked, 3 oz	2
● tilapia, cooked, 3 oz	1
● tilapia, farm-raised, cooked, 3 oz	1
● tilapia, farm-raised, uncooked, 4 oz	1
● tilapia, uncooked, 4 oz	1
● trout, cooked, 3 oz	3
● trout, rainbow, uncooked, 4 oz	3
trout, rainbow, wild, cooked, 3 oz	2
● tuna, bluefin, cooked, 3 oz	3
● tuna, bluefin, uncooked, 4 oz	3
tuna, canned, in oil, drained, 3 oz	3
● tuna, canned, in water, drained, 3 oz	1
● tuna, cooked, 3 oz	1
● tuna, uncooked, 4 oz	1
● tuna, yellowfin, cooked, 3 oz	1
● tuna, yellowfin, uncooked, 4 oz	1
● turbot, European, cooked, 3 oz	2
● turbot, European, uncooked, 4 oz	2
● whitefish, cooked, 3 oz	3
whitefish, smoked, 2 oz	1
● whitefish, uncooked, 4 oz	3
● whiting, cooked, 3 oz	1
● whiting, uncooked, 4 oz	1
● yellowtail, cooked, 3 oz	3
● yellowtail, uncooked, 4 oz	3
Fish amandine	
8 oz	17

Fish and chips

5 oz fish fillet with 20 chips (French fries)	17

Fish sticks

4" x 1" x ½", frozen, prepared, 1 (1 oz)	2
4" x 2" x ½", frozen, prepared, 1 (2 oz)	5
breaded, 4 (2 ½ oz)	5

Fish, baked, stuffed

7 oz	11

Fish, battered

fillet, prepared without fat, 3 oz	6

Fish, breaded

fillet, light, prepared without fat, 3 ¾ oz	4
fillet, prepared without fat, 3 ¾ oz	7

Fish, breaded and fried

breaded with flour, 8 oz	12
catfish, channel, 3 oz	5
croaker, Atlantic, 3 oz	5

Fish, breaded or battered and fried

fillet, family-style, restaurant-type, 8 oz	13
fillet, fast food, 3 oz	6

Fish, fried

without flour, 6 oz	13

Fish, grilled

fillet, with garlic butter, 3 ¾ oz	2
○ fillet, with lemon pepper, 3 ¾ oz	2

Five-spice chicken

breast, 4 ½ oz	7
leg, 6 oz	9

Flan (caramel custard)

½ cup	11
dry mix, ½ cup	9
prepared from dry mix, with reduced-fat (2%) milk, ½ cup	4
prepared from dry mix, with whole milk, ½ cup	4

Flatbread

1 (¾ oz)	2
chapati, 1 piece (¾ oz)	3
Indian (navajo), 1 piece (5 ⅓ oz)	17
injera, 1 (1 ½ oz)	2
lavash, 1 (2 oz)	8
lefse, 1 (4 ½ oz)	8
naan, 1 (3 oz)	6
paratha, 1 (1 ¼ oz)	5
puris, 1 (1 ½ oz)	4

Flauta

beef, 4 oz	14
chicken, 4 oz	13
pork, 4 oz	13

Flaxseed meal

ground, ¼ cup	3

Flour

bread, ¼ cup	3
cake, ¼ cup	4
chickpea (besan), ¼ cup	3
coconut, 1 tsp	0
corn (masa), white or yellow, ¼ cup	3
rice, brown, ¼ cup	4
rice, white, ¼ cup	4
rye, ¼ cup	4
wheat, white, self-rising, ¼ cup	3
wheat, white, tortilla mix, enriched, ¼ cup	3
white, ¼ cup	3
whole-wheat, ¼ cup	3
whole-wheat, white, ¼ cup	3

Fondue

cheese, 7 ⅔ oz	17

Frankfurger/hot dog on roll

chili cheese dog, restaurant-type, 1 (5 oz)	12
chili dog, 8 ½ oz	12
plain, 1 (3 ½ oz)	10
plain, fast food, 1 (3 ½ oz)	8
with chili, fast food, 1 (4 oz)	9

Frankfurter roll or bun

1 (2 oz)	5
○ light, 1 (1 ½ oz)	2
mixed grain, 1 (1 ½ oz)	4
○ reduced-calorie, 1 (1 ½ oz)	2

Frankfurter/hot dog

beef or pork, fat-free, 1 (1 ¾ oz)	1
beef or pork, low-fat, 1 (1 ¾ oz)	3
beef or pork, regular, 1 (2 oz)	6
beef or pork, with cheese, 1 piece (2 oz)	7
beef, low-fat, 1 (2 oz)	5
chicken, 1 (2 oz)	4
Meat & Poultry, 1 (1 ¾ oz)	5
meatless, 1 (2 ½ oz)	4
turkey, 1 (2 oz)	4
turkey with cheese, 1 piece (2 oz)	7
turkey, fat-free, 1 (1 ½ oz)	1
turkey, light, 1 (2 oz)	4

Franks (pigs) in blankets

1 oz	9
frozen, 1 (½ oz)	2

Freekeh

○ uncooked, 1 tsp	0

French fries

20 (5 ½ oz)	13
family-style, restaurant-type, 6 oz	16
fast food, 4 oz	11
frozen, prepared without fat, 3 oz	4

French toast

2 slices (4 ½ oz)	11
cinnamon swirl, with sausage, frozen breakfast, 5 ½ oz	13
frozen, 2 slices (4 oz)	7
sticks, fast food, 1 slice (1 oz)	3
sticks, frozen, 3 (2 ½ oz)	8
with butter, fast food, 2 slices (4 ¾ oz)	12

Fried rice

Chinese, without meat, restaurant-type, 4 ¾ oz	7
plain, 1 cup	11
Thai, kho-phat, 1 cup	11
with beef, 1 cup	11
with chicken, 1 cup	11
with chicken or pork, frozen, ½ cup	4
with pork, 1 cup	10
with shrimp, 1 cup	10

Fritters

apple, restaurant-type, 1 (4 oz)	16
conch, 2 (1 ¾ oz)	3
corn, 4 oz	7
vegetable, 7 oz	14

Frog legs

fried, 1 oz	4

Frosting/icing

chocolate, creamy, dry mix, 1 oz	3
chocolate, creamy, prepared from dry mix with margarine, 1 Tbsp	2
chocolate, creamy, prepared with butter from dry mix, 1 Tbsp	4
chocolate, creamy, ready-to-eat, 1 Tbsp	4
cream cheese-flavor, ready-to-eat, 1 Tbsp	7
decorating, 1 Tbsp	4
glaze, prepared from recipe, 1 oz	6
sour cream-flavor, ready-to-eat, 1 Tbsp	8
store-bought, reduced-fat, 1 Tbsp	3
store-bought, regular, 1 Tbsp	3
vanilla, creamy, prepared from dry mix, 1 oz	4
vanilla, creamy, prepared from dry mix with margarine, 1 Tbsp	2
vanilla, creamy, prepared with butter from dry mix, 1 Tbsp	10

vanilla, creamy, ready-to-eat, 1 Tbsp	3
white, fluffy, dry mix, ⅛ package (1 oz)	6
white, fluffy, prepared with water from dry mix, 1 Tbsp	2
Frozen yogurt	
bar, chocolate-covered, 1 (3 oz)	6
chocolate, ½ cup	6
chocolate, soft-serve, ½ cup	4
fat-free, no sugar added, ½ cup	3
fat-free, sweetened with sugar, ½ cup	5
low-fat, ½ cup	5
Fruit butter	
1 Tbsp	2
Fruit cocktail	
canned, in extra heavy syrup, ½ cup	7
canned, in heavy syrup, ½ cup	5
canned, in light syrup, ½ cup	4
○ canned, in water	0
○ canned, no sugar added	0
Fruit compote	
½ cup	8
Fruit cup	
○ restaurant-type, unsweetened	0
Fruit juice bar	
frozen, 1 (2 ¾ oz)	4
frozen, no sugar added, 1 (1 ¾ oz)	0
Fruit juice cup	
frozen, 1 (6 ½ oz)	10
Fruit juices and drinks	
apple cider, 8 fl oz	4
apple juice, frozen concentrate, undiluted, 8 fl oz	27
apple juice, unsweetened, 8 fl oz	6
apple-grape juice, 8 fl oz	7
apple-grape-pear juice, 8 fl oz	7

cranberry juice cocktail, frozen concentrate, undiluted, 2 fl oz	8
cranberry juice cocktail, low-calorie, 8 fl oz	3
cranberry juice cocktail, regular, 8 fl oz	8
cranberry juice, unsweetened, 8 fl oz	7
cranberry-apple drink, 8 fl oz	9
cranberry-apple drink, low-calorie, 8 fl oz	3
cranberry-apricot drink, 8 fl oz	9
cranberry-grape drink, 8 fl oz	4
drink mix, powdered, prepared, 8 fl oz	5
fruit punch, 8 fl oz	7
fruit punch, frozen concentrate, prepared, 8 fl oz	3
fruit punch, frozen concentrate, undiluted, 8 fl oz	14
grape drink, 8 fl oz	9
grape juice, 8 fl oz	9
grape juice, 8 fl oz	9
grapefruit juice, 8 fl oz	5
grapefruit juice, canned, sweetened, 8 fl oz	7
grapefruit juice, frozen concentrate, unsweetened, undiluted, 8 fl oz	23
grapefruit-mango juice, 8 fl oz	6
mango juice, 8 fl oz	8
nectar, any type, 8 fl oz	8
orange juice, 8 fl oz	6
orange juice, frozen concentrate, unsweetened, prepared, 8 fl oz	6
orange juice, frozen concentrate, unsweetened, undiluted, 8 fl oz	19
orange-apricot drink, 8 fl oz	7
orange-grapefruit juice, 8 fl oz	6
pineapple juice, 8 fl oz	7
pineapple-grapefruit drink, 8 fl oz	7
pineapple-orange drink, 8 fl oz	7

○ No Count	SmartPoints™ value
pomegranate juice, 8 fl oz	9
prune juice, 8 fl oz	10
tangerine juice, 8 fl oz	6
vegetable and fruit juice drink, reduced-calorie, 8 fl oz	0
Fruit leather	
1 oz	5
bar, 1 (¾ oz)	4
bar, with cream, 1 (¾ oz)	4
Fruit salad	
canned, in extra heavy syrup, ½ cup	7
canned, in heavy syrup, ½ cup	6
canned, in juice, ½ cup	3
canned, in light syrup, ½ cup	4
● canned, in water	0
● fresh, frozen, cooked, or canned, without added sugar	0
grape and apple, with yogurt and candied walnuts, 5 ⅔ oz	8
tropical, canned, in passionfruit juice, ½ cup	4
Fruit tart	
tarte aux fruits, 1 slice (5 ½ oz)	18
with custard, individual, 7 ½ oz	24
Fruit, mixed	
frozen, sweetened with sugar, ½ cup	4
Fudge	
with or without nuts, 1 piece (1" x 2") or 1 oz	6
Funnel cake	
1 (11 oz)	33

G

Garlic paste	
1 Tbsp	0
Gefilte fish/whitefish and pike	
gefilte fish, 3 oz	2
whitefish and pike, store-bought, 3 oz	3

○ No Count	SmartPoints™ value
Gelatin dessert	
dry mix, with sugar substitute, ½ cup	4
fruit-flavored, sugar-free, prepared from dry mix, ½ cup	0
fruit-flavored, sweetened with sugar, ½ cup	4
Gelatin, unflavored	
dry, 1 Tbsp	0
gelatin-fruit mold, ½ cup	4
General Tso's chicken	
homemade, 1 cup	19
restaurant-type, 3 pieces (1 ¾ oz)	5
Ginger	
pickled, 1 Tbsp	1
root, fresh, 1 Tbsp	0
Ginger chicken	
1 cup	**8**
Ginger, crystalized	
1 piece (1 tsp)	1
Gingerbread	
1 piece (2 ½ oz)	10
Gnocchi	
any type, frozen, 5 ½ oz	10
cheese, 6 ½ oz	17
potato, 4 oz	7
potato, refrigerated, 5 oz	8
spinach, 7 oz	19
Goat	
● cooked, 3 oz	2
● uncooked, 4 oz	2
Goat masala	
1 cup	5
Goose	
cooked, with skin, without bone, 3 oz	7
cooked, without skin and bone, 3 oz	4

Goulash
beef, 1 cup	11
Hungarian, 1 cup	11

Graham cracker crumbs
2 Tbsp	2

Grape leaves
○ fresh, frozen, cooked, or canned, without added sugar or oil	0

Grapefruit
canned, in light syrup, ½ cup	5
○ fresh, frozen, cooked, or canned, without added sugar	0
sections, in juice, ½ cup	3

Grapes
canned, Thompson seedless, in heavy syrup, ½ cup	6
○ fresh, frozen, cooked, or canned, without added sugar	0

Gravy
au jus, canned, 1 cup	1
au jus, canned, 2 Tbsp	0
au jus, dry mix, 2 Tbsp	2
beef, canned, ¼ cup	1
beef, canned, 2 Tbsp	0
beef, instant, dry mix, ¼ oz	1
brown, 2 Tbsp	2
brown, dry mix, 2 Tbsp	1
chicken, canned, 2 Tbsp	1
chicken, dry mix, 2 Tbsp	2
cream, 2 Tbsp	3
fat-free, canned, ½ cup	1
fat-free, canned, 2 Tbsp	0
giblet, 2 Tbsp	1
meat or poultry, low-sodium, prepared, 1 Tbsp	0
meat or poultry, low-sodium, prepared, ¼ cup	1
mushroom, canned, ½ cup	1
mushroom, canned, 2 Tbsp	0
mushroom, dry mix, ½ cup	1
mushroom, dry mix, 2 Tbsp	0

onion, dry mix, 1 cup	2
pork, dry mix, 2 Tbsp	6
sausage, 2 Tbsp	3
sausage, canned, 2 Tbsp	2
turkey, canned, 2 Tbsp	0
turkey, canned, 2 Tbsp	0
turkey, dry mix, 1 cup	1

Green bean casserole
8 oz	9

Green rice
1 cup	8

Greens
○ baby, mixed	0
○ beet, fresh, frozen, cooked, or canned, without added sugar or oil	0
○ mustard, fresh, frozen, cooked, or canned, without added sugar or oil	0
seasoned with bacon or salt pork, 1 cup	6
○ turnip, fresh, frozen, cooked, or canned, without added sugar or oil	0

Guava
○ fresh, frozen, cooked, or canned, without added sugar	0

Gum, chewing
sugarless, 1 piece	0
sweetened with sugar, 1 piece	0

Gyoza
1 (⅔ oz)	1

H

Halvah
1 piece (1 ¾ oz)	8
store-bought, 1 ½ oz	8

Ham
chopped, 3 oz	6
chopped, canned, 3 oz	6
cooked, lean, 3 oz	2

○ No Count	SmartPoints™ value
cooked, regular, 3 oz	3
extra lean (approximately 4% fat), canned, 3 oz	2
extra lean (approximately 4% fat), canned, roasted, 3 oz	2
extra lean (approximately 5% fat), 3 oz	3
● honey, smoked, 2 oz	1
minced, 3 oz	7
patties, 3 oz	9
patties, grilled, 3 oz	10
roasted, lean only, 3 oz	2
serrano, 1 oz	2
● spiral slice, lean, roasted, 3 oz	2
steak, extra lean, 3 oz	2
Ham hocks	
smoked, 4 oz	6
Ham, glazed, with pineapple	
4 oz ham with ½ pineapple slice	8
Hamburger dinner in a box	
prepared, 7 oz	10
Hamburger on bun	
double patty, plain, fast food, 1 (4 ¼ oz)	11
double patty, with condiments, fast food, 1 (7 ½ oz)	19
double, large patty, with condiments and vegetables, fast food, 1 (8 oz)	16
double, large patty, with condiments, vegetables and mayonnaise, fast food, 1 (13 oz)	31
fast food, 1 small (2 ¾ oz)	7
large, fast food with condiments, 1 (6 oz)	14
large, plain, fast food, 1 (4 ¾ oz)	13
microwave, 1 (1 ½ oz)	4
plain (without mayonnaise, lettuce, and tomato), 1 (4 ½ oz)	11
single, large patty, with condiments and vegetables, fast food, 1 (7 ⅔ oz)	16

○ No Count	SmartPoints™ value
single, with condiments, fast food, 1 (3 ½ oz)	8
small, with condiments and vegetables, fast food, 1 (4 oz)	8
triple patty, with condiments, fast food, 1 (9 oz)	21
Hamburger roll or bun	
1 (2 oz)	5
● light, 1 (1 ½ oz)	2
mixed grain, 1 (1 ½ oz)	4
Haroset	
1 Tbsp	1
Hash	
corned beef, canned, 3 oz	4
pork, 5 ¾ oz	7
roast beef, canned, 3 oz	5
Hazelnut and chocolate spread	
2 Tbsp	11
Hazelnuts	
¼ cup	7
dry-roasted, ¼ cup	6
Hearts of palm (palmetto)	
● ½ cup	0
Herring	
chopped, 3 oz	5
fillets, store-bought, 3 oz	4
in cream sauce, store-bought, 2 oz	5
in wine sauce, store-bought, 2 oz	3
kippered, 3 oz	4
pickled, 3 oz	7
Hibachi chicken	
1 cup	6
Hibachi shrimp	
1 cup	4
Hibachi steak	
1 cup	9
Hibachi vegetables	
1 cup	4

Hominy

●	canned, ½ cup	2
●	whole, cooked, 1 cup	4
	1 Tbsp	4

Honey

1 Tbsp	4

Honey bun

glazed, 2 ¼ oz	10

Honeydew

● fresh, frozen, cooked, or canned, without added sugar	0

Horchata

dry mix, unprepared, 1 oz	5

Horned melon

● fresh, frozen, cooked, or canned, without added sugar	0

Horseradish

prepared, 1 Tbsp	0

Hot chocolate

homemade, with whipped topping, 8 fl oz	14
homemade, without whipped topping, 8 fl oz	13

Hot cocoa

instant, fat-free, prepared, sweetened with sugar, 8 fl oz	2
instant, fat-free, sugar-free, dry mix, 1 Tbsp	1
instant, regular, prepared, 8 fl oz	4
instant, sugar-free, prepared, 8 fl oz	3

Hot cross bun

1 (2 ¼ oz)	9

Huevos rancheros

2 eggs with 2 tortillas	19

Huli huli chicken

breast, with skin and bone, 7 ½ oz	13
drumstick, with skin and bone, 2 oz	3
thigh, with skin and bone, 3 oz	6

Hummus

2 Tbsp	2
store-bought, 2 Tbsp	2

Hunan beef

hunan beef, 1 cup	11

Hush puppies

1 ½ oz	5
fast food, 1 (¾ oz)	2
frozen, prepared without fat, 2 oz	4

Hush puppy mix

⅓ cup	4

I

Ice cream

chocolate, ½ cup	7
chocolate, rich, ½ cup	9
chocolate, soft-serve, ½ cup	9
fat-free, no sugar added, ½ cup	3
fat-free, sweetened with sugar, ½ cup	3
French vanilla, soft-serve, ½ cup	9
fried, ½ cup	17
gelato, ½ cup	7
green tea, ½ cup	6
light, any flavor except chocolate, no sugar added, ½ cup	4
light, chocolate, ½ cup	6
light, chocolate, no sugar added, ½ cup	5
light, chocolate, soft-serve, ½ cup	6
light, sweetened with sugar, ½ cup	6
light, vanilla, ½ cup	6
light, vanilla, soft-serve, ½ cup	4
premium, ½ cup	13
regular, ½ cup	8
spumoni, ½ cup	13
strawberry, ½ cup	7

Ice cream (cont'd)

● No Count	SmartPoints™ value
vanilla, ½ cup	7
vanilla, fat-free, ½ cup	3
vanilla, rich, ½ cup	13
Ice cream bar	
chocolate- or caramel-covered, with nuts, 1 (1 ¾ oz)	9
chocolate-covered, 1 (1 ¾ oz)	8
chocolate-covered, with crisp rice, 1 (2 oz)	9
chocolate-covered, with crisp rice, no sugar added, 1 (1 ½ oz)	5
Ice cream cone only	
cake or wafer, 1 (1 oz)	4
plain or sugar, 1 (⅓ oz)	1
Ice cream in cone	
light, vanilla, soft-serve, fast food, 3 ⅔ oz	8
sundae cone, 1 (3 ½ oz)	15
Ice cream nuggets	
with crunch coating, 26 pieces (3 ⅓ oz)	17
Ice cream sandwich	
1 (2 ½ oz)	7
cookie-type, 1 (3 oz)	8
light, vanilla, 1 (2 ½ oz)	5
light, vanilla, no sugar added, 1 (2 ½ oz)	5
Ice cream soda	
8 fl oz	14
Ice cream sundae	
6 ½ oz	21
banana split, 14 oz	32
bananas Foster, 2 scoops ice cream, ½ banana, and ⅓ cup sauce	31
caramel, fast food, 5 ½ oz	10
hot fudge, fast food, 5 ½ oz	9
strawberry, fast food, 5 ½ oz	9

● No Count	SmartPoints™ value
Ice pop	
fruit-flavored, 1 (1 ¾ oz)	2
Ices, Italian	
restaurant-type, ½ cup	2
Imperial roll	
2 oz	5
Italian casserole (ground beef, pasta and cheese over rolls)	
1 cup	22

J

Jalapeño poppers	
1 (1 ½ oz)	5
Jalapeños, stuffed	
prepared without fat, store-bought, 2 oz	7
Jam	
1 Tbsp	3
apricot preserves, sugar-free, 1 Tbsp	0
apricot preserves, sugar-free, ¼ cup	1
blueberry preserves, sugar-free, 1 Tbsp	0
blueberry preserves, sugar-free, ¼ cup	1
cherry preserves, sugar-free, 1 Tbsp	0
cherry preserves, sugar-free, ¼ cup	1
reduced-sugar, 1 Tbsp	1
Jambalaya	
chicken, with rice, 1 ½ cups	13
fish, with rice, 1 ½ cups	13
Jambalaya mix	
1 ½ oz	4
JapChae	
beef, 1 cup	9
chicken, 1 cup	10
pork, 1 cup	11

	SmartPoints™ value
Jelly	
1 Tbsp	3
Jerk chicken breast	
without skin, 1 large breast (5 ¾ oz)	3
Jerky	
beef sticks, smoked, 1 (⅔ oz)	4
Jerusalem artichokes (sunchokes)	
O fresh, frozen, cooked, or canned, without added sugar or oil	0
Jicama	
O fresh, frozen, cooked, or canned, without added sugar or oil	0
Johnny cake	
3 (5 oz)	22

K

	SmartPoints™ value
Kabobs	
beef, 3 oz	5
chicken, 4 ¾ oz	4
fish, 4 ¾ oz	4
lamb, 4 ¾ oz	9
Kale	
O fresh, frozen, cooked, or canned, without added sugar or oil	0
Kalua pig	
3 oz	3
Kasha (buckwheat groats)	
O cooked, 1 cup	4
O uncooked, 2 oz	5
Kasha varnishkes	
1 cup	8
Kashmiri (lamb meatballs)	
3 ⅔ oz	13
Katsu	
ahi, 4 oz	5
chicken, 4 oz	5
pork, 4 oz	7

	SmartPoints™ value
Ketchup	
1 Tbsp	1
low-sodium, 1 Tbsp	1
Kibbe	
baked, 1 piece (⅓ oz)	1
uncooked, 3 oz	6
Kielbasa	
3 oz	9
fully cooked, grilled, 3 oz	10
fully cooked, pan-fried, 3 oz	10
Polish, turkey and beef, smoked, 3 oz	6
pork and beef, nonfat dry milk added, 3 oz	9
turkey, uncooked, 1 oz	1
Kim chee	
½ cup	1
King ranch chicken casserole	
1 cup	10
Kishke	
¾ oz	3
Kiwifruit	
O fresh, frozen, cooked, or canned, without added sugar or oil	0
Knish	
potato, 3 ½" square	9
potato, store-bought, 4 ½ oz	15
Knockwurst	
3 oz	9
Kofta (vegetable balls without sauce)	
3 oz	8
Kohlrabi	
O fresh, frozen, cooked, or canned, without added sugar or oil	0
Korean barbecue beef	
4 oz	7
Korean barbecue short ribs	
4 oz	9

Complete A-Z Food List

Korean barbeuce chicken thighs

5 oz	14

Korma

chicken, 1 cup	16
lamb, 1 cup	18
vegetable, 1 cup	14

Kreplach

boiled, 2 (2 ⅔ oz)	8
fried, 2 (2 ¾ oz)	9

Kugel (pudding)

lukschen (noodle) store-bought, 4 oz	7
lukschen (noodle), with fruit, 6 ½ oz	12
lukschen (without fruit), 5 ½ oz	7
potato, 6 oz	6
potato, store-bought, 3 ½ oz	6

Kumquats

O	fresh, frozen, cooked, or canned, without added sugar	0

Kung pao

beef, 1 cup	11
chicken, 1 cup	9
pork, 1 cup	12
shrimp, 1 cup	10

L

Lamb

	leg, cooked, 3 oz	6
O	leg, cooked, lean, trimmed, 3 oz	3
	leg, lean and fat, uncooked, 4 oz	7
O	leg, uncooked, lean, trimmed, 4 oz	2
	loin, cooked, 3 oz	8
	loin, cooked, trimmed, 3 oz	4
	loin, uncooked, trimmed, 4 oz	10
	rib, cooked, 3 oz	10
	rib, uncooked, lean and fat, 4 oz	14
	shoulder, cooked, 3 oz	9
	shoulder, uncooked, 4 oz	9

Lamb chop

O	baby, cooked, 3 oz	3
O	baby, uncooked, 4 oz	3
O	cooked, 3 oz	4
O	uncooked, 4 oz	4

Lamb masala

lamb masala, 1 cup	6

Lamb, ground

cooked, 3 oz	7
lean, cooked, 3 oz	7
lean, uncooked, 4 oz	11
uncooked, 4 oz	11

Lard

1 Tbsp	5

Lasagna

cheese, with tomato sauce, 10 oz	13
chicken, 7 oz	8
vegetable, 7 ½ oz	10
vegetarian, with cheese, 10 oz	15
vegetarian, with cheese and spinach, 10 ½ oz	13
with meat, 7 ½ oz	9
with meat sauce, 7 ½ oz	8

Latte

O	made with fat-free milk, 8 fl oz	3
	made with low-fat (1%) milk, 8 fl oz	4
	made with reduced-fat (2%) milk, 8 fl oz	4
	made with whole milk, 8 fl oz	5

Latte, chai tea

made with fat-free milk, 8 fl oz	4
made with reduced-fat (2%) milk, 8 fl oz	6

Lechon asado (roast pork)

lechon asado (roast pork), 3 oz	4

Leeks

O	fresh, frozen, cooked, or canned, without added sugar or oil	0

Lemon
○ fresh	0
peel (zest), 1 Tbsp	0

Lemon curd
1 Tbsp	3

Lemon grass chicken
1 cup	9

Lemon juice
canned or bottled, unsweetened, 8 fl oz	2
fresh, 1 Tbsp	0

Lemonade
8 fl oz	6
drink mix, powder, 1 Tbsp	3
drink mix, powder, low-calorie, 1 packet (2 g)	0
drink mix, powder, low-calorie, prepared, 8 fl oz	0
drink mix, powder, prepared, 8 fl oz	6
frozen concentrate, prepared, 8 fl oz	6
frozen concentrate, undiluted, 1 fl oz	4

Lentils
○ cooked, ½ cup	3
○ dried, ¼ cup	4
urad dal, prepared, ½ cup	3

Lettuce
○ celtuce (stem lettuce)	0
○ fresh, frozen, cooked, or canned, without added sugar or oil	0

Lime
peel (zest), 1 Tbsp	0

Lime juice
canned or bottled, unsweetened, 8 fl oz	2
lime, fresh, 1 Tbsp	0

Limeade
8 fl oz	8
frozen concentrate, undiluted, 2 fl oz	7

Linguine
with red clam sauce, 1 cup linguine with ½ cup sauce	9
with white clam sauce, 1 cup linguine with ½ cup sauce	11

Liver
○ beef, cooked, 3 oz	3
○ beef, uncooked, 4 oz	3
chicken, cooked, 1 ½ oz	1
chopped, 3 oz	5

Liver with bacon
3 oz	7

Liver with onions
3 oz	4

Lo mein
beef, 1 cup	11
chicken, 1 cup	10
pork, 1 cup	10
shrimp, 1 cup	10
vegetable, 1 cup	9

Lobster Cantonese
7 ½ oz	9

Lobster newberg
10 oz	20

Lobster thermidor
1 cup	20

Lomi lomi salmon
½ cup	2

Luncheon meat
beef, jellied, 2 oz	1
beef, thin sliced, 2 oz	1
bratwurst, 2 oz	6
braunschweiger, 2 oz	7
chicken breast, deli-type, sliced, ½ oz	0

● No Count	SmartPoints™ value
chicken breast, deli-type, sliced, 2 oz	1
chicken breast, fat-free, mequite flavor, sliced, 2 oz	0
chicken breast, fat-free, mequite flavor, sliced, 3 oz	1
chicken breast, roasted, fat-free, sliced, 2 oz	0
chicken breast, roasted, fat-free, sliced, 3 oz	1
chicken roll, 2 oz	1
Dutch loaf, pork, beef, 2 oz	5
● fat-free, 2 oz	0
● fat-free, 3 oz	1
ham and cheese, loaf or roll, 2 oz	4
ham, 11% fat, sliced, regular, 2 oz	2
ham, 96% fat-free, pre-packaged, water added, 2 oz	1
honey ham, lean, deli-sliced, 2 oz	2
lean (3 g fat or less per oz), 2 oz	1
liverwurst, 2 oz	6
mother's loaf, pork, 2 oz	5
olive loaf, 2 oz	4
peppered loaf, 2 oz	2
pickle and pimiento loaf, 2 oz	5
regular (4 g fat or more per oz), 2 oz	7
roast beef, deli-type, 2 oz	2
turkey breast, 2 oz	1
● turkey breast, low-sodium, deli-type, 2 oz	1
turkey ham, 2 oz	2
turkey roll, 2 oz	2
turkey, deli-type, sliced, 2 oz	1
turkey, white, rotisserie, deli-type, 2 oz	1
turkey-ham, extra lean, sliced, deli-type, 2 oz	1

M

● No Count	SmartPoints™ value
Macadamia nuts	
dry-roasted, ¼ cup	8
shelled, ¼ cup	8
Macaroni	
all shapes, regular, uncooked, 2 oz	6
cooked, 1 cup	5
manicotti shells, uncooked, 2 oz	6
vegetable, cooked, 1 cup	5
vegetable, uncooked, 2 oz	6
● whole-wheat, cooked, 1 cup	5
● whole-wheat, uncooked, 2 oz	5
Macaroni and cheese	
1 cup	14
canned, 14 ¾ oz	10
family-style, restaurant-type, 7 ½ oz	11
frozen, 7 ½ oz	12
in a cup, unprepared, 1 container (2 oz)	8
package mix, prepared, 1 cup	13
Macaroni and cheese, Bahamian	
1 cup	13
Malai kofta (vegetable balls in cream sauce)	
7 oz	14
Malanga	
● cooked or uncooked, ½ cup	3
Malted milk	
chocolate, added nutrients, powder, 2 Tbsp	8
chocolate, added nutrients, powder, prepared with whole milk, 8 fl oz	11
natural, added nutrients, powder, 2 Tbsp	2
natural, added nutrients, powder, prepared with whole milk, 8 fl oz	10

Complete A-Z Food List

Mango

dried, ¼ cup	5
○ fresh, frozen, cooked, or canned, without added sugar	0

Manicotti

cheese, with tomato sauce, frozen, 10 oz	14
cheese, without sauce, frozen, 5 ½ oz	9
with meat sauce, 2 pieces with ½ cup sauce (12 oz)	20
with tomato sauce, 2 pieces with ½ cup sauce (12 oz)	17

Margarine

blend, margarine-butter, 1 Tbsp	4
fat-free, 1 Tbsp	0
fat-free, ¼ cup	1
reduced-calorie, 1 Tbsp	3
regular, 1 Tbsp	4
soft, 1 Tbsp	4
spread, margarine-like (approximately 40% fat), 1 Tbsp	2

Marinade

soy, 1 Tbsp	1

Marmalade

1 Tbsp	3
low-sugar, 1 Tbsp	1

Marshmallows

1 (¼ oz)	1
mini, 10 (¼ oz)	1

Marzipan

1 Tbsp	3

Masala dosa

with filling, 7 ¾ oz	16
without filling, 5 ⅓ oz	14

Matzo

egg, 1 oz	3
egg and onion, 1 oz	3
plain, 1 oz	3
whole-wheat, 1 oz	3

Matzo brei

3 oz	7

Matzo cake meal

¼ cup	3

Matzo farfel

store-bought, ½ oz	2

Matzo meal

¼ cup	3

Mayonnaise

fat-free, 1 Tbsp	1
imitation, low-calorie, 2 Tbsp	1
imitation, soybean, 1 Tbsp	1
imitation, soybean, without cholesterol, 1 Tbsp	2
light, 2 Tbsp	3
low-calorie, 2 Tbsp	3
reduced-calorie, 1 Tbsp	2
regular, 1 Tbsp	3

Meal replacement/supplement bar for weight loss

1 (1 oz)	5

Meal replacement/supplement drinks

8 fl oz	10
breakfast powder, instant, 1 Tbsp	1

Meal replacement/supplement drinks for weight loss

prepared from powder using fat-free milk, or canned, 8 fl oz	8

Meat substitute

soy burger, 1 (2 ½ oz)	3
○ soy crumbles, meatless, ½ cup	1
textured vegetable protein, 3 oz	5
vegetarian breakfast link, sausage-type, 1 ½ oz	3
vegetarian breakfast patty, sausage-type, 1 ½ oz	1
vegetarian breakfast strips, 1 (¼ oz)	1
vegetarian burger, black bean, frozen, 1 (1 ½ oz)	3

Complete A-Z Food List

○ No Count	SmartPoints™ value
○ vegetarian burger, fat-free, frozen, 1 (2 ¾ oz)	1
vegetarian burger, frozen, 1 (2 ¾ oz)	3
○ vegetarian burger, with 2 g fat or less, 1 (3 oz)	2
vegetarian chicken patty, frozen, 1 (3 oz)	3
vegetarian chicken pieces (nugget-style), frozen, 2 ¾ oz	4
vegetarian deli slices, frozen, 2 ¾ oz	1
vegetarian frankfurter, fat-free, frozen, 1 (2 ½ oz)	1
vegetarian frankfurter, regular, frozen, 1 (3 oz)	2
○ vegetarian ground meat, frozen, ½ cup	1
vegetarian luncheon meats, 1 ½ oz	1
vegetarian meatloaf, 3 oz	4
vegetarian sausage, frozen, 1 ⅓ oz	2
Meatballs	
Swedish, 4 oz	12
Swedish, with noodles, frozen, 1 cup	10
with sauce, 2 meatballs and ½ cup Italian tomato sauce	15
without sauce, 1 (1 ¾ oz)	6
without sauce, frozen, 3 oz	8
Meatloaf	
4 oz	8
Melba toast or rounds	
1 oz	3
Melon balls	
○ fresh, frozen, cooked, or canned, without added sugar	0
Milk	
○ buttermilk, fat-free, 8 fl oz	3
buttermilk, low-fat (1%), 8 fl oz	4

○ No Count	SmartPoints™ value
buttermilk, reduced-fat (2%), 1 cup	6
buttermilk, whole, 8 fl oz	7
○ fat-free (skim), 8 fl oz	3
low-fat or light (1%), 8 fl oz	4
reduced-fat (2%), 8 fl oz	5
whole, 8 fl oz	7
Milk shake	
chocolate, fast food, 8 fl oz	12
chocolate, thick, 8 fl oz	14
dairy, reduced-calorie, 1 packet (¾ oz)	3
strawberry, fast food, 8 fl oz	13
vanilla, fast food, 8 fl oz	11
vanilla, thick, 8 fl oz	13
Milk, chocolate	
fat-free, 8 fl oz	7
low-fat (1%), 8 fl oz	8
reduced-fat (2%), 8 fl oz	8
regular, 8 fl oz	10
Milk, condensed	
sweetened with sugar, 1 Tbsp	3
sweetened with sugar, fat-free, 2 Tbsp	6
Milk, dry	
nonfat, instant, powder, ¼ cup	2
whole, ¼ cup	7
Milk, evaporated	
fat-free, 8 fl oz	8
low-fat, 8 fl oz	9
whole, 8 fl oz	15
Milk, filled	
8 fl oz	7
Milk, goat	
8 fl oz	7
Milk, oat	
any flavor, 8 fl oz	6
Milk, soy	
fat-free, chocolate, 8 fl oz	4
○ fat-free, plain, 8 fl oz	3

	flavored, 8 fl oz	5
○	low-fat, 8 fl oz	4
	original, vanilla, 8 fl oz	4
○	regular, plain, 8 fl oz	3
○	unflavored, 8 fl oz	3
○	unsweetened, 8 fl oz	2

Millet

○	cooked, 1 cup	6
○	uncooked, 2 oz	6

Miso paste

	1 Tbsp	1
	light, 1 Tbsp	1

Mochi

	1 piece (1 ¼ oz)	4
	butter, 1 piece (2 ¾ oz)	12

Molasses

	1 Tbsp	3
	blackstrap, 1 Tbsp	3
	light, 1 Tbsp	3

Mongolian beef

	1 cup	9

Moo goo gai pan

	1 cup	8

Moo shoo

	chicken, ½ cup with 2 pancakes	9
	pork, ½ cup with 2 pancakes	9
	tofu, ½ cup with 2 pancakes	10

Moose

○	cooked, 3 oz	1
○	uncooked, 4 oz	1

Moussaka

	8 ¼ oz	17

Mousse

	chocolate, ½ cup	22
	crème caramel, ½ cup	7

Muffin

	any type other than those listed here, 1 large (3" diameter) or 3 ¾ oz	10

	any type other than those listed here, store-bought, 1 large (4 oz)	17
	banana-walnut, restaurant-type, 1 (5 oz)	23
	blueberry, reduced-fat, restaurant-type, 1 (5 oz)	17
	blueberry, store-bought, 1 (2 oz)	5
	blueberry, toaster-type, 1 (1 oz)	3
	chocolate chip, restaurant-type, 1 (5 oz)	22
	corn, prepared from dry mix, 1 (1 ¾ oz)	6
	corn, restaurant-type, 1 (5 oz)	16
	corn, store-bought, 1 (2 oz)	6
	corn, toaster-type, 1 (1 oz)	4
	cranberry-orange, restaurant-type, 1 (5 oz)	19
	fat-free, store-bought, 1 (2 oz)	5
	oat bran, 1 (2 oz)	5
	orange, 1 (2 oz)	9
	pumpkin, restaurant-type, 1 (5 oz)	18
	wheat bran, with raisins, toaster-type, 1 (1 ¼ oz)	4

Muffin mix

	blueberry, 1 oz	5
	corn, dry mix, 1 ½ oz	6

Mung dal

	mung dal, 1 cup	8

Mushrooms

	breaded, prepared without fat, 7 (3 oz)	4
○	dried or reconstituted	0
○	fresh, frozen, cooked, or canned, without added sugar or oil	0
	marinated, ½ cup	3

Mushrooms, stuffed

	4 (2 ¾ oz)	5

Mussels Marinière

	4 mussels with 3 Tbsp sauce	7

Complete A-Z Food List

		SmartPoints™ value
○ No Count		

Mustard

1 Tbsp	0
honey, 1 Tbsp	2
honey-dijon, 1 Tbsp	1

N

Nachos

beef, 8 ½ oz	19
cheese, 3 oz	12
cheese and bean, 6 ½ oz	14
chicken, 8 ½ oz	16
with cheese and jalapeño peppers, fast food, 7 oz	21
with cheese sauce, ½ cup tortilla chips with ¼ cup sauce	8
with cheese, beans, ground beef, and peppers, fast food, 9 oz	19
with cheese, beans, ground beef, and tomatoes, fast food, 7 ¾ oz	15
with cheese, fast food, 2 ¾ oz	9

Napoleon

1 slice (6 oz)	23

Nectarine

○ fresh, frozen, cooked, or canned, without added sugar or oil	0

Noodles

cellophane, cooked, 1 cup	6
cellophone, uncooked, 2 oz	6
chow mein, packaged, 2 oz	9
egg, cooked, 1 cup	6
egg, no yolk, uncooked, 2 oz	6
egg, spinach, cooked, 1 cup	6
egg, spinach, uncooked, 2 oz	6
egg, uncooked, 2 oz	6
○ egg, whole-wheat, uncooked, 2 oz	5
fried, 1 cup	8
lasagna, no cook, 2 oz	6
lasagna, uncooked, 2 oz	6

		SmartPoints™ value
○ No Count		

○ lasagna, whole-wheat, uncooked, 2 oz	5
Oriental (bean thread), cooked, 1 cup	7
Oriental potato noodles (dang myeon), 2 oz	6
ramen, cooked, 1 cup	6
ramen, fresh, uncooked, 1 ½ oz	6
rice, cooked, 1 cup	5
rice, uncooked, 2 oz	6
soba, with sauce, 1 cup	13

Noodles and sauce mix

prepared, ½ cup	5

Noodles, Japanese

soba, cooked, 1 cup	3
soba, uncooked, 2 oz	5
somen, cooked, 1 cup	6
somen, uncooked, 2 oz	6
udon, uncooked, 2 oz	6

Nopales

○ fresh, frozen, cooked, or canned, without added sugar or oil	0

Nut butter

almond, 2 Tbsp	6
cashew, 2 Tbsp	6

Nuts, mixed

dry-roasted, ¼ cup	6
oil-roasted, ¼ cup	7
shelled, ¼ cup	6

O

Oil

almond, 1 Tbsp	4
any type, vegetable, 1 Tbsp	4
apricot kernel, 1 Tbsp	4
avocado, 1 Tbsp	4
beluga, 1 Tbsp	5
butter, 1 Tbsp	6
canola, 1 Tbsp	4

chili, 1 Tbsp	4
coconut, 1 Tbsp	7
corn, 1 Tbsp	4
flaxseed, 1 Tbsp	4
grapeseed, 1 Tbsp	4
olive, 1 Tbsp	4
peanut, 1 Tbsp	4
safflower, 1 Tbsp	4
sesame, 1 Tbsp	4
sesame, dark, 1 Tbsp	4
sesame, toasted, 1 Tbsp	4
soybean, partially hydrogenated, 1 Tbsp	4
sunflower, 1 Tbsp	4
walnut, 1 Tbsp	4

Okra

○ fresh, frozen, cooked, or canned, without added sugar or oil	0

Okra, breaded

frozen, prepared without fat, 3 oz	3

Okra, fried

7 oz	12

Olives

black, ripe, canned, 4 jumbo	1
black, ripe, canned, 4 large	1
black, ripe, canned, 4 super colossal	2
black, ripe, canned, 6 small	1
green, pickled, canned or bottled, 6 (½ oz)	1
oil-cured, 1 oz	4
pimiento-stuffed, 4	1

Omelet

cheese, 1 (2-egg)	11
ham and cheese, 1 (2-egg)	12
ham and cheese, restaurant-type, 1 (9 ½ oz)	18
herb or plain, 1 (2-egg)	8
vegetable, 1 (2-egg)	10
vegetable, restaurant-type, 1 (11 ⅔ oz)	18

Onion

○ fresh, frozen, cooked, or canned, without added sugar or oil	0

Onion flakes, dehydrated

1 Tbsp	0

Onion rings

breaded, frozen, prepared without fat, 10 large (2 ½ oz)	10
family-style, restaurant-type, 10 oz	31
fast food, 4 oz	16
fried, 3 oz	9
frozen, unprepared, 3 oz	8

Onion, blooming

4 ¾ oz	8

Orange

○ blood orange	0
○ fresh, frozen, cooked, or canned, without added sugar	0
peel (zest), 1 Tbsp	0
○ sections	0

Orange chicken

1 cup	15

Orange, Mandarin

canned, in juice, ½ cup	3
canned, in light syrup, ½ cup	5
○ fresh, frozen, cooked, or canned, without added sugar	0

Orange-ginger beef

1 cup	18

Osso bucco

10 oz	13

Oysters Rockefeller

2 oz	4

Oysters, fried

5 oz	9
breaded or battered, fast food, 5 oz	11

P

Pad si-iew (stir-fried beef with noodles)

1 cup	8

Pad Thai (Thai rice noodles with chicken and shrimp)

1 cup	12

Paella

1 cup	9

Pajun (Korean green onion and shrimp pancake)

7 oz	10

Pakora

vegetable, 1 (1 ¾ oz)	4

Pancake

and sausage on a stick, 3 (6 oz)	23
any type, frozen, 3 (3 ¾ oz)	8
any type, prepared from mix, 3 (4" diameter) or 4 oz	6
buttermilk, with butter and syrup, restaurant-type, 3 (9 oz)	25
Chinese, 1 (1 oz)	2
fast food, 3 (5 ¼ oz)	13
mini, frozen, without syrup, 3 (¾ oz)	2
prepared from incomplete dry mix, 3 (4 oz)	7
prepared from incomplete whole-wheat dry mix, 3 (4 ⅔ oz)	8
prepared from scratch, 3 (4" diameter) or 6 oz	13
with butter and syrup, fast food, 3 (12 ¼ oz)	25

Pancake mix

complete, ⅓ cup	5
incomplete, ⅓ cup	4
incomplete, buckwheat, ⅓ cup	4
incomplete, whole-wheat, ⅓ cup	4

Pancetta

2 oz	17

Pancit canton (sautéed egg noodles)

5 oz	7

Paneer, jalfrezi

7 oz	9

Paneer, mutter

1 cup	15

Paneer, palak

1 cup	17

Paneer, saag

1 cup	8

Papaya

O	fresh, frozen, cooked, or canned, without added sugar	0

Parsnips

O	cooked or canned, ½ cup	2
O	uncooked, ½ cup	2

Passionfruit

O	fresh, frozen, cooked, or canned, without added sugar	0

Pasta

	brown rice, cooked, 1 oz	1
O	brown rice, uncooked, 2 oz	6
	corn, cooked, 1 cup	5
	corn, uncooked, 2 oz	6
	fresh, refrigerated, plain, cooked, 1 cup	8
	fresh, refrigerated, plain, uncooked, 3 oz	6
	fresh, refrigerated, spinach, cooked, 1 cup	8
	fresh, refrigerated, spinach, uncooked, 3 oz	7
	homemade, made with egg, cooked, 1 cup	8
	homemade, made without egg, cooked, 1 cup	8
	regular, any shape other than those listed here, cooked, 1 cup	5
	regular, any shape other than those listed here, uncooked, 2 oz	6

No Count		SmartPoints™ value
○	whole-wheat, any shape other than those listed here, cooked, 1 cup	5
○	whole-wheat, any shape other than those listed here, uncooked, 2 oz	5
Pasta primavera		
	with cream sauce, 1 cup pasta with ¾ cup sauce	20
	with marinara sauce, 1 cup pasta with ¾ cup sauce	7
Pasta shells, stuffed		
	stuffed with ricotta cheese, without sauce, frozen, 5 ¼ oz	6
Pasta with garlic and oil		
	5 ⅔ oz	9
Pastelitos de carne (Cuban meat pastry)		
	1 (2 ½ oz)	13
Pastitsio		
	10 oz	19
Pastrami		
	beef, 3 oz	3
○	beef, 98% fat-free, 2 oz	1
	made from turkey, 2 oz	2
Pâté		
	chicken liver, canned, 1 Tbsp	1
	fish, store-bought, 2 oz	4
	liver, 3 oz	5
	meat, store-bought, 1 Tbsp	2
Pâté de foie gras		
	duck liver, canned, 1 Tbsp	2
	goose liver, smoked, 1 Tbsp	2
Pea shoots		
○	fresh, frozen, cooked, or canned, without added sugar or oil	0
Peach		
	canned, in extra light syrup, ½ cup	2
	canned, in heavy syrup, ½ cup	6
	canned, in light syrup, ½ cup	4

No Count		SmartPoints™ value
	dried halves, ¼ cup	5
	dried, stewed, sweetened with sugar, ½ cup	8
	dried, stewed, without added sugar, ¼ cup	3
○	fresh, frozen, cooked, or canned, without added sugar	0
	frozen, sweetened with sugar, 1 cup	14
	spiced, canned, in heavy syrup, ½ cup	5
Peach Melba		
	½ cup ice cream with 2 peach halves and raspberry sauce	15
Peanut butter		
	chunky, 2 Tbsp	6
	reduced-fat, smooth, 2 Tbsp	6
	reduced-sodium, 2 Tbsp	6
	smooth, 2 Tbsp	6
	with omega-3, creamy, 2 Tbsp	6
Peanuts		
	¼ cup	6
	cooked, shelled, ¼ cup	4
	dry-roasted, ¼ cup	7
	honey, reduced-fat, ¼ cup	3
	oil-roasted, ¼ cup	6
	uncooked, ¼ cup	6
Pear		
○	Asian	0
○	canned, in extra light syrup, ½ cup	2
	canned, in heavy syrup, ½ cup	5
	canned, in light syrup, ½ cup	4
	dried, ¼ cup	7
	dried, stewed, with added sugar, ½ cup	11
	dried, stewed, without added sugar, ½ cup	9
○	fresh, frozen, cooked, or canned, without added sugar	0
	poached, 6 oz	13

Pear (cont'd)

No Count	SmartPoints™ value
prickly	0
puree, prune, 2 Tbsp	4
Peas	
baby, frozen, ½ cup	2
green, canned, drained solids, ½ cup	2
green, canned, solids and liquids, ½ cup	2
green, cooked, ½ cup	2
green, frozen, cooked, ½ cup	2
green, frozen, unprepared, ½ cup	2
green, uncooked, ½ cup	2
Peas and rice	
Bahamian-style, 1 cup	12
Jamaican, 1 cup	12
Peas, black-eyed	
canned, ½ cup	3
cooked, ½ cup	3
fresh, uncooked, ¼ cup	1
Peas, snow (Chinese pea pods)	
fresh, frozen, cooked, or canned, without added sugar or oil	0
Peas, split	
cooked, ½ cup	3
dry, ¼ cup	4
Peas, sugar snap	
fresh, frozen, cooked, or canned, without added sugar or oil	0
Pecans	
chopped, ¼ cup	6
halves, ¼ cup	6
oil-roasted, ¼ cup	6
pecans, dry-roasted, ¼ cup	6
Pectin	
desserts, rennin, tablets, unsweetened, 1 package (⅓ oz)	0
Peking duck	
2 oz duck with 1 piece duck skin and 3 pancakes	13

No Count	SmartPoints™ value
Penne alla vodka	
1 cup pasta with ½ cup sauce	12
Pepper steak	
6 oz	16
Pepperoncini	
fresh, frozen, cooked, or canned, without added sugar or oil	0
Pepperoni	
2 oz	9
turkey, 1 oz	2
Peppers	
ancho, dried, 1 (¼ oz)	0
chopped green chillis, canned, ½ cup	0
fresh, frozen, cooked, or canned, without added sugar or oil	0
peppers, chipotle, in adobo sauce, canned, ½ cup	3
Peppers, roasted red	
packed in water	0
Persimmon	
fresh, frozen, cooked, or canned, without added sugar	0
Pheasant	
breast, uncooked, without skin and bone, 4 oz	2
cooked, 3 oz	5
leg, uncooked, without skin and bone, 1 (3 ¾ oz)	2
Phyllo (fillo) dough	
1 sheet (⅔ oz)	2
wheat, 1 sheet (⅔ oz)	2
mini, 2 (¼ oz)	1
Pickles, sweet	
¼ cup	3
Pickles, unsweetened	
dill	0
dill gherkins	0
dill, kosher, sandwich slices	0
dill, low-sodium	0

sour	0
sour, low-sodium	0

Pico de gallo

○ fresh, frozen, cooked, or canned, without added sugar or oil	0

Pie crust

any type, ¾ oz	3
any type, refrigerated or frozen, baked, ⅛ of 9" one-crust pie (⅔ oz)	3
chocolate cookie type, prepared from recipe, 1 oz	5
graham cracker, 1 ⅓ oz	9
graham cracker, prepared from recipe, 1 oz	6
graham cracker, reduced-fat, ⅛ of 9" one-crust pie (¾ oz)	4
prepared from dry mix, baked, ⅔ oz	3
prepared from recipe, ¾ oz	4
ready-to-bake, frozen, ⅛ of 9" one-crust pie (¾ oz)	3

Pie crust mix

¼ package (2 ½ oz)	12

Pie filling

fruit, canned, ¼ cup	3
fruit, light, canned, ¼ cup	2
pumpkin, canned, ¼ cup	4

Pie, dessert

apple, prepared from recipe, 1 slice (5 ½ oz)	16
apple, store-bought, 1 slice (4 ½ oz)	12
banana cream, prepared from mix, no-bake type, 1 slice (3 ¼ oz)	10
banana cream, prepared from recipe, 1 slice (5 oz)	15
blueberry, prepared from recipe, 1 slice (5 oz)	14
blueberry, store-bought, 1 slice (4 oz)	10
cherry, prepared from recipe, 1 slice (6 ⅓ oz)	19
cherry, store-bought, 1 slice (4 oz)	12
chocolate cream, store-bought, 1 slice (3 ½ oz)	17
chocolate mousse, prepared from mix, no-bake type, 1 slice (3 ½ oz)	11
coconut cream, prepared from mix, no-bake type, 1 slice (3 ⅓ oz)	11
coconut cream, store-bought, 1 slice (1 ¾ oz)	7
coconut custard, 1 slice (6 oz)	17
coconut custard, store-bought, 1 slice (3 ⅔ oz)	12
cream, with or without fruit, frozen, 1 slice (4 ¾ oz)	15
custard, 5 ½ oz	14
egg custard, store-bought, 1 slice (3 ¾ oz)	8
fruit, any type, frozen, 1 slice (4 ½ oz)	13
fruit, fast food, 1 slice (3 ½ oz)	13
fruit, fried, 1 (4 ½ oz)	16
fruit, one-crust, ⅛ of 9" diameter	13
fruit, two-crust, ⅛ of 9" diameter	18
key lime, 5 ⅓ oz	25
key lime, store-bought, 1 slice (4 ½ oz)	22
lemon meringue, prepared from recipe, 1 slice (4 ½ oz)	16
lemon meringue, store-bought, 1 slice (4 oz)	13
meringue, ⅛ of 9" diameter	21
meringue, any type, frozen, 5 oz	16
mince, frozen, 4 ¼ oz	12
mince, prepared from recipe, 1 slice (5 ¾ oz)	21
mincemeat, with meat, 5 ⅓ oz	24

● No Count	SmartPoints™ value
peach, 1 slice (4 oz)	9
pecan, 1 slice (4 ⅓ oz)	21
pecan, frozen, 1 slice (4 ½ oz)	23
pecan, prepared from recipe, 1 slice (4 ⅓ oz)	16
pecan, store-bought, 1 slice (4 oz)	18
pumpkin, 1 slice (6 ½ oz)	17
pumpkin, frozen, 1 slice (5 oz)	13
pumpkin, prepared from recipe, 1 slice (5 ½ oz)	14
pumpkin, store-bought, 1 slice (4 ⅔ oz)	13
rhubarb, 1 slice (6 oz)	21
vanilla cream, prepared from recipe, 1 slice (4 ½ oz)	13
Pierogies	
cabbage, 2 (2 ⅓ oz)	9
cheese, 2 (2 ½ oz)	10
meat, 2 (2 ½ oz)	10
potato, 2 (2 ½ oz)	10
potato and cheese or onion, low-fat, frozen, 4 ½ oz	5
potato and cheese, frozen, 4 oz	5
Pignolias (pine nuts)	
¼ cup	6
dried, ¼ cup	6
Pigs' feet	
pickled, store-bought, 3 oz	3
Pimientos	
● canned	0
Pineapple	
● canned, chunks, in juice, drained	0
● canned, crushed, in juice, drained	0
● canned, sliced, in juice, drained	0
● canned, spears, in juice, drained, 1 spear	0
● fresh, frozen, cooked, or canned, without added sugar	0

● No Count	SmartPoints™ value
pineapple rings, canned, in juice, ½ cup	4
pineapple, canned, in heavy syrup, ½ cup	6
pineapple, canned, in juice, ½ cup	4
pineapple, canned, in light syrup, ½ cup	4
pineapple, crushed, canned, in juice, ½ cup	4
pineapple, dried, rings, 1 oz	4
pineapple, frozen chunks, sweetened, 1 cup	13
Pistachio nuts	
dry-roasted, shelled, ¼ cup	5
Pita	
pocketless, 1 (2 oz)	5
white, 1 (1 oz)	2
whole-wheat, 1 (1 oz)	2
Pita chips	
1 oz	4
whole-wheat, 1 oz	3
Pizza	
14" pie, cheese and pepperoni, regular crust, restaurant-type, 1 slice (⅛ pie)	10
14" pie, cheese and pepperoni, thick crust, restaurant-type, 1 slice (⅛ pie)	11
14" pie, cheese and pepperoni, thin crust, restaurant-type, 1 slice (⅛ pie)	9
14" pie, cheese and sausage, regular crust, restaurant-type, 1 slice (⅛ pie)	11
14" pie, cheese and sausage, thick crust, restaurant-type, 1 slice (⅛ pie)	12
14" pie, cheese and sausage, thin crust, restaurant-type, 1 slice (⅛ pie)	9
14" pie, cheese, meat, and vegetable, regular crust, restaurant-type, 1 slice (⅛ pie)	11

14" pie, cheese, regular crust, restaurant-type, 1 slice (⅛ pie)	9
14" pie, cheese, stuffed crust, restaurant-type, 1 slice (⅛ pie)	11
14" pie, cheese, thick crust, restaurant-type, 1 slice (⅛ pie)	10
14" pie, cheese, thin crust, restaurant-type, 1 slice (⅛ pie)	8

Pizza bagel

mini, any type, 3 oz	6

Pizza crust dough

mix, ¼ cup	5
refrigerated, frozen or ready-made, 1 oz	3
whole-wheat, refrigerated, 2 oz	3

Pizza, frozen

pepperoni, 5 oz	13
pieces, prepared without fat, 3 oz	7
supreme, 5 oz	12
vegetable, frozen, 5 oz	9

Pizza, frozen, single serving

cheese, 6 ¾ oz	16
pepperoni, 6 ¾ oz	14
sausage, 7 oz	13
supreme, 7 ¼ oz	15

Pizza, one-meat topping

deep-dish, restaurant-type, 1 slice (⅛ pie)	10
thin crust, restaurant-type, 1 slice (2 ¾ oz)	6

Pizza, Sicilian

cheese, 1 slice (3 oz)	6

Plantain

baked or boiled, 1 cup	8
fried, ½ cup	4
uncooked, 1 medium (6 ⅓ oz)	10

Plantain chips

1 oz	5

Plátanos maduros (fried sweet plantains)

½ cup	4

Plum

● fresh, frozen, cooked, or canned, without added sugar	0
purple, canned, in heavy syrup, 1	2
purple, canned, in juice, 1	2
purple, canned, in light syrup, 1	2

Poi

● ½ cup	4

Poke (Hawaiian fish salad)

ahi, ½ cup	1
tako, ½ cup	2

Polenta

● cooked, ½ cup	4
● dry mix, instant, ¼ cup	4
● in tube, ready-to-eat, 1 oz	1

Pomegranate

● fresh, frozen, cooked, or canned, without added sugar	0
● seeds	0

Pomelo (pummelo)

● fresh, frozen, cooked, or canned, without added sugar	0

Popcorn

buttered, popped, 2 cups	5
butter-flavored, popped, 1 cup	1
caramel-coated, popped, with peanuts, 2 cups	15
caramel-coated, popped, without peanuts, 2 cups	23
cheese-flavored, popped, 2 cups	4
light, butter-flavored, popped, 2 cups	2
light, caramel-coated, popped, 2 cups	11
light, cheese-flavored, popped, 2 cups	4
● light, microwave-popped, 2 cups	2
light, plain, popped, 2 cups	2
movie, without butter, 2 cups	3

Popcorn (cont'd)

● No Count	SmartPoints™ value
oil popped, microwave, regular flavor, 1 cup	2
oil popped, white, 1 cup	2
● plain, air-popped, 2 cups	2
● plain, microwave-popped, 2 cups	3
plain, oil popped, 1 cup	1
plain, popped, packaged, 2 cups	3
● reduced-fat (94% fat-free), microwave-popped, 2 cups	2
● white, air-popped, 2 cups	2
Popcorn cake	
mini, 1	0
other than plain or butter-flavored, 1 (½ oz)	2
plain or butter-flavored, 1 (⅓ oz)	1
Popover	
1 (1 ½ oz)	3
Pork	
backribs, cooked, barbecued, 1 rib (3 ¼ oz)	10
backribs, lean and fat, cooked, 1 rib (2 ½ oz)	6
backribs, lean and fat, uncooked, 4 oz	7
barbecue, 8 ½ oz	9
center, loin, lean and fat, cooked, 3 oz	4
center, loin, lean and fat, uncooked, 4 oz	6
● center, loin, lean only, cooked, 3 oz	3
chop, center, loin, uncooked, 4 oz	4
● chop, cooked, lean, without bone, 3 oz	3
● chop, lean, boneless, trimmed, uncooked, 4 oz	3
country-style ribs, cooked, 3 oz	6
country-style ribs, uncooked, 4 oz	6
leg, cooked, 3 oz	6
leg, lean and fat, uncooked, 4 oz	8

● No Count	SmartPoints™ value
leg, lean only, uncooked, 4 oz	3
leg, trimmed, cooked, 3 oz	4
loin, center rib, lean and fat, cooked, 3 oz	6
loin, lean and fat, cooked, 3 oz	5
loin, lean and fat, uncooked, 4 oz	5
● loin, lean only, uncooked, 4 oz	4
loin, trimmed, cooked, 3 oz	4
● pork, center loin, lean only, raw, 4 oz	3
shoulder, lean and fat, cooked, 3 oz	6
shoulder, lean and fat, uncooked, 4 oz	7
shoulder, lean only, cooked, 3 oz	5
● shoulder, lean only, uncooked, 4 oz	3
sirloin, cooked, 3 oz	5
sirloin, lean and fat, uncooked, 4 oz	4
● sirloin, lean only, cooked, 3 oz	3
● sirloin, lean only, uncooked, 4 oz	3
spareribs, lean and fat, cooked, 3 oz	10
spareribs, lean and fat, uncooked, 4 oz	10
● stomach, cooked, 3 oz	3
● tenderloin, lean only, cooked, 3 oz	2
● tenderloin, lean only, uncooked, 4 oz	2
● top loin, lean only, cooked, 3 oz	3
Pork and beans	
canned, 4 ½ oz	4
Pork in barbecue sauce	
frozen, 2 oz	4
Pork rinds (skins)	
barbecue-flavor, 1 oz	4
plain, 1 oz	4
Pork with cashews	
1 cup	13

No Count	SmartPoints™ value
Pork, ground	
72% lean/28% fat, cooked, 3 oz	10
84% lean/16% fat, cooked, 3 oz	7
84% lean/16% fat, uncooked, 4 oz	7
◖ 96% lean, cooked, 3 oz	2
◖ 96% lean, uncooked, 4 oz	2
cooked, 3 oz	7
uncooked, 4 oz	10
Pot pie	
any type, fast food, 14 oz	25
beef, chicken, or turkey, frozen, 7 oz	15
chicken, homemade, 8 ⅓ oz	15
Pot sticker (filled wonton)	
pork or vegetable, frozen, 1 ½ oz	3
vegetarian, fried, 4 (3 oz)	4
vegetarian, steamed, 4 (3 oz)	4
Potato	
◖ baby, cooked, 1 (4 ¾ oz)	4
◖ baby, uncooked, ½ cup	2
◖ baked, plain, 1 (6 oz)	5
baked, topped with cheese sauce and broccoli, fast food, 12 oz	15
◖ bliss, cooked, 6 oz	5
◖ bliss, uncooked, ½ cup	2
◖ boiled, ½ cup	2
◖ canned, drained, ½ cup	2
◖ new, cooked, 6 oz	5
◖ new, uncooked, ½ cup	2
◖ red, cooked, ½ cup	2
◖ red, uncooked, 1 medium (7 ½ oz)	4
shoestring, canned, ½ cup	5
◖ uncooked, ½ cup	2
◖ white, cooked, ½ cup	2
◖ white, whole, uncooked, ½ cup	2
◖ whole, frozen, uncooked, ½ cup	2
◖ whole, new, canned, drained, ½ cup	2

No Count	SmartPoints™ value
◖ whole, new, canned, with liquid, ½ cup	2
◖ with 1 tsp olive oil, ¾ cup	3
◖ Yukon gold, uncooked, ½ cup	2
Potato chips	
baked, 1 oz	3
barbecue-flavor, 1 oz	5
cheese-flavor, 1 oz	5
fat-free, 1 oz	2
light, 1 oz	5
lightly salted, 1 oz	5
plain, 1 oz	5
reduced-calorie, 1 oz	4
reduced-fat, 1 oz	4
reduced-fat, 1 oz	4
regular, 1 oz	5
sour-cream-and-onion-flavor, 1 oz	5
Potato flakes	
dry, ¼ cup	1
Potato latkes	
6 ⅓ oz	8
Potato mix	
flavored, prepared, ½ cup	4
Potato pancake mix	
2 oz	6
Potato pancakes	
3 ¼ oz	3
frozen, 2 oz	3
Potato puffs	
appetizer pastry, frozen, 1 (1 oz)	2
frozen, prepared, 10 (2 ¾ oz)	5
Potato skins	
"loaded, " frozen, 2 (4 oz)	8
◖ frozen, plain, unprepared, 1 ⅓ oz	1
with cheese, bacon, and sour cream, 1 (3 ½ oz)	7
Potato sticks	
1 oz	5

O No Count	SmartPoints™ value

Potato, baked

stuffed with bacon and cheese, 1 (9 ⅔ oz)	17
stuffed with vegetables and cheese, 1 (13 ⅓ oz)	16
with cheese sauce and bacon, fast food, 1 (10 ½ oz)	16
with cheese sauce and chili, fast food, 1 (14 oz)	17
with cheese sauce, fast food, 10 ⅓ oz	17
with sour cream and chives, fast food, 1 (10 ½ oz)	15
with vegetables and cheese, fast food, 13 oz	14

Potatoes O'Brien

frozen, prepared without fat, 4 ¼ oz	3
home-prepared, ½ cup	2

Potatoes au gratin

11 oz	21
prepared from dry mix with water, whole milk, and butter, 4 ¾ oz	5

Potatoes au gratin mix

unprepared, 1 ¾ oz	5

Potatoes, garlic mashed

½ cup	7

Potatoes, hash brown

family-style, restaurant-type, ½ cup	8
fast food, 1 patty (1 ¾ oz)	5
O frozen, uncooked, 3 ¾ oz	2
frozen, with butter sauce, unprepared, 6 oz	8
patty, frozen, prepared without fat, 1 (1 oz)	2

Potatoes, home-fried

1 cup	7

Potatoes, mashed

½ cup	4
dehydrated, prepared from flakes with whole milk and butter, 1 cup	8
fast food, 2 ¾ oz	2

O No Count	SmartPoints™ value

Potatoes, stuffed

with cheese, 5 ½ oz	7
with sour cream and chives, 5 ½ oz	6

Poutine

20 French fries with 2 oz cheese and ½ cup sauce	23

Preserves

1 Tbsp	3
low-sugar, 1 Tbsp	1

Pretzels

Bavarian, 1 oz	3
chocolate-covered, 1 oz	6
Philadelphia (soft), 1 oz	2
rods, 1 oz	3
salted or unsalted, 1 oz	3
soft, 1 oz	3
twists, 1 oz	3
whole-wheat, 1 oz	3
yogurt-covered, 1 oz	6

Profiterole

1 (1 ½ oz)	5

Prosciutto

2 oz	6

Prosecco

5 fl oz	4

Protein drink

powder, 1 Tbsp	1

Prunes

¼ cup	5
canned, in heavy syrup, ½ cup	7
stewed, with added sugar, ½ cup	9
stewed, without added sugar, ½ cup	6

Pubhouse battered halibut

3 ⅓ oz	4

Pudding

banana, instant, prepared from dry mix with whole milk, ½ cup	8
banana, prepared from dry mix with whole milk, ½ cup	8

banana, ready-to-eat, ½ cup	7
bread, ½ cup	12
chocolate prepared from dry mix with reduced-fat (2%) milk, ½ cup	8
chocolate, prepared from fat-free, sugar-free, instant dry mix with fat-free milk, ½ cup	3
chocolate, prepared from dry mix with whole milk, ½ cup	7
chocolate, prepared with fat-free milk, ½ cup	7
corn, home-prepared, ½ cup	6
lemon, ready-to-eat, ½ cup	4
plum, ½ cup, with 1 Tbsp sauce	20
prepared from fat-free, sugar-free mix with fat-free milk, ½ cup	3
pudding, any flavor other than those listed here, ½ cup	7
ready-made, ½ cup	7
ready-made, reduced-calorie, ½ cup	5
tapioca, ½ cup	5
tapioca, prepared from dry mix with reduced-fat (2%) milk, ½ cup	6
tapioca, prepared from dry mix with whole milk, ½ cup	7
tapioca, ready-to-eat, ½ cup	6
vanilla, prepared from dry mix with reduced-fat (2%) milk, ½ cup	4
vanilla, prepared from dry mix with whole milk, ½ cup	8
vanilla, prepared from fat-free, sugar-free, instant dry mix with fat-free milk, ½ cup	2
vanilla, prepared with fat-free milk, ½ cup	8
vanilla, ready-to-eat, ½ cup	3

Pudding mix

banana, ¼ package (¾ oz)	4
banana, fat-free, sugar-free, instant, ¼ package (⅓ oz)	1
banana, instant, ¼ package (¾ oz)	5
butterscotch, fat-free, sugar-free, instant, ¼ package (⅓ oz)	1
chocolate, ¼ package (¾ oz)	5
chocolate, fat-free, instant, ¼ package (½ oz)	1
chocolate, fat-free, sugar-free, instant, ¼ package (⅓ oz)	1
tapioca, ¼ package (¾ oz)	4
vanilla, ¼ package (¾ oz)	5
vanilla, fat-free, ¼ package (¾ oz)	2
vanilla, fat-free, sugar-free, instant, ¼ package (¼ oz)	1
vanilla, instant, ¼ package ¼ package (¾ oz)	6

Puff pastry

frozen, ready-to-bake, 1 shell (1 ½ oz)	9

Puff pastry shell

frozen, baked, 1 (1 ½ oz)	7

Pulled pork

in barbecue sauce, 8 ¾ oz	15

Pumpkin

○ fresh, frozen, cooked, or canned, without added sugar or oil	0
○ puree	0

Pumpkin butter

1 Tbsp	2

Pupusas con frijoles

restaurant-type, 1 (4 ½ oz)	9

Pupusas con queso

restaurant-type, 4 oz	10

Pupusas del cerdo

restaurant-type, 4 ⅓ oz	8

Complete A-Z Food List

Complete A-Z Food List

Q

Quail

○ breast, uncooked, without skin and bone, 4 oz	2
cooked, 3 oz	5
uncooked, with skin, without bone, 4 oz	5
○ uncooked, without skin and bone, 4 oz	3

Quenelles

8 (5 oz)	20

Quesadilla

beef, ½ of 6" diameter (4 oz)	9
cheese, ½ of 6" diameter (2 ¼ oz)	8
chicken, ½ of 6" diameter (3 ¾ oz)	8
vegetable, ½ of 6" diameter (3 ½ oz)	8
with chicken, fast food, 6 ⅓ oz	17

Quiche

appetizer, frozen, any type, 1 (¾ oz)	2
crab, frozen, 5 oz	18
quiche, vegetable, frozen, 5 oz	14
vegetable, ⅛ of 9" pie (6 ¼ oz)	14

Quiche Lorraine

1 (4 ⅓ oz)	16
frozen, 5 ½ oz	16

Quinoa

○ cooked, 1 cup	6
○ uncooked, 2 oz	6

R

Rabbit

○ domesticated, cooked, 3 oz	3
○ domesticated, uncooked, 4 oz	3
○ wild, cooked, 3 oz	2
○ wild, uncooked, 4 oz	2

Radicchio

○ fresh, frozen, cooked, or canned, without added sugar or oil	0

Radish

○ fresh, frozen, cooked, or canned, without added sugar or oil	0

Raisins

¼ cup	6
yogurt-covered, 2 oz	12

Raita

1 cup	7

Rajmah

1 cup	7

Raspberries

canned, in heavy syrup, ½ cup	7
○ fresh, frozen, cooked, or canned, without added sugar	0
frozen, sweetened with sugar, 1 cup	14

Ratatouille

1 cup	3

Ravioli

beef or chicken, without sauce, frozen, 4 oz	8
beef, breaded, frozen, 4 oz	7
beef, in meat sauce, canned, 8 ¾ oz	8
cheese filled, canned, 8 ½ oz	7
cheese, breaded, frozen, 4 oz	10
cheese, low-fat, 4 oz	6
cheese, with tomato sauce, 15 oz	23
cheese, without sauce, 8 ¾ oz	18
cheese, without sauce, frozen, 4 oz	8
cheese, without sauce, store-bought, 5 oz	10
meat, with tomato sauce, 13 oz	20
meat, without sauce, 7 oz	16
meat, without sauce, store-bought, 4 oz	9

	SmartPoints™ value
mushroom, without sauce, 4 ½ oz	9
vegetable and cheese, without sauce, store-bought, 4 oz	8
Red snapper Veracruz	
11 ¾ oz	11
Relish	
cranberry-orange, canned, ¼ cup	4
pickle, hot dog, ¼ cup	2
pickle, sweet, ¼ cup	3
Rhubarb	
cooked, with sugar, ½ cup	8
○ fresh, frozen, cooked, or canned, without added sugar	0
Rice	
arborio, 2 oz	6
basmati, uncooked, 2 oz	6
○ black, cooked, 1 cup	5
○ brown, cooked, 1 cup	6
○ brown, instant, uncooked, 2 oz	6
○ brown, medium-grain, cooked, 1 cup	6
○ brown, medium-grain, uncooked, 2 oz	6
○ brown, quick-cooking, 2 oz	6
○ brown, uncooked, 2 oz	6
Chinese, white, steamed, restaurant-type, 1 cup	6
jasmine, cooked, 1 cup	6
jasmine, uncooked, 2 oz	6
sushi, ½ cup	4
white, cooked, 1 cup	6
white, glutinous, cooked, 1 cup	5
white, glutinous, uncooked, 2 oz	6
white, long-grain, instant, cooked, 1 cup	6
white, long-grain, instant, uncooked, 2 oz	6
white, medium-grain, cooked, 1 cup	7

	SmartPoints™ value
white, medium-grain, uncooked, 2 oz	6
white, short-grain, cooked, 1 cup	7
white, short-grain, uncooked, 2 oz	6
white, uncooked, 2 oz	6
white, with pasta, cooked, 1 cup	7
○ wild, cooked, 1 cup	5
○ wild, uncooked, 2 oz	5
Rice bowl	
with chicken, frozen, prepared, 12 oz	13
Rice cake	
brown rice, buckwheat, 1 (⅓ oz)	1
brown rice, plain, 1 (⅓ oz)	1
buckwheat, 1 (⅓ oz)	1
corn, 1 (⅓ oz)	1
mini, cheddar, 1	0
multigrain, 1 (⅓ oz)	1
plain, 1 (⅓ oz)	1
sesame seed, 1 (⅓ oz)	1
Rice drink/rice beverage	
chocolate, 8 fl oz	8
fat-free, 8 fl oz	4
plain, 8 fl oz	5
Rice mix	
flavored, any type, prepared, ½ cup	5
long-grain and wild, unprepared, 2 oz	5
with black beans, prepared, 8 ½ oz	7
with red beans, prepared, 8 ½ oz	7
Rice pilaf	
1 cup	8
dry mix, unprepared, 2 oz	5
Rice pudding	
½ cup	7
arroz con leche, restaurant-type, 10 oz	18

Complete A-Z Food List

Complete A-Z Food List

○ No Count	SmartPoints™ value
kheer (Indian rice pudding), 7 ¾ oz	13
prepared from dry mix, with reduced-fat (2%) milk, ½ cup	8
prepared from dry mix, with whole milk, ½ cup	8
ready-to-eat, ½ cup	8
Rice pudding mix	
¼ package (1 oz)	5
Risotto	
1 cup	15
Risotto mix	
Milan-style risotto mix, 2 oz	6
Rogan josh	
1 cup	13
Roll dough	
crescent, reduced-fat, 1 piece (1 oz)	3
Rolls	
bollilo, 1 (3 ½ oz)	9
crescent dinner, store-bought, 1 (1 oz)	4
dinner, 1 (2 oz)	5
dinner, egg, 1 (1 ¼ oz)	3
dinner, oat bran, 1 (1 oz)	2
dinner, rye, 1 (1 ½ oz)	3
dinner, wheat, 1 (1 oz)	2
dinner, whole-wheat, 1 (1 ½ oz)	4
French, 1 (1 ⅓ oz)	3
hard, 1 (2 oz)	5
high fiber (3 g or more dietary fiber per roll), 1 (2 oz)	5
kaiser, restaurant-type, 1 (2 oz)	5
○ light, 1 (1 ½ oz)	2
pumpernickel, (2" square x 2" high), 1 (1 oz)	2
Ropa vieja	
6 ½ oz	10
Runza	
1 (5 ½ oz)	11

○ No Count	SmartPoints™ value
Rutabagas	
○ fresh, frozen, cooked, or canned, without added sugar or oil	0

S

Saag gosht	
8 ¼ oz	6
Saganaki	
1 piece (2 ¾ oz)	10
Salad	
Caesar, 3 cups	8
carrot and raisin, ½ cup	12
chef's, fast food, 11 ½ oz	7
chef's, with dressing, 4 cups	11
chef's, without dressing, 4 cups	8
chicken, ½ cup	6
chicken Caesar, grilled, restaurant-type, 6 ½ oz	9
chicken, grilled, without dressing, fast food, 1 (12 oz)	5
chicken, Oriental, 2 cups	6
chicken, restaurant-type, ½ cup	7
chicken, southwestern grilled, restaurant-type, 13 ¼ oz	6
chicken, store-bought, ½ cup	8
chicken-macaroni, 1 cup	7
cobb, without dressing, 3 cups	12
conch, 1 cup	2
cordon bleu, chicken, 6 ¾ oz	13
egg, ½ cup	9
fattoush, 2 cups	7
garden, restaurant-type, 6 oz	3
Greek, restaurant-type, 1 (12 ½ oz)	13
Greek, with dressing, 3 cups	11
Greek, without dressing, 3 cups	4
green papaya, with pork and shrimp, 1 cup	4
green papaya, without meat, 1 cup	3

lobster, ½ cup	4
macaroni, ½ cup	8
macaroni, store-bought, ½ cup	7
○ mixed greens	0
Niçoise, without dressing, 4 cups	9
Niçoise, with dressing, 4 cups	21
pasta, ½ cup	5
pasta, prepared from dry mix, 3 ¼ oz	5
pasta, store-bought, ½ cup	3
potato, ½ cup	6
potato, German, ½ cup	4
potato, store-bought, 4 oz	4
potato, with egg, ½ cup	7
salmon, kippered, with mayonnaise, store-bought, 2 oz	7
seafood, store-bought, ½ cup	8
seaweed, ½ cup	2
shrimp, ½ cup	4
○ side, without dressing, fast food	0
spinach, with dressing, 2 cups	8
taco, fast food, 7 oz	9
taco, with chili con carne, fast food, 1 ½ cups	10
taco, with shell, without dressing, fast food, 16 ½ oz	22
taco, without shell and dressing, fast food, 14 oz	12
Thai beef, 1 cup	18
Thai chicken, 2 cups	13
Thai seafood, 2 cups	12
three-bean, ½ cup	7
three-bean, canned, without oil, ½ cup	4
tomato and mozzarella, without dressing, 2 large tomato slices with 2 oz cheese	7
○ tossed, without dressing	0
tuna, ½ cup	5
tuna, store-bought, ½ cup	7

tuna-macaroni, 1 cup	6
turkey cobb, restaurant-type, 11 ⅓ oz	11
vegetable, tossed, with pasta and seafood, without dressing, fast food, 14 ¾ oz	11
vegetable, with cheese and egg, without dressing, fast food, 1 ½ cups	3
vegetable, with chicken, without dressing, fast food, 7 ⅔ oz	2
vegetable, with shrimp, without dressing, fast food, 1 ½ cups	2
vegetable, with turkey, ham, and cheese, without dressing, fast food, 1 ½ cups	8
Waldorf, ½ cup	8
whitefish, store-bought, 2 oz	6
yogurt and cucumber, ½ cup	2
Salad dressing	
bacon and tomato, 2 Tbsp	3
balsamic vinaigrette, fat-free, 2 Tbsp	1
balsamic vinaigrette, low-fat, 1 Tbsp	1
blue cheese, 2 Tbsp	5
blue cheese, fat-free, 2 Tbsp	1
blue cheese, light, 2 Tbsp	3
buttermilk, light, 2 Tbsp	2
Caesar, fat-free, 2 Tbsp	2
Caesar, low-calorie, 2 Tbsp	2
Caesar, regular, 2 Tbsp	6
coleslaw, 2 Tbsp	5
coleslaw, reduced-fat, 2 Tbsp	5
creamy, fat-free, 2 Tbsp	1
creamy, reduced-calorie, 2 Tbsp	3
creamy, regular, 2 Tbsp	5
dijonnaise, 2 Tbsp	1
dry mix, garlic-flavored, 1 oz	3
French, diet, 2 Tbsp	3
French, fat-free, 2 Tbsp	2

Complete A-Z Food List

Complete A-Z Food List

No Count	SmartPoints™ value
French, home recipe, 2 Tbsp	6
French, reduced-calorie, 2 Tbsp	3
French, reduced-fat, 2 Tbsp	3
French, regular, 2 Tbsp	5
French, store-bought, 2 Tbsp	6
ginger, 2 Tbsp	3
gluten-free light balsamic vinaigrette, 2 Tbsp	2
green goddess, 2 Tbsp	5
home recipe, cooked, 2 Tbsp	2
honey-mustard, 2 Tbsp	5
honey-mustard, fat-free, 1 Tbsp	2
Italian-type (not creamy), diet, 2 Tbsp	1
Italian-type (not creamy), fat-free, 2 Tbsp	1
Italian-type (not creamy), reduced-calorie, 2 Tbsp	2
Italian-type (not creamy), reduced-fat, store-bought, 2 Tbsp	1
Italian-type (not creamy), regular, 2 Tbsp	3
mayonnaise-type, 2 Tbsp	3
peppercorn, store-bought, 2 Tbsp	5
poppy seed, creamy, 2 Tbsp	5
raspberry vinaigrette, fat-free, 2 Tbsp	2
red wine vinaigrette, fat-free, 2 Tbsp	1
red wine vinaigrette, low-fat, 2 Tbsp	2
roquefort cheese, low-calorie or light, 2 Tbsp	1
Russian, 2 Tbsp	4
Russian, low-calorie, 2 Tbsp	2
sesame seed, 2 Tbsp	5
sesame-ginger, light, 1 Tbsp	1
spray-style, any type, 10 sprays	1
Thousand Island, 2 Tbsp	5
Thousand Island, diet (10 calories per tsp), 2 Tbsp	2

No Count	SmartPoints™ value
Thousand Island, fat-free, 2 Tbsp	2
vinaigrette, 2 Tbsp	5
vinaigrette, fat-free, 2 Tbsp	1
vinaigrette, low-fat, 2 Tbsp	1
vinegar and oil, home recipe, 2 Tbsp	5
Salad spread	
ham, 1 oz	2
Salami	
beef, 2 oz	5
beef and pork, 2 oz	6
beerwurst, beef, 3 oz	8
beerwurst, pork, 3 oz	7
beerwurst, pork and beef, 3 oz	8
pork and beef, Italian, dry sliced, 50% less sodium, 2 oz	6
pork and beef, less sodium, 2 oz	8
pork, dry or hard, 2 oz	7
pork, Italian, 2 oz	8
turkey, 2 oz	2
Salisbury steak	
5 ¾ oz	14
with gravy, frozen, 4 ¾ oz	7
Salmon patty	
3 oz	3
Salsa	
black bean and corn, 2 Tbsp	1
con queso, store-bought, 2 Tbsp	2
● fat-free	0
● gluten-free, fat-free	0
mango, 2 Tbsp	1
peach, 2 Tbsp	1
pineapple, 2 Tbsp	1
● salsa verde, fat-free	0
Salsify (vegetable oyster)	
● fresh, frozen, cooked, or canned, without added sugar or oil	0
Samosa	
1 (1 oz)	4

Sandwich

bacon, lettuce, and tomato, 9 oz	16
bacon, lettuce, and tomato, restaurant-type, 9 ⅓ oz	22
bagel, with cream cheese and lox, 6 ½ oz	17
bagel, with egg, sausage, cheese, and condiments, fast food, 7 ¾ oz	21
bagel, with ham, egg, and cheese, fast food, 6 ¾ oz	15
barbecued beef brisket, 15 ½ oz	44
barbecued pulled chicken, 14 ⅓ oz	20
barbecued pulled pork, 10 ¾ oz	20
barbeque beef, frozen, 5 oz	14
biscuit, with ham, fast food, 4 oz	14
biscuit, with sausage, fast food, 4 oz	14
chicken fillet with cheese, fast food, 8 oz	21
chicken fillet, plain, fast food, 6 ½ oz	17
chicken salad, 9 ½ oz	20
chicken salad, on reduced-calorie bread, 5 ½ oz	9
chicken salad, on regular bread, 5 ½ oz	11
chicken, fried, fast food, 7 oz	14
club, 8 ¾ oz	20
club, crispy chicken, with bacon, tomato, cheese, lettuce, and mayonnaise, 9 ½ oz	21
club, grilled chicken, with cheese, bacon, lettuce, tomato, and mayonnaise, 9 ½ oz	17
crispy chicken fillet, with lettuce and mayonnaise, fast food, 5 ⅓ oz	13
croque-monsieur, 6 ½ oz	15
Cuban, ½ (6 ½" x 3" x 4") or 5 ¾ oz	14

egg and cheese, fast food, 5 oz	11
egg salad, 6 oz	15
fish and cheese, fried, fast food, 6 ½ oz	17
fish fillet, frozen, 4 ½ oz	12
fish, with tartar sauce and cheese, fast food, 4 ¾ oz	11
fish, with tartar sauce, fast food, 7 ¾ oz	17
grilled cheese, restaurant-type, 4 oz	20
grilled cheese, with bacon, 4 ¾ oz	24
grilled chicken breast on bun, 6 ⅓ oz	11
grilled chicken fillet, with lettuce, tomato, and spread, fast food, 8 oz	10
grilled chicken, fast food, 7 oz	10
grilled chicken, frozen, 4 ¼ oz	9
grilled ham and cheese, restaurant-type, 5 oz	23
grinder, 2 ¾ oz	8
gyro, 11 ¼ oz	20
ham and cheese, 4 oz	12
ham and cheese, fast food, 5 oz	11
ham and Swiss cheese, restaurant-type, 9 oz	10
ham, egg, and cheese, fast food, 5 oz	11
hero, 11 oz	8
hoagie, 2 ¾ oz	8
lobster roll, 4 oz	6
lobster salad, 4 ½ oz	10
Monte Cristo, 3 ¾ oz	9
muffuletta, 11 oz	27
open-face roast beef, with gravy, 5 ¾ oz	12
panini, chicken, 8 oz	13
panini, ham and cheese, 7 ½ oz	15
panini, turkey, restaurant-type, 10 ½ oz	21

No Count	SmartPoints™ value
panini, vegetable, 13 oz	14
peanut butter and jelly, 3 ¼ oz	11
peanut butter and jelly, restaurant-type, 4 ⅓ oz	15
philly cheese steak, 9 oz	17
poor boy, 2 ¾ oz	8
poor boy, oyster, 8 ¾ oz	22
poor boy, shrimp, 8 ¾ oz	22
Reuben, 8 oz	24
roast beef, 7 ½ oz	10
roast beef with cheese, fast food, 6 oz	15
roast beef, plain, fast food, 5 oz	10
shrimp salad, 4 ½ oz	9
sloppy Joe, 6 oz	10
steak, fast food, 7 oz	12
submarine, 2 ¾ oz	8
submarine, with cold cuts, fast food, 8 oz	15
submarine, with roast beef, fast food, 7 ½ oz	12
submarine, with tuna salad, fast food, 9 oz	17
toasted cheese, 3 ¾ oz	12
tuna melt, 5 ⅔ oz	11
tuna salad, 6 ¼ oz	12
turkey, 4 oz	7
turkey and cheese sub, 6", no mayonnasie, restaurant-type, 8 ⅔ oz	11

Sangria

5 fl oz	5

Sashimi

No Count	
all varieties except salmon or mackerel, 2 oz	1
mackerel, 2 oz	3
salmon, 2 oz	2

Satay

beef, with peanut sauce, 2 skewers with ¼ cup sauce	15
beef, without peanut sauce, 2 skewers (3 oz)	5
chicken, with peanut sauce, 2 skewers with ¼ cup sauce	12
chicken, without peanut sauce, 2 skewers (3 oz)	2

Sauce

a la vodka, ½ cup	5
Alfredo sauce, ½ cup	14
Alfredo sauce, light, ½ cup	8
Alfredo sauce, light, store-bought, ½ cup	7
Alfredo sauce, regular, store-bought, ½ cup	14
arrabbiata, ½ cup	4
barbecue, 2 Tbsp	3
barbecue, low-sodium, 2 Tbsp	3
béarnaise, 2 Tbsp	6
béarnaise, store-bought, 2 Tbsp	5
black bean, 2 Tbsp	2
bolognese, ½ cup	7
brown, Chinese, 1 Tbsp	1
cheese, 2 Tbsp	2
cheese, ready-to-serve, 2 Tbsp	2
cheese, store-bought, 2 Tbsp	2
chili, green, 2 Tbsp	0
chili, red, 2 Tbsp	1
chipotle, canned, 2 Tbsp	1
clam, red, ¼ cup	2
clam, red, store-bought, ¼ cup	1
clam, white, ¼ cup	3
clam, white, store-bought, ¼ cup	2
curry, Hawaiian-style, 1 Tbsp	2
curry, store-bought, 1 Tbsp	1
donair, 2 Tbsp	4
duck, 1 Tbsp	2
enchilada, canned, 2 Tbsp	0
fish, ready-to-serve, ¼ cup	1
hoisin, 1 Tbsp	2
hollandaise, 2 Tbsp	6
hollandaise, store-bought, 1 Tbsp	1
horseradish, store-bought, 1 Tbsp	2

hot, 1 Tbsp	0
hot chili pepper, canned, 1 Tbsp	0
hot dog, 2 Tbsp	1
hot, Asian, 1 Tbsp	0
kung pao, 1 Tbsp	2
marinara, fat-free, jarred, ½ cup	2
marinara, homemade, ½ cup	3
marinara, low-sodium, ½ cup	3
marinara, store-bought, ½ cup	3
meat, ½ cup	6
mole poblano, 2 Tbsp	3
mole, store-bought, 2 Tbsp	2
mornay, 2 Tbsp	3
nam prik, 1 Tbsp	0
nuoc cham, 2 Tbsp	1
oyster, ¼ cup	1
pasta, bottled, any type, ½ cup	5
pasta, bottled, any type, reduced-fat, ½ cup	2
peanut, made from peanut butter and soy sauce, 1 Tbsp	2
peanut, spicy, 1 Tbsp	2
peanut, Thai, canned, 1 Tbsp	2
pepper, 2 Tbsp	0
pesto, ½ cup	19
pesto, reduced-fat, ¼ cup	8
pesto, store-bought, ½ cup	16
picadillo, 2 Tbsp	2
pizza, store-bought, 2 Tbsp	0
plum, 2 Tbsp	2
puttanesca, ½ cup	15
remoulade, 2 Tbsp	4
sambal oelek, 1 Tbsp	0
satay, 1 Tbsp	1
seafood cocktail, store-bought, ¼ cup	3
sloppy Joe, store-bought, 2 Tbsp	1
sofrito, 2 Tbsp	2
soy (shoyu), 1 Tbsp	0
soy (shoyu), low-sodium, 1 Tbsp	0

	spaghetti, bottled, any type, ½ cup	5
	spaghetti, bottled, any type, reduced-fat, ½ cup	3
	Spanish, 2 Tbsp	0
	sriracha, hot, 1 Tbsp	0
	steak, 1 Tbsp	1
	stir-fry, Asian, 1 Tbsp	1
	sweet and sour, 1 Tbsp	1
	sweet and sour, dehydrated, dry mix, 2 Tbsp	5
	taco, 2 Tbsp	1
	tamari, 2 Tbsp	0
	tartar, ¼ cup	5
	tartar, fat-free, ¼ cup	2
	teriyaki, 1 Tbsp	0
	teriyaki, reduced-sodium, 1 Tbsp	1
●	tomato, canned	0
●	tomato, canned, Spanish-style	0
	tomato, Italian, ½ cup	3
	tomato, with herbs and cheese, canned, ½ cup	2
●	tomato, with mushrooms, canned	0
●	tomato, with onions, canned	0
	tomato, with onions, green peppers, and celery, canned, ½ cup	3
●	tomato, with roasted garlic	0
●	tomato, with tomato tidbits, canned	0
	tzatziki, 2 Tbsp	1
	white, medium, 2 Tbsp	2
	white, thin, 2 Tbsp	1
	wine, 2 Tbsp	2
	Worcestershire, 1 Tbsp	1

Sauerbraten

3 oz beef with 2 Tbsp gravy	7

Sauerkraut

fresh or canned, without added sugar or oil	0

O No Count	SmartPoints™ value
Sausage	
50% vension, 50% beef, uncooked, 3 oz	5
50% vension, 50% pork, uncooked, 3 oz	5
60% venison, 40% pork, uncooked, 3 oz	4
andouille, 3 oz	6
beef, cooked, 3 oz	9
beef, fresh, cooked, 3 oz	9
beef, pre-cooked, 3 oz	13
berliner, pork and beef, 2 oz	4
blood pudding, 3 oz	12
boudin, store-bought, 3 oz	4
bratwurst, 1 (3 oz)	9
chicken and beef, smoked, 1 oz	3
chicken and beef, smoked, 2 oz	5
chicken, beef and pork, skinless, smoked, 2 oz	4
chicken, cooked, 3 oz	3
chicken, uncooked, 4 oz	4
honey roll, beef, 3 oz	4
Italian, pork, cooked, 3 oz	9
Italian, pork, uncooked, 4 oz	14
Italian, turkey, smoked, 2 oz	3
lamb, 3 oz	7
low-fat (1 g fat or less per oz), 3 oz	3
luncheon, pork and beef, 3 oz	7
meatless, 2 oz	4
mini, 3 oz	9
mortadella, beef and pork, 3 oz	9
patty, restaurant-type, 3 oz	9
Polish, 3 oz	10
Polish, beef with chicken, hot, 2 oz	5
Polish, pork and beef, smoked, 2 oz	6
pork and beef, smoked, 3 oz	9
pork and beef, with cheddar cheese, smoked, 2 oz	6
pork, cooked, 3 oz	9

O No Count	SmartPoints™ value
pork, smoked, 3 oz	9
summer, pork and beef, with cheddar cheese, 2 oz	8
thuringer or cervelat summer sausage, beef or pork, 3 oz	10
turkey, breakfast links, mild, 2 oz	4
turkey, fresh, cooked, 3 oz	4
turkey, fresh, uncooked, 4 oz	4
turkey, hot, smoked, 2 oz	3
turkey, Italian, sweet, uncooked, 3 ¾ oz	3
turkey, reduced-fat, brown and serve, cooked, 3 oz	4
Vienna, canned, beef and pork, 3 oz	7
Vienna, chicken, canned, 3 oz	7
Sausage biscuit	
fast food, 4 ⅓ oz	15
frozen, 2 oz	8
Sausage on a roll	
plain, 5 ½ oz	16
Scallion (green onion)	
○ fresh, frozen, cooked, or canned, without added sugar or oil	0
Scallion pancake	
1 (2 oz)	9
Scalloped potato mix	
dry mix, unprepared, 5 ½ oz	16
Scalloped potatoes	
½ cup	6
prepared from dry mix with water, whole milk, and butter, ½ cup	4
Scallops, breaded and fried	
3 oz	5
fast food, 3 oz	7
Scallops, fried	
3 oz	5
frozen, prepared without fat, 3 oz	6
Schaum torte	
with whipped cream, 1 oz	3
without whipped cream, 1 oz	2

Scone

blueberry, restaurant-type, 1 (4 ¼ oz)	17
chocolate, restaurant-type, 1 (4 ¼ oz)	20
cinnamon, restaurant-type, 1 (4 oz)	20
cranberry, restaurant-type, 1 (4 ¼ oz)	16
orange, restaurant-type, 1 (4 ¼ oz)	18
plain, 1 (1 ½ oz)	5
raspberry, restaurant-type, 1 (4 ¼ oz)	18

Scrapple

1" cube (3 oz)	6

Seafood crêpes

11 oz	17

Seafood mix

○ frozen, 4 oz	1

Seasoning mix

chili, dry, 1 Tbsp	1
fajita, dry, 1 tsp	0
taco, dry, 1 Tbsp	1

Seasonings, herbs, and spices, fresh

1 Tbsp	0

Seaweed

○ nori, 10 sheets	0

Seeds

chia, dried, ¼ cup	6
flaxseed, ¼ cup	7
pepitas, roasted, 1 Tbsp	1
pumpkin, roasted, ¼ cup	4
sesame, 1 tsp	1
sunflower, dry-roasted, ¼ cup	6
sunflower, oil-roasted, ¼ cup	6
sunflower, toasted, ¼ cup	6

Seitan

2 oz	1

Sesame chicken

1 cup	11

Sesame noodles

1 cup	9

Shabu shabu

4 oz beef, 2 oz tofu, and 1 ½ cups vegetables	9

Shellfish

○ abalone, cooked, 3 oz	2
○ clams, canned, 3 oz	2
○ clams, cooked, 3 oz	2
○ clams, uncooked, 4 oz	1
○ crab, canned, 3 oz	1
○ crab, cooked, 3 oz	1
○ crab, uncooked, 4 oz	1
○ crayfish, cooked, 3 oz	1
○ crayfish, uncooked, 4 oz	1
○ lobster, cooked, 3 oz	1
○ lobster, in the shell, steamed, 1 ¼ pounds	1
○ lobster, spiny, cooked, 3 oz	2
○ lobster, spiny, uncooked, 4 oz	2
○ lobster, uncooked, 4 oz	1
○ mussels, cooked, shelled, 3 oz	3
○ mussels, uncooked, in shell, 4 oz	2
○ octopus, cooked, 3 oz	2
○ octopus, uncooked, 4 oz	1
○ oysters, canned, 3 oz	1
○ oysters, cooked, 3 oz	2
○ oysters, uncooked, 4 oz	2
○ scallops, cooked, 3 oz	1
○ scallops, uncooked, 4 oz	1
○ shrimp, canned, 3 oz	1
○ shrimp, cooked, 3 oz	1
○ shrimp, frozen, 3 oz	1
○ shrimp, uncooked, 4 oz	2
○ squid, cooked, 3 oz	1
○ squid, uncooked, 4 oz	2

Complete A-Z Food List

No Count	SmartPoints™ value
Shephard's pie	
9 ¾ oz	12
Sherbet	
any flavor, ½ cup	6
Sherry	
dry, 3 ½ fl oz	5
sweet, 3 ½ fl oz	7
Shish kebob	
4 ¾ oz	9
Shortening, vegetable	
1 Tbsp	5
Shoyu chicken	
3 oz	7
Shrimp Cantonese	
7 ½ oz	9
Shrimp creole	
store-bought, 1 cup	5
without rice, 1 cup	6
Shrimp puffs	
1 (1 ½" round) or ⅓ oz	1
Shrimp remoulade	
3 ¾ oz	10
Shrimp scampi	
3 ½ oz	12
Shrimp toast	
1 oz	3
Shrimp, barbecued	
3 oz	15
Shrimp, breaded	
butterfly, frozen, prepared without fat, 3 oz	7
popcorn, frozen, prepared without fat, 3 oz	7
Shrimp, breaded and fried	
3 oz	5
family-style, restaurant-type, 6 oz	15
fast food, 3 pieces (1 ⅓ oz)	4
Shrimp, fried	
3 oz	5

No Count	SmartPoints™ value
Shrimp, stuffed	
broiled, 3 oz	12
fried, 9 ½ oz	10
Shumai	
fried, 1 (2" diameter) or ¾ oz	2
steamed, 1 (2" diameter) or ¾ oz	2
Smoke, liquid	
2 Tbsp	0
Smoothie	
prepared, 8 fl oz	6
Snack mix	
Oriental, low-fat, store-bought, 1 oz	3
Oriental, rice-based, 1 oz	4
reduced-fat, store-bought, 1 oz	4
store-bought, 1 oz	4
Texas trash (cereal and nut mix), 1 oz	4
Snow cone	
1 (1 cup)	6
Soft drink, carbonated	
any flavor other than those listed here, sweetened with sugar, 8 fl oz	7
any flavor, diet, 8 fl oz	0
club soda, 8 fl oz	0
cola, 8 fl oz	5
cream, 8 fl oz	8
ginger ale, 8 fl oz	5
lemon-lime, 8 fl oz	6
pepper-type, 8 fl oz	6
root beer, 8 fl oz	6
seltzer, plain or flavored, no sugar added, 8 fl oz	0
tonic water, 8 fl oz	5
Sopaipillas	
2 (1 oz)	3
Sorbet	
any flavor, ½ cup	5

Soufflé

cheese, 1 cup	7
fruit, ½ cup	5
spinach, home prepared, 1 cup	9

Soup, beef

beef and mushroom, chunky, low-sodium, canned, ready-to-serve, 1 cup	6
beef and vegetable, canned, ready-to-serve, 1 cup	4
○ beef and vegetable, reduced-sodium, canned, ready-to-serve, 1 cup	3
beef stroganoff, canned, chunky, 1 cup	8
beef, canned, chunky, ready-to-serve, 1 cup	5
beef, canned, prepared with water, 1 cup	2
beef-mushroom, canned, condensed, ½ cup	2
beef-mushroom, canned, condensed, prepared with equal volume water, 1 cup	2
beef-noodle, canned, condensed, ½ cup	3
beef-noodle, canned, condensed, prepared with equal volume water, 1 cup	3
beef-noodle, dehydrated, dry form, 1 packet (⅓ oz)	1
beef-noodle, dehydrated, prepared with water, 1 cup	1
beef-vegetable, canned, prepared with water, 1 cup	2
chili, canned, condensed, prepared with equal volume water, 1 cup	5
chili-beef, canned, condensed, ½ cup	5
mushroom with beef stock, canned, condensed, ½ cup	3
mushroom with beef stock, canned, condensed, prepared with equal volume water, 1 cup	3

oxtail, 1 cup	2
oxtail, dehydrated, prepared with water, 1 cup	2
oxtail, Hawaiian-style, 1 cup	6
tomato-beef with noodle, canned, condensed, ½ cup	4
tomato-beef with noodle, canned, condensed, prepared with equal volume water, 1 cup	4
vegetable with beef broth, canned, condensed, ½ cup	3
vegetable with beef broth, canned, condensed, prepared with equal volume water, 1 cup	2
vegetable-beef, canned, prepared with water, 1 cup	2
vegetable-beef, dehydrated, prepared with water, 1 cup	2
○ Vietnamese beef noodle, 1 cup	3

Soup, chicken

chicken and stars, canned, prepared with water, 1 cup	2
chicken enchilada, 1 cup	6
chicken gumbo, 1 cup	7
chicken gumbo, canned, condensed, ½ cup	2
chicken gumbo, canned, condensed, prepared with equal volume water, 1 cup	2
○ chicken stock, homemade, 1 cup	3
chicken with dumplings, canned, condensed, ½ cup	3
chicken with dumplings, canned, condensed, prepared with equal volume water, 1 cup	3
chicken with matzo balls, 1 cup	4
chicken with matzo balls, canned, ready-to-serve, 1 cup	5
chicken with rice, canned, condensed, ½ cup	3
chicken with rice, canned, prepared with water, 1 cup	2
chicken with tortilla strips and shredded cheese, 1 cup	6

◐ No Count	SmartPoints™ value
chicken with wild rice, canned, prepared with water, 1 cup	2
chicken without matzo balls (broth only), 1 cup	1
chicken, canned, chunky, ready-to-serve, 1 cup	5
chicken-mushroom, canned, condensed, ½ cup	4
chicken-mushroom, canned, condensed, prepared with equal volume water, 1 cup	4
chicken-noodle, 1 cup	3
chicken-noodle with meatballs, canned, chunky, ready-to-serve, 1 cup	3
chicken-noodle, canned, chunky, ready-to-serve, 1 cup	3
chicken-noodle, canned, condensed, ½ cup	2
chicken-noodle, canned, prepared with water, 1 cup	2
chicken-noodle, dehydrated, dry form, 1 packet (⅓ oz)	1
chicken-noodle, dehydrated, prepared with water, 1 cup	2
chicken-noodle, in a cup, dehydrated, unprepared, 1 container (⅓ oz)	1
◉ chicken-noodle, low-sodium, canned, condensed, prepared with equal volume water, 1 cup	2
◉ chicken-noodle, reduced-sodium, ready-to-serve, 1 cup	3
chicken-rice, canned, chunky, ready-to-serve, 1 cup	3
chicken-rice, dehydrated, dry form, 1 packet (½ oz)	2
chicken-rice, dehydrated, prepared with water, 1 cup	2
chicken-vegetable with potato and cheese, chunky, ready-to-serve, 1 cup	6
chicken-vegetable, canned, chunky, ready-to-serve, 1 cup	2

◐ No Count	SmartPoints™ value
chicken-vegetable, canned, condensed, ½ cup	2
chicken-vegetable, dehydrated, dry form, 1 packet (⅓ oz)	1
chicken-vegetable, in a cup, dehydrated, unprepared, 1 container (1 oz)	3
cream of chicken, canned (made with fat-free milk), 1 cup	5
cream of chicken, canned (made with low-fat (1%) milk), 1 cup	6
cream of chicken, canned (made with whole milk), 1 cup	7
cream of chicken, canned, condensed, ½ cup	4
cream of chicken, canned, condensed, prepared with equal volume water, 1 cup	4
cream of chicken, dehydrated, dry form, 1 packet (⅔ oz)	3
cream of chicken, dehydrated, prepared with water, 1 cup	4
cream of chicken, low-fat, canned (made with fat-free milk), 1 cup	4
cream of chicken, low-fat, canned (made with low-fat (1%) milk), 1 cup	5
cream of chicken, reduced-sodium, canned, condensed, ½ cup	2
hot and spicy, 1 cup	3
knefla, 1 cup	8
Thai chicken-coconut, 1 cup	12
vegetable-chicken, low-sodium, canned, condensed, prepared with equal volume water, 1 cup	5
Soup, seafood	
asparagus-crab, 1 cup	2
bouillabaisse, 1 cup	4
chowder, Manhattan clam, 1 cup	5
chowder, Manhattan clam, canned, chunky, ready-to-serve, 1 cup	4

chowder, Manhattan clam, canned, condensed, ½ cup	3
chowder, Manhattan clam, canned, prepared with water, 1 cup	3
chowder, Manhattan clam, dehydrated, dry form, 1 packet (⅔ oz)	2
chowder, Manhattan clam, restaurant-type, 1 cup	5
chowder, New England clam, 1 cup	6
chowder, New England clam, canned (made with fat-free milk), 1 cup	4
chowder, New England clam, canned (made with low-fat (1%) milk), 1 cup	5
chowder, New England clam, canned (made with whole milk), 1 cup	6
chowder, New England clam, canned, condensed, ½ cup	3
chowder, New England clam, canned, ready-to-serve, 1 cup	6
chowder, New England clam, dehydrated, dry form, 1 packet (¾ oz)	3
chowder, New England clam, low-fat, canned (made with fat-free milk), 1 cup	4
chowder, New England clam, low-fat, canned (made with low-fat (1%) milk), 1 cup	5
chowder, New England clam, low-sodium, canned, ready-to-serve, 1 cup	5
chowder, New England clam, restaurant-type, 1 cup	11
cioppino, 1 cup	6
crab, canned, ready-to-serve, 1 cup	2
cream of shrimp, canned, condensed, ½ cup	3

cream of shrimp, canned, condensed, prepared with equal volume reduced-fat (2%) milk, 1 cup	6
cream of shrimp, canned, condensed, prepared with equal volume water, 1 cup	3
escarole, canned, ready-to-serve, 1 cup	1
gumbo, with rice, store-bought, 1 cup	5
lobster bisque, 1 cup	7
lobster bisque, canned, made with fat-free milk, 1 cup	4
lobster bisque, canned, made with low-fat (1%) milk, 1 cup	5
lobster bisque, canned, made with whole milk, 1 cup	6
lobster bisque, restaurant-type, 1 cup	16
oyster stew, canned (made with fat-free milk), 1 cup	4
oyster stew, canned (made with low-fat (1%) milk), 1 cup	4
oyster stew, canned (made with whole milk), 1 cup	6
oyster stew, canned, condensed, ½ cup	2
oyster stew, canned, condensed, prepared with equal volume water, 1 cup	2
seafood gumbo, 1 cup	5

Soup, turkey

turkey, chunky, ready-to-serve, 1 cup	3
turkey, chunky, ready-to-serve, 1 cup	3
turkey-noodle, canned, prepared with water, 1 cup	4
turkey-vegetable, canned, condensed, ½ cup	2
turkey-vegetable, canned, condensed, prepared with equal volume water, 1 cup	2

Complete A-Z Food List

Soup, vegetable and other

	SmartPoints™ value
avgolemono, 1 cup	4
baked potato, restaurant-type, 1 cup	8
bean and bacon, canned, prepared with water, 1 cup	5
bean and ham, canned, prepared with water, 1 cup	8
bean with bacon, dehydrated, dry form, 1 packet (1 oz)	3
bean with bacon, dehydrated, prepared with water, 1 cup	3
bean with frankfurters, canned, condensed, ½ cup	5
bean with frankfurters, canned, condensed, prepared with equal volume water, 1 cup	5
bean with ham, canned, chunky, ready-to-serve, 1 cup	7
bean with ham, reduced-sodium, canned, 1 cup	6
bean with pork, canned, condensed, ½ cup	5
bean with pork, canned, condensed, prepared with equal volume water, 1 cup	5
black bean, canned, condensed, ½ cup	3
black bean, canned, condensed, prepared with equal volume water, 1 cup	3
black bean, canned, ready-to-serve, 1 cup	6
black bean, homemade, 1 cup	3
black bean, in a cup, dehydrated, unprepared, 1 container (2 oz)	6
black bean, restaurant-type, 1 cup	7
borscht, 1 cup	6
borscht, low-calorie, store-bought, 1 cup	1
borscht, store-bought, 1 cup	5
broccoli-cheese, 1 cup	11

	SmartPoints™ value
broccoli-cheese, canned (made with fat-free milk), 1 cup	6
broccoli-cheese, canned (made with low-fat (1%) milk), 1 cup	6
broccoli-cheese, canned (made with whole milk), 1 cup	7
broccoli-cheese, low-fat, canned (made with fat-free or low-fat (1%) milk), 1 cup	4
cabbage, 1 cup	2
cauliflower, dehydrated, prepared with water, 1 cup	2
cheddar cheese, 1 cup	14
cheddar cheese, canned (made with fat-free milk), 1 cup	5
cheddar cheese, canned (made with low-fat (1%) milk), 1 cup	5
cheddar cheese, canned (made with whole milk), 1 cup	7
cheese, canned, condensed, ½ cup	4
cheese, canned, condensed, prepared with equal volume water, 1 cup	6
cheese, canned, condensed, prepared with equal volume whole milk, 1 cup	9
cherry, 1 cup	7
chowder, corn, in a cup, dehydrated, unprepared, 1 container (1 oz)	4
cream of asparagus, canned, condensed, ½ cup	3
cream of asparagus, canned, condensed, prepared with equal volume water, 1 cup	3
cream of asparagus, canned, condensed, prepared with equal volume whole milk, 1 cup	5
cream of asparagus, dehydrated, dry mix, 1 packet (2 oz)	7
cream of asparagus, dehydrated, prepared with water, 1 cup	2
cream of broccoli, 1 cup	11

Food	SmartPoints™ value
cream of broccoli, canned (made with fat-free milk), 1 cup	5
cream of broccoli, canned (made with low-fat (1%) milk), 1 cup	6
cream of broccoli, canned (made with whole milk), 1 cup	7
cream of broccoli, low-fat, canned (made with fat-free milk), 1 cup	5
cream of broccoli, low-fat, canned (made with low-fat (1%) milk), 1 cup	5
cream of celery, canned (made with fat-free milk), 1 cup	5
cream of celery, canned (made with low-fat-milk), 1 cup	5
cream of celery, canned (made with whole milk), 1 cup	6
cream of celery, canned, condensed, ½ cup	3
cream of celery, canned, condensed, prepared with equal volume water, 1 cup	3
cream of celery, dehydrated, prepared with water, 1 cup	2
cream of celery, low-fat, canned (made with fat-free milk), 1 cup	4
cream of celery, low-fat, canned (made with low-fat (1%) milk), 1 cup	4
cream of mushroom, 1 cup	14
cream of mushroom, canned (made with fat-free milk), 1 cup	6
cream of mushroom, canned (made with low-fat (1%) milk), 1 cup	7
cream of mushroom, canned (made with whole milk), 1 cup	8
cream of mushroom, canned, condensed, ½ cup	4
cream of mushroom, canned, condensed, prepared with equal volume water, 1 cup	3

Food	SmartPoints™ value
cream of mushroom, low-fat, canned (made with fat-free milk), 1 cup	4
cream of mushroom, low-fat, canned (made with low-fat (1%) milk), 1 cup	5
cream of mushroom, low-sodium, canned, ready-to-serve, 1 cup	5
cream of mushroom, reduced-sodium, canned, condensed, 1 cup	5
cream of onion, canned, condensed, ½ cup	4
cream of onion, canned, condensed, prepared with equal volume water, 1 cup	3
cream of onion, canned, condensed, prepared with equal volume whole milk, 1 cup	6
cream of potato, canned (made with fat-free milk), 1 cup	4
cream of potato, canned (made with low-fat (1%) milk), 1 cup	5
cream of potato, canned (made with whole milk), 1 cup	6
cream of potato, canned, condensed, ½ cup	3
cream of potato, restaurant-type, 1 cup	6
cream of tomato, 1 cup	7
cream of vegetable, dehydrated, dry form, 1 packet (⅔ oz)	3
cream of vegetable, dehydrated, prepared with water, 1 cup	3
● egg drop, homemade, 1 cup	1
egg drop, restaurant-type, 1 cup	2
French onion au gratin, 1 cup	11
● gazpacho, 1 cup	5
gazpacho, canned, prepared with water, 1 cup	1
gazpacho, canned, ready-to-serve, 1 cup	1
green pea, canned, condensed, ½ cup	5

Complete A-Z Food List

● No Count	SmartPoints™ value
green pea, canned, condensed, prepared with equal volume water, 1 cup	5
green pea, dehydrated, dry form, 1 packet (1 oz)	3
green pea, dehydrated, prepared with water, 1 cup	4
hot and sour, homemade, 1 cup	3
hot and sour, restaurant-type, 1 cup	2
Italian wedding, 1 cup	6
leek, dehydrated, dry form, 1 packet (2 ¾ oz)	9
lentil, 1 cup	5
lentil with ham, canned, ready-to-serve, 1 cup	4
lentil, in a cup, dehydrated, unprepared, 1 container (2 oz)	6
lentil-vegetable, 1 cup	5
minestrone, 1 cup	7
minestrone, canned, chunky, ready-to-serve, 1 cup	4
minestrone, canned, condensed, ½ cup	2
minestrone, canned, condensed, prepared with equal volume water, 1 cup	2
minestrone, dehydrated, dry form, 1 packet (⅔ oz)	2
minestrone, low-fat, canned, prepared with water, 1 cup	3
minestrone, reduced-sodium, canned, ready-to-serve, 1 cup	4
miso, 1 cup	2
mulligatawny, 1 cup	9
mushroom, dehydrated, prepared with water, 1 cup	3
mushroom-barley, 1 cup	5
mushroom-barley, canned, condensed, ½ cup	2
mushroom-barley, canned, condensed, prepared with equal volume water, 1 cup	2
nebeyaki udon, 1 cup	3

● No Count	SmartPoints™ value
onion, canned, condensed, ½ cup	2
onion, dehydrated, dry form, 1 packet (1 ⅓ oz)	3
onion, dehydrated, dry form, ¼ packet (⅓ oz)	1
onion, dehydrated, prepared with water, 1 cup	1
Oriental, in a cup, dehydrated, unprepared, 1 container (1 oz)	3
pasta e fagioli, 1 cup	7
pasta with vegetables, canned, prepared with water, 1 cup	3
pea, low-sodium, canned, condensed, prepared with equal volume water, 1 cup	5
pepperpot, canned, condensed, ½ cup	3
pepperpot, canned, condensed, prepared with equal volume water, 1 cup	3
Persian noodle, store-bought, 1 cup	5
Persian pomegranate, store-bought, 1 cup	8
petite marmite, 1 cup	4
pigeon pea and dumpling, 1 cup	8
Portuguese bean, 1 cup	7
● potato, frozen, 7 ½ oz	3
potato-leek, in a cup, dehydrated, unprepared, 1 container (1 oz)	4
pozole (pork and hominy soup), 1 cup	5
pozole (pork and hominy soup), canned, 1 cup	4
ramen noodle, dehydrated, dry form, 1 packet (3 oz)	13
ramen noodle, low-fat, dehydrated, dry form, 1 packet (3 oz)	6
red beans and rice, in a cup, dehydrated, unprepared, 1 container (2 oz)	5
saimin, 1 cup	6

	SmartPoints™ value
○ sambhar (Indian lentil soup), 1 cup	4
split pea, 1 cup	4
split pea with ham, canned, chunky, ready-to-serve, 1 cup	6
split pea with ham, canned, prepared with water, 1 cup	5
split pea with ham, condensed, ½ cup	5
split pea, frozen, 1 package (7 ½ oz)	3
split pea, in a cup, dehydrated, unprepared, 1 container (2 oz)	5
suimono, 1 cup	2
Thai coconut-ginger, canned, ready-to-serve, 1 cup	8
tom yum kung, 1 cup	2
tomato, 1 cup	5
tomato bisque, canned, condensed, ½ cup	4
tomato bisque, canned, condensed, prepared with equal volume water, 1 cup	4
tomato bisque, canned, condensed, prepared with equal volume whole milk, 1 cup	6
tomato, canned (made with fat-free milk), 1 cup	5
tomato, canned (made with low-fat (1%) milk), 1 cup	6
tomato, canned (made with whole milk), 1 cup	7
tomato, canned, condensed, 1 cup	4
tomato, canned, condensed, prepared with equal volume reduced-fat (2%) milk, 1 cup	6
tomato, canned, prepared with water, 1 cup	3
tomato, dehydrated dry, 1 packet (¾ oz)	2
tomato, dehydrated, prepared with water, 1 cup	3

	SmartPoints™ value
tomato, dehydrated, prepared with water, 1 cup	4
tomato, reduced-sodium, canned, condensed, ½ cup	3
tomato-rice, canned, condensed, ½ cup	4
tomato-rice, canned, condensed, prepared with equal volume water, 1 cup	4
tomato-vegetable, dehydrated, dry form, 1 packet (1 ⅓ oz)	4
○ tomato-vegetable, dehydrated, prepared with water, 1 cup	2
tortilla, 1 cup	8
turtle, 1 cup	3
vegetable, 1 cup	3
vegetable, canned, chunky, ready-to-serve, 1 cup	3
vegetable, canned, prepared with water, 1 cup	2
vegetable, dehydrated, dry form, 1 packet (1 ¾ oz)	5
vegetable, low-sodium, canned, condensed, ½ cup	3
○ vegetable, low-sodium, canned, condensed, prepared with equal volume water, 1 cup	3
vegetarian vegetable, canned, condensed, ½ cup	3
vegetarian vegetable, canned, condensed, prepared with equal volume water, 1 cup	2
vegetarian vegetable, in a cup, dehydrated, unprepared, 1 container (2 oz)	5
vichyssoise, 1 cup	4
wonton, restaurant-type, 1 cup	2
○ yogurt and cucumber, 1 cup	4
Souvlaki	
chicken, 1 large or 2 small skewers (4 ½ oz)	4
lamb, 1 large or 2 small skewers (4 ¾ oz)	9

Complete A-Z Food List

	SmartPoints™ value
○ No Count	

Souvlaki in pita

| chicken, 6 ½ oz | 9 |
| lamb, 6 ½ oz | 11 |

Soy chips

| 1 oz | 3 |

Soybean nuts

| ¼ cup | 3 |

Soybeans

○ cooked, ½ cup	4
○ dry, ¼ cup	5
○ green, cooked, ½ cup	3
○ green, uncooked, ¼ cup	2
roasted, 1 cup	20

Spaetzle

| 1 cup | 14 |

Spaghetti

regular, cooked, 1 cup	5
regular, uncooked, 2 oz	6
spinach, cooked, 1 cup	5
spinach, uncooked, 2 oz	6
○ whole-wheat, cooked, 1 cup	5
○ whole-wheat, uncooked, 2 oz	5

Spaghetti and meatballs

| family-style, restaurant-type, 1 ¼ pounds | 31 |

Spaghetti bolognese

| 1 cup spaghetti with ½ cup sauce | 14 |

Spaghetti carbonara

| 1 cup | 16 |

Spaghetti, with marinara sauce

| 1 cup spaghetti with ½ cup sauce | 10 |

Spaghetti, with meat sauce

| 1 cup spaghetti with ½ cup sauce | 13 |
| frozen, 10 oz | 7 |

	SmartPoints™ value
○ No Count	

Spaghetti, with tomato sauce

| with meatballs, 1 cup spaghetti with ½ cup sauce and 2 meatballs | 22 |
| with meatballs, canned, 8 ¾ oz | 8 |

Spam musubi

| 4 oz | 9 |

Spanakopita

| 1 (3" square) or 1 cup | 13 |
| frozen, 1 piece (1 oz) | 5 |

Spanish rice

| canned, 1 cup | 4 |
| homemade, 1 cup | 7 |

Spareribs, barbecued

| 4 (4" long each) | 12 |
| Chinese, 2 (4" long each) | 5 |

Spinach

| ○ baby, uncooked | 0 |
| ○ fresh, frozen, cooked, or canned, without added sugar or oil | 0 |

Spinach, creamed

| restaurant-type, ½ cup | 8 |

Spoon bread

| 1 cup | 15 |

Sports drink

| 8 fl oz | 4 |

Spring roll

beef or pork, 1 (2 ½ oz)	7
chicken, 1 (2 ½ oz)	5
lumpia (Filipino spring rolls), 1 (4 ½" x 1" x 1 ½") or 2 ½ oz	6
shrimp, 1 (2 ½ oz)	5
Thai, 1 (4 ½" long) or 2 ½ oz	5
Vietnamese, fresh, 1 (1 ¾ oz)	2
Vietnamese, fried, 1 (4 ½" long) or 2 ½ oz	5
Vietnamese, sauce for dipping, 2 Tbsp	0

Spring roll wrapper

lumpia (Filipino spring roll) wrapper, 1 oz ... 2

Sprouts

○ fresh, frozen, cooked, or canned, without added sugar or oil ... 0

○ mung bean, stir-fried, ½ cup ... 1

Squash

○ spaghetti, fresh, frozen, cooked, or canned, without added sugar or oil ... 0

○ summer, all varieties, fresh, frozen, cooked, or canned, without added sugar or oil ... 0

○ winter, all varieties, fresh, frozen, cooked, or canned, without added sugar or oil ... 0

Squid, fried

3 oz ... 3

Starfruit (carambola)

○ fresh, frozen, cooked, or canned, without added sugar ... 0

Stew

bean and lentil stew (dal maharani), 1 cup ... 9

beef, 7 ⅓ oz ... 5

beef, canned, 1 cup ... 7

beef, frozen, 1 cup ... 5

Brunswick, 1 cup ... 4

burgoo, 1 cup ... 5

caribou, 1 cup ... 2

carne guisado (Cuban beef stew), 1 cup ... 6

chicken, canned, 8 ½ oz ... 7

Irish brown, 1 cup ... 8

lamb, 1 cup ... 6

menudo, 10 oz ... 7

menudo, canned, 8 ½ oz ... 6

vegetarian, 1 cup ... 6

Sticky rice with mango

1 cup mango with ½ cup rice ... 21

Stir-fried vegetables

○ frozen, unprepared, 3 oz ... 1

with beef, 1 cup ... 5

with chicken, 1 cup ... 3

with oil or sauce, 5 ½ oz ... 5

with pork, 1 cup ... 4

○ without oil or sauce, 1 cup ... 1

Stir-fry, broccoli

5 ½ oz ... 5

Stir-fry, with garlic or black bean sauce

beef, 1 cup ... 8

chicken, 1 cup ... 8

pork, 1 cup ... 9

shrimp, 1 cup ... 7

Stock

○ beef, homemade, 1 cup ... 1

chicken, store-bought, 1 cup ... 0

○ fish, homemade, 1 cup ... 1

Strawberries

canned, in heavy syrup, ½ cup ... 7

dried, ¼ cup ... 4

○ fresh, frozen, cooked, or canned, without added sugar ... 0

sweetened with sugar, 1 cup ... 12

Strawberry drink

powder, prepared with whole milk, 8 fl oz ... 11

Stromboli

2 ¾ oz ... 6

Strudel

any type, 1 piece (6 oz) ... 19

apple, 1 piece (2 ½ oz) ... 8

Stuffed cabbage

11 oz ... 9

Stuffed peppers

with beef and rice, 7 ¾ oz ... 13

with beef, in tomato sauce, frozen, 7 oz ... 7

○ No Count | SmartPoints™ value

Stuffing

½ cup	6
bread, prepared from dry mix, ½ cup	6
cornbread, prepared from dry mix, ½ cup	6

Stuffing mix

bread, 1 oz	3
cornbread, 1 oz	3

Succotash

○	cooked, 1 cup	7
○	frozen, cooked, ½ cup	2
○	frozen, unprepared, ½ cup	2
○	with whole-kernel corn, canned, ½ cup	2

Sugar Substitute

1 tsp	0
aspartame, 1 packet	0
saccharin, 1 packet	0
stevia leaf, 1 packet	0

Sugar, brown

dark, packed or unpacked, 1 tsp	1
granulated, 1 tsp	1
light, packed or unpacked, 1 tsp	1

Sugar, confectioners' (powdered)

1 tsp	1

Sugar, maple

1 tsp	1

Sugar, sucanat

1 tsp	1

Sugar, superfine

1 tsp	1

Sugar, white

granulated, 1 tsp	1

Sukiyaki

with sauce, 2 cups with ¼ cup sauce	15

Summer squash casserole

7 ½ oz	12

○ No Count | SmartPoints™ value

Sunflower seed butter

1 Tbsp	3

Sunomono

½ cup	1

Surimi (imitation seafood)

○	4 oz	3

Sushi

cone, 3 oz	4
inari, 3 oz	4
kappa maki (cucumber roll), 6 pieces (1" diameter x 1" thick)	3
maki (vegetables and rice rolled with seaweed), 1 piece (¾ oz)	1
nigiri (sliced raw fish over rice), 4 pieces (1 ½" diameter x ¾" thick)	2
nigiri uni (sea urchin), 4 pieces (2" long x ¾" wide)	3
nigiri, albacore (white tuna), 4 pieces (2" long x ¾" wide)	3
nigiri, amaebi (sweet shrimp), 4 pieces (2" long x ¾" wide)	3
nigiri, ebi (cooked shrimp), 4 pieces (2" long x ¾" wide)	3
nigiri, hamachi (yellowtail), 4 pieces (2" long x ¾" wide)	3
nigiri, ika (squid), 4 pieces (2" long x ¾" wide)	3
nigiri, ikura (salmon roe), 4 pieces (2" long x ¾" wide)	3
nigiri, kani (crab), 4 pieces (2" long x ¾" wide)	3
nigiri, maguro (tuna), 4 pieces (2" long x ¾" wide)	3
nigiri, masago (smelt roe), 4 pieces (2" long x ¾" wide)	3
nigiri, saba (mackerel), 4 pieces (2" long x ¾" wide)	3
nigiri, sake (fresh salmon), 4 pieces (2" long x ¾" wide)	3
nigiri, smoked salmon, 4 pieces (2" long x ¾" wide)	3
nigiri, tai (red snapper), 4 pieces (2" long x ¾" wide)	3

	SmartPoints™ value
nigiri, tairagai (scallops), 4 pieces (2" long x ¾" wide)	3
nigiri, tako (octopus), 4 pieces (2" long x ¾" wide)	3
nigiri, unagi (fresh water eel), 4 pieces (2" long x ¾" wide)	3
nori maki (raw fish and rice rolled with seaweed), 4 pieces (1 ½" diameter x ¾" thick)	3
roll, Alaskan, 2 pieces (1" high x 1 ¾" diameter)	4
roll, California, 4 pieces (1" high x 1 ¾" diameter)	5
roll, Philadelphia, 2 pieces (1" high x 1 ¾" diameter)	4
roll, rainbow, 4 pieces (1 ½" diameter x ¾" thick)	3
roll, shrimp tempura, 6 pieces (1 ½" diameter x 1" thick)	10
roll, spider, 6 pieces (2" diameter x 1" thick)	10
roll, tuna, 4 pieces (1 ½" diameter x ¾" thick)	3
roll, tuna, spicy, 6 pieces (2" diameter x 1" thick)	7
roll, vegetable tempura, 6 pieces (1 ½" diameter x 1" thick)	6
roll, yellowtail, 6 pieces (1 ½" diameter x 1" thick)	3
unagi maki, 4 pieces (1 ½" diameter x ¾" thick)	3
uni maki, 4 pieces (1 ½" diameter x ¾" thick)	3
Sweet and sour	
beef, 1 cup	16
chicken, 1 cup	15
pork, 1 cup	17
shrimp, 1 cup	15
Sweet potato	
○ baked, ½ cup	4
candied, ½ cup	8
canned, in syrup, ½ cup	5

	SmartPoints™ value
canned, in syrup, drained, ½ cup	4
○ canned, mashed, 9 oz	9
○ canned, vacuum pack, ½ cup	4
○ cooked, cubed, ½ cup	3
○ cooked, mashed, ½ cup	6
○ frozen, cooked, ½ cup	4
○ frozen, unprepared, ½ cup	2
○ uncooked, ½ cup	2
Sweet potato pie	
6 ¾ oz	16
Sweet potato puffs	
frozen, unprepared, 3 oz	5
Sweet roll	
1 (4 oz)	9
cheese, 1 (2 ⅓ oz)	9
cinnamon, made from refrigerated dough, with frosting, 1 (1 oz)	4
cinnamon, made from refrigerated dough, with frosting, baked, 1 (1 oz)	4
pecan-swirl, store-bought, 1 (1 oz)	5
store-bought, 1 (2 oz)	9
Sweetbreads	
○ cooked, 3 oz	2
Swiss chard	
○ fresh, frozen, cooked, or canned, without added sugar or oil	0
Syrup	
agave nectar, ¼ cup	15
chocolate, ¼ cup	11
chocolate, fudge-type, ¼ cup	12
corn, dark, ¼ cup	15
corn, light, ¼ cup	15
dietetic, 1 Tbsp	0
flavored, ¼ cup	10
grenadine, 1 Tbsp	3
high fructose corn, ¼ cup	9

Complete A-Z Food List

Syrup (cont'd)

● No Count	SmartPoints™ value
maple, ¼ cup	12
pancake, low-calorie, ¼ cup	5
pancake, regular, ¼ cup	8
pancake, with butter, ¼ cup	12
sorghum, ¼ cup	15
table blend, ¼ cup	10
Szechuan chicken	
frozen, 7 oz	9
Szechuan pork hotpot	
8 oz	7

T

● No Count	SmartPoints™ value
Tabouli	
½ cup	6
Taco	
beef, 1 (3 ½ oz)	7
breakfast, 1 (3 ¾ oz)	7
chicken, 1 (3 ½ oz)	6
fish, 1 (4 ⅓ oz)	5
hard, dinner kit in a box, prepared, 2 (5 ½ oz)	9
hard, fast food, 1 (3 oz)	5
pork, 1 (3 ½ oz)	5
soft, dinner kit in a box, prepared, 2 (5 ½ oz)	12
soft, fast food, 1 (3 ½ oz)	4
Taco salad shell	
store-bought, 2 large (2 oz)	8
store-bought, 2 small (1 ½ oz)	6
Taco shell	
store-bought, 2 (1 ½ oz)	6
Tahini (sesame butter)	
2 Tbsp	6
Tamago-yaki (omelet roll)	
1 (1 ½ oz)	2
Tamale	
2 (6 ¾ oz)	13
beef, canned, 2 (4 oz)	5
beef, frozen, 1 (1 ½ oz)	3
chicken, canned, 1 (2 oz)	3

● No Count	SmartPoints™ value
chicken, frozen, 1 (2 oz)	3
corn, restaurant-type, 5 ¾ oz	11
pork, frozen, 1 (1 ½ oz)	3
pork, restaurant-type, 5 oz	8
Tamale pie	
1 cup	16
Tandoori chicken	
breast, without skin, 4 ½ oz	4
thigh, without skin, 1 (3 oz)	4
Tandoori fish	
¾ cup	5
Tandoori shrimp	
¾ cup	3
Tangelo	
● fresh, frozen, cooked, or canned, without added sugar	0
Tangerine	
canned (mandarin oranges), in light syrup, ½ cup	5
● fresh, frozen, cooked, or canned, without added sugar	0
● satsuma Mandarin	0
Taquito	
beef, 1 (5 ½" x 1 ½") or 3 oz	5
chicken, 1 (5 ½" x 1 ½") or 3 oz	3
frozen, 1 (1 oz)	2
Taro	
● cooked, ½ cup	3
Tart shell	
1 (2 oz)	10
store-bought, 1 (1 ½ oz)	10
Tater tots	
cooked, 3 oz	5
Tea	
black, decaffeinated or regular, without sugar, 8 fl oz	0
Earl Grey, 1 cup	0
herb, chamomile, brewed, 8 fl oz	0
sweetened with sugar, 8 fl oz	5
tea, decaffeinated or regular, sweetened, 8 fl oz	5

Complete A-Z Food List

Tea smoked duck

2 oz	3

Tea, iced

diet, peach, 8 fl oz	0
instant, sweetened with sugar, 1 Tbsp	5
instant, unsweetened, 1 Tbsp	0
unsweetened, 1 fl oz	0

Tea, instant

artificially sweetened, lemon flavored, prepared, 8 fl oz	0
sweetened with sugar, lemon flavor, prepared, 8 fl oz	5
unsweetened, prepared, 8 fl oz	0

Tempeh (fermented soybean cake)

¼ cup (1 ½ oz)	2

Tempura

shrimp, 3 ¾ oz	13
vegetable, 4 ½ oz	10

Tempura batter mix

⅓ cup	4

Teppan yaki (mixed grill of beef, chicken, shrimp, and vegetables)

1 ½ cups	13

Teriyaki

beef, 5 ½ oz	8
chicken, 5 ½ oz	6
fish other than salmon, 5 ½ oz	5
salmon, 5 ½ oz	9
tofu, 5 ½ oz	5

Tetrazzini

chicken, 1 ½ cups	18
turkey, 1 ½ cups	19

Thai chicken with basil

without skin and bone, 3 ¾ oz	4

Thai chili beef (neua pad prik)

1 cup	6

Thai coffee or tea

8 fl oz	16

Thai crisp noodles

1 cup	11

Thai green chicken curry (gaeng kheow wan gai)

1 cup	13

Thai grilled beef (nuea nam tok)

½ cup on lettuce leaves	6

Thai seafood cakes (haw mok thalay)

¾ cup	14

Tiramisu

1 piece (2 ¼" square)	15
restaurant-type, 1 piece (4 ¾ oz)	20

Toaster pastry

brown sugar-cinnamon, 1 oz	4
fruit, 1 (1 ¾ oz)	8
fruit, frosted, 1 (1 ¾ oz)	8
low-fat, 1 (1 ¾ oz)	8

Tofu

	aburage, bean curd, fried, 3 oz	8
○	extra firm, 3 oz	2
○	firm, light, 3 oz	1
○	firm, regular, 3 oz	1
	fried, 3 oz	6
○	silken, 3 oz	1
○	silken, light, 3 oz	1
	smoked, 3 oz	5
○	soft, regular, 3 oz	1

Tofu, agedashi

fried, 5 oz	7

Tofu, frozen

nondairy dessert, 3 oz	11

Tomatillo

○	fresh, frozen, cooked, or canned, without added sugar or oil	0

Tomato

○	canned, crushed, in tomato puree	0
○	canned, with green chilies	0

Complete A-Z Food List

● No Count	SmartPoints™ value
● fresh, frozen, cooked, or canned, without added sugar or oil	0
● Italian-style, canned	0
Tomato juice	
canned, 8 fl oz	2
Tomato paste	
canned, ¼ cup	2
Tomato puree	
● canned	0
Tomato-clam juice	
clam-tomato, 8 fl oz	4
Tomatoes, dried	
● not packed in oil	0
packed in oil, drained, ½ cup	4
Tomatoes, fried green	
2 slices (4 ¾ oz)	6
Tonkatsu	
beef, 3 ½ oz	8
chicken, 3 ½ oz	7
pork, 3 ½ oz	10
Tortellini	
beef, chicken, or pork without sauce, frozen, 3 ¼ oz	8
cheese, without sauce, 3 oz	7
cheese, without sauce, frozen, 3 ¾ oz	9
cheese, without sauce, store-bought, 4 ¼ oz	9
meat, without sauce, 3 oz	5
meat, without sauce, store-bought, 4 ½ oz	10
mushroom, without sauce, frozen, 3 ¼ oz	10
sausage, without sauce, frozen, 3 ¼ oz	11
spinach, with cheese, without sauce, store-bought, 4 oz	10
vegetable and cheese, without sauce, 3 ¾ oz	9
with cheese filling, fresh, refrigerated, store-bought, ¾ cup	7

● No Count	SmartPoints™ value
Tortilla	
corn, 1 (¾ oz)	2
● corn, reduced-fat, 2 (1 ½ oz)	3
flour, 1 medium (1 oz)	3
flour, 1 (8")	5
flour, burrito-size wheat, 1 large (2 oz)	3
flour, fat-free, 1 (½ oz)	1
multigrain, 1 (8")	5
whole-wheat, 1 (1 ¼ oz)	2
whole-wheat, 96% fat-free, 1 (7-8") or 1 ½ oz	4
Tortilla chips	
1 oz	4
baked, blue corn, 10 chips (1 oz)	3
baked, low-fat, 1 oz	3
light, 1 oz	4
nacho cheese, 1 oz	5
nacho cheese, low-fat, made with fat substitute, 1 oz	3
nacho cheese-flavor, light, 1 oz	4
plain, white corn, 1 oz	4
plain, yellow corn, 1 oz	4
ranch-flavor, 1 oz	4
reduced-fat, 1 oz	4
taco flavor, 1 oz	4
Tortoni	
2 ½ oz)	12
Tostada	
beef, 1 (8 ¼ oz)	13
chicken, 1 (8 ¼ oz)	11
with beans and cheese, fast food, 1 (5 oz)	7
with beans, beef, and cheese, fast food, 1 (8 oz)	12
with beef and cheese, fast food, 1 (5 ⅔ oz)	11
with guacamole, fast food, 2 (9 ¼ oz)	13

Tostada shell

corn, 1 (½ oz)	2
store-bought, 1 (½ oz)	2

Tourtière (Canadian meat pie)

4 ¾ oz	11

Trail mix

1 oz	5
tropical, 1 oz	5
with chocolate chips, 1 oz	5

Trifle

½ cup	5

Tuna steak, grilled

○ frozen, 3 oz	1

Tuna-noodle casserole

7 ¾ oz	10

Turkey

canned, 3 oz	3
diced, light and dark meat, seasoned, 3 oz	2
fryer-roaster, with skin, without bone, cooked, 3 oz	2
meat only, roasted, 3 oz	2
roast, seasoned, light and dark meat, roasted, 3 oz	3
with gravy, frozen, 3 oz	1

Turkey breast

○ from whole bird, without skin, raw, 4 oz	1
○ smoked, 3 oz	2
with skin, without bone, cooked, 3 oz	3
○ without skin and bone, cooked, 3 oz	1
○ without skin or bone, uncooked, 4 oz	1

Turkey breast, ground

○ 99% fat-free, cooked, 3 oz	1
○ 99% fat-free, uncooked, 4 oz	1
○ uncooked, 4 oz	2

Turkey burger

frozen, prepared, 3 oz	4

Turkey drumstick

with skin, without bone, cooked, 3 oz	4
without skin and bone, cooked, 3 oz	2
without skin, with bone, uncooked, 4 oz	2

Turkey leg

with skin, without bone, cooked, 3 oz	4

Turkey neck

cooked, 3 oz	2

Turkey patty

breaded, battered, fried, 3 oz	7
○ fat-free, cooked, 3 oz	1

Turkey thigh

pre-basted, roasted, with skin and bone, 3 oz	3
with skin and bone, cooked, 3 oz	4
without skin, with bone, uncooked, 4 oz	2

Turkey wing

meat and skin, cooked, 3 oz	4

Turkey, dark meat

with skin and bone, uncooked, 4 oz	4
with skin, without bone, cooked, 3 oz	4
without skin and bone, cooked, 3 oz	2

Turkey, ground

85% lean/15% fat, pan-broiled crumbles, 3 oz	6
85% lean/15%, uncooked, 3 oz	4
93% lean/7% fat, cooked, 3 oz	4
93% lean/7% fat, pan-broiled crumbles, 3 oz	4
93% lean/7% fat, uncooked, 4 oz	3

Complete A-Z Food List

○ No Count	SmartPoints™ value
regular, cooked, 3 oz	5
regular, uncooked, 4 oz	4
Turkey, light meat	
with skin and bone, uncooked, 4 oz	3
○ without skin and bone, cooked, 3 oz	1
○ without skin, with bone, uncooked, 4 oz	1
Turnips	
○ fresh, frozen, cooked, or canned, without added sugar or oil	0
Turnover	
fruit, any type, 1 (3 ½ oz)	9
fruit, any type, fast food, 1 (4 oz)	13
Twice-cooked pork	
3 oz	6
Tzimmes	
vegetable, 6 ½ oz	6

V

○ No Count	SmartPoints™ value
Veal	
○ cubed, lean only, cooked, 3 oz	2
○ cubed, lean only, uncooked, 4 oz	2
leg (top round), lean and fat, cooked, 3 oz	3
leg (top round), lean and fat, pan-fried, breaded, 3 oz	4
leg (top round), lean only, pan-fried, breaded, 3 oz	3
○ leg (top round), lean only, uncooked, 4 oz	1
leg, cooked, 3 oz	3
leg, trimmed, cooked, 3 oz	3
○ leg, trimmed, uncooked, 4 oz	1
leg, uncooked, 4 oz	2
loin, cooked, 3 oz	6
loin, lean and fat, uncooked, 4 oz	5
loin, lean only, raw, 4 oz	2
○ loin, trimmed, cooked, 3 oz	3
○ loin, trimmed, uncooked, 4 oz	2

○ No Count	SmartPoints™ value
rib, cooked, 3 oz	5
rib, lean only, cooked, 3 oz	3
rib, lean only, uncooked, 4 oz	2
rib, uncooked, 4 oz	5
shank, cooked, 3 oz	3
○ shank, lean and fat, uncooked, 4 oz	2
○ shank, lean only, cooked, 3 oz	2
○ shank, lean only, uncooked, 4 oz	2
shoulder, cooked, 3 oz	4
shoulder, lean and fat, uncooked, 4 oz	3
○ shoulder, lean only, raw, 4 oz	2
shoulder, trimmed, cooked, 3 oz	3
○ shoulder, trimmed, uncooked, 4 oz	2
sirloin, cooked, 3 oz	5
○ sirloin, lean only, uncooked, 4 oz	2
○ sirloin, lean, cooked, 3 oz	3
Veal and peppers	
9 ⅔ oz	11
Veal chop	
cooked, 3 oz	6
lean, cooked, 3 oz	4
lean, uncooked, 4 oz	2
uncooked, 4 oz	5
Veal cutlet	
breaded, fried, 4 oz	8
cooked, 3 oz	3
○ uncooked, 4 oz	2
Veal marsala	
10 oz	17
Veal parmigiana	
with sauce, 5 oz veal with ½ cup Italian tomato sauce	14
without sauce, 5 ½ oz	12
Veal piccata	
5 ¾ oz	12
Veal scaloppine	
4 ½ oz	8

Veal, breast

cooked, 3 oz	6
lean and fat, cooked, 3 oz	6
lean and fat, uncooked, 4 oz	7
trimmed, cooked, 3 oz	4
trimmed, uncooked, 4 oz	7

Veal, ground

ground, cooked, 3 oz	3
ground, uncooked, 4 oz	6

Vegetable burger on bun

restaurant-type, 7 oz	14

Vegetable chips

1 oz	4
sweet potato, 1 oz	5
taro, 1 oz	5
yucca (cassava), 1 oz	5

Vegetable juice

carrot, canned, 8 fl oz	4
low-sodium, canned, 8 fl oz	2
mixed, 8 fl oz	2

Vegetable pulao

5 oz	5

Vegetable-fruit juice blend

100% vegetable and fruit blend, 8 fl oz	6
cold-pressed, detox-type, vegetable and fruit, 8 fl oz	4
cold-pressed, greens, vegetable and fruit, 8 fl oz	3

Vegetables, creamed

except corn, ½ cup	2

Vegetables, fried

3 oz	5

Vegetables, in sauce

frozen, ½ cup	2

Vegetables, mixed

○	Asian, frozen, unprepared	0
○	canned, drained solids, ½ cup	1
	carrots and parsnips, ½ cup	1

○	frozen, unprepared, ½ cup	1
○	oven-roasted, with 1 tsp olive oil, 1 cup	2
○	peas and carrots, canned, solids and liquids, ½ cup	1
○	peas and carrots, cooked, ½ cup	1
○	peas and carrots, uncooked, ½ cup	1
○	peas and onions, canned, solids and liquids, ½ cup	1
○	peas and onions, cooked, ½ cup	1
○	sautéed, with 1 tsp olive oil, 1 cup	2

Vegetables, pot-roasted

with pan drippings, ½ cup	3

Vegetables, sautéed

½ cup	5

Venison

○	cooked, 3 oz	2
○	uncooked, 4 oz	2

Venison, ground

cooked, 3 oz	4
uncooked, 4 oz	4

Vietnamese beef balls (thit bo vien)

6 (1 ½ oz)	2

Vietnamese chao tom (shrimp mousse over sugar cane)

3 ½ oz	2

Vietnamese chicken curry

1 cup	11

Vindaloo

chicken, 7 ¾ oz	7
lamb, 8 ¼ oz	20
pork, 8 ¼ oz	9

Vinegar

1 Tbsp	0

Vitello tonnato

7 ½ oz	17

Complete A-Z Food List

W

Waffle

any type, frozen, 2 (2 ½ oz)	6
any type, low-fat, frozen, 2 (4" round or square) or 2 ½ oz	5
Belgian, frozen (2-3"), 2 (2 oz)	5
Belgian, restaurant-type, without butter or toppings, 1 (7-8")	14
made from mix (2-4"), 2 (1 ½ oz)	5
made from mix (7" round), 1 (2 ½ oz)	7
mini, frozen, 2 (¾ oz)	2
whole-grain, frozen, 2 (2 ½ oz)	5

Waffle stick

frozen, 2 (2 oz)	5

Walnuts

¼ cup	6
black, dried, ¼ cup	5
chopped, ¼ cup	6
glazed, 1 oz	5

Wasabi paste

prepared, 1 Tbsp	1

Wasabi powder

1 Tbsp	1

Water chestnuts

○ fresh, frozen, cooked, or canned, without added sugar or oil	0

Watercress

○ fresh, frozen, cooked, or canned, without added sugar or oil	0

Watermelon

○ fresh, frozen, cooked, or canned, without added sugar or oil	0

Wheat berries

○ cooked, 1 cup	5

Wheat germ

2 Tbsp	1
crude, 2 Tbsp	1
toasted, 2 Tbsp	1

Wiener schnitzel

3 oz	10

Wine

light, 5 fl oz	2
red, 5 fl oz	4
white, 5 fl oz	4
white, late harvest, 5 fl oz	5

Wine cooler

5 fl oz	4

Wine spritzer

8 fl oz	3

Wine, cooking

marsala, 2 Tbsp	1
rice, 1 Tbsp	1
sherry, 5 fl oz	5

Wine, dessert

dry, 3 ½ fl oz	5
sweet, 3 ½ fl oz	7

Wine, non-alcoholic

5 fl oz	0

Wonton

boiled, 6 (6 oz)	7
fried, 6 (4 oz)	13

Wonton wrapper

5 (1 ½ oz)	3

Wrap

chicken Caesar, restaurant-type, 10 ½ oz	18
lettuce, beef, 1 (3 oz)	2
lettuce, chicken, 1 (3 oz)	2
spinach, 1 (2 ½ oz)	6

Wrapper

rice paper, 1 (½ oz)	1

Complete A-Z Food List

Y

Yaki-soba

beef, ½ cup noodles with ½ cup beef and vegetables	5
chicken, ½ cup noodles with ½ cup chicken and vegetables	5
pork, ½ cup noodles with ½ cup pork and vegetables	6

Yakitori

7 ½ oz	7

Yam

canned, in syrup, ½ cup	5
○ cooked, ½ cup	2

Yeast

baker's, active dry, ¼ oz	0
baker's, compressed, 1 cake (⅔ oz)	0

Yogurt drink

1 cup	9
mango lassi, 1 cup	7

Yogurt parfait

fruit and yogurt, restaurant-type, 8 ½ oz	10

Yogurt, fat-free

flavored (vanilla, lemon, coffee), sweetened with sugar, 1 cup	7
fruit-flavored, sweetened with sugar, 1 cup	11
○ plain, 1 cup	5

Yogurt, Greek

○ fat-free, plain, 1 cup	3
○ fat-free, vanilla, 1 cup	5
low-fat, plain, 1 cup	4
low-fat, vanilla, 1 cup	9

Yogurt, light

○ 1 cup	5

Yogurt, low-fat

flavored (vanilla, lemon, coffee), sweetened with sugar, 1 cup	10
fruit-flavored, sweetened with sugar, 1 cup	12
plain, 1 cup	6

Yogurt, soy

flavored, ¾ cup	7
○ plain, ¾ cup	4

Yogurt, tofu

1 cup	7

Yogurt, whole milk

whole milk, plain, 1 cup	6

Yorkshire pudding

5 oz	9

Yosenabe

2 cups	4

Yucca

yucca, raw (cassava), ½ cup	5

Z

Zabaglione

½ cup	7

Zeppole

1 (3 oz)	9

Ziti, baked

with meat, 1 cup	13
without meat, 1 cup	9

Zucchini

○ fresh, frozen, cooked, or canned, without added sugar or oil	0
○ Italian-style, canned, ½ cup	1

Zucchini, breaded

prepared without fat, 6 pieces (3 oz)	6

Zuppa di pesce

2 cups	10

Zuppa Inglese

½ cup	16

Zwieback

1 oz	4

Complete A-Z Food List

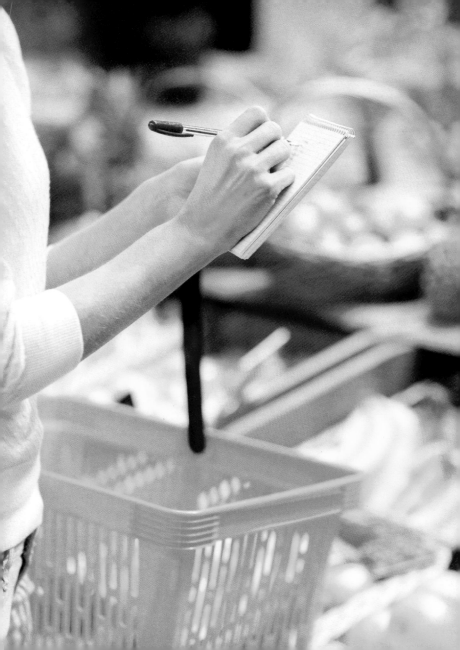

Brand Name

food list

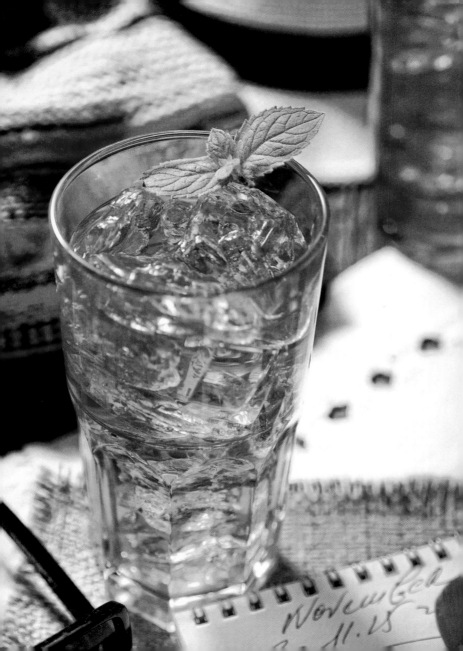

beverages

Alcoholic Beverages

Absolut

Vodka, 1 ½ fl oz	3

Agave Loco

Rum chata, 1 ½ fl oz	6

Bacardi Superior

Puerto Rican rum, 1 ½ fl oz	3

Captain Morgan

Spiced rum, original, 1 ½ fl oz	3

Crown Royal

Regal apple flavored whisky, 1 ½ fl oz	3

Fireball

Red hot cinnamon whiskey, 1 ½ fl oz	4

Grey Goose

Vodka, 1 ½ fl oz	3

Jack Daniel's Old No. 7 Brand

Tennessee whiskey, 1 fl oz	3

Jose Cuervo

Margarita, golden, 1 ½ fl oz	2
Margarita, light, classic lime, 1 ½ fl oz	1

Kahlúa

Liqueur, imported, 1 ½ fl oz	4

Malibu

Caribbean rum with natural coconut flavor, 1 ½ fl oz	3

Margaritaville

Margarita, skinny, 4 fl oz	3

Red Lobster

Martini (vodka), 1 serving (70.6 g)	5

Seagram's

7 crown blended whiskey, 1 ½ fl oz	3

Skyy

Vodka, 1 ½ fl oz	3

Alcoholic Malt Beverages

Seagram's Escapes

Malt beverage, flavored, peach fuzzy navel, 1 bottle (331 ml)	9
Malt beverage, flavored, strawberry daiquiri, 1 bottle (331 ml)	9
Malt beverage, Jamaican me happy, 1 bottle (331 ml)	9

Smirnoff

Malt mixed drink, premium, signature screwdriver, 1 bottle (331 ml)	11

Smirnoff Ice

Malt beverage, 1 bottle (331 ml)	11
Malt beverage, premium, green apple bite, 1 bottle (331 ml)	11
Malt beverage, premium, raspberry burst, 1 bottle (331 ml)	11

Beer & Ale

Blue Moon

Ale, Belgian white, 1 bottle (355 ml)	5
Ale, pale moon, 12 fl oz	5

Bud Light

Beer, 12 fl oz	4
Beer (12 pack bottles), 1 bottle (354 ml)	3
Beer, lime, 12 fl oz	3
Beer, platinum, 12 fl oz	5
Chelada beer & clamato with salt and lime, 12 fl oz	5

Busch

Light beer, 12 fl oz	3

Corona Extra

Beer, 1 can (355 ml)	5

Corona Light

Beer, 12 fl oz	3

Coronita Extra

Beer, 1 bottle (207 ml)	3

Beverages

Dos Equis XX

Beer, lager especial, 1 bottle (355 ml)	5

Fat Tire

Ale, amber new Belgium, 1 bottle (355 ml)	5
Fat tire draft beer, 14 fl oz	6

Full Moon Seasonal Collection

Ale, summer honey wheat, 1 bottle (355 ml)	5

Goose Island

Ale, 312 urban wheat, 1 bottle (355 ml)	5

Grolsch

Blonde lager, 12 fl oz	4

Heineken

Beer, lager, 1 bottle (355 ml)	5
Beer, lager, light, 1 bottle (354 ml)	3

Henry Weinhard's

Hefeweizen, 12 fl oz	4
Lager, dark, classic, 12 fl oz	5
Pale ale, Indian, 1 can or bottle (340.19 g)	6

Lagunitas Brewing

India pale ale, 12 fl oz	5

Land Shark

Lager, island style, 1 bottle (355 ml)	5

Leinenkugel's

Beer, summer shandy, 1 bottle (355 ml)	5
Sunset wheat beer, 12 fl oz	5

Michelob

Beer, ultra amber, 12 fl oz	4

Miller

Beer, lite, 12 fl oz	3
Blue moon Belgian white, 1 can or bottle (340.19 g)	5
George Killian's Irish red, 1 can or bottle (340.19 g)	5

Henry Weinhard's woodland pass ipa, 1 can or bottle (340.19 g)	6
High life light, 1 can or bottle (340.19 g)	3
Mgd 64, 12 fl oz	2

Miller Genuine Draft Light

Beer, draft light, 1 bottle (355 ml)	5

Miller Lite

Pilsner beer, 1 can (354 ml)	3

Modelo Especial

Beer, especial, 1 bottle (355 ml)	5

Natural Light

Beer, 1 can (354 ml)	3

Newcastle

Ale, brown, 1 bottle (355 ml)	5

RedBridge

Beer, gluten-free sorghum, 12 fl oz	4

Redds

Ale, apple, 1 bottle (355 ml)	5

Sam Adams

Beer, light, 12 oz	4
Draft beer, 14 fl oz	6

Samuel Adams

Lager, Boston, 1 bottle (355 ml)	5
Lager, winter, 1 bottle (355 ml)	5

Samuel Adams Seasonal Brew

Lager, Octoberfest, 1 bottle (355 ml)	5

Shiner Bock

Beer, 1 bottle (355 ml)	5

Shock Top

Ale, Belgian white, 1 bottle (355 ml)	5

Shock Top Seasonal Collection

Ale, pumpkin wheat, 1 bottle (355 ml)	5

Sierra Nevada

Pale ale, 1 bottle (355 ml)	5

Stella Artois

Premium lager beer, 1 bottle (336 ml)	5

Beverages

	SmartPoints™ value

Yuengling

Draft beer, 14 fl oz	5
Lager, light, 1 bottle (355 ml)	3
Lager, traditional, original amber, 1 bottle (355 ml)	5

Cider, Hard

Angry Orchard

Apple ginger hard cider, 12 fl oz	8
Crisp apple hard cider, 12 fl oz	9
Golden hard cider, 12 fl oz	9
Traditional dry hard cider, 12 fl oz	8

Crispin

Hard apple cider, honey crisp, 12 fl oz	8
Hard apple cider, natural, brut, 12 fl oz	6
Hard apple cider, the saint, 12 fl oz	6
Hard apple cider, imported classic English dry cide, 1 can (500 ml)	12

Michelob Ultra

Beer, light cider, 12 fl oz	5

Stella Artois Cidre

Cider, premium, 12 fl oz	7

Strongbow

Cider, England's dry, 12 fl oz	6

Woodchuck

Hard cider, amber, 12 fl oz	9
Hard cider, granny smith, 12 fl oz	7
Hard cider, pear, 12 fl oz	7

Cocktail Mix

Mr. & Mrs. T

Bloody mary mix, bold & spicy, 4 fl oz	2
Bloody mary mix, original, 5 fl oz	1

V8

Original bloody mary mix, 5 fl oz	2

Zing Zang

Bloody mary mix, 3 fl oz	1

	SmartPoints™ value

Cocoa & Chocolate Drinks

Archer Farms

Sea salt caramel hot cocoa mix, 1 packet (28 g)	6

Cafe Escapes

K-cups, hot cocoa, dark chocolate, 1 pack (15 g)	3
K-cups, hot cocoa, milk chocolate flavored, 1 portion pack (15 g)	3

Carnation

Malted milk, chocolate, 3 Tbsp	4
Malted milk, original, 3 Tbsp	4

CytoSport

Chocolate flavor genuine muscle milk mix, 1 scoop (75 g)	4

Dagoba Drinking Chocolate

Organic authentic cacao powder mix, 1 Tbsp	3

FLAVIA®

Dove® hot chocolate, 1 serving (20 g)	4

Ghirardelli Chocolate

Hot cocoa, premium, double chocolate mix, 3 Tbsp	7

Glucerna

Rich chocolate flavor shake, 8 fl oz	6

GNC Total Lean

Lean shake, Swiss chocolate, 2 scoops (48 g)	5

Godiva

Hot cocoa, dark chocolate, 4 Tbsp	8

Great Value

Hot cocoa mix, milk chocolate flavored, ¼ cup	7

Grove Square

Hot cocoa (single serve cup), 1 (15 g)	3

Horizon Organic

Chocolate organic lowfat milk, 1 container (236 ml)	7

Kellogg's Breakfast To Go

Milk chocolate shake, 1 bottle (296 g)	7

Kroger

Hot cocoa mix, Dutch, fat free, milk chocolate, 1 packet (8 g)	1
Hot cocoa mix, Dutch, milk chocolate, 1 packet (15 g)	2
Hot cocoa mix, Dutch, with mini-marshmallows, packet, 1 packet (21 g)	4

Land O' Lakes Cocoa Classics

Hot cocoa mix, arctic white, 1 envelope (35 g)	8
Hot cocoa mix, caramel & chocolate, 1 envelope (35 g)	8
Hot cocoa mix, chocolate supreme, 1 envelope (35 g)	8
Hot cocoa mix, French vanilla & chocolate, 1 envelope (35 g)	8
Hot cocoa mix, mint & chocolate, ¼ cup dry	8
Raspberry and chocolate hot cocoa mix, 1 envelope (35 g)	8

Maxwell House International Latte

Beverage mix, cafe-style, mocha, 1 ⅓ Tbsp	3
Beverage mix, peppermint mocha, 1 ⅓ Tbsp	3

Nestlé

Hot cocoa mix, 1 packet (20 g)	4
Hot cocoa mix, dark chocolate flavor, 1 envelope (26 g)	5
Hot cocoa mix, mini marshmallows, with rich chocolate flavor, 1 envelope (20 g)	4
Hot cocoa mix, rich milk chocolate flavor, 1 envelope (20 g)	4
Rich milk chocolate fat free hot chocolate mix, 1 envelope (28 g)	1

Nestlé Abuelita

Mexican style instant hot chocolate mix, 1 envelope (28 g)	6

Nestlé Nesquik

Chocolate flavor no sugar added powder drink mix, 2 Tbsp	1
Drink mix, chocolate flavor, 2 Tbsp	3

ON Gold Standard

100% casein, chocolate supreme, 1 scoop (33 g)	1

Ovaltine

Malt mix, classic, 4 Tbsp	4
Rich chocolate drink mix, 2 Tbsp	2

Safeway Kitchens

Hot cocoa mix, rich chocolate flavor, fat free, 1 envelope (8 g)	1

ShopRite

Hot cocoa mix, instant, milk chocolate flavor, reduced calorie, fat free, 1 envelope (15 g)	2

Slim Fast 3-2-1 Plan

Shake mix, chocolate royale, 1 scoop (26 g)	4

Starbucks

Hot cocoa mix, double chocolate, 1 envelope (28 g)	6
Hot cocoa mix, salted caramel, 1 envelope (28 g)	6
Hot cocoa mix, toasted marshmallow, 1 envelope (28 g)	5

Stephen's

Hot cocoa, gourmet, milk chocolate, 3 Tbsp	8

Swiss Miss

Candy cane hot cocoa mix with peppermint marshmallows, 1 envelope (21 g)	5
Caramel cream hot cocoa mix, 1 envelope (28 g)	6
Dark chocolate hot cocoa mix, 1 envelope (35 g)	8
Hot cocoa mix with calcium, no sugar added and marshmallows, 1 envelope (15 g)	2
Hot cocoa mix, fat free with calcium, 1 envelope (19 g)	3

Beverages

Beverages

SmartPoints™ value

Hot cocoa mix, French vanilla, 1 envelope (16 g)	2
Hot cocoa mix, great start cocoa, 1 envelope (28 g)	6
Hot cocoa mix, marshmallow madness, 1 envelope (34 g)	7
Hot cocoa mix, rich chocolate, 1 envelope (28 g)	6
Marshmallow hot cocoa mix, 2 Tbsp	4
Milk chocolate hot cocoa mix, 3 Tbsp	5
Sensible sweets diet hot chocolate mix, 1 envelope (8 g)	1
Sensible sweets fat free hot chocolate mix, 1 envelope (16 g)	2
Sensible sweets no sugar added hot chocolate mix, 1 envelope (16 g)	3
Simply cocoa dark chocolate flavor hot cocoa mix, 1 envelope (27 g)	5
Swiss Miss Classics	
Hot cocoa mix, marshmallow lovers, 1 envelope (26 g)	5
Hot cocoa mix, milk chocolate flavor, 1 envelope (21 g)	4
Hot cocoa mix, with marshmallows, 2 Tbsp	4
Milk chocolate hot chocolate k-cup, 1 K-cup pack	3
Swiss Miss Sensible Sweets	
No sugar added milk chocolate hot cocoa mix, 1 envelope (16 g)	3
Swiss Miss Simply Cocoa	
Hot cocoa mix, milk chocolate flavor, 1 envelope (24 g)	5
Trader Joe's	
European sipping chocolate, 3 Tbsp	5
Organic hot cocoa mix, 1 packet (28 g)	5

SmartPoints™ value

Coconut Milk

A Taste of Thai	
Coconut milk, lite, ⅓ cup	3
Silk Pure Coconut	
Coconutmilk, unsweetened, 1 cup	2
Coconutmilk, vanilla, 1 cup	5
Original coconut milk, 1 cup	4
Simple Truth	
Coconut milk, 1 cup	4
So Delicious	
Coconut milk beverage unsweetened vanilla, 1 cup	2
Coconut milk beverage, dairy free, unsweetened vanilla, 1 cup	3
Coconut milk beverage, original, 1 cup	3
Coconut milk beverage, vanilla, 1 cup	5
Coconut milk, beverage, unsweetened, 1 cup	3
Coconut milk, cultured, Greek style, strawberry, 1 container (170 g)	6
Coconut milk, cultured, Greek style, vanilla, 1 container (170 g)	6
Coconut milk, cultured, plain, 4 oz	4
Coconut milk, cultured, vanilla, 4 oz	5
Unsweetened coconut milk beverage, 1 cup	2
Unsweetened cultured coconut milk, 4 oz	3
Thai Kitchen	
Coconut milk, lite, ⅓ cup	3
Trader Joe's	
Coconut milk vanilla, 1 cup	5
Original unsweetened coconut milk, 1 cup	3
Unsweetened coconut milk beverage, 1 cup	3
Unsweetened coconut milk beverage, 8 fl oz	3

Coconut Water

Bai 5 Antioxidant Infusions

Molokai coconut, 8 fl oz	0

C2O

Coconut water, pure, 8 fl oz	3

Coco Café

Coconut water, cafe latte, espresso, 1 container (330 g)	7

Evolution Fresh

Juice blend, pineapple coconut water, 8 fl oz	4

Goya

Coconut water, 1 cup	4

Harmless Harvest

Coconut water, 100% raw, 1 bottle (235 ml)	3

O.N.E.

Coconut water, 8 fl oz	2

SoBe Lifewater

Coconut water beverage, pacific coconut, 8 fl oz	2

Trader Joe's

Organic coconut water, ½ container (240 ml)	2

Vita Coco

Coconut water, with peach & mango, 1 bottle (330 ml)	5
Pure coconut water, 1 container (330 ml)	4
Pure coconut water, lemonade flavored, 8 fl oz	4

Zico

Coconut water, pure premium, 8 oz	3
Premium chocolate flavored coconut water, 8 fl oz	4

Coffee & Cappuccino

Archer Farms Savor Everyday

Vanilla bean creme brulee coffee k cup, 1 (10 g)	0

Bolthouse Farms Perfectly Protein

Mocha cappuccino coffee beverage, 8 fl oz	8
Salted caramel latte, 8 fl oz	6

Cafe Escapes

Cafe caramel, 1 serving (15 g)	3
Cafe caramel k cups, 1 k cup	3
Cafe vanilla, 1 serving (14 g)	3
Cafe vanilla k cups, 1 k cup	4
K-cups, coffee, cafe mocha, 1 k-cup	3
Vue cups, cafe caramel, 1 vue cup (16 g)	4

Caffe D'Vita

Cappuccino, instant premium, mocha, 1 Tbsp	3
Cappuccino, premium instant, Irish cream, 1 Tbsp	3
Cappuccino, premium instant, sugar free, mocha, 2 tsp	2

Caffe Vergnano 1882 Espresso

Limited edition cafe pumpkin spice k cups, 1 (14 g)	3

Califia Farms

Pure cafe latte iced coffee with almond milk, 8 fl oz	4
Pure iced mocha coffee with almond milk, 8 fl oz	4

Donut House Collection

Coffee, iced, k-cup packs, medium roast, sweet & creamy regular, 1 k-cup pack	5

Donut House Collection Keurig Brewed

Donut house coffee light roast k-cups, 1 k-cup	0

Donut Shop

K-cup, sweet and creamy regular iced coffee, 1 k-cup pack	5

Beverages

Beverages

	SmartPoints™ value
K-cup, extra bold, medium roast coffee, 1 cup	0
K-cups, medium roast, coconut mocha coffee, 1 cup	0
Dunkin' Donuts	
Coffee, ground, French vanilla, 1 cup	0
Coffee, ground, original blend, 1 cup	0
Original blend medium roast ground coffee, 6 fl oz	0
Dunkin' Donuts Bakery Series	
Chocolate glazed donut flavored ground coffee, 1 serving (5 g)	0
Eight O'Clock	
Hazelnut coffee k cups, 1 single serve cup (9.5 g)	0
FLAVIA®	
Cappuccino-latte swirl, 1 serving (13 g)	2
Folgers	
100% Colombian med-dark roast ground coffee, brewed, 6 fl oz	0
Black silk dark roast ground coffee, brewed, 6 fl oz	0
Breakfast blend mild roast ground coffee, 6 fl oz	0
Cappuccino, French vanilla, 8 oz	4
Classic roast coffee crystals, 1 serving (2 g)	0
Coffee singles, 1 bag	0
Coffee, ground, French roast, med-dark, 1 cup	0
Coffee, medium, classic roast, 1 cup	0
Folgers Classic Roast	
Medium roast ground coffee, 6 fl oz	0
Folgers Flavors	
French vanilla ground coffee, brewed, 6 fl oz	0

	SmartPoints™ value
Folgers Gourmet Selections	
Caramel drizzle flavored coffee k cup, 1 k-cup	0
K-cups, coffee, flavored, caramel drizzle, 1 cup	0
Mocha swirl coffee k cups, 1 (10 g)	0
Mocha swirl coffee pod, 1 k-cup	0
Vanilla biscotti flavored coffee k cup, 1 k-cup	0
Folgers Simply Smooth	
Decaf medium ground coffee, 1 serving (2 g)	0
General Foods International	
Coffeehouse beverage mix, cafe francais, 1 ⅓ Tbsp	3
Coffeehouse beverage mix, cafe vienna, 1 ⅓ Tbsp	4
Coffeehouse beverage mix, French vanilla cafe, 1 ⅓ Tbsp	3
Coffeehouse beverage mix, hazelnut cafe, 1 ⅓ Tbsp	4
Coffeehouse beverage mix, sugar free, French vanilla cafe, 1 ⅓ Tbsp	1
Coffeehouse beverage mix, sugar free, Suisse mocha cafe, decaffeinated, 1 ⅓ Tbsp	1
Coffeehouse beverage mix, Suisse mocha cafe, 1 ⅓ Tbsp	3
General Foods International On The Go	
Coffee house drink mix, artificially flavored, vanilla latte, 1 packet (13 g)	3
Gevalia	
2 step vanilla latte (1 cup and froth packet), 1 cup & froth pack	5
2 step vanilla latte cup and froth packet, 1 cup & froth pack	5
Cappuccino, 2-step, 1 coffee cup (27 g)	5
Caramel macchiato, 2-step, single serve, 8 fl oz	5

	SmartPoints value
Mocha latte, 2-step, 1 serving (169 g)	4
Gevalia Kaffe	
Cappuccino k cup with froth packet, 1 k-cup	5
Caramel macchiato k cup and froth packet, 1 serving (29 g)	5
Mocha latte k cup with froth packet, 1 k-cup	4
Gloria Jean's Coffees	
Butter toffee medium roast coffee k-cups, 6 fl oz	0
Hazelnut medium roast coffee k-cups, 1 k-cup	0
Macadamia cookie flavored coffee k-cups, 1 k-cup	0
Mudslide flavored coffee k-cups, 1 k-cup	0
Great Value	
Cappuccino, instant, French vanilla, 3 Tbsp	6
Green Mountain Coffee	
Breakfast blend k-cups, 1 k-cup	0
Caramel vanilla cream flavored k cup, 1 k-cup	0
Hazelnut flavored light roast coffee k-cups, 1 k-cup	0
Hazelnut k-cup coffee, 1 (9.35 g)	0
K-cups, coffee, breakfast blend, light roast, 1 cup	0
K-cups, coffee, flavored, light roast, French vanilla, 1 cup	0
K-cups, coffee, light roast, caramel vanilla cream, 1 cup	0
Pumpkin spice coffee k-cups, 1 k-cup	0
Pumpkin spice flavored k cup, 1 k-cup	0
Green Mountain Coffee Keurig Brewed	
Nantucket blend medium roast coffee k-cups, 1 k-cup	0

	SmartPoints value
Grove Square	
French vanilla cappuccino mix, 1 single serve cup (15 g)	4
Hills Bros.	
Drink mix, cappuccino, double mocha, 3 Tbsp	6
Drink mix, cappuccino, English toffee, 3 Tbsp	6
Drink mix, cappuccino, fat free, French vanilla, 2 Tbsp	3
Drink mix, cappuccino, French vanilla, 3 Tbsp	6
Drink mix, cappuccino, sugar free, French vanilla, 2 Tbsp	2
Drink mix, skinny latte, fat free French vanilla, 3 Tbsp	5
International Delight	
Iced coffee, caramel macchiato, 1 cup	7
Iced coffee, mocha, 1 cup	7
Iced coffee, sweet & creamy light, mocha, 1 cup	5
Iced coffee, sweet & creamy light, vanilla, 1 cup	5
International Delight Light	
Iced coffee, 1 cup	5
Kahlúa	
Original flavored light roast coffee k-cups, 1 k-cup	0
Kellogg's Special K	
Breakfast shake, protein, coffee house vanilla cappuccino, 1 bottle (296 ml)	7
Keurig Cinnabon	
Classic cinnamon roll k-cups, 1 (9.4 g)	0
Kroger	
Cappuccino drink mix, French vanilla, 1 cup	4
Cappuccino drink mix, hazelnut, 1 cup	4
Caramel cappuccino single serve drink mix, 1 (15 g)	4

Beverages

SmartPoints™ value

SmartPoints™ value

Maxwell House

Breakfast blend ground coffee, 6 fl oz	0
Instant coffee, 6 fl oz	0
Master blend light ground coffee, 1 Tbsp	0
Original roast coffee, 6 fl oz	0
Original roast ground coffee, 6 fl oz	0

Maxwell House Cafe Collection

Coffee, 100% arabica, single serve cups, medium roast, house blend, 1 cup	0

Maxwell House International Latte

Beverage mix, cafe-style, vanilla bean, 1 ⅓ Tbsp	3
Beverage mix, cafe-style, vanilla caramel, 1 ⅓ Tbsp	3

McCafe

Medium roast coffee k-cup packs, 1 (9.75 g)	0

Nescafé Taster's Choice

Coffee, gourmet instant, original, 1 cup	0
French roast instant coffee, 1 tsp	0
Instant coffee beverage, gourmet, hazelnut, 1 packet (2 g)	0

Nestlé Nescafé

Instant coffee mix & French vanilla flavored coffee-mate creamer, 2 Tbsp	5

Private Selection

Coffee drink mix, instant, sugar free, French vanilla, 4 tsp	1

Safeway Select

K-cups, cappuccino, caramel, 1 cup	4

San Francisco Bay OneCup

Coffee, premium gourmet, single serve, French roast, 1 cup	0

Senseo

Ground coffee pods, with coffee creamer, cappuccino, 1 pod (13 g)	2

Skinny Cow

Creamy cappuccino creamy iced coffee drink, 1 bottle (236 ml)	6
Mocha latte creamy iced coffee drink, 1 bottle (236 g)	6
Vanilla latte creamy iced coffee drink, 1 bottle (236 g)	6

Starbucks

Bottled mocha lite frappuccino coffee drink (13.7 fl oz bottle), 1 bottle (405 ml)	6
Caramel flavored k-cup ground coffee, 1 k-cup	0
Caramel flavored premium iced coffee beverage, 1 cup	3
Cinnamon dolce coffee k-cups, 1 (10 g)	0
Coffee drink, frappuccino, 8 fl oz	8
Coffee, iced, 2% milk, caramel, 1 bottle (325 g)	6
Espresso beverage, chilled, skinny caramel macchiato, 8 fl oz	3
Espresso beverage, chilled, skinny vanilla latte, 8 fl oz	3
Iced coffee and milk, 1 bottle (330 g)	6
Lightly sweetened premium iced coffee beverage, 1 cup	3
Low calorie iced coffee and milk, 1 bottle (330 g)	2
Mocha coffee k-cups, 1 (10 g)	0
Unsweetened premium iced coffee beverage, 1 cup	0
Vanilla coffee k-cups, 1 (10 g)	0
Vanilla flavored coffee k-cup, 1 k-cup	0
Vanilla iced coffee, 1 bottle (325 ml)	6
Vanilla iced coffee and milk, 1 bottle (325 ml)	6

Starbucks Discoveries

Chilled espresso beverage, caffe mocha, 8 fl oz	6
Chilled espresso beverage, caramel macchiato, 8 fl oz	6
Chilled espresso beverage, vanilla latte, 8 fl oz	6
Espresso beverage, chilled, peppermint mocha, 8 fl oz	6

Starbucks Doubleshot

Coffee drink, premium, espresso & cream, 1 can (190 ml)	7

Starbucks Doubleshot Light

Coffee drink, premium, espresso & cream, 6 ½ fl oz	3

Starbucks Frappuccino

Chilled coffee drink, caramel, 1 bottle (405 g)	14
Chilled vanilla coffee drink, 1 bottle (281 ml)	10
Coffee drink, chilled, 1 bottle (281 ml)	10
Coffee drink, chilled, caramel, 1 bottle (281 ml)	10
Coffee drink, light, vanilla, 1 bottle (281 ml)	4
Coffee drink, vanilla, 1 bottle (281 g)	10
Mocha coffee drink, 1 bottle (114 ml)	9
Mocha coffee drink, 1 bottle (281 ml)	9
S'mores chilled coffee drink, 1 bottle (45 ml)	14

Starbucks Via

Caffeè mocha latte, 1 packet (37 g)	7

Starbucks Via Latte

Coffee beverage, specialty, caffe mocha, 1 packet (37 g)	7
Peppermint mocha coffee beverage mix, 1 packet (40 g)	8
Vanilla latte specialty coffee beverage, 1 packet (31 g)	6

Starbucks Via Ready Brew

Coffee, iced, ½ packet (13 g)	3
Coffee, instant, extra bold, Italian roast, decaf, 1 cup	0
Coffee, instant, iced, caramel, ½ packet (14 g)	3
Iced coffee lightly sweetened mix, ½ packet (13.3 g)	3

Tassimo Cafe Collection

Coffee, latte, 1 disc (8 g)	2

Tassimo Gevalia

Coffee, cappuccino, 1 disc (8 g)	3
Coffee, latte macchiato, caramel flavored, 1 disc (6 g)	3

Trader Joe's

100% instant Colombian decaf coffee, 6 fl oz	0
Cold brew coffee concentrate, 6 fl oz	0
Instant coffee packets (all dressed up with cream and sugar), 1 packet (12 g)	3

Van Houtte

French vanilla flavored medium roast coffee k-cups, 1 k-cup	0
Raspberry chocolate truffle coffee, 1 k-cup	0

Fruit Juices & Drinks

Alpine

Instant drink mix, spiced apple cider, 1 pouch (21 g)	5
Instant drink mix, spiced apple cider, sugar free, 1 pouch (4 g)	0

Apple & Eve

100% naturally cranberry juice, 8 fl oz	7

Bai 5 Antioxidant Infusions

Brasilia blueberry, 8 fl oz	0
Costa Rica clementine, 8 fl oz	0
Ipanema pomegranate, 8 fl oz	0
Malawi mango, 8 fl oz	0
Sumatra dragonfruit, 8 fl oz	0

Beverages

SmartPoints™ value

SmartPoints™ value

BluePrint

Juice beverage, cold pressed, 1 bottle (473 ml)	6
Juice beverage, cold pressed, beet apple carrot lemon ginger, 1 bottle (473 ml)	10
Juice beverage, cold pressed, lemon cayenne agave, 1 bottle (473 ml)	7

Bragg

Apple cider vinegar drink, organic, apple-cinnamon, 8 fl oz	1

Capri Sun

100% juice, fruit punch, 1 pouch (236 ml)	5
Juice drink blend, pacific cooler, 1 pouch (177 g)	4

Cheribundi

Juice, tart cherry, tru cherry, 8 fl oz	7

Coconut Dream

Coconut drink, original, unsweetened, 1 cup	3

Crush Singles To Go!

Drink mix, orange, ½ packet (1.3 g)	0

Crystal Light

Beverage, raspberry ice, 8 fl oz	0
Drink mix, energy, citrus, ½ packet (2 g)	0
Drink mix, energy, sugar free, wild strawberry, 1 serving (2 g)	0
Drink mix, energy, wild strawberry, ½ packet (2 g)	0
Drink mix, fruit punch, ½ packet (1 g)	0
Drink mix, strawberry orange banana, ⅛ packet (2 g)	0
Drink mix, sugar free, natural cherry pomegranate, unprepared, 1 serving (2 g)	0
Drink mix, sunrise classic orange, ½ packet (2 g)	0

Crystal Light Energy

Drink mix, grape, ½ packet (2 g)	0
Drink mix, peach mango, ½ packet (1 g)	0

Crystal Light On The Go

Drink mix, energy, citrus, ½ packet (1.6 g)	0
Drink mix, fruit punch, ½ packet (1 g)	0

Crystal Light On The Go Antioxidant

Drink mix, natural cherry pomegranate flavor, ½ packet (2 g)	0

Crystal Light Pitcher Packs

Concord grape flavor drink mix, ⅛ packet (1 g)	0

Cuties

Juice, clementine mandarin blend, 8 fl oz	6

Dole

100% juice, orange peach mango, 8 fl oz	7
100% juice, orange strawberry banana, 8 fl oz	7
100% juice, pineapple, 8 fl oz	7
100% juice, pineapple orange, 8 fl oz	7
100% juice, pineapple orange banana, 8 fl oz	7
Juice, pineapple, 8 fl oz	8

Dynamic Health

Juice concentrate, tart cherry, 2 Tbsp	4

Eden Organic

Cherry juice, tart, 8 oz	7

Emergen-C

Raspberry flavored fizzy drink mix with vitamins, 1 packet (9.1 g)	1

Emergen-C 1,000 mg Vitamin C

Super orange flavored fizzy drink mix, 1 packet (8.8 g)	1
Tangerine flavored fizzy drink mix, 1 packet (9.4 g)	1

Evolution Fresh

Juice blend, vegetable and fruit sweet greens and lemon, 8 fl oz	2
Juice blend, vegetable and fruit, essential greens with lime, 8 fl oz	1
Orange juice, 8 fl oz	7

Florida's Natural

100% juice, grapefruit, premium, original ruby red, 8 fl oz	5
100% juice, orange, premium, no pulp, calcium & vitamin D, 8 fl oz	6
Grapefruit juice, original ruby red, 8 fl oz	5
Juice, orange, most pulp, growers style, 8 fl oz	6
Juice, orange, no pulp, 8 fl oz	6
Juice, orange, with pulp, home squeezed style, calcium & vitamin D, 8 fl oz	6
Orange juice, 8 fl oz	6
Orange juice, no pulp, calcium & vitamin D, 8 fl oz	6
Orange juice, no pulp, original, 8 fl oz	6
Orange juice, premium, no pulp, 8 oz	6
Premium orange juice, 8 fl oz	6
Premium pure Florida orange juice, 1 bottle (296 ml)	9

Florida's Natural Fit & Delicious

Valencia orange juice beverage with calcium and vitamin D, 8 fl oz	3

Florida's Natural Growers' Pride

Orange juice, country style with juicy bits of orange, 8 fl oz	7

Florida's Natural Premium

100% juice, orange, with pulp, 8 fl oz	6

Gatorade G Series Pro

Thirst quencher, 02 perform, lemon-lime, 12 fl oz	5

Gatorade G2

Thirst quencher, 02 perform, mixed berry, 1 bottle (355 ml)	2

Glaceau Vitaminwater Zero

Revive fruit punch, 1 bottle (591 g)	0

Good Belly

Probiotic juice drink, plus multi-vitamins, blueberry acai flavor, 1 bottle (80 ml)	3

Good Belly Plus

Probiotic juice drink, plus multi-vitamins, pomegranate blackberry flavor, 1 bottle (80 ml)	3

Good Belly Straight Shot

Probiotic drink, plain flavor, value pack, 1 bottle (80 ml)	1

Great Value

100% juice, apple, no sugar added, 8 fl oz	7
Juice cocktail, light apple, 8 oz	4

Green Mountain Naturals

Hot apple cider, 1 k-cup	4
Hot apple cider k-cups, 1 k-cup	4

Hawaiian Punch

Juice drink, fruit juicy red, 8 fl oz	4

Hawaiian Punch Singles to Go!

Drink mix, sugar free, fruit juicy red, ½ packet (1 g)	0
Drink mix, sugar free, wild purple smash, ½ packet (1 g)	0

Herbalife

Beverage mix, peach mango, 2 scoops (19.5 g)	1
Beverage mix, wild berry, 2 scoops (20 g)	1

Hi C Blast

Flavored fruit drink, orange, 8 oz	8

HomeMaker

Orange juice, 100% Florida, original, 8 fl oz	6

Beverages

SmartPoints™ value

Honest Kids

Juice drink, organic, super fruit punch, 1 pouch (200 ml)	2

Izze Esque

Juice beverage, sparkling black raspberry flavored, 1 bottle (355 g)	4

Kevita

Daily cleanse lemon cayenne drink sparkling probiotic drink, 8 fl oz	0
Probiotic drink, sparkling, lemon ginger, ½ bottle (240 ml)	2

Kool Aid

Drink mix, sugar sweetened, cherry, 1 serving (19 g)	4

Kroger

Apple juice, 8 fl oz	7
Lite orange juice, 8 fl oz	2
Orange juice, calcium, 8 fl oz	5
Orange juice, homestyle, 8 fl oz	5
Orange juice, original, 8 fl oz	5

Lakewood Organic

100% juice blend, tart cherry, 8 fl oz	6

Mamma Chia

Blackberry hibiscus chia vitality beverage, 1 bottle (296 ml)	5

Martinelli's

Sparkling cider, 8 fl oz	8

Martinelli's Gold Medal

Sparkling cider, 8 oz	8

Meijer

Orange juice, original, light, 8 fl oz	3

Metamucil

Orange flavor multi-health fiber, 1 rounded Tbsp	2

Minute Maid

100% apple juice, 1 box (177 ml)	5
100% juice, orange, calcium & vitamin D, pure squeezed, no pulp, 8 fl oz	6
100% juice, orange, original, 8 fl oz	6

SmartPoints™ value

100% juice, pulp free, orange, 8 fl oz	3
100% orange juice, 8 fl oz	6
Juice beverage, cranberry apple raspberry, 8 fl oz	7
Juice beverage, cranberry grape, 8 fl oz	9
Juice beverage, light, pure squeezed, orange, 8 fl oz	3
Juice, orange, 1 bottle (295 ml)	8
Orange juice, 1 bottle (295 ml)	8
Orange juice, original, calcium & vitamin D, 8 fl oz	6
Orange juice, original, low pulp, calcium & vitamin D, 8 oz	6
Orange juice, pure squeezed, no pulp, 8 fl oz	6
Orange juice, pure squeezed, some pulp, 8 fl oz	6

Minute Maid Just 15 Calories

Fruit punch, 8 fl oz	1

Minute Maid Light

Fruit drink, light mango passion, 8 fl oz	1
Orange juice beverage, light, pure squeezed, no pulp, 8 fl oz	3

Minute Maid Light 15 Calories

Peach fruit drink with tea, 8 fl oz	1

Minute Maid Low Acid

Premium 100% orange juice, 8 fl oz	6

Minute Maid Premium

Fruit punch, 8 fl oz	7
Orange juice, pulp free, 8 fl oz	6

Minute Maid Premium Light

Orange juice beverage, low pulp, 8 fl oz	3

Mio

Liquid water enhancer, orange tangerine, ½ tsp	0

Monster

Energy juice, khaos, 8 fl oz	4

Mott's

100% apple juice, 8 fl oz	7
100% apple juice, original, 8 fl oz	7
100% juice, apple, 1 bottle (473 ml)	7

Mott's For Tots

Fruit juice plus purified water, apple, 8 fl oz	4

Mott's Plus

Juice beverage, apple, light, 8 oz	4

Mountain Dew Kick Start

Sparkling juice beverage, energizing, black cherry, 1 can (473 ml)	5
Sparkling juice beverage, energizing, pineapple orange mango, 1 can (355 ml)	4
Sparkling juice beverage, energizing, strawberry kiwi, 1 can (355 ml)	4

Naked

100% juice, kale blazer, 8 fl oz	5
100% juice, o-j, 8 fl oz	6

Naked Juice

Mighty mango, 1 (296 ml)	10

Naked Super Food

Food-juice, green machine, 8 fl oz	7

Northland

100% juice, cranberry pomegranate, 8 fl oz	8

Ocean Spray

100% cranberry juice, 8 fl oz	7
100% cranberry juice no sugar added, 8 fl oz	7
100% juice, apple, 8 fl oz	6
100% juice, cranberry, 1 cup	7
100% juice, cranberry & raspberry, 1 cup	8
100% juice, no sugar added, cranberry concord grape flavor, 8 fl oz	8
100% juice, no sugar added, cranberry pomegranate flavor, 8 fl oz	7
100% juice, no sugar added, ruby red grapefruit, 8 fl oz	6
100% juice, no sugar added, white grapefruit, 8 fl oz	5
100% juice, orange, 8 fl oz	6
100% juice, pink grapefruit, 8 oz	6
Cranberry juice cocktail, light, from concentrate, 8 fl oz	2
Cran-grape juice drink, 8 fl oz	7
Juice beverage, diet, cranberry, 1 cup	0
Juice beverage, diet, cranberry grape, 8 fl oz	2
Juice beverage, diet, cranberry pomegranate, 8 fl oz	0
Juice cocktail, cranberry, 1 bottle (295 ml)	8
Juice drink, cran-apple, 1 cup	8
Juice drink, cranberry pomegranate, 1 cup	7
Juice drink, cranberry, light, 8 fl oz	3
Juice drink, cran-cherry, 1 cup	7
Juice drink, cran-mango, 8 fl oz	7
Juice drink, cran-raspberry, 8 fl oz	7
Juice drink, diet cranberry with a hint of lime, 1 cup	0
Juice drink, diet, cran-mango, 8 fl oz	0
Juice drink, grapefruit, ruby red, 1 cup	7
Juice drink, light, cran-pomegranate, 8 fl oz	2
Juice drink, white cran-strawberry, 8 fl oz	7
Light cranberry juice cocktail, 8 fl oz	2

Ocean Spray Diet

Juice beverage, blueberry, 1 cup	0
Juice beverage, blueberry pomegranate, 1 cup	0

Beverages

SmartPoints™ value

	SmartPoints™ value
Juice beverage, cranberry grape spray, 12 fl oz	1
Juice beverage, sparkling cranberry, 1 can (248 ml)	1
Ocean Spray Light	
Cranberry and concord grape juice drink, 1 cup	3
Juice drink, cranberry, 1 cup	3
Juice drink, cran-raspberry (64 oz container, "light"), 8 fl oz	2
Juice drink, ruby red, 1 cup	2
Juice, cran-raspberry, 8 oz	2
Odwalla Superfood	
Fruit juice drink, micronutrient, 8 oz	7
Old Orchard	
Juice cocktail blend, cranberry, 8 oz	2
Juice cocktail, apple, 8 fl oz	1
Old Orchard Healthy Balance	
Juice cocktail, grape, 8 fl oz	2
Pom Wonderful	
Juice, pomegranate juice, 8 fl oz	8
R.W. Knudsen	
Juice, just cranberry, 8 fl oz	3
Juice, organic, just tart cherry, 8 fl oz	7
Sambazon	
Juice blend, organic, acai, original blend, 8 fl oz	8
San Pellegrino	
Sparkling beverage, blood orange, 1 can (330 ml)	8
Sparkling beverage, grapefruit, 1 can (330 ml)	9
Simply All Natural	
Mixed berry juice drink, 8 fl oz	6
Tropical juice drink, 8 fl oz	6
Simply Apple	
Apple juice, pure pressed, 8 fl oz	7

	SmartPoints™ value
Simply Cranberry	
Cranberry juice cocktail, 1 bottle (340 ml)	12
Simply Grapefruit	
Grapefruit juice, pulp free, original, 8 fl oz	5
Simply Orange	
100% high pulp orange juice, 8 fl oz	6
Juice blend, 100%, with mango, 8 oz	6
Juice blend, 100%, with pineapple, 8 fl oz	6
Juice blend, with banana, pulp free, 8 fl oz	6
Juice blend, with tangerine, pulp free, 8 fl oz	6
Orange juice pulp free calcium and vitamin D, 1 bottle (400 ml)	10
Orange juice, country stand, calcium, medium pulp, 8 fl oz	6
Orange juice, high pulp, 8 fl oz	6
Simply Orange Calcium & Vitamin D Pulp Free	
100% orange juice, 1 bottle (340 ml)	9
Simply Orange Pulp Free	
100% orange juice, 1 bottle (340 ml)	9
100% orange juice blend with mango, 1 bottle (340 ml)	9
Snapple	
Diet juice drink, low calorie, cranberry raspberry, diet, 1 cup	1
Soda Stream	
Drink mix, sparkling, crystal light, fruit punch, 1 capful (10 ml)	0
Starbucks Via Ready Brew Refreshers	
Instant beverage, very berry hibiscus, ½ packet (10 g)	2

Beverages

Sunny D

Orange flavored citrus punch, 1 bottle (199 ml)	6
With calcium, smooth California style, 8 fl oz	8

Sunsweet

Juice, prune, 8 fl oz	8
Prune juice cocktail, light, 8 fl oz	4
Prune juice, with pulp, 8 fl oz	7

Sunsweet PlumSmart

Juice cocktail, plum, light, 8 fl oz	3

Tampico

Punch, citrus, 8 fl oz	7

Trader Joe's

100% pure Florida orange juice with extra pulp, 8 fl oz	6
Fresh squeezed orange juice, 1 cup	6
Green cold pressed juice, 1 bottle (450 ml)	4
Organic orange juice, 8 fl oz	6

Tree Top

100% juice, apple, 8 fl oz	7

Tropicana

100% juice, apple, 10 fl oz	8
100% juice, orange, 10 fl oz	7
100% juice, orange, with calcium, 8 fl oz	6
100% pure orange juice, antioxidant advantage, no pulp, 8 fl oz	6
Juice, orange, no pulp, original, 8 fl oz	6
Juice, ruby red grapefruit, 8 fl oz	5
No pulp orange juice with calcium and vitamin D, 8 fl oz	6
Orange juice, low acid, 8 fl oz	6
Original no pulp pure premium orange juice, 8 fl oz	6

Tropicana Essentials

Orange juice, fiber, some pulp, 8 fl oz	6
Orange juice, no pulp, 8 fl oz	6

Tropicana Farmstand

100% juice, fruit & vegetable, pomegranate blueberry, 8 fl oz	7

Tropicana Light 'n Healthy

Orange juice, with pulp, 8 fl oz	3

Tropicana Pure Premium

100% juice, orange, homestyle, some pulp, 8 fl oz	6
100% juice, orange, no pulp, 12 fl oz	9
100% juice, orange, no pulp calcium + vitamin D, grab and go, 8 fl oz	6
100% juice, orange, no pulp original, 8 fl oz	6
100% juice, orange, no pulp, calcium + vitamin D, 8 fl oz	6
100% juice, orange, premium, no pulp, calcium + vitamin D, 8 fl oz	6
100% juice, orange, some pulp, 8 fl oz	6
100% juice, orange, some pulp homestyle, 8 fl oz	6
Juice, calcium + vitamin D, orange, lots of pulp, 8 fl oz	6
Juice, orange, lots of pulp, 8 fl oz	6
Light orange juice beverage, calcium, light 'n healthy, 8 oz	3
Orange juice, 100% pure Florida, no pulp, 14 fl oz	10
Orange juice, 100%, no pulp, calcium & vitamin D, 8 fl oz	6
Orange juice, grovestand, lots of pulp, 8 fl oz	6

Tropicana Trop50

Juice beverage blend, pomegranate blueberry, 8 fl oz	3
Juice beverage blend, red orange, 8 fl oz	3
Juice beverage, orange with vitamins, calcium + vitamin D, 8 fl oz	3
Juice beverage, orange with vitamins, no pulp, 8 fl oz	3

Beverages

Beverages

	SmartPoints™ value
Juice beverage, orange with vitamins, some pulp, 8 fl oz	3
Juice beverage, orange, no pulp, 8 fl oz	3
Juice beverage, orange, no pulp calcium + vitamin D, 12 fl oz	4
Juice beverage, orange, some pulp, 8 fl oz	3
Juice beverage, raspberry acai, 8 fl oz	3
Orange juice, calcium + vitamin D, no pulp, 8 fl oz	3
V8 Original	
Vegetable juice with a hint of lime, 8 fl oz	2
V8 Splash	
Diet juice beverage, berry blend, 8 oz	1
Diet juice beverage, tropical blend, 8 oz	1
Flavored beverage, fruit medley, 8 oz	5
V8 V-Fusion	
100% juice, vegetable & fruit, strawberry banana, 8 fl oz	6
V8 V-Fusion + Energy Diet	
Cranberry raspberry flavored juice beverage, 8 fl oz	1
V8 V-Fusion 100% Juice	
Black cherry apple vegetable and fruit juice, 8 fl oz	6
Welch's	
100% grape juice, 8 fl oz	9
Concord grape juice, light, 8 fl oz	2
Grape juice, 8 fl oz	10
White grape juice, 8 fl oz	9
Welch's Light	
Juice beverage, concord grape, 8 fl oz	3
Welch's Sparkling	
Juice cocktail, red grape, 8 fl oz	9
Juice cocktail, white grape, 8 fl oz	9

Lemonade & Limeade

	SmartPoints™ value
Country Time	
Lemonade, 8 fl oz	6
Crystal Light	
Beverage, lemonade, 8 fl oz	0
Drink mix, natural lemonade, ½ packet (2 g)	0
Drink mix, natural pink lemonade flavor, ½ packet (2 g)	0
Crystal Light Liquid	
Blackberry lemonade flavored drink mix, ½ tsp	0
Strawberry lemonade flavored drink mix, ½ tsp	0
Crystal Light On The Go	
Drink mix, natural lemonade, ½ packet (2 g)	0
Drink mix, natural pink lemonade, ½ packet (2 g)	0
Drink mix, raspberry lemonade, ½ packet (1 g)	0
Mike's	
premium, hard black cherry lemonade, 1 bottle (331 ml)	11
premium, hard cranberry lemonade, 1 bottle (331 ml)	11
premium, hard lemonade, 1 bottle (331 ml)	11
premium, hard strawberry lemonade, 1 bottle (331 ml)	11
premium, lite, hard lemonade, 1 bottle (331 ml)	5
Mike's Lite	
Black cherry hard lemonade, 11 fl oz	5
Hard lemonade, 11 ¼ fl oz	4
Minute Maid	
Lemonade, 1 can (355 ml)	9
Pink lemonade, 8 fl oz	6
Minute Maid Just 15 Calories	
Lemonade, 8 fl oz	1
Minute Maid Light	
Lemonade, 1 can (355 ml)	0

Mountain Dew Kick Start

Sparkling juice beverage, energizing, limeade, 1 can (473 ml)	5

Ocean Spray

Juice, cran-lemonade, 1 cup	7

Ocean Spray Diet

Juice, cran-lemonade, 1 cup	0

Simply Lemonade

Lemonade, 1 bottle (340 ml)	10
Lemonade with raspberry, 1 bottle (340 ml)	9
Lemonade, with blueberry, 8 fl oz	6

Simply Limeade

Limeade, 8 fl oz	7

Sparkling Ice

Lemonade, raspberry, 8 fl oz	0
Lemonade, strawberry, 8 fl oz	0

Starbucks Via Ready Brew Refreshers

Instant beverage, strawberry lemonade, ½ packet (10 g)	2

True Lemon

Drink mix, lemonade, raspberry, 1 packet (3 g)	0

Smoothies

Bolthouse Farms

100% fruit juice smoothie multi-v goodness, 1 cup	7
100% fruit smoothie + boosts, amazing mango, 8 fl oz	9
100% fruit smoothie + boosts, strawberry banana, 8 fl oz	7
Berry boost fruit smoothie, 8 fl oz	6
Breakfast smoothie, peach parfait, 8 fl oz	8
Fruit smoothie, amazing mango, 8 fl oz	9
Fruit smoothie, blue goodness, 8 fl oz	8
Fruit smoothie, c-boost, 8 fl oz	8

Green goodness fruit smoothie, 8 fl oz	8
Multi-v goodness 100% fruit juice smoothie, 8 fl oz	7
Strawberry banana fruit smoothie, 8 fl oz	7

Concord Foods

Banana smoothie mix, 1 ½ Tbsp	4
Smoothie mix, chocolate banana, 1 ½ Tbsp	1
Smoothie mix, strawberry, 1 Tbsp	4

Danimals

Banana split flavored smoothie, 1 bottle (93 ml)	3
Strawberry explosion flavored smoothie, 1 bottle (93 ml)	3

Dole

Peach mango fruit smoothie, 4 oz	5

Dole Shakers

Smoothie, fruit, mixed berry, 4 oz	4
Smoothie, fruit, strawberry, 4 oz	4
Smoothie, fruit, strawberry banana, 4 oz	4
Yellow power fruit and veggie smoothie mix, 1 container (106 g)	3

Evolution Fresh

Smoothie, fruit and juice blend, 8 oz	7
Smoothie, fruit puree and juice blend, super green, 8 fl oz	7

Jamba

Smoothies, fruit & veggie, green fusion, ½ pouch (113 g)	3

Kellogg's Special K

Red berries breakfast shake, 1 bottle (296 ml)	7

Lifeway

Blueberry lowfat kefir cultured milk smoothie, 1 cup	6
Kefir cultured milk smoothie, lowfat, blueberry, 1 cup	6
Kefir cultured milk smoothie, lowfat, madagascar vanilla, 1 cup	6

Beverages

Beverages

	SmartPoints™ value
Kefir cultured milk smoothie, lowfat, mango, 1 cup	6
Kefir cultured milk smoothie, lowfat, peach, 1 cup	6
Kefir cultured milk smoothie, lowfat, plain, 1 cup	4
Kefir cultured milk smoothie, lowfat, plain, unsweetened, 1 cup	4
Kefir cultured milk smoothie, lowfat, raspberry, 1 cup	6
Kefir cultured milk smoothie, lowfat, strawberry, 1 cup	6
Naked	
100% fruit & veg juice smoothie, berry veggie, 8 fl oz	6
100% fruit & veg juice smoothie, orange carrot, 8 fl oz	7
100% juice smoothie, berry blast, 8 fl oz	7
100% juice smoothie, boosted, blue machine, 8 fl oz	9
100% juice smoothie, boosted, green machine, 8 fl oz	7
100% juice smoothie, boosted, power-c machine, 8 fl oz	6
100% juice smoothie, boosted, red machine, 8 fl oz	8
100% juice smoothie, mighty mango, 8 fl oz	8
100% juice smoothie, strawberry banana, 10 fl oz	8
All natural juice smoothie, mighty mango, 8 fl oz	6
Green machine juice smoothie, 10 fl oz	9
Protein and greens protein juice smoothie no sugar added, 8 fl oz	8
Protein juice smoothie, protein zone double berry, 8 fl oz	9
Protein zone protein juice smoothie no sugar added, 8 fl oz	9
Naked No Sugar Added	
Banana chocolate protein juice smoothie, 8 fl oz	10

	SmartPoints™ value
Odwalla	
Fruit smoothie blend, mango tango, 8 oz	8
Strawberry banana juice smoothie blend, 1 bottle (450 ml)	12
Odwalla C Monster	
Fruit smoothie blend, vitamin C, strawberry c, 8 oz	8
Odwalla Super Protein	
Protein drink, soymilk, chocolate protein, 8 fl oz	7
Odwalla Superfood	
Premium original fruit smoothie blend, 8 fl oz	7
Sambazon	
Smoothie packs, the original, acai berry + guarana, 1 pack (100 g)	5
Smoothie packs, unsweetened, pure acai berry, 1 pack (100 g)	3
Six Star Pro Nutrition	
Mixed berry instant protein moothie, 1 scoop (34 g)	2
Suja Essentials	
Fruit & vegetable juice smoothie, organic, mighty greens, 1 bottle (354 ml)	5
Trader Joe's	
Very green 100% juice smoothie, 1 cup	7
Vega	
Choc-a-lot protein smoothie, 1 scoop (26 g)	2

Soft Drinks, Carbonated

	SmartPoints™ value
7Up	
Soda, 8 fl oz	6
Soda, cherry, 12 fl oz	9
Soda, diet, 8 fl oz	0
A&W Ten	
Root beer, 8 fl oz	0

Barq's

Root beer, 12 fl oz	10
Root beer, diet, 8 fl oz	0

Big Red

Soda, 1 bottle (591 ml)	15

Canada Dry

Ginger ale, 1 can (221 ml)	5
Ginger ale, caffeine free, 1 can (354 ml)	8
Ginger ale, cranberry, 8 fl oz	6
Ginger ale, diet, 1 can (355 ml)	0
Ginger ale, diet, cranberry, 1 cup	0
Soda, ginger ale, 1 can (355 ml)	1

Canada Dry Ten

Ginger ale, 12 fl oz	1

Cheerwine

Soft drink, legend, 1 bottle (355 ml)	10

Clear Choice Ice

Sparkling water beverage, flavored, black raspberry, 8 fl oz	0

Coca-Cola

Cola, 1 bottle (251 ml)	6
Cola, cherry, 8 fl oz	6
Cola, original formula, sixer, 1 can (355 ml)	9
Cola, vanilla, 8 fl oz	16

Coca-Cola Classic

Caffeine free cola, 1 can (355 ml)	9

Coca-Cola Life

Reduced calorie cola, 1 can (355 ml)	6

Crush

Diet orange soda, 1 can (355 ml)	0
Orange soda, 1 can (355 ml)	10
Soda, grape, 12 fl oz	10

Diet Rite Pure Zero

Cola, 8 fl oz	0

Fanta

Soda, grape, 8 oz	8
Soda, orange, 12 fl oz	10
Soda, strawberry, 8 fl oz	8

IBC

Root beer, 1 bottle (354 ml)	10

Izze

Juice beverage, sparkling apple, fortified, 1 can (248 ml)	5
Juice beverage, sparkling blackberry, 1 bottle (355 g)	7
Juice beverage, sparkling clementine, 8 fl oz	5
Juice beverage, sparkling grapefruit, 8 fl oz	5

Izze Fortified

Juice beverage, sparkling blackberry, 1 can (248 ml)	5
Juice beverage, sparkling clementine, 1 can (248 ml)	5

La Croix

Sparkling water, coconut flavored, 1 can (355 ml)	0

Live Soda

Soda, kombucha, revive rootbeer, 12 fl oz	4

Maid-Rite Beverages

Diet Mountain Dew, 1 serving (623.68 g)	0

Mello Yello Zero

Soda, citrus flavored, 1 can (355 ml)	0

Monster

Energy drink, lo-carb, 8 fl oz	1
Energy drink, lo-carb, monster mini's, 1 can (96 ml)	1
Lo-carb energy supplement, 8 fl oz	1

Mountain Dew Code Red

Soda, 8 fl oz	7
Soda, cherry flavor, 8 fl oz	7

Beverages

SmartPoints™ value

	SmartPoints™ value
Mountain Dew Distortion	
Soda, lime blasted dew, 1 can (355 ml)	11
Mr. Pibb	
Cola, 8 fl oz	6
Mug	
Root beer, 8 oz	7
Pepsi Max	
Cola, zero calorie, 8 fl oz	0
Pepsi Next	
Cola, 60 calories per can, 1 can (355 ml)	4
Pibb Xtra	
Cola, 8 fl oz	6
San Pellegrino	
Aranciata rossa blood orange sparkling beverage, 1 can (330 ml)	8
Sparkling beverage, lemon, limonata, 1 bottle (200 ml)	5
Sparkling lemon beverage, limonata, 1 can (55 ml)	8
Seagram's	
Ginger ale, 12 fl oz	6
Sierra Mist	
Diet lemon lime soda, 1 can (355 ml)	0
Lemon lime soda caffeine free, 1 can (355 ml)	7
Soda, diet, cranberry splash, 1 can (355 ml)	0
Sierra Mist Natural	
Soda, lemon-lime, 8 fl oz	6
Sparkling Ice	
Sparkling water, crisp apple, 8 fl oz	0
Sparkling water, peach nectarine, 8 fl oz	0
Talking Rain Sparkling Ice	
Cherry limeade sparkling beverage, 8 fl oz	0
Strawberry watermelon sparkling beverage, 8 fl oz	0

	SmartPoints™ value
Vernor's	
Ginger soda, 8 oz	6
Ginger soda, diet, 12 fl oz	0

Soy, Rice, Hemp, Almond & Chai Drinks

Almond Breeze	
Almond milk, unsweetened original, 1 cup	1
Almond Breeze Unsweetened	
Vanilla almond coconut blend, 1 cup	2
Friendly Farms Original	
All natural almond milk, 8 fl oz	3
Silk	
Unsweetened original almondmilk, 1 cup	1
Simple Truth	
Vanilla almond milk, 1 cup	3
Whole Foods 365 Everyday Value	
Organic unsweetened almond milk, 8 fl oz	1
8th Continent	
Soymilk, original, 1 cup	2
Almond Breeze	
Hint of honey almondmilk, 1 cup	2
Hint of honey vanilla almondmilk, 1 cup	3
Vanilla almondmilk, 1 bottle (295 ml)	5
Almond Breeze Reduced Sugar	
Original almondmilk, 1 cup	1
Vanilla almondmilk, 1 cup	3
Almond Breeze Unsweetened	
Almond coconut milk blend, 1 cup	2
Chocolate almondmilk, 1 cup	1
Vanilla almond coconut milk blend, 1 cup	2
Vanilla almondmilk, 1 cup	1

Archer Farms Savor Everyday	
Chai latte tea drink mix k cup, 1 (14 g)	3
Big Train	
Spiced chai, 3 Tbsp	7
Vanilla chai, 3 Tbsp	7
Bigelow	
Chai tea, spiced, decaffeinated, 8 fl oz	0
BluePrint	
Cashew milk, non-dairy, cashew vanilla cinnamon agave, 1 bottle (473 ml)	11
Bolthouse Farms Perfectly Protein	
Chai tea, vanilla, 8 fl oz	7
Bolthouse Farms Protein Plus	
Chocolate protein shake, 8 fl oz	9
Vanilla protein shake, 8 fl oz	8
Breeze	
Vanilla almond coconut blend, 1 cup	3
Cafe Escapes	
Chai latte k-cup packs, 1 k-cup	3
Vue cups, coffee, chai latte, 1 vue cup (14 g)	4
Califia Farms Pure	
Almondmilk, creamy original, 8 fl oz	2
Almondmilk, unsweetened, 8 fl oz	1
Almondmilk, vanilla, 8 fl oz	2
Calnaturale Svelte	
Protein shake, organic, cappuccino, 11 fl oz	5
Protein shake, organic, French vanilla, 11 fl oz	5
Celestial Seasonings	
Chai tea, india spice, 1 tea bag	0
Celestial Seasonings Tea House Chai	
Chai tea, honey vanilla white tea, 1 tea bag	0
Coffee-Mate	
Coffee creamer, soy, French vanilla, 1 Tbsp	2

Friendly Farms	
Chocolate flavored almond milk, 8 fl oz	6
Full Circle	
Almond milk, rich & creamy, vanilla, 1 cup	4
Giant/Stop & Shop	
Unsweetened vanilla almond milk, 1 cup	1
Good Karma	
Flax milk, unsweetened, original, 1 cup	1
Flax milk, unsweetened, vanilla, 8 fl oz	1
Great Value	
Original soymilk, 1 cup	3
Original unsweetened almondmilk, 1 cup	1
Soymilk, organic, vanilla, 1 cup	3
Vanilla flavored almondmilk, 1 cup	4
Grove Square	
Chai latte k-cup, 1 single serve cup (15 g)	4
H-E-B	
Almond milk, vanilla, 1 cup	4
Hills Bros.	
Drink mix, cappuccino, sugar free, double mocha, 2 Tbsp	2
International Delight Chai Tea	
Vanilla chai latte, 1 cup	7
Kirkland Signature	
Organic vanilla soy milk, 1 cup	3
Organic vanilla soymilk, 1 fl oz	0
Lipton	
Tea, delight, chai, k-cup packs, 1 k-cup	2
Lucerne Farms	
Unsweetened original almond milk, 1 cup	1
Unsweetened vanilla almond milk, 1 cup	1

Beverages

SmartPoints™ value

Nutiva

Hemp protein, hi-fiber, bulk pack, 3 Tbsp	1

O Organics

Almond milk, original, 8 fl oz	3
Almond milk, vanilla, 8 fl oz	5
Rice milk, whole grain, organic, plain, 1 cup	4
Soy beverage, vanilla, 1 cup	3
Soymilk, light, organic, vanilla, 1 cup	3

Oregon Chai The Original

Chai tea latte mix, 1 packet (30 g)	7

Pacific Chai

Chai latte, spice, 2 Tbsp	5
Chai latte, vanilla, 2 Tbsp	5

Pacific Natural Foods

Non-dairy beverage, all natural, hemp milk, original, 1 cup	6

Pacific Natural Foods - Organic

Non-dairy beverage, almond, low fat, original, 1 cup	2

Pacific Natural Foods - Organic Almond

Non-dairy beverage, almond, original, unsweetened, 1 cup	1
Non-dairy beverage, almond, vanilla, unsweetened, 1 cup	1

Rice Dream

Rice drink, original, 1 cup	5

Rice Dream Heartwise

Rice drink, original, 1 cup	5

ShopRite

Rice milk, organic, original, 1 cup	5

Silk

Almond coconut blend beverage, 8 fl oz	2
Almond coconut blend, unsweetened, 1 cup	1
Almondmilk, protein plus fiber, original, 1 cup	3

SmartPoints™ value

Almondmilk, protein plus fiber, vanilla, 1 cup	4
Cashewmilk, original, 1 cup	3
Cashewmilk, unsweetened, no sugar added, 1 cup	1
Chocolate light soymilk, 1 cup	4
Dark chocolate almondmilk, 1 cup	5
Light vanilla soymilk, 1 cup	2
Original almond milk, 1 cup	3
Original soymilk, 1 cup	3
Soymilk, chocolate, 1 cup	6
Soymilk, light, original, 1 cup	2
Soymilk, plain, dha omega-3, 1 cup	4
Soymilk, unsweetened, 1 cup	2
Soymilk, very vanilla, 1 container (240 ml)	5
Unsweetened organic soymilk, 1 cup	2
Vanilla almondmilk, 1 cup	5
Vanilla soymilk, 1 cup	4

Silk Organic

Soymilk, organic, vanilla, 1 cup	4

Silk Pure Almond

Almondmilk, dark chocolate, 1 container (236 ml)	6
Almondmilk, original, unsweetened, 1 cup	1
Almondmilk, vanilla, 1 container (236 ml)	4
Almondmilk, vanilla, unsweetened, 1 cup	1
Light original almond milk, 1 cup	2
Light, vanilla almond milk, 1 cup	3
Original almondmilk, 1 cup	3

Simple Truth

Almond milk, 1 cup	3
Chocolate almond milk, 1 cup	3
Unsweetened almond milk, 1 cup	1

Simple Truth Organic

Soy milk, vanilla, 8 fl oz	4

So Delicious

Cashew milk, unsweetened, 1 cup	1

So Delicious Almond Plus

Almondmilk, dairy free, original, 1 cup	3
Almondmilk, dairy free, unsweetened, 1 cup	1
Almondmilk, dairy free, vanilla, 1 cup	3

Soy Dream

Soy milk, enriched, vanilla, 8 fl oz	4

Soy Slender

Soymilk, chocolate, 1 cup	2
Soymilk, vanilla, 1 cup	2

Stash

Chai spice black tea, 1 tea bag	0

Tassimo Twinings of London

Coffee, latte, chai tea, 1 disc (6 g)	4

Tazo

Black tea latte concentrate, spiced, organic chai, 4 fl oz	4
Black tea, chai, decaf, filterbags, 1 cup	0
Black tea, organic, chai, filterbags, 1 cup	0
Chai, ½ cup	4
Chai latte black tea concentrate, ½ cup	4
Decaf chai, 4 oz	4
Pumpkin spice chai latte, ½ cup	5
Vanilla caramel latte chai black tea concentrate, ½ cup	4

Trader Joe's

Low fat, vanilla soy milk, 1 cup	4
Original almond milk, 1 cup	3
Salted caramel chai tea latte mix, 1 scoop (40 g)	7
Spicy chai latte, 3 Tbsp	7

Trader Joe's Organic

Unsweetened soy milk, 1 cup	2

Twinings of London

Chai latte k-cup packs, 1 k-cup	3
Chai tea, 8 fl oz	0

Wegman's Food You Feel Good About

Almondmilk, organic, original, unsweetened, 1 cup	1
Almondmilk, organic, vanilla, 1 cup	4

West Soy

Soy milk, unsweetened, 1 cup	2
Soymilk, organic, unsweetened, 1 cup	2
Soymilk, unsweetened, vanilla, 1 cup	2

Whole Foods 365 Everyday Value

Unsweetened soy milk, 8 fl oz	2

Whole Foods 365 Organic

Vanilla almond milk, 8 fl oz	5

Sports & Energy Drinks

5-Hour Energy

Extra strength energy shot, 1 bottle (57 ml)	0

ABB Pure Pro

Protein shake, chocolate, 1 bottle (354 ml)	2

AMP

Energy drink, boost cherry, 8 fl oz	4

Atkins Day Break

Shake, creamy chocolate, 11 fl oz	4

Bai 5 Antioxidant Infusions

Congo pear beverage, 8 fl oz	0

Bai5 Bubbles Sparkling Antioxidant Infusions

Bolivia black cherry, 1 can (340 ml)	0
Peru pineapple, 1 can (340 ml)	0

Bing Bing

Energizing beverage, energy, 1 can (355 ml)	2

Beverages

Beverages

	SmartPoints™ value
Bolthouse Farms Protein Plus	
Blended coffee protein shake, 8 fl oz	8
Protein shake, blended coffee, 8 fl oz	8
Protein shake, mango, 8 fl oz	7
Protein shake, vanilla, 8 fl oz	8
Calnaturale Svelte	
Organic chocolate protein shake, 11 fl oz	6
Designer	
Protein shake, chocolate, 1 bottle (311 ml)	2
EAS AdvantEdge Carb Control	
Chocolate fudge shake, 11 fl oz	2
French vanilla shake, 11 fl oz	2
Rich dark chocolate shake, 11 fl oz	2
EAS Myoplex Lite	
French vanilla protein shakes, 1 shake (330 ml)	4
EAS Myoplex Original	
Protein shakes, chocolate fudge, 17 fl oz	6
Ensure	
Shake, high protein, creamy milk chocolate, 1 bottle (414 ml)	5
Shake, high protein, homemade vanilla, 1 bottle (414 ml)	5
Gatorade	
Strawberry lemonade thirst quencher beverage, 12 fl oz	5
Gatorade Fierce	
Blue cherry thirst quencher, 12 fl oz	5
Gatorade G Series	
02 perform lemon lime thirst quencher, 12 fl oz	5
02 perform tropical cooler thirst quencher, 12 fl oz	5
Blue cherry fierce thirst quencher 02 perform, 1 bottle (591 ml)	8
Frost glacier cherry thirst quencher beverage, 1 bottle (355 ml)	5

	SmartPoints™ value
Frost glacier freeze perform thirst quencher, 8 fl oz (355 ml)	5
Fruit punch flavor thirst quencher, 1 bottle (355 ml)	5
Fruit punch thirst quencher, 12 fl oz	5
Glacier cherry gatorade frost thirst quencher, 1 bottle (355 ml)	5
Orange thirst quencher, 1 bottle (355 ml)	5
Thirst quencher, 02 perform, fierce grape, 12 fl oz	5
Thirst quencher, 02 perform, frost glacier freeze, 12 fl oz	5
Thirst quencher, 02 perform, frost riptide rush, 8 fl oz	3
Thirst quencher, 02 perform, frost, glacier cherry, 12 fl oz	5
Thirst quencher, 02 perform, lemon-lime, 8 fl oz	3
Gatorade G2	
02 perform tropical blend thirst quencher, 8 fl oz	1
Mixed berry low calorie 02 perform thirst quencher, 1 bottle (355 ml)	2
Thirst quencher, 02 perform, grape, 1 bottle (355 ml)	2
Thirst quencher, tropical punch, 1 bottle (355 ml)	2
Gatorade G2 Series	
Thirst quencher, 02 perform, glacier freeze, 1 serving (6 g)	1
Glaceau	
Vitamin water, squeezed lemonade, 1 bottle (591 g)	7
Glaceau Vitaminwater Zero	
Vitamin water, power-c, dragonfruit, 1 bottle (591 g)	0
GTs Enlightened	
Kombucha, organic raw, bilberry no. 9, 8 fl oz	1
Kombucha, organic raw, citrus, 8 fl oz	1

	SmartPoints™ value
Kombucha, organic raw, gingerade, 8 fl oz	1
Kombucha, organic raw, hibiscus no. 7, 8 fl oz	1
Kombucha, organic raw, multi-green, 8 fl oz	1
Kombucha, organic raw, original, 8 fl oz	1
GU	
Energy gel, strawberry banana, 1 package (32 g)	3
Joint Juice	
Glucosamine + chondroitin drink, cran pomegranate, 1 bottle (237 ml)	1
Kellogg's Special K Protein	
Shake, French vanilla, 1 bottle (296 ml)	7
Metamucil	
Multi-health fiber powder orange smooth, made with real sugar, 1 Tbsp	2
Multi-health fiber powder orange smooth, sugar free, 1 Tbsp	1
Monster	
Beverage, rehab, tea + orangeade + energy, 8 oz	1
Energy drink, assault, 8 fl oz	6
Energy drink, energy, ultra sunrise, 8 fl oz	0
Energy drink, zero ultra, 8 fl oz	0
Rehab tea and pink lemonade energy drink, 8 fl oz	1
Ultra blue energy drink, 8 fl oz	0
Ultra red energy drink, 8 fl oz	0
Monster Energy	
Zero ultra beverage, 8 fl oz	0
Zero ultra drink, 8 fl oz	0
Monster Java	
Energy supplement, coffee + energy, loca moca, 8 fl oz	5
Energy supplement, coffee + energy, mean bean, 8 fl oz	5

	SmartPoints™ value
Monster Rehab	
Energy drink, green tea + energy, 8 oz	1
Energy drink, tea + lemonade + energy, 8 fl oz	1
Muscle Milk Genuine Light	
Nutritional shake, chocolate, 8 fl oz	2
Myoplex Lite	
Protein shake, chocolate fudge, 11 fl oz	4
Naturade Vegan Smart	
Nutritional shake, all-in-one, vanilla, 2 scoops (43 g)	4
Nos	
Energy drink, high performance, charged citrus, 1 can (473 ml)	13
Ocean Spray Cran Energy	
Energy juice drink, cranberry, raspberry, 1 cup	2
Powerade Ion4	
Fruit punch sport drink, 1 bottle (355 ml)	5
Mountain berry blast sports drink, 1 bottle (355 ml)	5
Sports drink, melon, 12 fl oz	5
Pure Protein	
Shake, rich chocolate, 1 bottle (325 ml)	2
Red Bull	
Energy drink, the red edition, 1 can (250 ml)	7
Energy drink, the silver edition, 1 can (250 ml)	7
Energy shot, sugar free, 1 bottle (59 ml)	0
The red edition cranberry energy drink, 1 can (355 ml)	9
Red Bull Total Zero	
The cherry edition energy drink, 1 can (355 ml)	0
The orange edition energy drink, 1 can (355 ml)	0

Beverages

Beverages

	SmartPoints™ value
Rockstar	
Perfect berry energy drink, 8 fl oz	0
Rockstar Freeze	
Pina colada energy drink, 8 fl oz	8
Rockstar Pure Zero	
Energy drink, zero calorie, punched, 8 fl oz	0
Energy drink, zero calorie, silver ice, 8 fl oz	0
Rockstar Recovery	
Energy/hydration, non-carbonated energy/tea/lemonade, 8 fl oz	0
Slim Fast 3-2-1 Plan	
Shakes, creamy milk chocolate, 1 bottle (295 ml)	8
Shakes, French vanilla, 1 bottle (295 ml)	7
Shakes, rich chocolate royale, 1 bottle (295 ml)	8
Shakes, vanilla cream, low carb diet, 1 bottle (325 ml)	4
SoBe Lifewater	
Hydration beverage, nutrient enhanced, acai raspberry, 8 fl oz	0
Hydration beverage, nutrient enhanced, blood orange mango, 8 fl oz	0
Starbucks	
Doubleshot, energy, white chocolate, 1 can (443 ml)	9
Starbucks Doubleshot	
Energy coffee drink, premium, vanilla light, 8 fl oz	3
Starbucks Refreshers	
Blueberry acai sparkling green coffee energy beverage, 1 can (355 ml)	5
Energy drink, sparkling green coffee, raspberry pomegranate, 1 can (355 ml)	3
Energy drink, sparkling green coffee, strawberry lemonade, 1 can (355 ml)	3

	SmartPoints™ value
Synergy	
Kombucha, organic & raw, gingerade, 8 fl oz	2
Synergy Enlightened	
Black chia kombucha, 8 fl oz	3
Cherry chia, 8 fl oz	3
Kambucha, guava goddess, 8 fl oz	2
Kambucha, mystic mango, 8 fl oz	3
Kambucha, strawberry serenity, 8 fl oz	2
Kombucha, grape chia, 8 fl oz	3
Kombucha, organic & raw, cosmic cranberry, 8 fl oz	1
Kombucha, organic & raw, trilogy, 8 fl oz	1
Kombucha, passionberry bliss, 8 fl oz	2
Kombucha, raspberry chia, 8 fl oz	2
V8	
Vanilla protein shakes, 1 bottle (296 ml)	8
V8 V-Fusion	
Energy beverage blend, orange pineapple, 8 fl oz	3
Energy drink, vegetable & fruit, peach mango flavored, 1 can (237 ml)	3
Energy drink, vegetable & fruit, pomegranate blueberry flavored, 1 can (237 ml)	3
V8 V-Fusion + Energy Diet	
Strawberry lemonade flavored juice beverage, 8 fl oz	1
Yakult	
Probiotic drink, light, nonfat, 1 bottle (80 ml)	1

Tea & Iced Tea

	SmartPoints™ value
Arizona	
Green tea, with ginseng and honey, 8 fl oz	4
Iced tea with lemon flavor, 8 fl oz	6
Iced tea, diet, lemon, 8 fl oz	0

Iced tea, diet, peach, 8 fl oz	0
Sweet tea, 8 fl oz	6
Barry's Tea	
Tea bags, Irish breakfast, 1 tea bag	0
Bigelow	
Green tea, bags, 8 fl oz	0
Green tea, chai, 8 fl oz	0
Green tea, jasmine green, bags, 8 fl oz	0
Green tea, naturally decaffeinated, bags, 8 fl oz	0
Green tea, pure green, 8 oz	0
Green tea, with lemon, naturally decaffeinated, bags, 8 fl oz	0
Green tea, with mint, 1 tea bag	0
Green tea, with pomegranate, 8 fl oz	0
Green tea, with pomegranate, bags, 8 fl oz	0
Herb tea, mint medley, 1 tea bag	0
Tea, English breakfast, 8 oz	0
Tea, French vanilla, decaffeinated, bags, 8 fl oz	0
Tea, herb plus probiotics, lemon ginger, tea bags, 1 tea bag	0
Tea, lemon lift, decaffeinated, bags, 8 fl oz	0
Tea, plantation mint, 8 fl oz	0
Brisk	
Iced tea, lemon flavor, 8 fl oz	5
Iced tea, raspberry flavor, 12 fl oz	4
Cafe Bustelo Cool	
Cafe con leche, 1 can (237 ml)	6
Carrington Tea	
Tea, peppermint, 1 bag	0
Celestial Seasonings	
Green tea, antioxidant, with white tea, 1 tea bag	0
Green tea, decaf, 1 tea bag	0
Green tea, decaf, with white tea, 1 tea bag	0

Green tea, honey lemon ginseng, with white tea, 1 tea bag	0
Herbal tea, caffeine free, 1 tea bag	0
Herbal tea, caffeine free, bengal spice, 1 tea bag	0
Herbal tea, caffeine free, cinnamon apple spice, 1 tea bag	0
Herbal tea, caffeine free, country peach passion, 1 tea bag	0
Herbal tea, caffeine free, honey vanilla chamomile, 1 tea bag	0
Herbal tea, caffeine free, lemon zinger, 1 tea bag	0
Herbal tea, caffeine free, sleepytime vanilla, 1 tea bag	0
Herbal tea, chamomile, 1 tea bag	0
Herbal tea, cinnamon apple spice, 1 tea bag	0
Herbal tea, fruit tea sampler, 1 tea bag	0
Herbal tea, lemon zinger, 1 tea bag	0
Herbal tea, mandarin orange spice, 1 tea bag	0
Herbal tea, peppermint, 1 tea bag	0
Herbal tea, raspberry zinger, 1 tea bag	0
Herbal tea, sleepytime, 1 tea bag	0
Herbal tea, wild berry zinger, 1 tea bag	0
Organic tea, green tea, 1 tea bag	0
Celestial Seasonings Keurig Brewed	
Sleepytime herbal tea k-cups, 1 k-cup	0
Celestial Seasonings Sleepytime	
Herbal tea, caffeine free, 1 tea bag	0
Crystal Light	
Beverage, iced tea, 8 oz	0
Drink mix, green tea, peach mango, unprepared, 1/8 packet (1 g)	0
Drink mix, green tea, raspberry, 1/2 packet (2 g)	0
Drink mix, iced tea, 1/8 packet (1 g)	0

Beverages

Beverages

	SmartPoints™ value
Drink mix, iced tea, natural lemon, ½ packet (1 g)	0
Drink mix, iced tea, raspberry, ⅛ packet (1 g)	0
Drink mix, peach iced tea, ½ packet (1 g)	0
Iced tea beverage, 8 fl oz	0
Soft drink, low calorie, peach tea, 8 oz	0
Tea mix, iced tea, raspberry, 8 fl oz	0
Crystal Light Metabolism	
Green tea beverage, peach mango, 8 fl oz	0
Crystal Light Pitcher Packs	
Sweet tea flavor drink mix, ⅛ packet (1 g)	0
Essensia	
Peppermint tea, 1 tea bag	0
Family	
Tea bags, oolong tea, 1 cup	0
Fuze	
Diet lemon iced tea, 12 fl oz	0
Iced tea, lemon, 12 fl oz	4
Lemon iced tea, 12 fl oz	4
Gold Peak	
Iced tea, diet, 8 fl oz	0
Iced tea, green, 8 fl oz	5
Iced tea, raspberry, 12 fl oz	8
Iced tea, sweet, 8 oz	5
Iced tea, sweet tea, 12 fl oz	8
Iced tea, unsweetened, 12 fl oz	0
Sweetened ice tea, 1 bottle (500 ml)	10
Good Earth	
Sweet & spicy tea & herb blend, 1 tea bag	0
Good Earth Sweet & Spicy	
Herbal tea blend, original, caffeine free, bags, 1 teabag	0
Tea & herb blend, original, bags, 1 tea bag	0

	SmartPoints™ value
Guayaki	
Yerba mate, organic, traditional tea bags, 1 bag	0
Honest Tea	
Green tea, honey green, 12 fl oz	3
Green tea, organic, honey, 8 fl oz	2
Half tea & half lemonade, organic, 8 fl oz	3
Tea, green, Moroccan mint, 8 fl oz	1
White tea, peach, 8 oz	2
Kirkland Signature	
Diet green tea with citrus, 8 fl oz	0
Kombucha Wonder	
Sparkling fermented tea, traditional kombucha, 7 oz	3
Lipton	
Black tea, black pearl, pyramid tea bags, 1 tea bag	0
Black tea, indulge, k-cup packs, 1 k-cup	0
Black tea, premium blend, 1 tea bag	0
Black tea, vanilla caramel truffle, pyramid tea bags, 1 tea bag	0
Citrus green tea, 1 bottle (591 ml)	8
Diet mixed berry green tea, 1 bottle (500 ml)	0
Green tea, 1 tea bag	0
Green tea with citrus, diet, 8 fl oz	0
Green tea, bags, 1 tea bag	0
Green tea, cranberry pomegranate, 1 tea bag	0
Green tea, decaffeinated, superfruit, blackberry and pomegranate, 1 tea bag	0
Green tea, diet, citrus, 8 fl oz	0
Green tea, honey lemon, 1 tea bag	0
Green tea, mint, tea bags, 1 tea bag	0
Green tea, mixed berry flavor, 1 tea bag	0

	SmartPoints™ value
Green tea, naturally decaffeinated, 1 tea bag	0
Green tea, orange, passionfruit & jasmine, 1 each (2 g)	0
Green tea, pure, 1 tea bag	0
Green tea, soothe, k-cup packs, 1 k-cup	0
Half & half, iced tea & lemonade, 8 fl oz	3
Half and half ice tea and lemonade, 1 bottle (500 ml)	6
Iced sweetened black tea k cups, 1 k-cup	3
Iced tea, lemon flavor, 8 fl oz	4
Iced tea, lemon, diet, 8 fl oz	0
Iced tea, sweet tea, 8 oz	5
Lemonade sparkling ice tea, 1 can (355 ml)	4
Peach flavor ice tea, 12 fl oz	4
Peach flavored iced tea, 1 bottle (591.4 ml)	7
Peach ice tea, 1 bottle (500 ml)	6
Peach sparkling ice tea, 1 can (355 ml)	4
Raspberry sparkling ice tea, 1 can (355 ml)	4
Sweet tea, iced, refresh, k-cup packs, 1 k-cup	3
Tea bags, 100% natural, 1 tea bag	0
Tea bags, decaffeinated, 1 tea bag	0
Tea bags, green tea, 1 tea bag	0
Tea beverage mix, milk tea, with milk & sugar, 1 packet (15 g)	3
Tea, 100% natural, iced tea brew, ¼ tea bag	0
Tea, bags, 1 tea bag	0
Tea, decaffeinated, bags, 1 tea bag	0
Tea, organic, green tea, 1 tea bag	0
White tea, with island mango & peach flavor, pyramid tea bags, 1 tea bag	0

	SmartPoints™ value
Lipton Brisk	
Ice tea, lemon, 1 each (288 ml)	8
Lemon ice tea, 1 can (355 ml)	8
Lipton PureLeaf	
Ice tea, diet, peach, 8 fl oz	0
Iced tea, unsweetened, 8 fl oz	0
Lipton Soothe	
Soothe green tea k cup, 1 k-cup pack	0
Lipton Superfruit	
Green tea, acai dragonfruit melon, bags, 1 tea bag	0
Green tea, purple acai and blueberry flavor, tea bags, 1 tea bag	0
Green tea, red goji and raspberry flavor, tea bags, 1 tea bag	0
Long Life	
Detox tea, 1 tea bag	0
Milo's	
Famous sweet tea, 8 fl oz	5
Tea, famous sweet, 8 fl oz	5
Mystic Chai	
Hot or cold spiced tea mix, 1 scoop (34 g)	6
Pure Leaf	
Tea, extra sweet, 8 fl oz	7
Tea, green tea, honey, 1 bottle (547 ml)	6
Tea, lemon, 8 fl oz	4
Tea, peach, 1 bottle (547 ml)	6
Tea, raspberry, 12 fl oz	7
Tea, real brewed, raspberry flavor, 8 fl oz	5
Tea, real brewed, unsweetened, 8 oz	0
Rishi	
Green tea, Japanese, matcha, 1 packet (2 g)	0
Salada	
100% green tea, traditional, 1 tea bag	0

Beverages

SmartPoints™ value

ShopRite Certified Organic

Tea bags, earl gray black, 1 tea bag	0

Snapple

All natural peach tea, 1 bottle (473 ml)	10
Diet iced tea, lemon, 1 can (340 ml)	0
Diet peach tea, 1 bottle (473 ml)	0
Green tea, diet, 8 oz	0
Green tea, diet, peach, 1 bottle (500 ml)	0
Half n half iced tea lemonade, 1 bottle (473 ml)	12
Iced tea, lemon, 8 fl oz	6
Lemon ice tea k-cup, 1 k-cup pack	2
Lemon tea, diet, 1 bottle (473 ml)	0
Lemonade iced tea, half & half, diet, 1 bottle (473 ml)	0
Peach iced tea k-cup packs, 1 k-cup pack	3
Tea, diet, raspberry, 1 cup	0
Tea, peach, 1 bottle (472 g)	10
Tropical tea, diet, bret's blend tea trop-a-rocka, 8 fl oz	0

Steaz Iced Teaz

Green tea, 100% natural, peach, 8 fl oz	2
Green tea, blueberry pomegranate acai, 8 fl oz	2

Sweet Leaf

Sweet tea, 8 fl oz	4

Teas' Tea

Green tea, jasmine, unsweetened, 8 fl oz	0
Green tea, pure, unsweetened, 8 fl oz	0

Teekanne

Tea, herbal wellness, relaxing, calming camomile, 1 tea bag	0

SmartPoints™ value

Tetley

Black tea, classic blend, 1 tea bag	0
Premium black tea, british blend, 1 bag	0
Tea bags, classic blend, naturally decaffeinated, black tea, 1 tea bag	0

Trader Joe's

Green tea, 1 tea bag	0
Original Irish breakfast tea, 1 tea bag	0
Peppermint tea, 1 tea bag	0

Tradewinds

Green tea, with honey, 8 fl oz	4
Sweet tea, 8 fl oz	5
Unsweet tea, 8 fl oz	0

Traditional Medicinals

Herbal tea, organic mother's milk, 1 cup	0
Herbal tea, organic, roasted dandelion root, caffeine free, 1 cup	0

Turkey Hill

Iced tea, diet, lemon flavored, 1 cup	0

Twinings of London

English breakfast tea, prepared, 6 fl oz	0
Green tea, 1 teabag	0

Yogi

Ginger tea bag, 1 teabag	0
Green tea kombucha, 1 cup	0

Vegetable Juices & Drinks

Biotta

Juice, beet, 8 fl oz	6

Bolthouse Farms

Daily greens 100% fruit & vegetable juice, 8 fl oz	5
Juice, 100% carrot, 8 fl oz	4

Campbell's

Juice, tomato, 1 can (163 ml)	1
Tomato juice, 8 fl oz	2
Tomato juice, low sodium, 8 fl oz	2

Beverages

Clamato

Tomato cocktail, 8 fl oz	3
Tomato cocktail, the original, 5 ½ fl oz	2

Naked

Kale blazer vegetable and fruit juice blend, 8 fl oz	5

Trader Joe's

100% juice carrot juice, 1 cup	4

V8

100% juice, vegetable & fruit, concord grape raspberry, 8 fl oz	8
100% juice, vegetable, high fiber, 8 fl oz	3
100% vegetable juice, low sodium, original, 5 ½ fl oz	1
100% vegetable juice, low sodium, spicy hot, 8 fl oz	2
Carrot mango veggie blend, 8 fl oz	3
Golden goodness veggie blend, 8 fl oz	3
Healthy greens veggie blend, 8 fl oz	3
Juice beverage, strawberry kiwi, 8 fl oz	4
Juice beverage, tropical blend, 8 fl oz	4
Original 100% vegetable juice, 8 fl oz	2
Purple power veggie blend, 8 fl oz	3
Spicy hot 100% vegetable juice, 8 fl oz	2
Vegetable juice, 8 fl oz	2

V8 Original

100% vegetable juice with a hint of black pepper, 8 fl oz	2

V8 Splash

Juice beverage, berry blend, 8 fl oz	4
Juice beverage, berry blend, diet, 8 fl oz	1

Juice beverage, mango peach, 8 fl oz	6
Juice beverage, tropical blend, diet, 8 fl oz	1

V8 V-Fusion

100% juice, vegetable & fruit, acai mixed berry, 8 fl oz	6
100% juice, vegetable & fruit, peach mango, 8 fl oz	7
100% juice, vegetable & fruit, pomegranate blueberry, 8 fl oz	6
100% vegetable & fruit juice, cranberry blackberry, 8 fl oz	6

V8 V-Fusion + Energy

Beverage blend, vegetable & fruit, peach mango, 1 can (237 ml)	3
Beverage blend, vegetable & fruit, pomegranate blueberry, 1 can (237 ml)	3

V8 V-Fusion Light

Acai mixed berry vegetable and fruit beverage blend, 8 fl oz	3
Beverage blend, vegetable & fruit, pomegranate blueberry, 8 fl oz	3
Peach mango beverage blend, 8 fl oz	3
Strawberry banana beverage blend, 8 fl oz	3

Wine & Wine Coolers

Arbor Mist

Merlot, blackberry, 8 fl oz	8
Moscato, mango strawberry, 8 fl oz	7
Moscato, pink, raspberry, 8 fl oz	7

Barefoot® Cellars

Cabernet sauvignon, 5 fl oz	4
Chardonnay, 5 fl oz	4
Merlot, 5 fl oz	4
Moscato, 5 fl oz	4
Pinot grigio, 5 fl oz	4
Pinot noir, 5 fl oz	4
Red wine, sweet, 5 fl oz	4
Sauvignon blanc, 5 fl oz	4

Beverages

Beverages

	SmartPoints™ value
Bella Sera	
Pinot grigio, 5 fl oz	4
Black Swan Wines	
Pinot grigio, 5 fl oz	4
Carlo Rossi	
Sangria, 6 fl oz	5
Castello del Poggio	
Moscato d'asti, 2010, 5 fl oz	6
Chateau Ste. Michelle	
Riesling 2010 columbia valley, 5 fl oz	4
Cupcake Vineyards	
Marlborough sauvignon blanc, 5 fl oz	3
Folie A Deux	
Sauvignon blanc, 5 fl oz	4
Franzia House Wine Favorites	
Sangria, fruity red, 5 fl oz	4
Franzia Vintner Select	
Chardonnay wine, 5 fl oz	4
Frontera	
Cabernet sauvignon merlot, chile, 2009, 5 fl oz	4
Gallo Family Vineyards	
Pinot grigio, 5 fl oz	4
Sauvignon blanc, 5 fl oz	4
White zinfandel, 5 fl oz	4
Kendall-Jackson Vintner's Reserve	
California chardonnay, winters reserve, 5 fl oz	4
Lost Vineyards	
Sangria, red wine, 8 fl oz	7
Main Street	
Cabernet sauvignon, 5 fl oz	4
Mark West	
Pinot noir 2011, 5 fl oz	4

	SmartPoints™ value
Menage a Trois	
2013 midnight dark red wine blend, 5 fl oz	4
Red wine, California, 2007, 5 fl oz	4
Montevina	
Moscato, 5 fl oz	4
White zinfandel, 5 fl oz	3
Redwood Creek Wine	
White zinfandel, 5 fl oz	4
Riunite	
Lambrusco, emilia, italia, 5 fl oz	4
Stella Rosa	
Sparkling wine, imperiale, 8 fl oz	9
Sutter Home	
Cabernet sauvignon, 5 fl oz	4
Chardonnay, 1 serving (147.85 ml)	4
Merlot, 5 fl oz	4
Moscato, 5 fl oz	4
Pinot grigio, 5 fl oz	4
White merlot, 5 fl oz	4
White zinfandel, 5 fl oz	3
White zinfandel, California, 5 fl oz	4
Trader Joe's Reserve	
Brut north coast sparkling wine, 5 ¼ oz	4
Woodbridge	
Cabernet sauvignon, California, 2001, 5 fl oz	4
Woodbridge Robert Mondavi	
2010 California chardonnay, 5 fl oz	3
Yellow Tail	
Moscato, vintage 2009, 5 fl oz	4
Shiraz wine, 6 fl oz	4

Wine, Sparkling

André	
Spumante, 4 fl oz	4

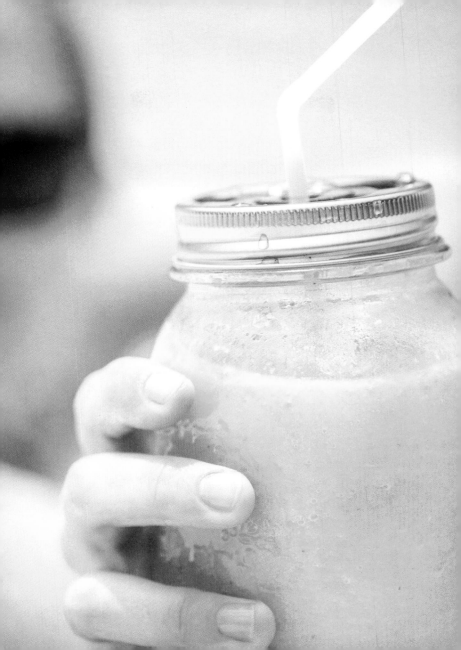

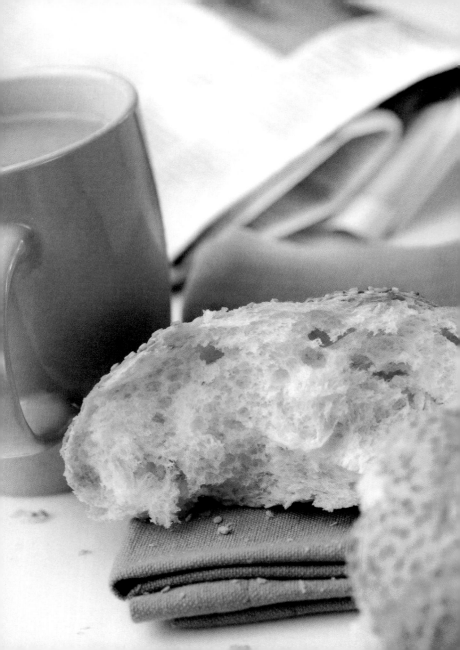

bread
& Baked Goods

Bagels

1st National Bagel

Bagels, plain, pre-sliced,
1 bagel (85 g)   6

Bagel House

Bagels, whole wheat, 1 bagel (83 g)   5

Daily Chef

Sliced mini plain bagel, 1 (57 g)   5

David's Deli

Everything bagel, 1 bagel (81 g)   6

French toast bagel, 1 bagel (81 g)   8

Franz

Bagels, premium, blueberry,
1 bagel (85 g)   7

Bagels, premium, cinnamon raisin,
1 bagel (85 g)   7

Bagels, premium, everything,
sliced, 1 bagel (85 g)   7

Bagels, premium, plain,
1 bagel (85 g)   6

Franz New York Bagel Boys

100% whole wheat sliced
premium bagels, 1 bagel (85 g)   6

Giant/Stop & Shop

Thin sliced everything bagels,
1 bagel (46 g)   3

Thin sliced whole wheat bagels,
1 bagel (46 g)   3

Kroger

Bagels, jumbo, whole wheat,
1 bagel (99 g)   7

Bagels, plain, 1 bagel (81 g)   6

Lender's

Bagels, blueberry, 1 bagel (81 g)   7

Bagels, New York style, plain,
1 bagel (93 g)   7

Bagels, onion, 1 bagel (104 g)   8

Bagels, plain, 1 bagel (26 g)   2

Bagels, pre-sliced, egg,
1 bagel (81 g)   6

Bagels, pre-sliced, onion,
1 bagel (57 g)   4

Bagels, pre-sliced, original,
100% whole wheat, 1 bagel (57 g)   4

Mini bagels, plain, pre-sliced,
1 bagel (57 g)   4

Original plain bagel, 1 bagel (57 g)   4

Lender's Bagel Shop Bagels

Bagels, 100% whole wheat,
1 bagel (81 g)   5

Bagels, cinnamon raisin swirl,
pre-sliced, 1 bagel (81 g)   7

Bagels, pre-sliced, onion,
1 bagel (81 g)   6

Blueberry bagel, 1 bagel (81 g)   7

Plain bagel, 1 bagel (81 g)   6

Martin's

Pre-sliced everything bagels,
1 bagel (95 g)   8

Meijer

Bagels, everything, 1 bagel (85 g)   6

Nature's Own

100% whole wheat bagel,
1 bagel (95 g)   6

100% whole wheat thin sliced
bagel, 1 bagel (46 g)   3

Bagels, thin sliced, cinnamon
raisin, 1 bagel (46 g)   4

Cinnamon raisin bagel,
1 bagel (95 g)   10

Original bagel, 1 bagel (95 g)   8

Plain thin sliced bagel,
1 bagel (46 g)   3

New York Bagel

Bagels, mini soft, 100% whole
wheat, 1 bagel (38 g)   3

Bagels, mini soft, plain,
1 bagel (38 g)   3

Oroweat

100% whole wheat bagels,
1 each (95 g)   7

Bagels, 100% whole wheat,
1 bagel (62 g)   5

Bread & Baked Goods

Pepperidge Farm

Bagel flats, cinnamon, 1 bagel flat (43 g)	3
Bagel flats, plain, 1 bagel flat (43 g)	3
Bagel, 100% whole wheat, 1 bagel (99 g)	8
Bagel, cinnamon raisin, 1 bagel (99 g)	9
Bagel, everything, 1 bagel (99 g)	8
Bagel, plain, 1 bagel (99 g)	8

Pepperidge Farm Mini

Bagel, brown sugar cinnamon, pre-sliced, 1 bagel (40 g)	4
Bagel, cinnamon raisin, pre-sliced, 1 bagel (40 g)	4
Bagel, plain, 1 bagel (40 g)	3
Bagels, whole grain, 100% whole wheat, 1 bagel (40 g)	3

Sara Lee Deluxe

Blueberry bagel, 1 bagel (95 g)	9
Cinnamon raisin bagel, 1 bagel (95 g)	9
Everything pre-sliced bagel, 1 bagel (95 g)	8
Plain bagel, 1 bagel (95 g)	7

Sara Lee Soft & Smooth

Whole grain blueberry mini bagel, 1 bagel (37 g)	3

Thomas'

Blueberry pre-sliced bagel, 1 bagel (95 g)	9
Cinnamon raisin pre-sliced bagel, 1 bagel (95 g)	8
Cinnamon swirl pre-sliced bagel, 1 bagel (95 g)	9
Everything pre-sliced bagel, 1 bagel (95 g)	8
Honey wheat pre-sliced bagel, 1 bagel (95 g)	8
Onion pre-sliced bagel, 1 bagel (95 g)	8

Plain made with whole grain pre-sliced bagel, 1 bagel (95 g)	8
Plain pre-sliced bagel, 1 bagel (95 g)	8

Thomas' Bagel Thins

100% whole wheat pre-sliced bagel, 1 bagel (46 g)	3
Cinnamon raisin pre-sliced bagel, 1 bagel (46 g)	4
Everything pre-sliced bagel, 1 bagel (46 g)	3
Oatmeal with cinnamon pre-sliced bagel, 1 bagel	3
Plain pre-sliced bagel, 1 bagel (46 g)	3

Thomas' Hearty Grains

100% whole wheat bagel, 1 bagel (95 g)	7

Thomas' Mini Bagels

100% whole wheat pre-sliced, 1 bagel (43 g)	3
Blueberry pre-sliced, 1 bagel (43 g)	4
Brown sugar cinnamon pre-sliced, 1 bagel (43 g)	4
Cinnamon raisin pre-sliced, 1 bagel (43 g)	4
Plain pre-sliced, 1 bagel (43 g)	4

Trader Joe's

100% whole wheat everything bagel slims, 1 bagel (46 g)	3
Plain mini bagels, 1 bagel (37 g)	3
Pretzel bagels, 1 bagel (85 g)	7
Whole wheat mini bagels, 1 (37 g)	3

Trader Joe's Bagel Shop

Everything bagels, 1 bagel (85 g)	7

Udi's

Bagel, gluten free, cinnamon raisin, 1 bagel (99 g)	9
Bagel, gluten free, whole grain, 1 bagel (99 g)	9
Bagel, plain, 1 bagel (99 g)	10

Udi's Gluten Free

Everything inside bagel, 1 bagel (99 g)	9

Bread & Baked Goods

Bread

Against the Grain Gourmet

Baguettes, original, ⅓ baguette (75 g)	8

Alexia Artisan Breads

Garlic baguette, twin pack, 2 pieces (43 g)	4

Alpine Valley Organic

Bread, honey whole wheat, 1 slice (28 g)	2
Bread, multi grain with omega-3, 1 slice (28 g)	2
Bread, sprouted honey wheat with flaxseed bread, 1 slice (28 g)	2

Alvarado St.

Bread, 100% sprouted whole wheat, fundamental fiber, 1 slice (43 g)	2
Bread, California style complete protein, 1 slice (34 g)	2
Bread, no salt!, sprouted multi-grain, 1 slice (34.1 g)	2
Bread, sprouted multi - grain, 1 slice (34.1 g)	2
Bread, sprouted rye seed, 1 slice (34 g)	2
Bread, sprouted sourdough, 1 slice (34.1 g)	2
Bread, sprouted whole wheat, 1 slice (38 g)	3
Essential flax seed bread, 2 slices (45 g)	3

Alvarado St. Diabetic Lifestyles

Bread, 1 slice (34 g)	2

Angelic Bakehouse

Sprouted honey wheat with raisins bread, 1 slice (28 g)	2
Sprouted seven grain bread, 1 slice (28 g)	2
Sprouted seven grain reduced sodium bread, 1 slice (28 g)	2
Sprouted wheat bread, 1 slice (28 g)	2

Arnold

Potato sandwich thins, 1 roll	3

Arnold Country

100% whole wheat bread, 1 slice (43 g)	3
Bread, sourdough, 1 slice (43 g)	3
Multi grain bread, 1 slice (43 g)	4
Oat bran bread, 1 slice (43 g)	3
Oatmeal bread, 1 slice (43 g)	4

Arnold Dutch Country

100% whole wheat bread, 1 slice (38 g)	3

Arnold Sandwich Thins

Flax and fiber roll, 1 roll (43 g)	3

Arnold, Brownberry, Oroweat Sandwich Thins

100% whole wheat no artificial sandwich thins, 1 roll	3
100% whole wheat sandwich thins, 1 roll	3
9 grain flax and fiber no artificial sandwich thins, 1 roll	3
Everything sandwich thins, 1 roll	3
Flax & fiber sandwich thins, 1 roll	3
Healthy multi grain sandwich thins, 1 roll	3
Honey wheat sandwich thins, 1 roll	3

Aunt Millie's

Bread, cracked wheat with whole grain, homestyle, 1 slice (34 g)	2
Bread, homestyle, 100% whole wheat, 1 slice (34 g)	2
Bread, homestyle, country buttermilk, 1 slice (34 g)	3
Butter top wheat bread, 1 slice (26 g)	2
Multi whole grain wheat bread 97% fat free, 2 slices (52 g)	4
Potato bread, split top, pre-priced, 1 slice (26 g)	2

Aunt Millie's 35 Calorie

Light 100% whole wheat bread, 2 slices (47 g)	2

Aunt Millie's Deluxe

Bread, wheat, 2 slices (57 g)	4
Bread, white, 2 slices (57 g)	4

Aunt Millie's Healthy Goodness

Bread, potato, 2 slices (52 g)	3
Bread, whole grain, white, 2 slices (45 g)	3

Aunt Millie's Hearth

Bread, 100% whole wheat, 1 slice (38 g)	3

Aunt Millie's Hearth Fiber for Life

Reduced calorie multi-grain bread, 1 slice (40 g)	2

Aunt Millie's Homestyle

Bread, enriched, Italian, seeded, 1 slice (34 g)	3

Aunt Millie's Swirl

Bread, cinnamon, 1 slice (35 g)	3
Bread, raisin, 1 slice (35 g)	3

Baby Bunny

Bread, ½ loaf, white enriched, 2 slices (48 g)	4

Bakers of Paris

Bread, sour dough, baguette, 2 oz	4

Beefsteak

Bread, hearty rye, seeded, 2 slices (50 g)	4
Bread, soft rye, no seeds, 2 slices (50 g)	4
Pumpernickel bread, 2 slices (57 g)	4
Seeded hearty rye bread, 2 slices (57 g)	4
Soft rye bread no seeds, 2 slices (57 g)	4

Berlin Natural Bakery

Bread, whole grain spelt, 1 slice (32 g)	2

Bimbo

Bread, 100% whole wheat, 2 slices (50 g)	4
Bread, honey wheat, 2 slices (52 g)	4
Bread, large white, 2 slices (57 g)	5

Bread, soft wheat, family, 2 slices (47 g)	3
Bread, soft white, small, 2 slices (41 g)	3
Bread, toasted, 1 slice (14 g)	2
Bread, toasted, double fiber, 1 slice (18 g)	2
Bread, whole grain, white, 2 slices (52 g)	4
Soft white bread, 2 slices (47 g)	4

Bob's Red Mill

Irish soda bread mix, 1 piece (43 g)	5

Bread for Life

Bread, sprouted, seven grain, 1 slice (34 g)	2

Breadsmith

Multigrain bread, 1 slice (45.7 g)	3

Brownberry All Natural

100% natural wheat bread, 1 slice (36 g)	3

Brownberry Bakery Light

100% whole wheat bread, 2 slices (45.4 g)	2

Brownberry Country

Honey whole wheat bread, 1 slice (43 g)	3

Brownberry Dutch Country

Premium potato bread, 1 slice (35 g)	3

Brownberry Health Full

Multigrain bread, 2 slices (46 g)	2

Brownberry Light 40 Calorie per Slice

Italian bread, 2 slices (43 g)	2

Brownberry Whole Grains

Bread, 100% whole wheat, 1 slice (43 g)	3
Bread, 12 grain, 1 slice (43 g)	3
Bread, health nut, 1 slice (43 g)	4
Bread, healthy multi-grain, 1 slice (43 g)	3
Bread, oatnut, 1 slice (43 g)	4
Double fiber bread, 1 slice (43 g)	3

	SmartPoints™ value
Bunny	
Bread, 100% whole wheat, original, 2 slices (50 g)	3
Bread, enriched, plantation, 1 slice (31 g)	2
Bread, giant, white enriched, 1 slice (28.3 g)	2
Bread, honey wheat, 1 slice (25.8 g)	2
Bread, original, large, white enriched, 1 slice (25.8 g)	2
Bread, thin sandwich, giant, white enriched, 1 slice (26.2 g)	2
Old fashioned bread, 1 slice (26 g)	2
Bunny Giant	
Original bread, 2 slices (49 g)	4
Bunny Soft-Twist	
Bread, white enriched, 2 slices (45.4 g)	3
Bunny Ultra-Soft	
Bread, whole grain white, 2 slices (56.7 g)	4
Butter Krust	
Extra thin sandwich bread, 2 slices (47 g)	4
Butternut	
Bread, 100% whole wheat, 2 slices (48 g)	3
Bread, all whole grain 100% whole wheat, 2 slices (57 g)	4
Bread, calcium fortified, large, 1 slice (26 g)	2
Bread, enriched, ½ loaf, 2 slices (48 g)	4
Bread, enriched, large, 1 slice (26 g)	2
Bread, honey wheat, 2 slices (45 g)	4
Butternut Ultra-Soft	
Bread, whole grain white, 2 slices (57 g)	4
Calandra's	
Bread, hearth oven baked panella, 1 each (45.2 g)	3

	SmartPoints™ value
California Goldminer	
Sourdough square bread, 2 oz	3
California Lavash	
Lavash, traditional, 1 sheet (56 g)	4
Lavash, whole grain, 1 sheet (56 g)	4
Canyon Bakehouse Gluten Free	
7 grain bread, 1 slice (34 g)	3
Mountain white bread, 1 slice (34 g)	3
Captain John Derst's	
Good old fashion bread, 1 slice (26 g)	2
Cinnabon	
Bread, cinnamon, 1 slice (38 g)	4
Bread, cinnamon, with cinnamon bursts, 1 slice (38 g)	4
Coast To Coast San Francisco Style	
Sliced bread, sourdough, 1 slice (43 g)	3
Cobblestone Bread Co.	
Brooklyn rye bread, 1 slice (32 g)	3
Cobblestone Mill	
Bread, New York style, Jewish rye, 1 slice (32 g)	2
New York style Jewish rye bread, 1 slice (31 g)	2
Spoleto Italian style bread, 1 slice (25 g)	2
Cole's	
Garlic bread, 1 serving (50 g)	6
Garlic bread, mini-loaf, 1 serving (45 g)	5
Garlic toast, pre-sliced, 1 piece (33.1 g)	4
Colombo	
Extra sour French bread, sliced, 1 each (40.7 g)	3
Colonial	
Sandwich bread, king thin, 2 slices (56.6 g)	4
Country Hearth	
12 grain bread, 1 each (42.5 g)	4
7 grain bread, 1 each (43 g)	3

Bread & Baked Goods

	SmartPoints™ value
Bread, 100% whole wheat, 1 slice (34 g)	2
Dakota style 12 grain bread, 1 slice (34 g)	3
Country Hearth Kid's Choice	
Wholegrain white bread, 2 slices (56 g)	4
Country Hearth Lite	
100% whole wheat bread, 2 slices (41 g)	2
Country Kitchen	
Bread, butter split wheat, 1 slice (28 g)	2
Hearty Canadian white, premium enriched bread, 1 slice (34.7 g)	2
Country Kitchen Light	
Enriched bread, Italian, pre-priced, 1 slice (27 g)	1
Oatmeal bread, 2 slices (42 g)	2
Wheat bread, 2 slices (42 g)	2
D'Italiano	
Italian bread, enriched, no seeds, 1 slice (29.8 g)	2
Italian bread, seeded, 1 slice (30 g)	2
Light Italian bread, sliced, 2 slices (45 g)	2
Duffy's	
Crumpets, 1 serving (44 g)	2
Ener G	
Tapioca loaf, light, 1 slice (19 g)	1
Eureka	
Bread, organic, grainiac, 1 slice (48 g)	4
Bread, organic, saaa-wheat!, 1 slice (48 g)	4
Bread, organic, seeds the day, 1 slice (48 g)	4
Grainiac organic sandwich bread, 1 slice (28 g)	2

	SmartPoints™ value
Saaa-wheat! organic sandwich bread, 1 slice (28 g)	2
Seeds the day organic sandwich bread, 1 slice (28 g)	3
Evangeline Maid	
Thin sandwich enriched bread, 2 slices (47 g)	4
Fabulous Flats	
Tandoori naan, 1 serving (63 g)	5
Tandoori naan, garlic, ¼ package (62 g)	5
Tandoori naan, whole grain, ½ flat (63 g)	5
Fantini	
Bread, enriched Italian, scali, with sesame, 2 slices (41.5 g)	3
Fiber One 100 Calorie	
Multigrain bread, 2 slices (50 g)	3
White bread, 2 slices (50 g)	3
Whole wheat thin sandwich roll, 1 (43 g)	3
Flatout	
Flatbread, lavash, pinwheel, classic white, party pack, 1 flatbread (77 g)	5
Flatout Foldit	
Flatbread, traditional white, 1 flatbread (43 g)	3
Food For Life	
7 sprouted grains bread, 1 slice (34 g)	2
Bread, sprouted 100% whole grain, cinnamon raisin, 1 slice (34 g)	3
Ezekiel 4:9 flax bread, 1 slice (34 g)	2
Sprouted grain bread, 1 slice (34 g)	2
Sprouted grain bread, cinnamon raisin, 1 slice (34 g)	3
Food For Life Ezekiel 4:9	
100% whole grain sprouted bread, 1 slice (34 g)	2
Bread, sprouted grain, low sodium, 1 slice (34 g)	2

	SmartPoints™ value
Bread, sprouted, sesame, organic, 1 slice (34 g)	2
Bread, sprouted 100% whole grain, 1 slice (34 g)	2
Cinnamon raisin 100% sprouted whole grain bread, 1 slice (34 g)	3
Food For Life Wheat & Gluten Free	
Bread, brown rice, 1 slice (42.5 g)	4
Francisco International	
Bread, sliced, extra sourdough, 1 slice (48.6 g)	4
Long sourdough bread, sliced, 1 ½ oz	3
Sweet French bread, sliced, 2 each (40.7 g)	3
Franz	
Bread, 100% whole wheat, 2 slices (45 g)	3
Bread, cracked wheat, 1 slice (30 g)	2
Bread, enriched, premium white, big, 1 slice (30 g)	2
Bread, gluten free, 7 grains, 1 slice (34 g)	3
Bread, gluten free, mountain white, 1 slice (34 g)	3
Bread, honey oat & nut, 1 slice (40 g)	4
Bread, organic twenty-four, thin sliced, 1 slice (28 g)	2
Bread, organic, twenty-four, 1 slice (45 g)	3
Bread, white, 2 slices (61 g)	4
Bread, whole grain white, 2 slices (68 g)	5
Franz Big Horn Valley	
Bread, organic, 100% whole wheat, 1 slice (43 g)	3
Franz Cannon Beach	
Bread, milk & honey, 1 slice (40 g)	3
Franz Columbia River	
Bread, made with whole grain, sweet dark, 1 slice (43 g)	4

	SmartPoints™ value
Franz McKenzie Farms	
Bread, old fashioned buttermilk, 1 slice (40 g)	3
Franz Oregon Trail	
Bread, 100% whole wheat, 1 slice (43 g)	3
Franz San Juan Island	
Bread, nine grain, 1 slice (43 g)	4
Bread, organic, nine grain, 1 slice (43 g)	3
Franz Willamette Valley	
Bread, organic, great seed, 1 slice (43 g)	3
Freihofer's	
Bread, 100% whole wheat, 1 slice (42.5 g)	3
100% whole wheat bread, stone ground, pre-priced, 1 slice (36 g)	3
Bread, 100% whole wheat, country double fiber, 1 slice (36 g)	2
Bread, country potato, 1 slice (36 g)	3
Bread, country white, 1 slice (36 g)	3
Split top wheat bread, 2 slices (52 g)	4
Freihofer's D'Italiano	
Italian bread, no seeds, 1 slice (32 g)	2
Fresh Bakery	
Bread, premium multigrain sandwich, 2 oz	6
Texas toast seasoned croutons, 2 Tbsp	1
Full Circle	
Bread, kalamata olive, 2 oz	4
Furlani	
Texas garlic toast, 1 slice (40 g)	5
Giant Lite	
Wheat bread, 2 slices (41 g)	2
Giant/Stop & Shop	
100% whole wheat bread, 2 slices (50 g)	4
Light Italian bread, 1 slice (28 g)	1

Bread & Baked Goods

Light multigrain bread,
2 slices (41 g) — 2

Light seeded rye bread,
1 slice (32 g) — 2

Light wheat bread, 2 slices (41 g) — 2

Multigrain thin sandwich roll,
1 roll (43 g) — 3

Whole wheat thin sandwich roll,
1 roll (43 g) — 3

Global Bakeries

No. 1 pita bread 14 Jack junior,
1 pita (57 g) — 3

Glutino Genius

Gluten free multigrain sandwich
bread, 1 slice (29 g) — 2

Golden Home

100% whole grain ultra thin pizza
crusts, 1 slice (45 g) — 4

Grandma Sycamore

Bread, home-maid, enriched
white, 1 slice (40 g) — 3

Bread, honey whole wheat,
1 slice (40 g) — 3

Bread, white, 1 slice (40 g) — 3

Great Value

100% whole wheat bread,
1 slice (27 g) — 2

Enriched sandwich bread,
1 slice (26 g) — 2

Hannaford

Bread, 12 grain, 1 slice (43 g) — 4

Healthy Choice

Hearty 7-grain bread, 1 slice (38 g) — 2

Healthy Life

Bread, 100% natural farmer's
12 grain, 1 slice (35 g) — 3

Bread, 100% natural whole
wheat, 1 slice (35 g) — 3

Bread, 100% whole grain rye,
sugar free, 2 slices (50 g) — 2

Bread, 100% whole wheat whole
grain, 2 slices (41 g) — 2

Bread, 100% whole wheat whole
grain, flaxseed, 2 slices (41 g) — 2

Bread, 100% whole wheat, southern
country style, 2 slices (56.7 g) — 3

Bread, Italian, 2 slices (41 g) — 2

Bread, white, 2 slices (41 g) — 2

Bread, whole grain, oat bran,
light, 2 slices (41 g) — 2

H-E-B Health Smart

Bread, 100% whole wheat,
1 slice (31 g) — 2

H-E-B Split Top

Bread, honey wheat, 1 slice (31 g) — 3

H-E-B Thin Rounds

Rolls, whole grain white,
pre-sliced, 1 roll (43 g) — 3

Heiner's

Bread, reduced calorie, 35,
hearty wheat, 2 slices (41.2 g) — 2

Heiner's 35

Bread, reduced calorie, vegetable
fiber, wheat, 2 slices (38 g) — 2

Hillbilly

Bread, old fashion, 1 slice (25.5 g) — 2

Hogan's

Soda bread mix, white Irish, 1 oz — 3

Holsum

Bread, wheat, light, 2 slices (45 g) — 2

Holsum Lite'r 35

Bread, wheat, 2 slices (41 g) — 2

Bread, white, 2 slices (41 g) — 2

Home Pride

Bread, 100% whole wheat,
2 slices (50 g) — 4

Bread, wheat, butter top,
1 slice (26 g) — 2

Bread, white, butter top,
1 slice (26 g) — 2

Innkeeper's Bed & Breakfast

Healthful 8 grain bread,
1 slice (54 g) — 6

SmartPoints™
value

SmartPoints™
value

IronKids

White bread, sliced, 1 slice (25.7 g)	2

J.J. Nissen

Bread, premium enriched, Canadian white, 1 slice (39 g)	3

Joseph's

Garlic and herb flatbread, 1 flatbread (56 g)	2
Lavash bread, flax, oat bran & whole wheat flour, ½ lavash (32 g)	1
Syrian bread, wheat, 1 pita (30.3 g)	2
Whole wheat bread, middle east, 1 ½ oz	3

Julian Bakery Paleo Bread

Gluten free bread, coconut, 1 slice (43 g)	1

King's Hawaiian

Bread, Hawaiian sweet, original, 1 slice (38 g)	5
Bread, sandwich, sliced, 1 slice (28 g)	4
Hawaiian sweet bread, 2 oz	6
Honey wheat rolls, 1 roll (31 g)	3

Kinnikinnick Gluten Free

Multigrain bread, 2 slices (57 g)	5

Kirkland Signature

Multigrain bread, 1 slice (53 g)	4
Split top wheat bread, 1 slice (34 g)	2

Kontos

Roghani nan, 1 loaf (80 g)	8

Kroger

Bread, classic garlic, 1 serving (50 g)	6
Enriched white sandwich bread, 2 slices (47 g)	4
Round top 100% whole wheat bread, 1 slice (28 g)	2
Round top white enriched bread, 1 slice (26 g)	2
Texas toast, garlic, 1 slice (50 g)	6

Texas toast, garlic 3-cheese, 1 slice (46 g)	5
Wheat sandwich bread, 2 slices (47 g)	4

Kroger Value

Enriched white bread, 2 slices (43 g)	4

Krusteaz

Cornbread mix, honey, fat free, ¼ cup	1

La Brea Bakery

Baguette, French demi, ½ baguette (57 g)	4
Bread, Italian boule round, 2 oz	4
French baguettes, take & bake, twin pack, ⅓ loaf (57 g)	4
Loaf, whole grain, 2 oz	5

Le Petit Francais

Baguettes, original French, 1 oz	2

Levy's

Bread, real Jewish rye, 1 slice (32 g)	2

Lewis Bunny

Special recipe honey wheat bread, 2 slices (45 g)	3

Libby's

Pumpkin bread kit, with icing, 1 slice (86 g)	11

L'Oven Fresh

100% whole wheat bread, 1 slice (45 g)	3
Bread, white, 2 slices (57 g)	4
Raisin cinnamon swirl bread, 1 slice (29 g)	3

Maier's

Bread, Italian wheat, 1 slice (31.5 g)	2
Bread, Italian, premium, 1 slice (32 g)	2
Bread, Italian, premium, seeded, 1 slice (32 g)	2

Market Pantry

Garlic Texas toast, 1 slice (42 g)	5

Bread & Baked Goods

Marketside

Savory garlic knots, 1 (37 g)	3

Martha White Cotton Country

Cornbread mix, buttermilk, 1 serving (34 g)	4

Martin's

100% whole wheat potato bread, 1 slice (35 g)	2
Enriched potato sandwich bread, 1 slice (32 g)	2

Martin's Swirl

Cinnamon raisin potato bread, 1 slice (28.35 g)	3

Mary Jane

Bread, giant enriched, 2 slices (48.6 g)	3

Matthews All Natural

Bread, whole wheat, 1 slice (31 g)	2

Meijer

Bread, light wheat, 2 slices (47 g)	2

Merita

Bread, enriched, 1 slice (26 g)	2
Old fashioned enriched bread, 1 slice (26 g)	2

Mestemacher

Bread, fitness, 1 piece (72 g)	3
Bread, sunflower seed, 1 piece (72 g)	4
Bread, whole rye, 1 piece (72 g)	3

Milton's

100% whole wheat bread, whole grains, 1 slice (50.4 g)	3
Bread, healthy whole grain, 1 slice (38 g)	3
Bread, multi-grain, 1 slice (43 g)	3
Healthy multi-grain bread, 1 slice (49 g)	4

Monks'

Bread, multigrain, 1 slice (28 g)	2
Bread, wholegrain wheat, 1 slice (28 g)	2

Mother's Butter Top

Bread, wheat, 1 slice (28.3 g)	2

Mrs. Baird's

Bread, 100% whole wheat, 2 slices (50 g)	4
Honey 7 grain recipe bread, 2 slices (57 g)	5
Honey wheat bread, 1 slice (30.9 g)	2
Whole grain white bread, 2 slices (57 g)	4

Mrs. Baird's Buttered Split Top

Wheat bread, 1 slice (26 g)	2

Natural Grain

Bread, 100% whole wheat, 1 slice (26 g)	1
Bread, double fiber, 1 slice (28 g)	1

Natural Ovens

Bread, hunger filler, 1 slice (36 g)	2
Bread, multi grain, 1 slice (36 g)	2

Natural Ovens Weight Sense

Bread, right wheat, 2 slices (45 g)	3

Nature's Harvest

Light 100% whole wheat bread, 2 slices (44 g)	2
Multigrain bread, 1 slice (28 g)	4
Whole grain white bread, 2 slices (52 g)	4

Nature's Harvest Whole Grains

100% stone ground whole wheat bread, 1 slice (40 g)	3
18 grains and seeds bread, 1 slice (40 g)	3
Honey wheatberry bread, 1 slice (40 g)	3

Nature's Own

Bread, 100% whole wheat, 2 slices (45 g)	3
Bread, 9-grain, enriched, 2 slices (45 g)	2
Bread, double fiber wheat, 1 slice (28 g)	1

Bread & Baked Goods

	SmartPoints™ value
Bread, enriched butterbread, 1 slice (31 g)	2
Bread, honey 7 grain, 1 slice (26 g)	2
Bread, honey wheat, enriched, 2 slices (45 g)	2
Bread, specialty, 100% whole wheat, 1 slice (43 g)	3
Bread, swirl, cinnamon raisin, 2 slices (56 g)	7
Bread, wheat, enriched, 2 slices (45 g)	2
Bread, white, enriched, 2 slices (45 g)	2
Bread, whole grain, 1 slice (43 g)	3
Butterbread bread, 1 slice (26 g)	2
Enriched bread, whitewheat, 1 slice (28 g)	2
Enriched bread, whitewheat sandwich, 1 slice (28 g)	2
Honey oat bread, 1 slice (26 g)	2
Honey wheat enriched bread, 1 slice (26 g)	2
Sugar free 100% whole wheat whole grain bread, 1 slice (25 g)	1
Nature's Own Premium Specially	
Bread, 12-grain, 1 slice (34 g)	3
Nature's Own Specialty	
Bread, 100% whole grain, 1 slice (43 g)	3
Bread, 100% whole wheat, with honey, 1 slice (43 g)	3
Bread, 12 grain, 1 slice (43 g)	3
Bread, healthy multi grain, 1 slice (28 g)	2
Nature's Own Whitewheat	
Whole grain enriched bread, 2 slices (52 g)	3
Nature's Promise Naturals	
Bread, multigrain, 1 slice (43 g)	3
Whole wheat bread, 1 slice (43 g)	3

	SmartPoints™ value
New York	
Garlic bread, pre-sliced, 2 slices (39.6 g)	5
Texas toast, cheese, 1 slice (48 g)	7
Texas toast, the original, five cheese, 1 slice (48 g)	6
Texas toast, the original, lite, 1 slice (40 g)	4
The original Texas toast with garlic, 1 slice (40 g)	5
New York Brand	
Lite Texas garlic toast, 1 slice (40 g)	4
New York Brand Soft Pull Aparts	
Garlic bread for sharing, 2 rolls (43 g)	5
O Organics	
Bread, whole grains, seeds & fiber, 1 slice (35 g)	2
Open Nature	
Bread, nuts & seeds, 1 slice (43 g)	3
Oroweat	
Bread, 100% whole wheat, 2 slices (50 g)	4
Bread, 100% whole wheat, whole grain, 1 slice (38 g)	3
Bread, 12 grain, 1 slice (38 g)	3
Bread, 7 grain, 1 slice (38 g)	3
Bread, country buttermilk, 1 slice (38 g)	3
Bread, country potato, 1 slice (38 g)	3
Bread, country white, 1 slice (38 g)	4
Bread, double fiber, 1 slice (38 g)	2
Bread, health nut, 1 slice (38 g)	3
Bread, healthy multi-grain, 1 slice (38 g)	3
Bread, honey wheat berry, 1 slice (34 g)	3
Bread, Jewish rye, 1 slice (28 g)	2
Bread, light, 100% whole wheat, 2 slices (45 g)	2

Bread & Baked Goods

Bread, original oatnut,
1 slice (38 g) — 3

Bread, premium Italian,
1 slice (32 g) — 2

Bread, Russian rye, 1 slice (28 g) — 2

Bread, whole grain & oat,
1 slice (38 g) — 3

Dill rye bread, 1 each (28 g) — 2

Schwarzwalder dark rye bread,
1 oz — 2

Oroweat Dutch Country

Bread, extra fiber, 1 slice (38 g) — 3

Oroweat HealthFull

Bread, 10 grain, 1 slice (38 g) — 2

Bread, multigrain, 1 slice (38 g) — 3

Bread, nutty grain, 1 slice (38 g) — 2

Oroweat Master's Best

Bread, winter wheat, 1 slice (32 g) — 3

Orowheat Dutch Country

Bread, 100% whole wheat,
1 slice (38 g) — 3

Oven Joy

Bread, enriched, wheat,
1 slice (28 g) — 2

Enriched wheat sandwich bread,
2 slices (48 g) — 2

Ozery Bakery Morning Rounds

Apple cinnamon toastable fruit
and grain buns, 1 bun (60 g) — 5

Pantry Essentials

Bread, enriched, wheat,
2 slices (45 g) — 3

Papa Pita

Thinwich, pre-sliced, 100% whole
wheat & honey, 1 thinwich (43 g) — 3

Thinwich, pre-sliced, Italian herb
& olive oil, 1 thinwich (43 g) — 3

Thinwich, pre-sliced, multi-grain
with flax seeds, 1 thinwich (43 g) — 2

Pepperidge Farm

Bread, garlic, 2 ½" slice — 6

Bread, garlic, five cheese,
2 ¼" slice — 6

Bread, Italian white, 1 slice (32 g) — 2

Bread, Jewish rye seeded,
1 slice (32 g) — 2

Bread, Jewish rye seedless,
1 slice (32 g) — 2

Bread, Jewish rye whole grain
seeded, 1 slice (32 g) — 2

Bread, oatmeal, 1 slice (25 g) — 2

Bread, white family size,
2 slices (53 g) — 5

Bread, whole grain, multi grain,
1 slice (43 g) — 4

Pepperidge Farm Carb Style

Bread, soft, 100% whole wheat,
1 slice (25.8 g) — 1

Pepperidge Farm Deli Swirl

Bread, rye and pump,
1 slice (32 g) — 2

Pepperidge Farm Farmhouse

Bread, 12 grain, 1 slice (43 g) — 4

Bread, hearty wheat, 1 slice (43 g) — 3

Bread, honey wheat sliced,
1 slice (43 g) — 4

Bread, multi-grain, 1 slice (43 g) — 4

Bread, oatmeal, 1 slice (43 g) — 4

Bread, potato, 1 slice (39 g) — 3

Bread, sourdough, 1 slice (43 g) — 3

Pepperidge Farm Light Style

Bread, 100% whole wheat,
3 slices (57 g) — 4

Bread, 7 grain, 3 slices (57 g) — 4

Bread, oatmeal, 3 slices (57 g) — 4

Pepperidge Farm Pumpernickel

Bread, dark pump, 1 slice (32 g) — 2

Pepperidge Farm Soft

Bread, seedless rye, 1 slice (32 g) — 2

Bread & Baked Goods

	SmartPoints™ value
Pepperidge Farm Stone Ground	
Bread, 100% whole wheat, 1 slice (25 g)	2
Pepperidge Farm Swirl	
Bread, 100% whole wheat cinnamon with raisins, 1 slice (28 g)	3
Bread, blueberry flavored, 1 slice (38 g)	4
Bread, brown sugar cinnamon flavored, 1 slice (38 g)	4
Bread, cinnamon, 1 slice (28 g)	3
Bread, French toast, 1 slice (33 g)	4
Bread, gingerbread flavored, 1 slice (28 g)	3
Bread, pumpkin spice, 1 slice (28 g)	3
Bread, raisin cinnamon, 1 slice (28 g)	3
Bread, strawberry, 1 slice (26 g)	3
Pepperidge Farm Texas Toast	
Bread, five cheese, 1 slice (45 g)	5
Bread, garlic, 1 slice (40 g)	5
Bread, mozzarella & Monterrey Jack, 1 slice (45 g)	4
Cheddar, 1 slice (45 g)	5
Pillsbury	
Bread Italian, country, ⅛ package (47 g)	3
Buttermilk biscuit dough, 1 biscuit	6
French loaf, crusty, 1 serving (52 g)	4
Pizza crust, artisan, with whole grain, 1 slice (65 g)	6
Pillsbury Simply	
Bread, rustic French, ⅛ package (47 g)	3
Private Selection	
Bread, 100% whole wheat, 1 slice (38 g)	3
Bread, multigrain, 1 slice (45 g)	4
Private Selection Sugar Free	
100% whole wheat bread, 1 slice (45 g)	3

	SmartPoints™ value
Publix	
Bread, enriched, white, large, 1 slice (26 g)	2
Bread, reduced calorie, wheat enriched, 2 slices (45 g)	2
Bread, wheat, 1 slice (26 g)	2
Texas toast, garlic, 1 slice (39 g)	5
Publix Premium	
Bread, 100% stoneground, whole wheat, 1 slice (28 g)	2
Bread, 100% whole wheat, 1 slice (43 g)	3
Bread, butter crust, 1 slice (26 g)	2
Bread, honey wheat, 1 slice (26 g)	2
Bread, Italian, 1 slice (40 g)	3
Bread, multi-grain, 1 slice (43 g)	3
Bread, reduced calorie, natural grain, 2 slices (47 g)	2
Rainbo Iron Kids	
Bread, 100% whole wheat, 2 slices (57 g)	4
Reese	
Crotons, premium, toasted, 2 Tbsp	1
Croutons, premium, seasoned, 2 Tbsp	1
Roma	
Bread, scali, sliced, 1 slice (23.6 g)	2
Roman Meal	
Bread, 100% whole grain, 1 slice (32 g)	2
Bread, honey split top, 2 slices (57 g)	4
Bread, multigrain, round top, 2 slices (57 g)	4
Bread, roman whole grain, 2 slices (85 g)	4
Bread, sandwich, 1 slice (28 g)	2
Bread, sandwich, thin sliced, 2 slices (56 g)	4
Roman Meal SunGrain	
Bread, 100% whole wheat, 2 slices (46 g)	3

Bread & Baked Goods

Rotella's

Bread, Italian, 2 slices (59 g)	3

Rotella's Italian Bakery

Bread, soft white sandwich, 2 slices (53 g)	4

Rubschlager

Bread, cocktail rye, 3 slices (31 g)	2

Rudi's

Bread, double fiber sandwich, 1 slice (37 g)	2
Bread, sandwich, cinnamon raisin, 1 slice (37 g)	3
Bread, sandwich, original, 1 slice (37 g)	3

Rudi's Gluten Free Bakery

Multigrain sandwich bread, 1 slice (37 g)	3

Rudi's Organic

Bread, 100% whole wheat, double fiber, 1 slice (45 g)	3
Bread, 7 grain with flax, 1 slice (40 g)	3
Bread, country morning white, 1 slice (43 g)	3
Bread, honey sweet whole wheat, 1 piece (41.6 g)	3
Bread, multigrain oat, 1 slice (41.6 g)	3
Bread, spelt, 1 slice (41 g)	3

Rudi's Organic Bakery

Bread, 100% whole wheat, 1 piece (41.6 g)	3

Rustic

Bread, hearth style hard crust, 1 slice (44 g)	3

S. Rosen's

Bread, bohemian style rye, thin sliced, unseeded, 2 slices (37.8 g)	3
Bread, rye, 1 slice (27 g)	2
Bread, rye with caraway seeds, thin sliced, 2 slices (37.8 g)	3

Sacramento Bake

Bread, sourdough, sliced, 1 slice (42 g)	2

Safeway Kitchens

100% whole wheat bread, 2 slices (45 g)	3
Bread, 100% whole wheat (24 oz), 1 slice (38 g)	3
Bread, 8 grain, 1 slice (43 g)	3
Bread, butter top wheat., 2 slices (56 g)	4
Bread, cinnamon raisin, 1 slice (25 g)	2
Bread, enriched, 15 grain, 1 slice (38 g)	3
Bread, enriched, butter top white, 2 slices (56 g)	4
Bread, oats & nuts, 1 slice (38 g)	3
Bread, sourdough, sliced long loaf, 1 slice (26 g)	2

Safeway Select Artisan

Bread, French, European style, 1 slice (45 g)	3

San Luis Sourdough

Bread, 1 slice (48.6 g)	4
Bread, deli, sourdough, 1 slice (45 g)	3
Bread, sourdough, cracked wheat, 1 slice (28 g)	2
Bread, sourdough, rosemary & olive oil, 1 slice (52 g)	4

Sara Lee

Bread, 100% whole wheat, 2 slices (57 g)	5
Bread, classic oats 'n honey, 2 slices (52 g)	4
Bread, honey wheat, 2 slices (57 g)	5
Bread, old fashioned white, 2 slices (49 g)	4
Bread, white, 2 slices (57 g)	5
Roll, sweet Hawaiian, 1 roll (35 g)	3

	SmartPoints™ value
Sara Lee 45 Calories & Delightful	
100% multi-grain bread, 2 slices (44 g)	2
100% whole wheat bread, 2 slices (45 g)	2
100% whole wheat with honey bread, 2 slices (44 g)	2
Healthy multi-grain bread, 2 slices (45 g)	2
Sara Lee Classic	
100% whole wheat bread, 1 slice (26 g)	2
Butter bread, 1 slice (26 g)	2
Honey wheat bread, 1 slice (26 g)	2
White bread, 2 slices (57 g)	5
Sara Lee Delightful	
45 calories wheat bread, 2 slices (45 g)	2
Sara Lee Hearty & Delicious	
100% whole wheat bakery bun, 1 bun (82 g)	6
100% whole wheat with honey bread, 1 slice (38 g)	3
12 grain bread, 1 slice (38 g)	3
Bread, healthy multi-grain, 1 slice (38 g)	3
Sara Lee Soft & Smooth	
100% whole wheat bread, 2 slices (57 g)	4
White bread made with whole grain, 2 slices (52 g)	4
Sara Lee Swirl	
Cinnamon with raisins bread, 1 slice (28 g)	3
Schar	
Bread, classic white, 1 slice (30 g)	3
Bread, deli-style, gluten-free, 1 slice (48 g)	4
Bread, multigrain, 1 slice (30 g)	2
Schmidt	
Bread, enriched, Italian, 1 slice (31 g)	2

	SmartPoints™ value
Schmidt Old Tyme	
Bread, 100% whole grain, 1 slice (31 g)	2
Bread, enriched, honey wheat, 1 slice (28 g)	2
Bread, split-top wheat, 1 slice (31 g)	2
Schwebel's	
Bread, enriched lite wheat, 2 slices (41 g)	2
Bread, enriched lite white, 2 slices (41 g)	2
Bread, enriched, giant, 1 slice (26 g)	2
Bread, sweet harvest wheat, 1 slice (27 g)	2
Bread, 'taliano, sliced Italian, 1 slice (26.7 g)	2
Seattle Baking	
Sourdough, cracked wheat, 1 slice (48.6 g)	3
Seattle International	
Bread, classic sourdough, 1 slice (28 g)	2
Seattle Sourdough Baking	
Bread, old town sourdough, 2 oz	3
Sliced sourdough, 1 slice (48.6 g)	3
ShopRite	
Bread, enriched, light, wheat, 2 slices (41 g)	2
Bread, light, hearth baked Jewish rye, no seeds, 1 slice (32 g)	2
Bread, light, hearth baked Jewish rye, seeded, 1 slice (32 g)	2
Bread, round top white, 2 slices (47 g)	4
Bread, sandwich white, 2 slices (47 g)	4
Bread, wheat, 1 slice (28 g)	2
Silva's Bakery	
Portuguese-Italian round bread, homemade, 2 oz	4

Silver Hills

Sprouted grain bread, 16 grain, 1 slice (41 g)	3
Sprouted grain breads, squirrelly, 1 slice (40 g)	3

Soft N Good

Bread, enriched white, giant, 2 slices (57 g)	5

Stroehmann Split Top

Wheat bread, 2 slices (50 g)	4

Sunbeam

Bread, enriched white, 2 slices (45 g)	3
Bread, enriched, sandwich, 1 slice (26 g)	2
Bread, enriched, Texas toast, 1 slice (38 g)	3
Giant enriched bread, 2 slices (49 g)	4
Honey wheat bread, 1 each (25.8 g)	2
Lite Italian bread, low fat, 2 pieces (45 g)	2
Old fashioned enriched bread, 1 slice (26 g)	2
Split top white bread, 1 slice (26 g)	2
Thin enriched white bread, 2 slices (41 g)	3

Sunbeam Bunny

Small enriched bread, 2 slices (46 g)	4

Sun-Maid

Bread, raisin, cinnamon swirl, 1 slice (32 g)	4

Tandoor Chef

Garlic naan, 1 piece (85 g)	6

Texas Toast

Bread, enriched, 1 slice (43 g)	3

Three Bakers

Bread, whole grain, 7 ancient grains, 2 slices (68 g)	6

Three Bakers

Bread, whole grain, rye style, 2 slices (68 g)	4
Bread, whole grain, white, 2 slices (68 g)	4

Trader Joe's

100% whole grain fiber bread, multigrain, 1 slice (43 g)	3
100% whole grain fiber bread, whole wheat, 1 slice (43 g)	3
Garlic naan, 1 piece (85 g)	6
Low calorie light wheat bread, 1 slice (28 g)	1
Multigrain country bread, 1 slice (34 g)	3
Panini slims sandwich bread, 1 panini (78 g)	6
Soft multigrain rustico bread, 1 slice (28 g)	2
Soft whole wheat bread, 1 slice (34 g)	2
Sprouted flourless whole wheat berry bread, 1 slice (34 g)	2
Sprouted multigrain bread, 1 slice (34 g)	2
Sprouted whole wheat fiber bread, 100% whole wheat, low fat, 1 slice (43 g)	2
Stone hearth baked sourdough loaf, 1 slice (50 g)	3
Tandoori naan, 1 piece (85 g)	7
Texas toast, 1 slice (45 g)	3
Tuscan pane oven baked classic Italian bread, 1 slice (57 g)	3

Trader Joe's Artisan Breads

Ciabatta, 2 oz	3

Turano

Italian bread, pane turano, 1 each (56.7 g)	4

Udi's

Bread, cinnamon raisin, 2 slices (60 g)	6
Bread, sandwich, white, 2 slices (57 g)	5

Bread & Baked Goods

	SmartPoints™ value
Bread, whole grain, 2 slices (57 g)	5
Gluten free millet chia bread, 2 slices (58 g)	4
Gluten free omega flax and fiber bread, 2 slices (58 g)	4
Ultimate Grains	
Bread, all natural, whole grain, multi-grain, 1 slice (43 g)	3
Vermont	
All natural bread, cinnamon raisin, 1 slice (32 g)	3
Bread, organic, soft wheat, 1 slice (40 g)	3
Bread, soft 10 grain, 1 slice (34 g)	2
Bread, soft white, 1 slice (34 g)	3
Bread, soft whole wheat, 1 slice (38 g)	2
Village Hearth Light	
12 grain bread, 2 slices (46 g)	2
Italian bread, 2 slices (43 g)	2
Wheat bread, 2 slices (46 g)	2
Vitalicious Energy Loaf	
Banana nut, 1 loaf (54 g)	4
Wal-Mart	
Texas garlic toast, 1 slice (40 g)	4
Wegman's	
Bread, homestyle, 1 slice (26 g)	2
Bread, lite, white, 2 slices (43 g)	2
Wegman's Food You Feel Good About	
Bread, giant, 1 slice (26 g)	2
Bread, Italiano, 100% whole wheat, 1 slice (31 g)	2
Bread, lite, wheat, 2 slices (42 g)	2
Bread, soft, 100% whole wheat, 2 slices (57 g)	5
Bread, white, 2 slices (60 g)	4
Multigrain bread, 1 slice (48 g)	3
Whole Foods	
Multigrain deli thins, 1 thin (43 g)	3
Whole Foods Organic	
7 grain sandwich bread, 1 slice (29 g)	2

	SmartPoints™ value
Wonder	
Bread, 100% whole grain, 2 slices (62 g)	5
Bread, 100% whole wheat, 1 slice (25 g)	1
Bread, light, wheat, 2 slices (45 g)	2
Bread, white, classic, 2 slices (50 g)	4
Bread, whole grain white, 2 slices (57 g)	3

Croutons

	SmartPoints™ value
Archer Farms	
Salad topping, crispy onion strings, 2 Tbsp	1
Salad topping, wonton strips salad topper, 2 Tbsp	1
Cardini's	
Croutons, Caesar, 2 Tbsp	1
Chatham Village	
Croutons, cheese & garlic, large cut, 2 Tbsp	1
Croutons, traditional cut, fat free, garlic & onion, 2 Tbsp	1
Croutons, traditional cut, garlic & butter flavored, 2 Tbsp	1
Garlic and butter croutons, 2 Tbsp	1
Traditional cut croutons, Caesar, 2 Tbsp	1
Traditional cut croutons, garden herb, 2 Tbsp	1
Chatham Village All Natural	
Croutons, large cut, sea salt & pepper, 2 Tbsp	1
Fresh Gourmet	
Croutons, focaccia, roasted garlic, 2 Tbsp	1
Croutons, premium, cheese & garlic, 6 croutons (7 g)	1
Croutons, premium, country ranch, 6 croutons (7 g)	1
Crunchy toppings for salads, wonton strips, garlic ginger, 2 Tbsp	1

Bread & Baked Goods

	SmartPoints™ value
Garlic Caesar fat free croutons, 6 croutons (7 g)	1
Organic seasoned croutons, 2 Tbsp	1
Premium croutons, butter & garlic, ¼ oz	1
Premium croutons, classic Caesar, 6 croutons (7 g)	1
Premium croutons, garden herb, 6 croutons (7 g)	1
Premium croutons, Italian seasoned, 6 croutons (7 g)	1
Premium croutons, multi-grain, parmesan Caesar, 6 croutons (7 g)	1
Premium croutons, parmesan ranch, 12 croutons (7 g)	1
Premium Italian seasoned croutons, 1 packet (14 g)	2
Texas toast cheddar croutons, 2 Tbsp	1
Wonton strips, authentic, 2 Tbsp	1

Fresh Gourmet Cornbread

Sweet butter premium croutons, 5 croutons (7 g)	1

Giant

Croutons, cheese & garlic, 6 croutons (7 g)	1
Croutons, Italian seasoned, 6 croutons (7 g)	1

Hy-Vee

Croutons, baked, cheese & garlic, premium large cut, 6 croutons (7 g)	1

Kroger

Croutons, homestyle, ceasar, 2 Tbsp	1
Croutons, homestyle, cheese & garlic, 2 Tbsp	1
Croutons, homestyle, ranch, 2 Tbsp	1
Croutons, jumbo, Texas toast butter & garlic flavored, ¼ cup	1

Kroger Homestyle

Croutons, seasoned herb, 2 Tbsp	1
Croutons, zesty Italian, 2 Tbsp	1

Marzetti

	SmartPoints™ value
Croutons, flavored large cut, garlic & butter, 2 Tbsp	1
Croutons, large cut, Caesar, 2 Tbsp	1
Croutons, large cut, cheese & garlic, 2 Tbsp	1
Croutons, large cut, ranch, 2 Tbsp	1
Croutons, fat free large cut, garlic & onion, 2 Tbsp	1

Meijer

Croutons, fat free, garlic & onion, 2 Tbsp	1
Croutons, seasoned, 2 Tbsp	1
Croutons, Texas toast, garlic & cheese, 2 Tbsp	1

Mrs. Cubbison's

Authentic wonton strips salad topping, 2 Tbsp	1
Croutons, butter & garlic, 2 Tbsp	1
Croutons, garlic & butter, 8 croutons (7 g)	1
Croutons, restaurant style, Caesar salad, 5 croutons (7 g)	1
Croutons, restaurant style, cheese & garlic, 5 croutons (7 g)	1
Croutons, restaurant style, classic seasoned, 5 croutons (7 g)	1
Croutons, restaurant style, fat free, seasoned, 2 Tbsp	1
Garlic and butter focaccia croutons, 2 Tbsp	1
Southwest flavor tortilla strips, 2 Tbsp	1

Mrs. Cubbison's Texas Toast Bread

Seasoned croutons, 2 Tbsp	1

New York The Original Texas Toast

Croutons, Caesar, 2 Tbsp	1
Croutons, cheese & garlic, 2 Tbsp	1
Croutons, garlic & butter flavored, 2 Tbsp	1
Croutons, sea salt & pepper, 2 Tbsp	1
Croutons, seasoned, 2 Tbsp	1

Bread & Baked Goods

	SmartPoints™ value
Olive Garden	
Garlic and romano seasoned croutons, 2 Tbsp	1
Olive Garden Signature Recipe	
Garlic and romano seasoned croutons, 2 Tbsp	1
Rothbury Farms	
Croutons, buttery garlic, 2 Tbsp	1
Croutons, cheese garlic, 2 Tbsp	1
Croutons, classic seasoned, 2 Tbsp	1
Croutons, fat free, seasoned, 2 Tbsp	1
Croutons, seasoned, 2 Tbsp	1
Croutons, seasoned, Italian style, 2 Tbsp	1
Texas Toast New York	
Asiago cheese croutons, 2 Tbsp	1
Cheddar bacon croutons, 2 Tbsp	1
Tuscan Garden Classics	
Cheese garlic gourmet restaurant style crouton, 2 Tbsp	1
Wegman's	
Croutons, twice baked, Caesar, 2 Tbsp	1
Croutons, twice baked, cheese & garlic, 2 Tbsp	1
Croutons, twice baked, fat free garlic & onion, 2 Tbsp	1
Croutons, twice baked, garlic, 2 Tbsp	1
Croutons, twice baked, lightly seasoned, 2 Tbsp	1
Croutons, twice baked, zesty Italian, 2 Tbsp	1

Danish, Sweet Rolls & Pastries

	SmartPoints™ value
Bimbo	
Conchas, 1 piece (60 g)	9
Sweet bread, semitas, 1 piece (60 g)	8
Churros	
Churros pastry stix, 1 churro (28.3 g)	4

	SmartPoints™ value
Cream Curls Bakery	
Cream puffs, mini, filled, 1 cream puff (18 g)	2
Delizza	
Cream puffs, Belgian mini, 6 cream puffs (75 g)	13
Entenmann's	
Danish twist, pecan, 1 serving (58 g)	10
Fresh Bakery	
Hot cross buns, 2 oz	6
Goya	
Pastries, guava, 1 pastry (43 g)	5
Pastries, guava & cream cheese, 1 pastry (43 g)	5
Immaculate Baking Co.	
Rolls, cinnamon, 1 roll (99 g)	13
Kontos	
Baklava, assorted, 1 oz	5
Kroger	
Cinnamon rolls, with icing, 1 roll (44 g)	6
Markets of Meijer Fresh	
Rolls, mini Danish, assorted, 1 roll (35 g)	4
Mila's European Bakery	
Cake roll, pumpkin, 2 oz	7
Ozery Bakery Morning Rounds	
Cranberry orange toastable fruit and grain buns, 1 bun (60 g)	5
Pillsbury	
Caramel rolls, 1 roll (49 g)	7
Cinnamon rolls with cinnabon cinnamon icing, 1 (44 g)	6
Cinnamon rolls, cream cheese icing, 1 roll (44 g)	6
Cinnamon rolls, reduced fat, with icing, 1 roll (44 g)	6
Pastries, fill & bake flaky, real apple turnovers, 1 pastry (57 g)	7

Pastries, fill & bake flaky, real cherry turnovers, 1 pastry (57 g)	7
Sweet rolls, orange, with icing, 1 roll (49 g)	6

Pillsbury Cinnabon

Bakery inspired cinnamon rolls (with topping and frosting), 1 serving (138 g)	19
Cinnamon rolls with icing, 1 roll with icing (44 g)	6
Rolls, flaky cinnamon, with butter cream icing, 1 roll (46 g)	7

Pillsbury Grands!

Cinnamon rolls, with cream cheese icing, 1 (99 g)	12
Cinnamon rolls, with icing, 1 roll with icing (99 g)	12

Pillsbury Grands! Flaky Supreme

Cinnamon rolls, with icing, 1 sweet roll (99 g)	15

Rhodes Bake-N-Serv

Cinnamon rolls, with cream cheese frosting, 1 roll with frost (89.8 g)	8

Super Bun

Cinnamon buns, 1 bun (57 g)	8

Tastykake Kandy Bar Kakes

Kandy bar kakes, peanut butter, 1 cake (48 g)	11

Trader Joe's

Mini café twists, 4 (26 g)	5

Upper Crust Bakery

Gourmet mini cinnamon rolls (serves 32), 1 serving (18 g)	3

Doughnuts

Clyde's

Donuts, apple cider, 2 oz	9

Duchess

Chocolate donuts, 6 donuts (227 g)	19

Entenmann's

Classic rich frosted donuts, 1 (55 g)	13
Donuts, cinnamon, snack size, 4 donuts (57 g)	11
Donuts, classic, pumpkin, 1 donut (57 g)	10
Rich frosted mini party donuts, 1 donut (33 g)	9

Entenmann's Pop'ems

Donuts, rich frosted, 3 pieces (62 g)	15
Powdered donuts, 4 donuts (57 g)	11

Franz

Donuts, old fashioned glazed, maple, 1 donut (57 g)	11

Hostess

Donettes, mini donuts, frosted devil's food, 4 donuts (57 g)	12
Donuts, mini, crunch, 6 donuts (113 g)	20
Donuts, mini, frosted, 6 donuts (85 g)	18
Powdered mini donuts, 4 donuts (60 g)	10

Katz

Donuts, chocolate frosted, 1 donut (65 g)	11

Kinnikinnick

Donuts, cinnamon sugar, 1 donut (45 g)	7

Krispy Kreme

Doughnuts, chocolate iced with kreme filling, 1 doughnut (85 g)	17
Original glazed doughnut, 1 doughnut (49 g)	8

Krispy Kreme Doughnuts

Doughnut holes, 5 pieces (54 g)	8

Krispy Kreme Doughnuts Krispy Juniors

Lemon mini cake doughnuts, 2 pieces (55 g)	9

Bread & Baked Goods

SmartPoints™ value

SmartPoints™ value

Little Debbie

Donut sticks, 2 donuts (78 g)	17
Donuts, coconut crunch, 6 donuts (92 g)	17
Donuts, mini frosted, 4 donuts (60 g)	13
Donuts, mini glazed, 4 donuts (60 g)	12
Donuts, mini powdered, 4 donuts (53 g)	10

Safeway Kitchens

Donut holes, glazed, old fashioned, 4 holes (48 g)	9
Donut holes, powdered, 5 holes (54 g)	9

Tastykake

Cinnamon mini donuts, 4 donuts (52 g)	10
Donuts, mini, powdered sugar, family pack, 4 donuts (52 g)	10
Donuts, mini, rich frosted, family pack, 4 donuts (59 g)	13
Salted caramel flavored mini donuts, 4 doughnuts (65 g)	12

Wegman's

Donut holes, glazed, 4 donut holes (57 g)	10
Donut holes, glazed chocolate, 4 donut holes (57 g)	10
Donut holes, sugared, 5 donut holes (58 g)	10
Donuts, mini, chocolate covered, 3 donuts (63 g)	15

English Muffins

Bays

English muffins, honey wheat, 1 muffin (57 g)	4
English muffins, multi-grain, 1 muffin (57 g)	4
English muffins, original, 1 muffin (57 g)	4
English muffins, sourdough, 1 muffin (57 g)	4

Fiber One

100% whole wheat English muffin, 1 muffin (57 g)	3
Multigrain English muffin, 1 muffin (57 g)	3

Food For Life

English muffins, 7-sprouted grains, ½ muffin (37.8 g)	2
English muffins, sprouted grain, ½ muffin (38 g)	2
English muffins, sprouted whole grain & seed, ½ muffin (38 g)	2
Multi seed gluten free English muffins, 1 muffin (85 g)	4

Food For Life Ezekiel 4:9

English muffins, cinnamon raisin, ½ muffin (37.8 g)	3

Food For Life Gluten free

Brown rice English muffins, ½ muffin (43 g)	4

Franz

100% whole wheat English muffins, 1 muffin (66 g)	4
English muffins, 100% whole wheat, 1 muffin (61.3 g)	3
English muffins, extra crisp, 1 muffin (61 g)	4
English muffins, extra sourdough, 1 muffin (61 g)	3
English muffins, old fashion raisin, 1 muffin (66 g)	5
English muffins, original, 1 muffin (61 g)	4
English muffins, premium, healthy multigrain, 1 muffin (61 g)	3
Original English muffin, 1 muffin (61 g)	3

Giant

English muffins, lite, 1 muffin (56.7 g)	2

Bread & Baked Goods

Giant/Stop & Shop

100% whole wheat English muffin, 1 muffin (56 g)	3
Light English muffin, 1 muffin (55 g)	2
Light multigrain English muffin, 1 muffin (57 g)	3

Glutino

English muffins, gluten free, 1 muffin (80 g)	6

Hannaford

English muffins, wheat, 1 muffin (57 g)	3

Healthy Life

English muffins, 100% whole wheat, 1 muffin (57 g)	3
English muffins, light, 1 muffin (57 g)	2
English muffins, light, multi-grain, 1 muffin (57 g)	2

Kroger

English muffins, original, 1 muffin (57 g)	4
English muffins, pre-split, sourdough, 1 muffin (56 g)	3
Sourdough English muffin, 1 muffin (57 g)	4

L'oven Fresh

pre-sliced English muffins, 1 muffin (57 g)	3

Master

English muffin toasting bread, 1 slice (30.3 g)	2
English muffins, 1 muffin (61 g)	3

Nature's Own

English muffins, 100% whole wheat, 1 muffin (57 g)	3
English muffins, original, 1 muffin (57 g)	4

Nature's Own 100 Calorie

English muffins, multi grain, 1 muffin (57 g)	3

Old Home

English muffin, sourdough, pre-split, 1 muffin (61.5 g)	4

Open Nature

English muffins, multi grain, 1 muffin (57 g)	3

Oroweat

English muffins, 100% whole wheat, 1 muffin (65 g)	5
English muffins, cinnamon raisin, sliced, 1 muffin (68.5 g)	6
English muffins, double fiber, 1 muffin (59 g)	4
English muffins, extra crisp, 1 muffin (59 g)	4
English muffins, fork-split, sourdough, 1 muffin (59 g)	4

Pepperidge Farm

English muffins, 100% whole wheat, pre-sliced, 1 muffin (56.7 g)	4
English muffins, original, pre-sliced, 1 muffin (56.7 g)	4

Rudi's Organic

English muffins, organic multigrain with flax, 1 (56.7 g)	4
English muffins, organic spelt, 1 (56.7 g)	3
English muffins, organic whole grain wheat, 1 (56.7 g)	3

Safeway Kitchens

English muffins, 100% whole wheat, 1 muffin (66 g)	4
English muffins, extra crisp, 1 muffin (57 g)	3
English muffins, sourdough, 1 muffin (57 g)	3

Sara Lee Original

English muffin made with whole grain, 1 muffin (66 g)	4

ShopRite

English muffins, fork split, light, 1 muffin (56 g)	2

Bread & Baked Goods

SmartPoints™ value

Thomas'

Banana bread English muffin, 1 muffin (61 g)	5
Cinnamon raisin English muffin, 1 muffin (61 g)	5
Corn English muffin, 1 muffin (61 g)	4
High fiber plain English muffin, 1 muffin (57 g)	3
Honey wheat English muffin, 1 muffin (57 g)	4
Pumpkin spice English muffin, 1 muffin (61 g)	5
Sourdough English muffin, 1 muffin (57 g)	4

Thomas' Double Protein

Oatmeal English muffin, 1 muffin (61 g)	4

Thomas' Light

Multigrain English muffin, 1 muffin (57 g)	3

Thomas' Original

English muffin, 1 muffin (57 g)	3
Sandwich size English muffin, 1 (92 g)	5
Whole grain English muffin, 1 muffin (57 g)	4

Thomas' Whole Grain

100% whole wheat English muffin, 1 muffin (57 g)	3

Total

100% whole wheat English muffins, 1 muffin (57 g)	3

Trader Joe's

Classic british muffins, 1 muffin (57 g)	4
Whole wheat british muffins, 1 muffin (57 g)	3

Vermont Bread Company

100% whole wheat English muffins, 1 muffin (61 g)	3

Village Hearth Light

English muffins, 1 muffin (47 g)	2

SmartPoints™ value

Wegman's

English muffins, lite, 1 muffin (57 g)	2

Flatbread & Pita

365

Naan, tandoori, whole wheat, 1 (85 g)	8

Arnold Pocket Thins

100% whole wheat flatbread, ½ flatbread (42 g)	3

Flatout

Flatbread, Italian herb, ½ flatbread (39.7 ml)	3
Flatbread, original, 1 each (79.4 ml)	6
Flatbread, thin crust, artisan pizza, rosemary & olive oil, 1 flatbread (48 g)	4

Flatout Foldit

5 grain flax artisan flatbread, 1 flatbread (43 g)	2
Artisan rosemary and olive oil flatbread, 1 flatbread (43 g)	3
Everything artisan flatbreads, 1 (43 g)	3
Flatbread, artisan, traditional country, 1 flatbread (51 g)	4
Hungry girl 100% whole wheat with flax flatbread, 1 flatbread (43 g)	2
Sliders, classic white, 3 pieces (60 g)	4

Flatout Healthy Grain

Flatbread wraps, harvest wheat, 1 flatbread (57 g)	3
Flatbread wraps, honey wheat, 1 flatbread (53 g)	3
Flatbread wraps, multi-grain with flax, 1 flatbread (53 g)	2

Flatout Hungry Girl Foldit

Flatbread, rosemary & olive oil, 1 flatbread (43 g)	3

Bread & Baked Goods

Flatout Light

Flatbread wraps, garden spinach, 1 flatbread (53 g)	2
Flatbread wraps, Italian herb, 1 flatbread (53 g)	2
Flatbread wraps, low fat, original, 1 flatbread (53 g)	2
Flatbread wraps, sundried tomato, 1 flatbread (53 g)	2

Flatout Soft Wraps

100% whole wheat flatbreads, 1 flatbread (53 g)	2

Flatout Thin Crust Flatbreads

Artisan pizza rustic white, 1 flatbread (48 g)	4
Artisan pizza spicy Italian, 1 flatbread (48 g)	4

Food For Life Ezekiel 4:9

Prophet's pocket bread, 1 piece (47 g)	2

Giant

Pita bread, white, 1 pocket (45.3 g)	3

Joseph's

Enriched syrian bread, middle east style, 1 pita (30.3 g)	2
Flax, oat bran & whole wheat pita bread, 1 pita (28 g)	1
Flax, oat bran and whole wheat flour pita bread, 1 pita (38 g)	1
Honey wheat flatbread, 1 flatbread (56 g)	3
Multi-grain flatbread, 1 flatbread (56 g)	2
Pita bread, ½ pita (39 g)	2

Joseph's Heart Friendly

Pita bread, 1 pita (40 g)	1

Kangaroo

Flat bread, Greek pita, 1 pita (74 g)	6
Pita pockets, original white, ½ pita (33 g)	3
Pita pockets, sliced halves, original white, ½ pita (34 g)	3
Pita pockets, sliced halves, whole wheat, ½ pita (34 g)	2
Pita pockets, whole wheat, ½ pita (33 g)	2
Pocket bread, pita, multi-grain, 1 pocket (35 g)	3
Salad pockets, original white, 1 pocket (37 g)	3
Salad pockets, whole wheat, 1 pocket (37 g)	2
Sandwich pockets, multi-grain, 1 pocket (37 g)	2

Kontos Taste of the Mediterranean

Flatbreads, pocket-less pita, traditional white, 1 loaf (79 g)	6

Mediterranean

Pita bread, white, 1 pita (57 g)	4
Pita bread, whole wheat, 1 pita (57 g)	4

Meijer Deli Style

Pitas, wheat, ½ pita (34 g)	2
Pitas, white, ½ pita (34 g)	2

Middle East

Bread, pita pocket, 2 oz	4
Bread, whole wheat pita pocket, 1 pita (57 g)	4

Oasis

Pita bread, Greek, ½ pita (38 g)	3

Opaa

Flatbreads, artisan-style, naan bread, 1 naan (98 g)	9

Oroweat Pocket Thins

Flatbread, 1 pocket (39 g)	3
Flatbread, 8 grain, 1 pocket (42 g)	3
Flatbread, Italian herb, 1 pocket (42 g)	3

Ozery Bakery Morning Rounds

Muesli toastable fruit and grain buns, 1 bun (60 g)	5

Ozery Bakery One Bun

Original multi grain thin sandwich buns, 1 bun (75 g)	6

Perfection Pastry

Pita bread, wheat, ½ pita (34 g)	2

Bread & Baked Goods

Pita Gourmet

Flat bread, white, ½ pita (42.5 g)	3
Flat bread, whole wheat, ½ pita (42.5 g)	4

Stonefire

Tandoor baked naan, 1 (69 g)	6

Thomas' Sahara

100% whole wheat regular size pita pocket, 1 loaf (57 g)	4
White bread regular size pita pocket, 1 loaf (57 g)	5

Toufayan

Flat bread, mediterranean style, wheat, 1 flatbread (79.4 g)	8
Flat bread, mediterranean style, white, 1 flatbread (79.4 g)	8
Low carb pita bread, 1 (57 g)	3
Multi grain pita bread, 1 loaf (56 g)	4
Pita bread, white, 1 loaf (56 g)	4
Pitettes, mini, hearth baked, whole wheat, 5 pieces (50 g)	4
Sweet onion pita, 1 (56 g)	4
Whole wheat pita bread, 1 loaf (57 g)	4

Toufayan Bakeries Pitettes

Whole wheat pita bread, 1 (28 g)	2

Toufayan Bakeries Small Pockets

100% whole wheat with multigrain pocket pita bread, 1 (43 g)	2

Trader Joe's

Middle Eastern flatbread, 1 (64 g)	5
Pita bread, 1 (29 g)	2

Turlock

Pita bread, whole grain, 1 pita (85 g)	4
Pita bread, whole wheat, 1 pita (85 g)	5

Wegman's

Pita bread, white, 1 pita (66.2 g)	4

Matzo

Gefen

Matzah, 1 piece (32 g)	3

Manischewitz

Matzos, thin, 1 matzo (26 o)	3
Matzos, unsalted, 1 oz	3

Yehuda

Matzo-style cracker, square, gluten free, 1 matzo (30 g)	4

Yehuda Matzos

Matzos, 1 piece (32 g)	3

Muffins & Muffin Mixes

All But Gluten

Gluten free blueberry muffin, 1 muffin (62 g)	9

Betty Crocker

Lemon poppy seed muffin and bread mix, ¼ cup (dry)	6
Muffin mix, banana nut, 1 serving (30 g)	5
Muffin mix, blueberry, 1 serving (30 g)	5
Muffin mix, chocolate chip, 1 serving (31 g)	5
Muffin mix, lemon poppy seed, 1 serving (31 g)	5
Quick bread mix, banana nut muffin, 3 Tbsp	4

Butterfly Bakery

Muffins, pumpkin, ½ muffin (51 g)	3

Duncan Hines Simple Mornings

Apple cinnamon premium muffin mix (serves 12), 1 serving mix (38 g)	6

Entenmann's

Chocolate chip muffins, 1 muffin (50 g)	8

Entenmann's Little Bites

Pumpkin muffins, 1 pouch (47 g)	8
Strawberry yogurt muffins, 1 pouch (47 g)	8

Fiber One

Blueberry premium muffin mix, ¼ CUP	6

Flax4Life

Muffins, flax, mini, chocolate brownie, 1 muffin (33 g)	5

Garden Lites

Veggie muffins, blueberry oat, 1 muffin (56 g)	5
Veggie muffins, carrot berry, 1 muffin (56 g)	5
Veggie muffins, zucchini banana chocolate chip, 1 muffin (56 g)	5
Veggie muffins, zucchini chocolate, 1 muffin (56 g)	5

Garden Lites Veggie Muffins

Zucchini chocolate muffins, 1 muffin (56 g)	5

Hostess

Mini blueberry muffins, 1 package (57 g)	7
Mini chocolate chip muffins, 1 package (46 g)	8

Jiffy

Vegetarian corn muffin mix, ¼ cup dry	6

Krusteaz

Blueberry swirl crumb cake and muffin mix with 1 tbsp topping, ¼ cup dry mix	7
Muffin mix, banana, ⅓ cup	6
Muffin mix, supreme, fat free, cranberry orange, 1 muffin (36 g)	6
Muffin mix, supreme, fat free, wild blueberry, 1 muffin (45 g)	6
Southern cornbread and muffin mix, ¼ cup dry	3

Little Debbie

Little muffins, blueberry, 1 pouch (47 g)	8
Little muffins, chocolate chip, 1 pouch (47 g)	8

Martha White

Chocolate chocolate chip muffin mix, ¼ cup dry	7

Otis Spunkmeyer

Banana nut muffin, ½ muffin (57 g)	9

Pillsbury Sugar Free

Deluxe cinnamon swirl quick bread and muffin mix (serves 14), 1 serving (33 g)	3

Safeway

Muffin, banana nut, 1 muffin (102 g)	17
Muffin, blueberry, 1 muffin (102 g)	17
Muffin, bran, 1 muffin (102 g)	16
Muffin, chocolate chip, 1 muffin (102 g)	20

Thomas' Hearty Muffins

Corn, 1 muffin (61 g)	4

Trader Joe's

Cranberry mango blueberry bran muffins, ½ muffin (68 g)	4
Protein power banana chocolate chunk muffins, 1 (57 g)	5
Pumpkin bread and muffin mix, ¼ cup	7

Udi's

Muffin tops, chocolate chip, 1 (57 g)	8
Muffins, blueberry, 3 oz	11

Udi's Gluten Free

Blueberry oat muffin-tops, 1 muffin top (57 g)	6

Vitalicious VitaMuffin

Deep chocolate vita muffin mix (serves 6), 1 serving (30 g)	4

Vitalicious VitaMuffin 100 Calories

Deep chocolate muffin, 1 muffin (55 g)	4

Bread & Baked Goods

	SmartPoints™ value
Vitalicious VitaTops	
Banana choco chip muffin top, 1 (55 g)	4
Chocolate chip muffin top, 1 vitatop (55 g)	4
Wild blueberry, 1 vitatop (55 g)	4
Vitalicious VitaTops 100 Calories	
Apple crumb muffin top, 1 vitatop (55 g)	4
Banana nut muffin top, 1 vitatop (55 g)	3
Carrot cake muffin top, 1 vitatop (55 g)	4
Chocolate peanut butter chip muffin top, 1 vitatop (55 g)	4
Cran bran muffin top, 1 vitatop (55 g)	4
Deep chocolate muffin top, 1 vitatop (55 g)	4
Fudgy peanut butter chip muffin top, 1 vitatop (55 g)	4
Golden corn muffin top, 1 vitatop (55 g)	4
Sugar free velvety chocolate muffin top, 1 vitatop (55 g)	3
Triple chocolate chunk muffin top, 1 vitatop (55 g)	4
VitaMuffin	
Muffin, blue bran, 1 muffin (55 g)	4
VitaMuffin VitaTops	
Deep chocolate muffin top, 1 (55 g)	4

Rolls & Buns

	SmartPoints™ value
Alexia	
Classic French rolls, 1 roll (42.5 g)	3
Dinner rolls, stone baked artisan, multi-grain, 1 roll (50 g)	4
Alexia Artisan Breads	
Italian style rolls, ciabatta, with rose mary and olive oil, 1 roll (42.5 g)	3
Roll, whole grain, 1 roll (43 g)	2

	SmartPoints™ value
Amoroso's	
Rolls, club, 1 roll (57 g)	4
Rolls, Italian, 1 roll (74 g)	5
Anzio & Sons	
Rolls, kaiser, 1 roll (56 g)	5
Arnold Sandwich Thins	
100% whole wheat roll, 1 roll (43 g)	3
Everything roll, 1 roll (43 g)	3
Flax and fiber roll, 1 roll (43 g)	3
Honey wheat rolls, 1 roll (43 g)	3
Multi-grain roll, 1 roll (43 g)	3
Aunt Hattie's Country Rolls	
Potato dinner roll, 1 roll (33 g)	3
Aunt Millie's	
Buns, enriched, onion, 1 bun (64 g)	6
Aunt Millie's Deli Style	
Sub buns, mini, 1 bun (66 g)	5
Aunt Millie's Slimwiches	
Buns, slim, pre-sliced, 100% whole wheat, 1 bun (42 g)	3
Buns, slim, pre-sliced, white with whole grain, 1 bun (42 g)	3
Big Marty's	
Rolls, large, 1 roll (63.8 g)	5
Bob Evans	
Rolls, white dinner, 1 roll (51 g)	6
Brownberry	
100% whole wheat sandwich thins, 1 roll (43 g)	3
Honey wheat sandwich thin, 1 roll (43 g)	3
Multi-grain sandwich thin, 1 roll (43 g)	3
Onion bun, 1 roll (64 g)	6
Brownberry Crustini	
Sandwich rolls, 1 roll (64 g)	5
Brownberry Stadium Style	
Crustini buns, 1 bun (64 g)	5

Butternut

Burger buns, 1 bun (43 g)	3

Calise & Sons

Rolls, bulkie, enriched, deli, 1 roll (61.3 g)	5
Torpedo rolls, 1 roll (75.5 g)	6

Chabaso Bakery

Ciabatta rolls, 2 oz	3
Ciabatta rolls, classic, 1 roll (57 g)	4

Cobblestone Bread Co.

Wheat grinders sub roll, 1 roll (90 g)	7
White grinder sub roll, 1 roll (90 g)	7

Damascus Bakeries Roll-Up

Flax flatbread, 1 roll up (57 g)	2

Deli Breads

Rolls, 1 roll (66.2 g)	6

D'Italiano Deli

Hero rolls, 1 roll (70.8 g)	5

Earth Grains

100% multi-grain thin bun, 1 bun (43 g)	3
100% whole wheat thin bun, 1 bun (43 g)	3

Eating Right For Calorie Counting

Sandwich slenders, multigrain, 1 bun (43 g)	3
Sandwich slenders, whole wheat, 1 bun (43 g)	3

Essential Everyday

Rolls, dinner, garlic, 1 roll (38 g)	3

Fantini

Bulkie rolls, enriched, 2 oz	5

Fiber One 90 Calorie

12 grain thin sandwich roll, 1 roll (43 g)	3

Food Club

Buns, deli-thin sandwich bread, multi-grain, 1 bun (43 g)	3
Garlic knots, hand tied, 1 garlic knot (34 g)	4

Pretzel rolls, soft, 1 roll (49 g)	4
Yeast rolls, parker house style, 1 roll (26 g)	3

Francisco International

Sandwich rolls, French, 1 roll (87 g)	7

Franz

Buns, bar-b-que, sesame, 1 bun (74 g)	6
Buns, mini, sliders, restaurant 24 pack, 1 bun (28 g)	2
Sliders buns, mini, restaurant style, 1 bun (28 g)	2

Fresh Bakery

Hoagie rolls, 1 roll (57 g)	5

Gonnella

Sub buns, 1 bun (71 g)	6

Great Value

Reduced fat crescent rolls, 1 serving (28 g)	3

Hannaford

Dinner roll dough, white, 1 roll (37.8 g)	3
Wheat sub rolls, 8-inch, 1 roll (70.8 g)	5

Healthy Life

Sandwich buns, light, wheat, 1 bun (43 g)	2
Sandwich buns, light, white, 1 bun (43 g)	2

Heiner's Sunny Buns

Buns, super deluxe, 1 bun (52 g)	4

Holsum

Buns, small, round rolls, enriched, 1 roll (33.1 g)	2

Johnsonville

Sausage rolls, 1 roll (71 g)	5

Kasanof's

Onion rolls, 1 roll (66.2 g)	5

King's Hawaiian

Hawaiian sweet roll (12 pack), 1 roll (28 g)	3
Rolls, honey wheat, 1 roll (28 g)	3

Bread & Baked Goods

	SmartPoints™ value
Rolls, sandwich, large, 1 roll (77 g)	10
Rolls, savory butter, 1 roll (28 g)	3
King's Hawaiian Original Hawaiian Sweet	
Mini sub rolls, 1 bun (57 g)	7
Klosterman	
Buns, onion, 1 bun (75 g)	6
Koffee Kup	
Grinder rolls, 1 roll (84 g)	7
Kroger	
100% whole wheat sliders, 1 bun (28 g)	2
Original yeast dinner roll dough, 1 roll (38 g)	3
Kroger Value	
Sandwich buns, 1 bun (43 g)	4
La Brea Bakery	
Dinner rolls, French, take & bake, 1 roll (57 g)	4
La Brea Bakery Take and Bake	
Telera sandwich roll, 1 roll (85 g)	6
Lewis Healthy Life	
100% whole wheat sandwich bun, 1 roll (57 g)	3
L'oven Fresh Sandwich Skinnys	
pre-sliced multigrain buns, 1 roll (43 g)	3
Maier's	
Enriched rolls, Italian style, steak, 1 roll (70.8 g)	6
Rolls, hoagie, Italian style, 1 roll (85 g)	7
Rolls, kaiser, Italian, 1 roll (56.8 g)	5
Martin's	
100% whole wheat potato roll, 1 roll (42 g)	3
Enriched dinner rolls, potato, 1 roll (35.4 g)	3
Long potato rolls, 1 roll (53 g)	4
Potato party rolls, 3 rolls (53 g)	4
Potato roll, 1 roll (53 g)	4

	SmartPoints™ value
Rolls, enriched hoagie rolls, unseeded, 1 roll (95 g)	6
Rolls, potato, sliced, sandwich, whole wheat, 1 roll (35.4 g)	2
Nature's Own	
100% whole wheat sandwich rounds, 1 roll (43 g)	3
Rolls, sandwich, honey wheat, 1 bun (53 g)	4
Sandwich rolls, 100% whole wheat, 1 roll (53 g)	4
Sandwich rounds, 100% whole grain, 1 roll (43 g)	3
Sandwich rounds, healthy multi-grain, 1 roll (43 g)	3
New French Bakery	
Ciabatta roll, 1 roll (57 g)	4
New York	
Ciabatta rolls, olde world, cheese, 1 slice (47 g)	5
Nickle's	
Kaiser buns, deli style, 1 bun (52 g)	5
Opaa	
Skinny buns, 100% whole wheat, 1 roll (40 g)	3
Skinny buns, multigrain, 1 bun (40 g)	3
Skinny buns, white whole grain, 1 bun (40 g)	3
Open Nature	
Sandwich rolls, 100% whole wheat, 1 bun (74 g)	5
Oroweat	
100% whole wheat sandwich thins, 1 roll (43 g)	3
Buns, country potato, sliced, 1 bun (74 g)	6
Sandwich thins, pre-sliced, whole grain white, 1 roll (43 g)	3
Steak rolls, specialty, 1 roll (71 g)	5

Bread & Baked Goods

Oroweat Naturals Sandwich Thins

9 grain pre-sliced roll, 1 roll (43 g)	3
Rolls, pre-sliced, 100% whole wheat, flax & fiber, 1 roll (43 g)	3

Oroweat Sandwich Thins

Rolls, pre-sliced, 1 roll (43 g)	3

Oroweat Select

Sandwich rolls, wheat, 1 roll (57 g)	5

Ozery Bakery One Bun

100 calorie whole wheat thin sandwich buns, 1 bun (40 g)	3

Papa Ciro's

Garlic knots, 1 knot (36 g)	3

Parisian Gold Reserve

Rolls, French bolillo, ½ roll (56.8 g)	4

Pepperidge Farm

Dinner rolls, stone baked artisan, French, 1 roll (50 g)	3

Pepperidge Farm 100 Calorie

Thin rolls, whole grain white, 1 roll (43 g)	3

Pepperidge Farm Bakery Classics

Bun, sliders golden potato, 1 bun (36 g)	3

Pepperidge Farm Classic

Roll, soft hoagie, 100% whole wheat, with sesame seeds, 1 roll (69 g)	5
Roll, soft hoagie, with sesame seeds, 1 roll (69 g)	6
Sandwich buns, mini, slider, 1 bun (36 g)	3
Sandwich buns, mini, wheat slider, 1 bun (36 g)	3
Sandwich buns, onion with poppy seeds, 1 roll (53 g)	4
Sandwich buns, with sesame seeds, 1 roll (46 g)	4

Pepperidge Farm Deli Flats

Thin rolls, 7 grain, 1 roll (43 g)	3
Thin rolls, soft 100% whole wheat, 1 roll (43 g)	3
Thin rolls, soft honey wheat, pre-sliced, 1 roll (43 g)	3

Perfection Deli

Buns, mini sub, 1 bun (66 g)	5

Pillsbury

Dinner rolls, 1 roll (40 g)	4
Dinner rolls, crescent, butter flake, 1 roll (28 g)	4
Dinner rolls, crescent, garlic butter, 1 roll (28 g)	4
Rolls, crescent, big & buttery, 1 roll (43 g)	6
Rolls, crescent, big & flaky, 1 roll (43 g)	6
Rolls, crescent, dinner reduced fat, 1 roll (28 g)	3

Pillsbury Crescent

Rolls, original, 1 roll (28 g)	4

Pillsbury Place 'N Bake

Crescent rounds, original, 1 roll (28 g)	4

Pretzilla

Buns, burger, soft pretzel, 1 bun (91 g)	8
Buns, mini, soft pretzel, 1 bun (40 g)	3
Buns, sausage, soft pretzel, 1 bun (74 g)	6

Rhodes

Rolls, warm-n-serv, crusty, 1 roll (57 g)	4

Rhodes Bake-N-Serv

Dinner rolls, white, 1 roll (37.8 g)	3
Rolls, white dinner, large, 1 roll (57 g)	5
White dinner rolls, 1 roll (37.8 g)	3
Rolls, soft dinner, 1 roll (57 g)	5

Bread & Baked Goods

SmartPoints™ value

Rudi's Organic	
100% whole wheat sandwich flatz, 1 roll (43 g)	3
Buns, 100% whole wheat, 1 bun (63.8 g)	5
S. Rosen's	
Rolls, French, 1 roll (64 g)	5
Sadie Rose Baking	
Buns, brioche, 1 bun (84 g)	7
Sara Lee	
Bun, honey wheat thin style, 1 bun (43 g)	3
Thin style buns made with whole grain white, 1 bun (43 g)	3
Sara Lee Classic	
Dinner roll, 1 roll (40 g)	4
Sara Lee Hearty & Delicious	
Center split deli roll, 1 roll (71 g)	5
White bakery bun, 1 bun (74 g)	7
Sara Lee Soft & Smooth	
White mini buns made with whole grain, 1 bun (35 g)	3
Schar	
Ciabatta rolls, multigrain, 1 roll (50 g)	4
Rolls, parbaked, ciabatta, 1 roll (50 g)	3
Schmidt	
Rolls, potato, sandwich, 1 roll (53.1 g)	4
Schmidt Old Tyme	
Rolls, sandwich, 100% whole wheat, 1 roll (53.1 g)	4
Schwebel's	
Buns, sandwich, enriched, 1 bun (42.5 g)	4
Buns, sandwich, lite, 1 bun (42 g)	3
Buns, sandwich, sweet harvest wheat, 1 bun (50 g)	4
Seattle International	
Hoagie rolls, French, 1 roll (85 g)	7

SmartPoints™ value

ShopRite Kosher	
Rolls, egg challah, 1 roll (61.3 g)	6
Sister Schubert's	
Rolls, soft pretzel, 1 roll (48 g)	4
Rolls, yeast, dinner, 1 roll (42.5 g)	5
Rolls, yeast, dinner, wheat, 1 roll (43 g)	5
Rolls, yeast, Parker house style, 2 rolls (41 g)	5
Sister Schubert's Warm & Serve	
Yeast rolls, parker house style, 2 rolls (41 g)	5
Specially Selected	
Pretzel buns, 1 roll (113 g)	9
Sunbeam	
Wheat sandwich bun, 1 bun (39 g)	2
Trader Joe's	
Multigrain slims sandwich bread, 1 roll (43 g)	3
Whole wheat slims sandwich bread, 1 roll (43 g)	3
Trader Joe's Artisan Breads	
Ciabatta rolls, 1 (57 g)	3
Turano	
Pre-sliced French rolls, 1 each (75.7 g)	5
Village Hearth Slender Rounds	
Multi-grain pre-sliced roll, 1 roll (43 g)	2
Wegman's	
Rolls, kaiser, 1 roll (66 g)	3
Rolls, mini, sliders, 1 roll (26 g)	2
Rolls, submarine, super soft, 1 roll (57 g)	4
Sub rolls, Italiano, 1 roll (99 g)	7
Whole Foods Bread & Circus Bakery	
Slider wheat buns, 1 roll (30 g)	2
Wimberger's	
Rolls, sour dough kaiser, 1 roll (44.9 g)	4

Bread & Baked Goods

Wonder

Brat buns, enriched, 1 roll (52 g)	4

Rolls & Buns, Hamburger & Hot Dog

Albertson's

Hotdog buns, sliced, 1 serving (43 g)	3

Angelic Bakehouse

Sprouted seven grain hamburger bun, 1 bun (57 g)	4

Aunt Hattie's

Potato hamburger bun, 1 bun (53 g)	4
Potato hot dog bun, 1 bun (53 g)	4

Aunt Millie's

Hamburger buns, deluxe, white, 1 bun (60 g)	4
Hamburger buns, homestyle, honey, 1 bun (60 g)	5

Aunt Millie's Hearth

Hamburger buns, Hawaiian, 1 bun (60 g)	5
Hamburger buns, whole grain, 1 bun (60 g)	4

Ball Park

Golden hot dog bun, 1 bun (47 g)	4
Hamburger buns, 1 bun (50 g)	4
Pre-sliced hot dog bun, 1 bun (46 g)	4

Bimbo

Hamburger buns, 100% whole wheat, 1 bun (57 g)	4

Brownberry Select

Hamburger rolls, 1 roll (57 g)	5

Bunny

Hamburger buns, enriched, 1 bun (43 g)	4
Hamburger buns, original, 1 bun (43 g)	3

Cottons

Lite wheat hamburger buns, 1 bun (42 g)	2

Equate Bread

Hot dog buns, 1 bun (39 g)	3

Franz

100% whole wheat hamburger bun, 1 bun (53 g)	4
Hamburger buns, enriched, 1 bun (53 g)	4
Hot dog buns, 100% whole wheat, 1 bun (50 g)	3
Hot dog buns, enriched, 1 bun (48 g)	4

Giant/Stop & Shop

Hamburger rolls, 1 roll (43 g)	4
Light enriched hamburger roll, 1 roll (43 g)	2
Light hamburger roll, 1 roll (43 g)	2
Light hot dog roll, 1 roll (43 g)	2

Great Valley

Hamburger buns, 1 serving (1 g)	3

Great Value

Hamburger buns, 1 bun (43 g)	4

Great Value 80 Calories

99% fat free hamburger bun, 1 roll (43 g)	2
99% fat free hot dog bun, 1 roll (43 g)	2

Healthy Life

Hot dog buns, wheat, light, 1 bun (43 g)	2
Hot dog buns, white, light, 1 bun (43 g)	2

Heiner's

Hamburger buns, enriched, sliced, 1 bun (49.5 g)	3

King's Hawaiian Original Hawaiian Sweet

Hamburger buns, 1 bun (45 g)	6
Hot dog buns, 1 bun (42 g)	5

Kroger

Hot dog buns, 1 bun (39 g)	3

L'oven Fresh

Hamburger buns, 1 bun (43 g)	3

	SmartPoints™ value

Meijer

Pretzel hamburger bun, 1 roll (85 g)	7
Wheat hamburger bun, 1 roll (44 g)	3
White hamburger bun, 1 roll (44 g)	3

Merita

Hamburger buns, lite, wheat, 1 bun (43 g)	2
Sliced enriched hamburger bun, 1 bun (43 g)	4

Nature's Own

Hot dog rolls, 100% whole wheat, 1 roll (46 g)	3
Hot dog rolls, honey wheat, 1 bun (46 g)	4
Whitewheat enriched sliced hamburger bun, 1 bun (50 g)	3

Nature's Own Butter Buns

Hamburger rolls, 1 bun (57 g)	4
Hotdog rolls, 1 bun (53 g)	4

Nature's Own Whitewheat

Hot dog buns, 1 bun (46 g)	3

Oroweat

Hamburger buns, 100% whole wheat, 1 bun (74 g)	6

Oroweat Select

Hot dog rolls, wheat, 1 roll (50 g)	4

Ozery Bakery One Bun

Whole wheat hot dog buns, 1 bun (50 g)	4

Pepperidge Farm

Buns, hot dog, top sliced, classic, 1 roll (50 g)	5

Pepperidge Farm Bakery Classics

Bun, hamburger, 100% whole wheat, 1 bun (51 g)	4
Bun, hamburger, golden potato, 1 bun (53 g)	5
Bun, hamburger, soft white, 1 bun (51 g)	4
Bun, hotdog, golden potato, 1 bun (50 g)	4

	SmartPoints™ value

Pepperidge Farm Classic

Buns, hot dog, side sliced, 1 roll (50 g)	4

Publix

Buns, hamburger, 1 bun (46 g)	4
Buns, hot dog, 1 bun (46 g)	4

Rudi's

Buns, hamburger, multigrain, 1 bun (74 g)	5

Safeway Kitchens

Hamburger buns, enriched, sesame, 1 bun (38 g)	3
Hamburger buns, giant, onion, 1 bun (66 g)	4

Sara Lee

Bun, white hamburger, 1 bun (43 g)	4
Premium white hamburger bun made with whole grain, 1 bun (43 g)	4

Sara Lee 80 Calories & Delightful

Wheat hamburger bun, 1 bun (43 g)	2
Wheat hot dog bun, 1 bun (43 g)	2

Sara Lee Hearty & Delicious

Heart healthy 100% whole wheat hamburger bun, 1 bun (82 g)	6
Sesame seed hamburger bun, 1 bun (74 g)	7

Sara Lee Soft & Smooth

100% whole wheat heart healthy hamburger bun, 1 bun (57 g)	4
Heart healthy wheat hamburger roll, 1 bun (43 g)	4
Heart healthy wheat hot dog bun, 1 bun (43 g)	4
Heart healthy whole wheat hamburger bun, 1 bun (57 g)	4
Hot dog bun made with whole grain, 1 bun (43 g)	4
White hamburger buns made with whole grain, 1 bun (43 g)	4

Schwebel's

Hot dog buns, lite, 1 bun (43 g)	2

ShopRite

Hot dog rolls, light, 1 roll (43 g)	2
Rolls, hamburger, light, enriched, 1 roll (42.5 g)	2

Stroehmann

Hamburger buns, 1 bun (39 g)	3

Stroehmann Dutch Country

Hamburger rolls, potato, 1 roll (53 g)	5

Sunbeam

Hot dog buns, enriched, 1 bun (43 g)	4

Trader Joe's

Whole wheat hamburger buns, 1 (43 g)	3

Udi's

Hot dog buns, classic, 1 bun (64 g)	5

Udi's Gluten Free

Hamburger buns, classic, 1 bun (77 g)	6
Wholegrain hamburger buns, 1 bun (81 g)	5

Village Hearth

Buns, hamburger, light Italian, 1 roll (46 g)	2

Wegman's

Rolls, sliced, hamburger, 1 roll (50 g)	4

Wonder

Hamburger bun, enriched, classic, 1 bun (43 g)	4
Hot dog bun, enriched, classic, 1 bun (43 g)	4

Wonder 80 Calorie

Hamburger bun, wheat, 1 bun (43 g)	3

Stuffing & Stuffing Mixes

Stove Top

Cornbread stuffing mix (serves 6), 1 serving (28 g)	3
Stuffing mix for chicken (serves 6), 1 serving (28 g)	3
Stuffing mix for pork (serves 6), 1 serving (28 g)	3
Stuffing mix for turkey (serves 6), 1 serving (28 g)	3
Stuffing mix, made with whole wheat, for chicken, unprepared, 1 serving (28 g)	3
Stuffing mix, traditional sage, unprepared, 1 serving (28 g)	3

Stove Top Everyday

Stuffing mix, for chicken, ⅓ pouch dry mix (28 g)	3
Stuffing mix, for turkey, ⅓ pouch dry mix (28 g)	3
Stuffing mix, homestyle herb, 1 cup dry	3

Taco Shells

Azteca

Salad shells, 1 tortilla (40 g)	7

Great Value

Taco shells, 2 shells (28 g)	4

Kroger

Taco shells, 2 taco shells (22 g)	3

La Tiara

Taco shells, 1 shell (6.6 g)	1

Old El Paso

Taco shells, crunchy, 3 shells (32 g)	5
Taco shells, crunchy white corn, 3 shells (32 g)	5
Taco shells, super stuffer, 2 shells (37 g)	6

Old El Paso Bold

Nacho cheese flavored taco shells, 2 taco shells (31 g)	6

Bread & Baked Goods

	SmartPoints™ value
Ortega	
Taco shells, white corn, 2 shells (28 g)	4
Taco shells, whole grain corn, 2 shells (28 g)	3
Taco shells, yellow corn, 2 shells (28 g)	4
Ortega Fiesta Flats	
Flat bottom taco shells, 2 (27 g)	4
Taco shells, flat bottom, yellow corn, 3 (30 g)	5
Taco Bell	
Crunchy taco shells, 3 taco shells (32 g)	5
Trader Jose's	
Taco shells, 2 shells (27 g)	4

Tortillas

	SmartPoints™ value
Azteca	
Soft taco size flour tortillas, 2 tortillas (48 g)	4
Ultragrain tortillas, 1 tortilla (38 g)	4
Benita	
Large flour tortillas, 1 tortilla (71 g)	8
Medium flour tortillas, 1 tortilla (49 g)	4
Small fajita flour tortillas, 1 tortilla (37 g)	2
Buena Vida	
Whole wheat tortillas, for low carb diets, 1 tortilla (32 g)	2
Calidad	
Corn tortillas, 2 tortillas (47 g)	3
Soft corn tortillas, 2 tortillas (47 g)	3
Tortillas, flour, soft taco, 1 tortilla (41 g)	4
Tostadas, 2 tostadas (33 g)	5
Charras	
Baked corn tostadas, 2 pieces (25 g)	2
Corn tostadas, 3 pieces (40 g)	7

	SmartPoints™ value
Chi-Chi's	
Flour tortilla, burrito size, 1 tortilla (60 g)	5
Tortilla, flour, fajita style, 1 tortilla (57 g)	5
Tortilla, white corn, soft taco, 1 tortilla (25.5 g)	2
Tortillas, cafe style, enchilada size, 1 tortilla (57 g)	5
Tortillas, fajita style, multi-grain, 1 tortilla (49 g)	4
Tortillas, flour, soft taco size, 1 tortilla (28 g)	3
Whole wheat fajita style tortillas, 1 tortilla (57 g)	5
Chi-Chi's 100 Calorie	
Fajita style tortilla, 1 (43 g)	3
Chipotle	
Flour tortilla (burrito size), 1 (1 g)	9
Don Pancho	
Tortillas, whole wheat, soft taco & wraps style, 1 tortilla (45 g)	4
El Milagro	
Tortillas, corn, 1 tortilla (24 g)	1
El Milagro Blancas	
Tortillas, corn, family pack, 1 tortilla (22 g)	1
Fit & Active	
Multi grain wraps, 1 wrap (53 g)	2
Food For Life	
Sprouted corn tortillas, 2 tortillas (47 g)	3
Sprouted grain tortillas, 1 tortilla (28 g)	2
Tortillas, brown rice, 1 tortilla (57 g)	4
Food For Life Ezekiel 4:9	
Sprouted grain tortillas, New Mexico style, 1 tortilla (57 g)	4
Frescados	
Flour tortilla burrito size, 1 tortilla (44 g)	4

Bread & Baked Goods

Guerrero

4.5" tortillas de maíz blanco (white corn tortillas), 3 tortillas (45 g)	3
6" tortillas de maíz blanco (white corn tortillas), 2 tortillas (50 g)	3
6" tortillas de maíz blanco (white corn tortillas), 2 tortillas (51 g)	3
6" tortillas de maíz estilo ranchero (yellow corn tortilla), 2 tortillas (51 g)	3
7" tortillas de maíz blanco (king size white corn tortilla), 1 tortilla (35 g)	2
8" tortillas de harina (soft taco flour tortilla), 1 tortilla (41 g)	4
8" tortillas de harina integral tortillas (whole wheat flour tortilla), 1 tortilla (41 g)	4
10" tortillas de harina caseras tortillas (flour burrito tortilla), 1 tortilla (70 g)	7
Tortillas de maíz blanco (white corn tortillas), 2 (54 g)	4
Tostadas caseras doraditas, 2 tostadas (32 g)	5
Tostadas, caseras amarillas, 2 tostadas (32 g)	5
Tostadas, nortenas clasicas, 2 tostadas (23 g)	4

Hy-Vee

Tortillas, whole wheat, 1 tortilla (57 g)	5

Joseph's

Oat bran and whole wheat flour tortilla, 1 tortilla (43 g)	2

Kroger

100% whole wheat soft taco size tortillas, 1 (45 g)	4
Tortillas, burrito size, flour, 1 tortilla (71 g)	6

Tortillas, fajita size, flour, 1 tortilla (33 g)	2
Tortillas, soft taco size, flour, 1 tortilla (50 g)	5
Tortillas, soft taco size, wheat, 1 tortilla (50 g)	4
White corn tortillas, 2 (45 g)	3

La Banderita

Extra large burrito grande flour tortilla, 1 tortilla (71 g)	7
Fajitas flour tortilla, 1 tortilla (31 g)	2
Fat free soft taco flour tortilla, 1 tortilla (39 g)	3
Flour tortilla (family pack), 1 tortilla (33 g)	2
Large soft taco flour tortilla, 1 tortilla (45 g)	4
Mini taco corn tortilla, 2 tortillas (36 g)	3
Tostadas, 1 tostada (11 g)	1
Whole wheat fajita flour tortilla, 1 tortilla (28 g)	3
Whole wheat soft taco tortilla, 1 tortilla (45 g)	4

La Banderita Carb Counter

Low carb tortilla, 1 (42 g)	3

La Banderita Low Carb

Soft taco tortilla, 1 tortilla (45 g)	2

La Banderita Xtreme Fiber

Soft taco flour tortilla, 1 tortilla (45 g)	1

La Tortilla

100 calorie 100% whole wheat tortilla, 1 tortilla (58 g)	3
Flour tortillas, original-style, burrito size, 1 tortilla (57 g)	5
Flour tortillas, original-style, soft taco size, 1 tortilla (43 g)	4
Tortillas, corn, hand made style, green chile, 1 tortilla (41 g)	2
Tortillas, white corn, 1 tortilla (41 g)	2
Tortillas, white corn, grande, 1 tortilla (72 g)	4

Bread & Baked Goods

	SmartPoints™ value
Tortillas, yellow corn, 1 tortilla (41 g)	2
Whole wheat low carb/low fat tortillas garlic and herb, 1 tortilla (37 g)	1
La Tortilla Low Carb High Fiber	
Traditional flour tortilla, 1 tortilla (42 g)	2
La Tortilla Smart & Delicious	
100 calorie traditional tortilla, 1 tortilla (58 g)	3
Large whole wheat gourmet tortilla, 1 tortilla (62 g)	2
Soft wraps, mini, fiesta, 1 wrap (29 g)	1
Tortillas low carb high fiber original made with whole wheat, 1 tortilla (37 g)	1
Tortillas, flour, light, 1 tortilla (39 g)	2
Tortillas, soft wraps, mini, multi-bran, 1 wrap (29 g)	1
La Tortilla Soft Wraps	
Tortillas, mini, white whole wheat, 1 wrap (29 g)	1
Mama Lupe's	
Low carb tortillas, 1 serving (36 g)	1
Marcela Valladolid	
Street taco white corn tortillas, 4 tortillas (47 g)	3
Maria and Ricardo's	
Tortillas, soft corn, yellow, handmade style, traditional size, 1 tortilla (41 g)	2
Tortillas, whole wheat, soft taco size, 1 tortilla (48 g)	4
Market Pantry	
Tortilla, flour, for burritos, 10-inch, 1 tortilla (70 g)	6
Meijer	
Tortillas, flour, fajita size, 8", 1 tortilla (57 g)	5
Tortillas, flour, soft taco size, 1 tortilla (28 g)	2

	SmartPoints™ value
Tortillas, flour, soft taco size, family pack, 1 tortilla (26 g)	2
Tortillas, whole wheat, fajita size, 8", 1 tortilla (57 g)	5
Mi Casa	
Tortillas, 100% whole wheat, 1 tortilla (45 g)	4
Tortillas, flour, fajita style, 1 tortilla (40 g)	4
Tortillas, flour, soft taco style, 1 tortilla (42.5 g)	4
Mi Rancho Organic	
Tortillas, corn, hand-crafted, 1 tortilla (33 g)	2
Mi Rancho Taco Sliders	
Tortillas, organic corn, 4 tortillas (59 g)	3
Mission	
100 % whole wheat soft taco flour tortilla, 1 tortilla (45 g)	4
Corn tortillas, 2 tortillas (55 g)	4
Flour tortilla fajita, 1 tortilla (36 g)	3
Flour tortillas, burrito size, 1 tortilla (67 g)	5
Flour tortillas, soft taco size, 1 tortilla (50 g)	5
Gluten free tortillas, 1 (49 g)	4
Large burrito flour tortilla, 1 tortilla (70 g)	6
Tortillas, artisan style, corn & whole wheat blend, 1 tortilla (36 g)	3
Tortillas, artisan style, multigrain, 1 tortilla (36 g)	4
Tortillas, flour, burrito, large, 1 tortilla (70 g)	7
Tortillas, flour, fajita grande, 1 tortilla (42 g)	4
Tortillas, flour, fajita, extra fluffy, 1 tortilla (32 g)	3
Tortillas, flour, homestyle, 1 tortilla (63 g)	6
Tortillas, flour, medium, 1 tortilla (49 g)	4

Bread & Baked Goods

	SmartPoints™ value
Tortillas, flour, medium, soft taco, 1 tortilla (49 g)	4
Tortillas, flour, multi-grain, medium, 1 tortilla (49 g)	5
Tortillas, flour, small, 1 tortilla (36 g)	3
Tortillas, flour, small, fajita, 1 tortilla (32 g)	3
Tortillas, white corn, 2 tortillas (61 g)	4
Tortillas, white corn, super size, 1 tortilla (33 g)	2
Tortillas, whole wheat, 96% fat free, medium, soft taco, 1 tortilla (49 g)	4
Tostadas, horneadas, 3 tostadas (37 g)	4
White corn tortillas, 2 tortillas (42 g)	3
Yellow corn tortillas, 2 tortillas (51 g)	3

Mission 96% Fat Free

Medium soft taco whole wheat tortillas, 1 tortilla (50 g)	4

Mission Carb Balance

Flour tortillas, fajita size, 2 each (28 g)	2
Large whole wheat tortilla burrito, 1 tortilla (70 g)	6
Medium soft taco flour tortillas, 1 tortilla (42.5 g)	4
Tortillas, flour, medium, soft taco, 1 tortilla (42 g)	4
Tortillas, flour, small fajita, 1 tortilla (28 g)	2
Wheat tortillas, fajita size, 1 each (28 g)	2
Whole wheat tortillas (small fajita size), 1 tortilla (28 g)	2

Mission Estilo Casero

Tostadas, 2 tostadas (32 g)	5

Mission Life Balance

Tortillas, whole wheat, medium, 1 tortilla (42 g)	4

Mission Restaurant Style

Flour tortillas, soft taco and burrito size, 1 tortilla (49.6 g)	4
White corn tortillas, 2 tortillas (52 g)	3

Nature's Promise Naturals

Whole wheat tortillas, 1 tortilla (45 g)	4

Old El Paso

Flour tortilla, 2 tortillas (46 g)	5
Flour tortillas, for soft tacos & fajitas, 2 tortillas (50 g)	5
Tortillas, flour, for burritos, 1 tortilla (39 g)	4
Tostada shells, 3 shells (32 g)	5

Old El Paso Stand 'n Stuff

Soft flour tortilla shell taco boats, 2 (47 g)	5

Ole

8 grain soft taco tortilla wrap, 1 tortilla (45 g)	3
Corn tortillas, 2 tortillas (52 g)	4
Corn tostadas, 3 tostadas (35 g)	5
Flour tortillas soft taco large, 1 tortilla (45 g)	3
Flour tortillas, burrito grande, large, 1 tortilla (71 g)	5
Flour tortillas, tortillas de harina, 1 tortilla (32 g)	2
Tortillas, flour, 1 tortilla (33 g)	2
Whole wheat tortilla wrap, 1 tortilla (45 g)	4

Ole Mexican Foods Xtreme Wellness!

Fat free flour tortilla wrap, 1 tortilla (45 g)	3
High fiber low carb tortilla wrap, 1 tortilla (45 g)	2
Spinach and herbs tortilla wrap, 1 tortilla (45 g)	2
Tomato basil tortilla wrap, 1 tortilla (45 g)	2

Bread & Baked Goods

	SmartPoints™ value
Ortega	
Tortillas, flour, 8-inch, 1 tortilla (40 g)	4
Tostada shells, 2 shells (27 g)	4
Whole wheat tortilla, 1 (45 g)	4
Pepito	
Flour tortilla, fajita size, 1 tortilla (28 g)	3
Reser's Fine Foods Baja Café	
Soft taco size flour tortillas, 1 tortilla (43 g)	3
Romero's	
Tortillas, 100% whole wheat grain flour soft regular taco size, 1 tortilla (38 g)	3
Tortillas, flour, casera style, regular/soft taco size, value pack, 1 tortilla (40 g)	3
Rudi's	
Tortillas, gluten-free, plain, 1 tortilla (32 g)	3
Rudi's Gluten Free	
Spinach tortillas, 1 tortilla (32 g)	3
Safeway Kitchens	
Tortillas, flour, medium taco size, 1 tortilla (41 g)	4
White corn tortillas, 2 tortillas (47 g)	3
Santa Fe Tortilla Company	
Homestyle whole grain tortillas, 1 tortilla (57 g)	2
Shurfresh	
Tortillas, flour, 6", 1 tortilla (28 g)	3
Tamxico's Lo - Carb	
Wheat tortillas, 1 tortilla (43 g)	2
Tia Rosa Specialties	
Tortillas, 100% whole wheat, soft taco size, 1 tortilla (38 g)	3

	SmartPoints™ value
Tortilla Land	
Flour tortillas, 1 tortilla (47 g)	4
Tortillas, uncooked, corn, 1 tortilla (40 g)	2
Uncooked flour tortilla, 1 piece (47 g)	4
Trader Joe's	
Brown rice tortillas, 1 (57 g)	4
Corn tortillas, 2 (52 g)	4
Flour tortillas, 1 (48 g)	5
Handmade 100% whole wheat flour tortillas, 1 (55 g)	4
Multigrain flour tortillas with whole grains, flax seed and oat bran, 1 tortilla (42 g)	2
Organic olive oil whole wheat wraps, 1 wrap (68 g)	4
Reduced carb whole wheat flour tortilla, 1 (28 g)	1
Wegman's	
Tortilla, taco, gordita style, 1 tortilla (35 g)	2
Tortillas, burrito, gordita style, flour, 1 tortilla (71 g)	5
Tortillas, whole wheat, 1 tortilla (75 g)	4

Wraps

	SmartPoints™ value
Cedar's	
Whole wheat wrap, 1 wrap (43 g)	2
Wraps, thin white, 1 piece (71 g)	5
Wraps, whole wheat, 1 wrap (71 g)	7
Don Pancho	
High fiber low carb wraps, 1 wrap (60 g)	2
Father Sam's Low Carb	
Wraps, wheat, 1 wrap (44 g)	2
Fiber One	
Vegetable garden wrap, 1 wrap (43 g)	2

Bread & Baked Goods

Fiber One 80 Calorie

Honey wheat wrap, 1 wrap (43 g)	2
Traditional white wrap, 1 wrap (43 g)	2

La Tortilla Smart & Delicious

Gourmet soft wraps, whole grain, white, 1 wrap (62 g)	2
Soft wraps, gourmet, tomato basil, 1 wrap (62 g)	2
Soft wraps, multi grain, 1 wrap (62 g)	2
Softwraps, gourmet, traditional, 1 wrap (62 g)	2
Wraps, gourmet, ivory teff, 1 wrap (66 g)	5

LiveGfree

Plain gluten free wrap, 1 wrap (52 g)	4

Melissa's

Won ton wraps, 4 pieces (28 g)	2

Mission

Garden spinach herb wrap, 1 tortilla (70 g)	7
Wraps, jalapeño cheddar, 1 tortilla (70 g)	6
Wraps, multi-grain, 1 tortilla (70 g)	7
Wraps, original, 1 tortilla (70 g)	7
Wraps, sun-dried tomato basil, 1 tortilla (70 g)	6
Yellow corn extra thin tortillas, 3 tortillas (38 g)	4

Nasoya

Won ton wraps, 8 wrappers (60 g)	4

Ole Mexican Foods Xtreme Wellness!

High fiber low carb tortilla wraps, 1 wrap (45 g)	2
Spinach & herbs tortilla wraps, 1 wrap (45 g)	2
Tomato basil tortilla wraps, 1 wrap (45 g)	2

Toufayan

Gluten free wraps, 1 wrap (52 g)	4
Low carb low sodium wrap, 1 wrap (57 g)	2
Wraps, plain, 1 wrap (57 g)	5
Wraps, wheat, 1 wrap (57 g)	5

Tumaro's Low-In-Carb

New York deli style everything wrap, 1 wrap (60 g)	2
New York deli style pumpernickel wrap, 1 wrap (60 g)	2
New York deli style sourdough wrap, 1 wrap (60 g)	2
Wraps, 9 grain with chia, 1 wrap (40 g)	1
Wraps, ancient grain, 1 wrap (40 g)	1
Wraps, garden veggie, 1 wrap (40 g)	1
Wraps, honey wheat, 1 wrap (40 g)	2
Wraps, multi-grain, 1 wrap (40 g)	1
Wraps, oat with flax, 1 wrap (40 g)	2
Wraps, premium white, 1 wrap (40 g)	1
Wraps, sundried tomato basil, 1 wrap (40 g)	1
Wraps, whole wheat, 1 wrap (40 g)	1

Wrap-itz

Sun dried tomato wraps, 1 tortilla (43 g)	3
Whole wheat wraps, 100% stoneground, 1 tortilla (43 g)	3

Bread & Baked Goods

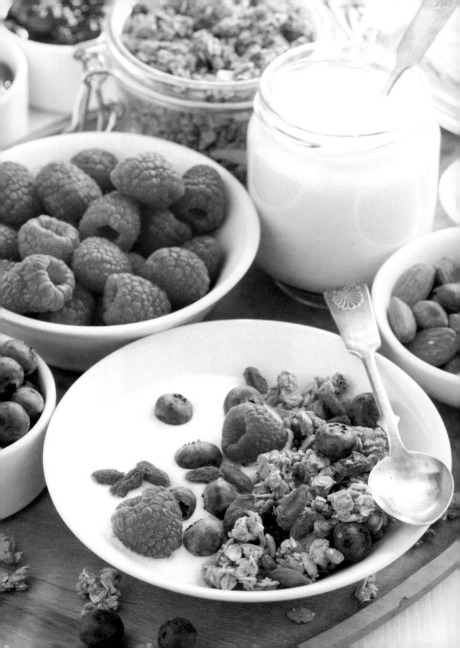

breakfast

Breakfast

Cereal, Hot

Active Lifestyle

Instant oatmeal, raisin, apple, & walnut, 1 pouch (45 g)	5

America's Choice

Oatmeal, instant, sugar free, maple 'n brown sugar, 1 packet (28 g)	3

Better Oats Oat Revolution!

Oats, steel cut, with flax, instant, apples and cinnamon, 1 container (55 g)	8
Oats, steel cut, with flax, instant, classic, 1 pouch (33 g)	4
Oats, steel cut, with flax, instant, maple and brown sugar, 1 container (55 g)	8
Oats, thick & hearty, with flax, instant, apples & cinnamon, 1 pouch (35 g)	5
Oats, thick & hearty, with flax, instant, maple & brown sugar, 1 pouch (43 g)	6
Seasonal blends instant oatmeal with chia, 1 pouch (35 g)	5

Better Oats OatFit

Oatmeal, instant, 100 calories, apples and cinnamon, 1 pouch (28 g)	3
Oatmeal, instant, 100 calories, cinnamon roll, 1 oz	3
Oatmeal, instant, 100 calories, maple and brown sugar, 1 pouch (28 g)	3

Better Oats Raw Pure & Simple

Organic multigrain hot cereal with flax, instant, bare, 1 pouch (42 g)	4
Organic quick oats, ½ cup	4

Bob's Red Mill

10 grain hot cereal, 100% stone ground, ¼ cup	5
Hot cereal, 7 grain, ¼ cup	4
Hot cereal, oat bran, ⅓ cup	3

Hot cereal, rolled whole grain, 5 grain, ⅓ cup	3
Oatmeal, scottish, ¼ cup	4
Rolled oats, extra thick, ½ cup	4
Rolled oats, extra thick whole grain, ½ cup dry	5
Rolled oats, extra thick, organic, ½ cup dry	5
Rolled oats, old fashioned, ½ cup dry	4
Rolled oats, organic, quick cooking, whole grain, ½ cup	5
Rolled oats, organic, whole grain, old fashioned, ½ cup dry	4
Rolled oats, quick cooking, ½ cup dry	4
Rolled oats, whole grain, old fashioned, organic, ½ cup	5
Steel cut oats, ¼ cup dry	5
Steel cut oats, organic, whole grain, ¼ cup	5

Bob's Red Mill Gluten Free

Hot cereal, mighty tasty, ¼ cup	4
Quick cooking oats, ½ cup dry	5
Rolled oats, whole grain, ½ cup dry	5

Bob's Red Mill Organic

Hot cereal, creamy rice, brown rice farina, ¼ cup	4
Oat bran, high fiber, ⅓ cup	3
Oats, steel cut, whole grain, ¼ cup	5

Chex Gluten Free

Oatmeal, gluten free, apple cinnamon, 1 pouch (45 g)	6
Oatmeal, gluten free, maple brown sugar, 1 pouch (45 g)	6
Oatmeal, original gluten free, ½ cup	4

Co Co Wheats

Hot cereal, coco wheats, ⅓ cup	5

Country Choice Organic

Hot cereal, multi grain, ½ cup	3
Oats, Irish style, ¼ cup dry	4
Oats, Irish style, steel cut, ¼ cup	4
Oats, oven toasted old fashioned, ½ cup	4
Oats, quick cook steel cut, 1 packet (40 g)	4

Cream of Wheat

Bananas and cream instant hot cereal, 1 packet (35 g)	5
Cinnabon instant hot cereal, 1 packet (35 g)	5
Maple brown sugar instant hot cereal, 1 packet (35 g)	5
Original 2 ½ minute cook time hot cereal, 3 Tbsp dry cereal	3
Original instant hot cereal, 1 packet (28 g)	3
Whole grain 2 ½ minute cook time hot cereal, 3 Tbsp	3

Dole Fruit & Oatmeal

Apples and brown sugar oatmeal, 1 container (92 g)	7
Blueberries and cream oatmeal, 1 container (92 g)	7
Peaches and vanilla walnut oatmeal, 1 container (92 g)	7

Earnest Eats

Cereal, hot & fit, American blend, ½ cup	5

Essential Everyday

Grits, cheese flavor, 1 packet (28 g)	3
Instant oatmeal, apples & cinnamon, 1 packet (35 g)	5
Instant oatmeal, fruit & cream variety pack, 1 packet (35 g)	5
Instant oatmeal, high fiber, cinnamon swirl, 1 packet (45 g)	5
Instant oatmeal, high fiber, maple & brown sugar, 1 packet (45 g)	5

Instant oatmeal, lower sugar, maple & brown sugar, 1 packet (34 g)	4
Instant oatmeal, maple & brown sugar, 1 packet (43 g)	6
Instant oatmeal, original flavor, 1 packet (28 g)	3
Instant oatmeal, raisins & spice, 1 packet (43 g)	6
Instant oatmeal, strawberries & cream, 1 packet (35 g)	5
Instant oatmeal, variety pack, 1 packet (28 g)	3
Oats, old fashioned, ½ cup	4
Oats, old fashioned, value size, ½ cup	4
Oats, quick - 1 minute, ½ cup	4
Quick 1 minute oats, ½ cup dry	4

Farina Original

Creamy hot wheat cereal, 3 Tbsp	4

Flahavans

Oatmeal, Irish steel cut, ¼ cup dry	4
Oatmeal, Irish steel cut, quick to cook, ⅓ cup dry	4

Giant/Stop & Shop

Honey nut instant oatmeal, 1 packet (43 g)	6
Maple and brown sugar flavored high fiber instant oatmeal, 1 packet (45 g)	5

Giant/Stop & Shop Sugar free

Apples and cinnamon instant oatmeal, 1 packet (28 g)	3
Maple and brown sugar instant oatmeal, 1 packet (28 g)	3

Giant/Stop & Shop Weight Control

Maple and brown sugar instant oatmeal, 1 packet (45 g)	4

Gluten Free Oats

Rolled oats, certified gluten free, ½ cup	4

Breakfast

SmartPoints™ value

Glutenfreeda

Instant oatmeal, apple cinnamon with flax, 1 ¾ oz	6
Instant oatmeal, natural, 1 package (50 g)	5

Good Food Made Simple

Oatmeal, fruit & berry, 8 oz	7
Oatmeal, vermont maple syrup, 1 container (227 g)	6
Unsweetened original oatmeal, 8 oz	4

Great Value

Apple cinnamon sugar free instant oatmeal, 1 packet (28 g)	3
Instant oatmeal, 1 packet (28 g)	3
Maple and brown sugar instant oatmeal, 1 packet (43 g)	6
Oven toasted quick oats, ½ cup dry	4
Sugar free instant oatmeal, 1 packet (28 g)	3

Great Value Morning Trio

Baked apple instant oatmeal (variety pack), 1 packet (43 g)	6

Hannaford

Oatmeal, instant, maple & brown sugar, 1 each (43 g)	6

Harry's Fresh Foods Organic

Oatmeal, steel cut, 1 container (284 g)	6

Hodgson Mill

Hot cereal, multi grain, with milled flaxseed & soy, ⅓ cup	4
Hot cereal, oat bran, ¼ cup	3

Hodgson Mill Premium

Cereal, steel cut oats, ¼ cup	4

Hy-Vee

Instant oatmeal, lower sugar, apples & cinnamon, 1 packet (31 g)	4
Instant oatmeal, maple & brown sugar, 1 packet (43 g)	6

SmartPoints™ value

Instant oatmeal, weight control, maple & brown sugar, 1 packet (45 g)	4
Oatmeal, instant, apples & cinnamon, 1 packet (35 g)	5
Oatmeal, instant, high fiber, maple & brown sugar, 1 packet (45 g)	5
Oatmeal, instant, lower sugar, maple & brown sugar, 1 packet (34 g)	4
Oatmeal, instant, regular flavor, 1 packet (28 g)	3

Jim Dandy

Enriched quick grits, ¼ cup	5

John McCann's

Irish oatmeal, steel cut, ¼ cup	4

Kashi Go Lean

Instant hot cereal, truly vanilla, 1 packet (40 g)	4
Instant hot cereal, with clusters, honey & cinnamon, 1 packet (40 g)	5

Kashi Heart to Heart

Instant oatmeal, apple cinnamon, 1 packet (43 g)	6
Instant oatmeal, golden brown maple, 1 package (43 g)	6

Kroger

Country grits, instant, cheddar cheese flavor, 1 pouch (28 g)	3
Instant country grits, natural butter flavor, 1 pouch (28 g)	3
Instant oatmeal, apple cinnamon, 1 pouch (31 g)	4
Lower sugar instant maple & brown sugar oatmeal, 1 pouch (33 g)	4
Maple & brown sugar instant oatmeal, 1 pouch (43 g)	6
Oatmeal, instant, apple cinnamon, 1 pouch (35 g)	5
Oats, 100% whole grain, ½ cup	4
Old fashioned oats, 100% whole grain, ½ cup	4

	SmartPoints™ value
Original instant grits, 1 packet (28 g)	3
Original instant oatmeal, 1 pouch (28 g)	3
Peaches and cream instant oatmeal, 1 pouch (35 g)	5
Strawberries and cream instant oatmeal, 1 pouch (35 g)	6
Kroger Morning Favorites	
Maple and brown sugar instant oatmeal, 1 packet (43 g)	6
Oatmeal, instant, lower sugar, variety pack, 1 pouch (33 g)	4
Lean Cuisine Morning Collection	
Apple cinnamon and almond oatmeal, 1 oatmeal (113 g)	7
Wild blueberry and pomegranate oatmeal, 1 bowl (170 g)	6
Malt-O-Meal	
Hot wheat cereal, maple & brown sugar, ¼ cup dry	6
Hot wheat cereal, quick cooking, chocolate, 3 Tbsp dry	4
Hot wheat cereal, quick cooking, original, 3 Tbsp	3
Maypo	
Maple oatmeal, instant, ½ cup	5
McCann's	
Irish oatmeal, instant, apples & cinnamon, 1 packet (35 g)	5
Irish oatmeal, instant, regular flavor, 1 packet (28 g)	3
Irish oatmeal, instant, sugar free, maple & brown sugar flavor, 1 packet (28.3 g)	3
Irish oatmeal, instant, varity pack, 1 each (28 g)	3
Irish oatmeal, quick cooking, ½ cup	4
Irish oatmeal, steel cut, ¼ cup	4
Quick & easy steel cut Irish oatmeal (unprepared), ¼ cup	4

	SmartPoints™ value
Meijer	
Instant oatmeal, apples & cinnamon, 1 packet (35 g)	5
Instant oatmeal, sugar free, maple & brown sugar, 1 packet (28 g)	3
Meijer Naturals	
Oats, old fashioned, ½ cup	4
Quick oats, ½ cup	4
Meijer Organics	
Oats, steel cut, ¼ cup dry	4
Mom's Best Naturals	
Quick oats, ½ cup dry	4
Mother's	
Cereal, oat bran, ½ cup	4
My Essentials	
Quick oats, ½ cup	4
Nature's Path Organic	
Instant hot oatmeal flax 'n oats, 1 packet (50 g)	7
Instant hot oatmeal, apple cinnamon, 1 packet (50 g)	7
Instant hot oatmeal, maple nut, 1 packet (50 g)	7
Instant hot oatmeal, optimum power, 1 packet (40 g)	5
Instant hot oatmeal, original, 1 packet (50 g)	5
Instant hot oatmeal, variety pack, 1 packet (50 g)	7
Oatmeal, brown sugar maple, with ancient grains, 1 packet (40 g)	5
Nature's Path Organic Gluten Free Selections	
Homestyle oatmeal, 1 packet (40 g)	5
Spiced apple oatmeal with flax, 1 packet (40 g)	6
Spiced apple with flax gluten free oatmeal, 1 packet (40 g)	6

Breakfast

Breakfast

	SmartPoints™ value
Nature's Promise Organics	
Oatmeal, organic instant, apple cinnamon, 1 packet (35 g)	5
Oatmeal, organic instant, maple, 1 packet (43 g)	6
Oatmeal, steel cut, Irish style, ¼ cup	4
Quick oats, organic, ½ cup dry	4
Open Nature	
Instant hot cereal, multi grain, maple brown sugar with pecans, 1 packet (42 g)	6
Instant hot cereal, multi grain, vanilla, almond and honey, 1 packet (42 g)	6
Oats, steel cut, quick cook, ¼ cup	4
Our Family	
Instant oatmeal, sugar free, maple & brown sugar, 1 packet (28 g)	3
Prairie Mills Old Fashioned	
Oats, steelcut pinhead, ½ cup	5
Private Selection Organic All Natural No Preservatives	
Instant oatmeal, 1 pouch (28 g)	3
Quaker	
Cereal, instant, multigrain instant, ½ cup dry	3
Cereal, instant, oat bran, ½ cup dry	4
Grits, instant, American cheese flavor, 1 packet (28 g)	3
Grits, instant, butter flavor, 1 packet (28 g)	3
Grits, instant, cheddar cheese flavored, 1 packet (28 g)	3
Grits, instant, country bacon flavored, 1 packet (28 g)	3
Grits, instant, original, 1 packet (28 g)	3

	SmartPoints™ value
Grits, instant, red eye gravy and country ham, 1 packet (28 g)	3
Instant oatmeal, bananas and cream, 1 packet (35 g)	5
Instant oatmeal, blueberries and cream, 1 packet (35 g)	5
Instant oatmeal, pumpkin spice, 1 packet (43 g)	6
Oatmeal, instant, 50% less sugar, cinnamon pecan, 1 package (40 g)	5
Oatmeal, instant, apples and cranberries, 1 packet (43 g)	6
Oatmeal, instant, brown sugar, with dinosaur eggs, 1 packet (50 g)	7
Oatmeal, instant, chocolate chip, 1 packet (35 g)	5
Oatmeal, instant, cinnamon and spice, 1 packet (43 g)	6
Oatmeal, instant, cinnamon roll, 1 packet (43 g)	6
Oatmeal, instant, honey bun, 1 packet (35 g)	5
Oatmeal, instant, maple and brown sugar classic recipe, 1 packet (43 g)	6
Oatmeal, instant, raisin date and walnut, 1 packet (37 g)	5
Oatmeal, instant, raisins and spice, 1 packet (43 g)	6
Oatmeal, instant, steel cut, blueberries & cranberries, 1 packet (46 g)	6
Oats, instant, original, 1 packet (28 g)	3
Oats, old fashioned, ½ cup	4
Oats, steel cut, quick 3 minute, ⅓ cup	5
Oats, steel cut, quick 3-minute, brown sugar & cinnamon, 1 packet (48 g)	7
Quaker Express	
Butter instant grits, 1 package (42 g)	4

Quaker Fruit & Cream

Peaches and cream instant oatmeal, 1 packet (35 g)	5
Strawberries and cream instant oatmeal, 1 packet (35 g)	5

Quaker High Fiber

Cinnamon swirl instant oatmeal, 1 packet (45 g)	5
Maple and brown sugar instant oatmeal, 1 packet (45 g)	5

Quaker Lower Sugar

Apples and cinnamon instant oatmeal, 1 packet (31 g)	4
Cinnamon and spice instant oatmeal, 1 packet (34 g)	4
Fruit and cream variety pack instant oatmeal, 1 packet (35 g)	4
Maple and brown sugar instant oatmeal, 1 packet (34 g)	4

Quaker Oatmeal Cups

Apples and cinnamon flavored instant oatmeal to go, 1 container (43 g)	6
Apples and cranberries flavored instant oatmeal to go, 1 container (51 g)	7
Golden brown sugar instant oatmeal, 1 cup	8
Honey and almonds flavored instant oatmeal, 1 cup	6
Maple and brown sugar instant oatmeal, 1 cup	7

Quaker Organic

Maple and brown sugar instant oatmeal, 1 packet (41 g)	6
Regular instant oatmeal, 1 packet (28 g)	3

Quaker Original

Quick instant grits, ¼ cup dry	4

Quaker Perfect Portions

Cinnamon oatmeal no sugar added, ½ cup	4
Maple instant oatmeal, ½ cup	4

Quaker Protein

Banana nut instant oatmeal, 1 packet (61 g)	8
Cranberry almond instant oatmeal, 1 packet (62 g)	8

Quaker Quick Oats

1 minute hot cereal, ½ cup	4

Quaker Real Medleys

Blueberry hazelnut oatmeal, 1 container (70 g)	9
Peach almond oatmeal, 1 container (75 g)	11
Summer berry oatmeal, 1 package (70 g)	9
Super grains banana walnut flavor oatmeal, 1 package (70 g)	10

Quaker Warm and Crunchy

Apple cinnamon granola, 1 packet (48 g)	7
Cranberry almond granola, 1 packet dry (51 g)	7
Honey almond granola, 1 packet dry (48 g)	7

Quaker Weight Control

Banana bread instant oatmeal, 1 packet (45 g)	4
Cinnamon instant oatmeal, 1 packet (45 g)	4
Maple and brown sugar instant oatmeal, 1 packet (45 g)	4

Raley's

Oats, steel cut, ¼ cup dry	4

Real Medley's

Cereal, instant, oatmeal, apple walnut, 1 package (75 g)	11
Cereal, instant, oatmeal, cherry pistachio, 1 package (73 g)	10

Roland

Oats, steel cut, ¼ cup	4

Roundy's

Apples and cinnamon instant oatmeal, 1 packet (31 g)	4

Breakfast

Breakfast

SmartPoints™ value

Safeway Kitchens

Instant oatmeal, apples & cinnamon, 1 packet (35 g)	5
Instant oatmeal, maple & brown sugar, 1 packet (43 g)	6
Instant oatmeal, original flavor, 1 packet (28 g)	3
Oatmeal, quick one minute, ½ cup	4
Oats, old-fashioned, ½ cup	4

ShopRite

Instant oatmeal, original, 1 packet (28 g)	3
Oatmeal, instant, apples & cinnamon, 1 packet (35 g)	5
Oats, old fashioned, ½ cup dry	4
Quick oats, ½ cup dry	4

ShopRite Certified Organic

Oats, Irish style, steel cut, ¼ cup	4

Simple Truth Organic

Maple and brown sugar flavor instant chia oatmeal, 1 pouch (42 g)	6
Natural maple and brown sugar flavored instant oatmeal, 1 pouch (40 g)	6

Simply Balanced

Hot cereal, organic, oat & quinoa blend, ¼ cup dry	3

Special K Nourish

Cinnamon raisin pecan hot cereal, 1 container (52 g)	7
Cranberry almond hot cereal, 1 container (52 g)	7
Hot cereal, maple brown sugar crunch, 1 container (52 g)	6
Maple brown sugar crunch hot cereal, 1 container (52 g)	6

The Silver Palate

Oatmeal, thick & rough, ⅓ cup dry	5

SmartPoints™ value

Trader Joe's

Heart healthy whole grain blueberry instant oatmeal, 1 packet (45 g)	6
Maple and brown sugar instant oatmeal, 1 pouch (43 g)	6
Multigrain triple berry instant hot cereal with flax & chia seeds, 1 packet (42 g)	7
Oatmeal complete maple brown sugar, 1 packet (50 g)	7
Organic cinnamon spice instant oatmeal, 1 packet (40 g)	4
Organic multigrain hot cereal, ½ cup	4
Organic oats & flax instant oatmeal, 1 packet (40 g)	5
Organic oats and flax instant oatmeal, 1 packet (40 g)	5
Pecan pumpkin instant oatmeal, 1 packet (45 g)	7
Quick cook steel cut oats, ¼ cup dry	4
Quinoa and steel cut oatmeal, 1 packet (227 g)	6
Rolled oats, ½ cup	4
Rolled oats, ½ cup dry	4
Steelcut oatmeal, 1 packet (227 g)	5

Umpqua Oats

Oatmeal, all natural, kick start, 1 container (77 g)	12

Umpqua Oats Kick Start

Super premium oatmeal, 1 container (77 g)	11

Wegman's

Oatmeal, instant, high fiber, cinnamon, 1 packet (45 g)	5
Oatmeal, instant, high fiber, maple & brown sugar, 1 packet (45 g)	5
Oatmeal, instant, maple & brown sugar, 1 packet (34 g)	4

Oatmeal, instant, weight control, cinnamon, 1 packet (45 g)	4
Oatmeal, instant, weight control, maple & brown sugar, 1 packet (45 g)	4

Wegman's Food You Feel Good About

Oatmeal, instant, apple & cinnamon, 1 packet (35 g)	5
Oatmeal, instant, maple & brown sugar, 1 packet (43 g)	6
Oatmeal, instant, organic, just oats, 1 packet (40 g)	4
Oatmeal, instant, organic, maple & spice, 1 packet (40 g)	5
Oatmeal, instant, regular flavor, 1 packet (28 g)	3
Oats, organic, steel cut, ¼ cup	4
Quick oats, ½ cup	4

Whole Foods 365 Everyday Value

Oatmeal, instant, apple cinnamon, 1 packet (40 g)	6
Cinnamon spice instant oatmeal, 1 package (40 g)	6
Steel cut oats, ¼ cup dry	4

Wild Oats Marketplace Organic

Instant oats & flax oatmeal, 1 packet (40 g)	5

Cereal, Ready-to-Eat

All-Bran

Cereal, original wheat bran, ½ cup	3
Cereal, wheat bran buds, ⅓ cup	3

All-Bran Complete

Cereal, wheat bran flakes, ¾ cup	3

Alpen

Muesli, no sugar added, ⅔ cup	7
Muesli, original, ⅔ cup	7

Alpha-Bits

Multigrain cereal, 1 cup dry	4

Anahola Granola

Original granola, ½ cup	8

Ancient Harvest

Quinoa flakes hot cereal, ⅓ cup dry	4

Arrowhead Mills

Cereal, puffed corn, 1 cup	2
Cereal, puffed kamut, organic, 1 cup	1
Cereal, puffed wheat, 1 cup	2
Organic flax seed meal, 2 Tbsp	2

Aurora Natural

Granola, cranberry vanilla, ½ cup	9
Granola, vanilla crunch, ⅔ cup	8

Back To Nature

Granola, classic, ½ cup	7
Granola, cranberry pecan, ½ cup	7
Granola, sunflower & pumpkin seed, ½ cup	7

Bakery On Main Gourmet Naturals

Granola, fruit & nut, extreme, ¾ cup	9

Barbara's Original

Cereal, multigrain spoonfuls, ¾ cup dry	4
Cereal, shredded oats, 1 ¼ cups	8

Barbara's Puffins

Cereal, cinnamon, ⅔ cup	3
Cereal, honey rice, ¾ cup	4
Cereal, multigrain, ¾ cup	4
Cereal, original, ¾ cup	3
Cereal, peanut butter & chocolate, ¾ cup	4

Basic 4

Cereal, 1 cup dry	8

Bear Naked

Granola, all natural, peak flax, oats and honey with blueberries, ¼ cup	4
Granola, chocolate elation, ¼ cup	5

Breakfast

Breakfast

	SmartPoints™ value
Granola, fruit and nutty, ¼ cup (dry)	5
Granola, honey and almond, ¼ cup	4
Granola, sea salt caramel apple, ¼ cup	4
Bear Naked 10 g Protein	
Granola, original, cinnamon, ¼ cup	4
Bear Naked Fit	
Granola, vanilla almond crunch, ¼ cup	4
Better Oats Mmm...Muffins	
Oatmeal, thick cut, blueberry muffin, 1 pouch (43 g)	6
Big G	
Cookies n' creme corn puffs, ¾ cup dry	4
Bob's Red Mill	
Granola, apple blueberry, ½ cup dry	6
Granola, honey oat, ½ cup dry	6
Granola, natural, ½ cup dry	6
Muesli, old country style, ¼ cup	4
Bob's Red Mill Gluten Free	
Muesli, ¼ cup dry	4
Cap'n Crunch	
Cereal, cinnamon roll crunch, 1 cup	6
Cereal, crunch berries, sweetened corn and oat, ¾ cup	5
Cereal, oops! all berries, 1 cup	6
Cereal, peanut butter crunch, sweetened corn and oat, ¾ cup	5
Cereal, sprinkled donut crunch, sweetened corn and oat, ¾ cup	5
Cereal, sweetened corn & oat, ¾ cup	5
Cap'n Crunch's Christmas Crunch	
Cereal, sweetened corn & oat, ¾ cup	5

	SmartPoints™ value
Cascadian Farm	
Cereal, fruitful o's, ¾ cup	4
Hearty morning fiber cereal, ¾ cup dry	6
Cascadian Farm Organic	
Apple crisp flavor granola with protein, ¾ cup	8
Berry cobbler granola, ½ cup	7
Berry vanilla puffs cereal, ¾ cup	4
Cereal, cinnamon crunch, 1 cup	4
Cereal, graham crunch, ¾ cup	4
Cereal, honey nut o's, 1 cup	4
Cinnamon crunch cereal, ¾ cup	4
Cinnamon raisin granola, ⅔ cup	9
Dark chocolate coconut protein granola, ¾ cup	9
Granola, French vanilla almond, ¾ cup	8
Granola, oats and honey, ⅔ cup	9
Maple brown sugar granola, ⅔ cup	8
Multi grain squares cereal, 1 cup	6
Purely o's cereal, 1 ¼ cups	3
Raisin bran cereal, 1 cup	7
Cascadian Farm Organic Ancient Grains	
Granola, with a touch of quinoa, spelt and kamut khorasan wheat, 1 cup	8
Cheerios	
Ancient grains cereal, ¾ cup	4
Chocolate flavored whole grain corn and oat cereal, ¾ cup dry	4
Honey nut medley crunch, ¾ cup	4
Original toasted whole grain oat cereal single serve cup, 1 container (39 g)	4
Cheerios Apple Cinnamon	
Naturally sweetened whole grain oat and corn cereal, ¾ cup dry	5

Cheerios Banana Nut

Sweetened corn and oat cereal flavored with real banana and natural banana and nut flavors, ¾ cup — 4

Cheerios Cinnamon Burst

Sweetened whole grain corn and oat cereal flavored with real cinnamon cereal, 1 cup — 5

Cheerios Dulce De Leche

Caramel flavored whole grain corn and oat cereal, ¾ cup dry — 4

Cheerios Frosted

Whole grain oat and corn cereal, ¾ cup dry — 4

Cheerios Honey Nut

Sweetened whole grain oat cereal with real honey and natural almond flavor, ¾ cup dry — 4

Cheerios Honey Nut

Sweetened whole grain oat cereal with real honey and natural almond flavor single serve container, 1 container (52 g) — 8

Cheerios Multi Grain

Peanut butter flavored whole grain toasted oats cereal, ¾ cup dry — 4

Cheerios Multi Grain Dark Chocolate Crunch

Chocolate flavored whole grain corn and oat cereal, ¾ CUP — 4

Cheerios Protein

Cinnamon almond flavored cereal, 1 ¼ cups — 8

Oats and honey cereal, 1 ¼ cups — 8

Chex

Cereal, apple cinnamon, gluten free, ¾ cup — 5

Cereal, honey nut, gluten free, ¾ cup — 5

Cereal, vanilla, gluten free, ¾ cup — 5

Cereal, wheat, ¾ cup — 5

Gluten free corn cereal, 1 cup — 4

Gluten free honey nut corn cereal, ¾ cup — 5

Gluten free honey nut granola mix, ⅔ cup — 9

Gluten free mixed berry almond granola, ⅔ cup — 10

Gluten free oven toasted rice cereal, 1 cup — 3

Gluten free rice cereal with natural chocolate flavor, ¾ cup — 5

Gluten free vanilla sweetened rice cereal, ¾ cup — 5

Chocolate Toast Crunch

Cereal, ¾ cup — 5

Cinnabon

Cereal, 1 cup — 5

Cinnamon Toast Crunch

Cereal, ¾ cup — 5

Cocoa Krispies

Chocolate flavored rice cereal, ¾ cup dry — 5

Rice cereal, ¾ cup — 5

Cocoa Pebbles

Sweetened rice cereal with real cocoa, ¾ cup — 5

Cocoa Puffs

Brownie crunch, ¾ cup — 4

Frosted puffs, reduced sugar, 1 cup — 4

Cookie Crisp

Cereal, ¾ cup — 4

Corn Pops

Sweetened corn cereal snack, 1 pouch (20 g) — 3

Crispix

Cereal, 1 cup — 4

Cereal, corn on one side, rice on the other, 1 cup — 4

Breakfast

Breakfast

	SmartPoints™ value
Crunchy Nut	
Cereal, golden honey nut flakes, ¾ cup	5
Daily Chef	
Swiss granola with raisins, hazelnuts and almonds, ½ cup	8
Enjoy Life Perky's	
Cereal, crunchy flax, original, ¾ cup	6
EnviroKidz Organic	
Cereal, gorilla munch, ¾ cup	4
EnviroKidz Organic	
Cereal, leapin' lemurs, peanut butter & chocolate, ¾ cup	4
Erewhon	
Cereal, crispy brown rice, gluten free, 1 cup	3
Essential Everyday	
Cereal, bran flakes, ¾ cup cereal	3
Cereal, oat squares, crunchy, ¾ cup cereal	4
Granola, with raisins & almonds, ⅔ cup	8
Fiber One	
Nutty clusters and almonds cereal, 1 cup	7
Original bran cereal, ½ cup	2
Raisin bran clusters cereal, 1 cup dry	7
Fiber One 80 Calorie	
Chocolate cereal, ¾ cup	3
Honey squares cereal, ¾ cup	3
Fiber One Protein	
Cranberry almond sweetened granola cereal, 1 cup	8
Maple brown sugar sweetened granola cereal, 1 cup	8
Fit & Active	
Low fat multigrain granola with raisins, ⅔ cup	7
Vanilla almond vitality cereal, ¾ cup	4

	SmartPoints™ value
Food For Life Ezekiel 4:9	
Cereal, almond, ½ cup	5
Cereal, cinnamon raisin, ½ cup	6
Cereal, golden flax, ½ cup	5
Cereal, original, ½ cup	5
French Toast Crunch	
Crispy sweetened corn cereal, ¾ cup	4
Froot Loops	
Sweetened multi-grain cereal, 1 cup	5
Froot Loops Treasures	
Breakfast cereal, 1 cup	5
Frosted Flakes	
Corn cereal cups, 1 container (60 g)	9
Frosted Mini-Wheats	
Big bite wholegrain cereal, 7 biscuits	7
Blueberry flavoured lightly sweetened whole grain cereal, 25 biscuits	7
Cereal, 21 pieces (54 g)	7
Cereal, bite-size, ¾ cups	3
Cereal, blueberry muffin, 24 biscuits	7
Cereal, blueberry muffin, bite size, 25 biscuits	7
Cereal, little bites, chocolate, 52 biscuits	7
Cereal, original, 21 biscuits	7
Cereal, touch of fruit in the middle, raisin, 24 biscuits	6
Maple brown sugar lightly sweetened wholegrain cereal, 25 pieces (55 g)	7
Raspberry mini wheats with touch of fruit in the middle, 1 cup dry	6
Strawberry flavored cereal, 25 biscuits	7

Frosted Mini-Wheats Crunch

Brown sugar cereal, 1 cup dry	7

Frosted Mini-Wheats Little Bites

Original lightly sweetened whole grain cereal, 1 cup	7

Frosted Mini-Wheats Organic

Cereal, whole grain wheat, 24 biscuits	7

Fruity Cheerios

Sweetened whole grain corn and oat cereal, ¾ cup dry	4

Fruity Pebbles

Cereal, sweetened rice, family size, ¾ cup	5
Fruit flavored sweetened rice cereal, ¾ cup	5

Golden Crisp

Cereal, ¾ cup	5

Grape-Nuts Fit

Cereal, cranberry vanilla, ⅔ cup	7

Great Grains

Cereal, whole grain, blueberry pomegranate, ¾ cup	7
Cereal, whole grain, protein blend, honey, oats & seeds, 1 cup	7
Protein blend cinnamon hazelnut cereal, 1 cup	7
Raisins dates and pecans cereal, ¾ cup	8
Super nutty granola, ½ cup	8

Great Grains Digestive Blend

Berry medley whole grain cereal, 1 cup	7
Cereal, whole grain, cinnamon hazelnut, 1 cup	7
Vanilla graham whole grain cereal, 1 cup	6

Great Grains Selects

Banana nut crunch cereal, 1 cup dry	8
Crunchy pecans cereal, ¾ cup	7

Great Value

Awake vanilla almond cereal, ¾ cup	4
Cereal, crunchy nuggets, ½ cup	6
Cereal, crunchy raisin bran, 1 cup	8
Cereal, raisin bran, 1 cup	8
Corn flakes cereal, 1 cup	3
Frosted shredded wheat cereal, 1 cup	6
Honey nut spins cereal, ¾ cup	5
Strawberry awake cereal, 1 cup	4
Toasted corn cereal, 1 cup	4
Toasted whole grain oat cereal, 1 cup	3

Heartland

Cereal, granola, low-fat, ½ cup	8
Cereal, granola, original, ½ cup	9

Honey Bunches of Oats

Cereal with almonds, double pack, ¾ cup	4
Cereal with real apples and cinnamon bunches, ¾ cup	4
Cereal with real tasty strawberries, ¾ cup dry	4
Cereal, crunchy cinnamon flavored granola, ⅔ cup	9
Cereal, fruit blends, peach & raspberry, ¾ cup	4
Cereal, honey roasted, ¾ cup	4
Cereal, honey roasted, family size, ¾ cup	4
Cereal, with almonds, ¾ cup	4
Cereal, with almonds, giant size, ¾ cup	4
Cereal, with banana bunches, ¾ cup	4
Cereal, with cinnamon bunches, ¾ cup	4
Cereal, with vanilla clusters and multi-grain flakes, 1 cup	8
Crunchy honey roasted cereal, ¾ cup	4

Breakfast

SmartPoints™ value

Nutty with pecan bunches cereal, ¾ cup	4
Protein granola with dark chocolate, ½ cup	8
Whole grain honey crunch cereal, 1 cup	8
Cereal, honey roasted, ⅔ cup	9
Honey Bunches of Oats Morning Energy	
Cereal, whole grain, chocolatey almond crunch, 1 cup cereal	8
Honey Comb	
Cereal, 1 ½ cups	5
Honey Smacks	
Cereal, 1 box (32 g)	6
Hy-Vee	
Cereal, shredded wheat, bite size, 1 cup	5
Jif	
Peanut butter cereal, ¾ cup	4
Kashi Cereal	
7 whole grain puffs, 1 cup	2
Berry fruitful cereal, 28 biscuits	6
Cereal squares, honey sunshine, ¾ cup	4
Cereal, 7 whole grain puffs, 1 cup	2
Cereal, berry blossoms, ¾ cup	4
Cereal, flakes, 7 whole grain, 1 cup	5
Cereal, honey puffs, 1 cup	4
Cereal, indigo morning, ¾ cup	4
Cereal, island vanilla, 27 biscuits	6
Cinnamon harvest organic whole wheat biscuits, 28 biscuits	6
Good friends original, 1 cup	6
Heart to heart, ¾ cup	4
Heart to heart cinnamon, ¾ cup	4
Honey sunshine, ¾ cup	4
Kashi u, 1 cup	7

SmartPoints™ value

Organic promise autumn wheat, 29 biscuits	6
Simply maize crispy cornflakes cereal, ¾ cup	4
Kashi Go Lean	
Cereal, 1 cup	5
Cereal, crunch, protein & high fiber, 1 cup	7
Naturally sweetened puff cereal, 1 cup	4
Vanilla graham clusters cereal, 1 cup	5
Kashi Go Lean Crisp!	
Cereal, toasted berry crumble, ¾ cup	6
Cinnamon crumble cereal, ¾ cup	6
Kashi Go Lean Crunch!	
Cereal, ¾ cup	6
Cereal, protein & high fiber, 1 container (45 g)	3
Cereal, protein & high fiber, 1 container (65 g)	8
Honey almond flax cereal, ⅔ cup	7
Multigrain cluster cereal, 1 cup	6
Naturally sweetened multigrain cluster cereal, 1 cup	6
Kashi Good Friends	
Cereal, toasted trio of flakes, twigs & granola, 1 cup	6
Kashi Heart to Heart	
Cereal, honey toasted, ¾ cup	4
Cereal, honey toasted oat, 1 container (40 g)	4
Cereal, oat, warm cinnamon, ¾ cup	4
Honey toasted oat, ¾ cup	4
Honey toasted oat cereal, ¾ cup	4
Oat flakes & blueberry clusters cereal, 1 cup	7
Warm cinnamon oat cereal, ¾ cup	4

Breakfast

Kashi Organic Promise

Raisin vineyard cereal, ¾ cup	6

Kellogg's

Apple Jacks cereal, 1 cup	5
Disney frozen cereal with snow and ice crystal marshmallows, 1 cup	5
Jif peanut butter flavored cereal, ¾ cup	4

Kind Healthy Grains

Fruit and nut clusters, ⅓ cup	3

Kind Healthy Grains

Maple quinoa clusters with chia seeds, ⅓ cup	4
Raspberry clusters with chia seeds, ⅓ cup	4

Kirkland Nature's Path Organic

Ancient grains granola with almonds, ¾ cup	9

Kix

Crispy corn puffs, 1 ¼ cups	4
Crispy corn puffs cereal, 1 ¼ cups	4

Krave

Cereal with chocolate flavored center, ¾ cup	5
Cereal, chocolate, 1 container (53 g)	9
Cereal, s'mores, ¾ cup	5
Cereal, with chocolate flavored center, ¾ cup	5
Cereal, with chocolate flavored center, double chocolate, ¾ cup	5

Kroger

Cereal, 100% natural, oats & honey, ½ cup	9
Cereal, 100% natural, oats, raisins & honey, ½ cup	9
Cereal, crispy rice, 1 ¼ cups	5
Cereal, frosted flakes, ¾ cup	5

Cereal, frosted wheat, original, 1 cup	7
Cereal, honey crisp medley, ¾ cup	4
Cereal, rice bitz, 1 ¼ cups	4
Cereal, shredded wheat, blueberry frosted, bite size, 1 cup	7
Cereal, shredded wheat, strawberry cream frosted, bite size, 1 cup	7
Chocolate toasted oats, ¾ cup	4
Frosted flakes sweetened corn cereal, ¾ cup	5
Granola, low fat, ⅔ cup	9
Honey crisp medley cereal, ¾ cup	4
Honey nut toasted oats cereal, ¾ cup	4
Muesli cereal (serves 7), 1 serving (55 g)	7
Raisin bran cereal, 1 cup	8

Life

Cereal, 1 box (31 g)	4
Cereal, cinnamon, ¾ cup	4
Cereal, maple & brown sugar, ¾ cup	4
Cereal, multigrain, original, ¾ cup	4
Cinnamon cereal, ¾ cup	4
Original multigrain cereal, ¾ cup	4

Low Fat Granola

Original multi-grain cereal, ½ cup	7
With raisins real, ⅔ cup	9

Lucky Charms

Cereal, ¾ cup	4
Cereal, swirled marshmallow charms, ¾ cup	4
Frosted toasted oat cereal with marshmallows, ¾ cup	4

Breakfast

Breakfast

	SmartPoints™ value
Malt-O-Meal	
Cereal, berry colossal crunch, ¾ cup	5
Cereal, frosted mini spooners, 1 cup	7
Cereal, golden puffs, ¾ cup	5
Cereal, honey & oats blender, ¾ cup	4
Cereal, marshmallow mateys, 1 cup	5
Frosted flakes sweetened flakes of corn cereal, ¾ cup	5
Millville	
Bran flakes, ¾ cup	3
Crunchy granola raisin bran, 1 cup	8
Honey crunch 'n oats cereal, ¾ cup	4
Honey nut crispy oats, ¾ cup dry	4
Multigrain crispy oats, 1 cup	4
Millville GetBalance	
Protein and high fiber multigrain cereal, 1 cup	5
Mini-Wheats	
Cereal, bite size, original, 1 container (71 g)	9
Cereal, little bites, chocolate, 52 biscuits	7
Cereal, little bites, frosted, chocolate, 42 biscuits	7
Cereal, little bites, original, 51 biscuits	7
Mom's Best Naturals	
Cereal, honey nut toasty o's, 1 cup	5
Cereal, oats & honey blend, ¾ cup	4
Cereal, sweetened wheat-fuls, 1 cup	7
Müeslix	
Whole grain cereal, ⅔ cup	8
Natural Nutrition	
Cereal, puffed brown rice, 1 cup	2

	SmartPoints™ value
Nature Valley	
Breakfast biscuits, honey, 4 biscuits	8
Cranberry apple crunch protein oatmeal, 1 container (73 g)	9
Mixed berry crunch protein oatmeal, 1 container (73 g)	10
Nature Valley Crunchy	
Oats and honey cereal, 1 cup	9
Nature Valley Protein	
Oats 'n dark chocolate crunchy granola, ½ cup	8
Oats 'n honey crunchy granola, ½ cup	7
Peanut butter granola, ½ cup	8
Nature's Path EnviroKidz Organic	
Cereal, koala crisp, ⅔ cup	4
Nature's Path Love Crunch	
Granola, aloha blend, ¼ cup	6
Granola, organic, fair trade dark chocolate macaroon, ¼ cup	6
Nature's Path Optimum	
Cereal, blueberry cinnamon flax, 1 cup	6
Nature's Path Organic	
Cereal, corn flakes, ¾ cup	4
Cereal, kamut puffs, eco-pac, 1 cup	1
Cereal, smart bran with psyllium & oatbran, ⅔ cup	3
Granola, premium organic, apple crumble, ¼ cup	5
Hemp plus granola, ¾ cup	9
Heritage ancient grains multigrain cereal, ¾ cup	3
Heritage flakes cereal, ¾ cup	4
Mesa sunrise cereal, ¾ cup	4
Optimum slim vanilla low fat cereal, 1 cup	6
Organic chia plus coconut chia granola, ¾ cup	10

Organic granola, premium organic, love crunch, dark chocolate & red berries, ¼ cup	5
Sunrise, crunchy vanilla, ⅔ cup	4
Vanilla almond flax plus granola, ¾ cup	9
Whole o's gluten free cereal, ⅔ cup	4

Nature's Path Organic Envirokidz

Cereal, peanut butter, panda puffs, ¾ cup	5
Corn puffs, gorilla munch, ¾ cup	4

Nature's Path Organic Flax Plus

Cereal, multibran flakes, ¾ cup	3
Cereal, pumpkin raisin crunch, ¾ cup	7
Cereal, red berry crunch, ¾ cup	7
Pumpkin flax granola (dry), 1 oz	5
Pumpkin flax granola cereal, ¾ cup	9

Nature's Path Organic Gluten Free Selections

Granola, honey almond with chia, ¼ cup	5
Granola, summer berries, ¼ cup	5
Sunrise crunchy cinnamon cereal, ⅔ cup	4
Sunrise crunchy honey cereal, ⅔ cup	4

Nature's Path Organic Love Crunch

Dark chocolate and red berries granola, ¼ cup	5

Nature's Path Organic Mesa Sunrise

Cereal, raisins, 1 cup	8

Nature's Path Organic Superfood

Breakfast cereal, qi'a, chia, buckwheat & hemp, cranberry vanilla, 2 Tbsp	4
Breakfast cereal, qi'a, chia, buckwheat & hemp, original flavor, 2 Tbsp	4

Nature's Promise Naturals

Vanilla almond granola, ½ cup	6

Newman's Own Sweet Enough

Cereal, flakes 'n strawberries, ¾ cup	4
Cereal, honey flax flakes, ¾ cup	4

Nutri-Grain

Fruit & oat harvest bar, hearty, country strawberry, 1 bar (50 g)	7

Oatmeal Crisp

Cereal, almond, 1 cup	9
Cereal, hearty raisin, 1 cup	9

Ola

Granola, handbaked, no nut vanilla, ⅓ cup	3

Open Nature

Granola, cranberry nut goodness, ⅔ cup	9
Granola, dark chocolate hazelnut heaven, ⅔ cup	9
Granola, honey nut dream, ½ cup	9
Granola, maple pecan deluxe, ⅔ cup	9
Granola, strawberry vanilla splendor, ¼ cup	4

Our Family Shredded Wheat

Ceral, frosted, bite size, 1 cup	7

Peanut Butter Toast Crunch

Cereal, ¾ cup	5

Product 19

Cereal, toasted corn, oats, wheat and rice., ¾ cup	2

Publix

Cereal, almonds & oats, ¾ cup	4

Puffed Wheat Essentials

Cereal, 1 ¼ cups	1

Purely Elizabeth

Granola, original, ⅓ cup	6
Granola, pumpkin fig, ⅓ cup	5

Breakfast

Breakfast

	SmartPoints™ value
Quaker Corn Bran Crunch	
Cereal, toasted corn, ¾ cup dry	3
Quaker Life	
Cereal, original (single serve), 1 container (65 g)	8
Cinnamon multigrain cereal, ¾ cup	4
Maple and brown sugar cereal, ¾ cup	4
Original multigrain cereal, ¾ cup	4
Quaker Oatmeal Squares	
Cereal, with a hint of cinnamon, 1 cup	7
Golden maple cereal, 1 cup	7
Honey nut cereal, 1 cup	7
Quaker Oh's	
Cereal, honey graham, ¾ cup dry	5
Quaker Puffed Rice	
Cereal, 1 cup	1
Quaker Real Medleys	
Cherry almond pecan multigrain cereal, ¾ cup	9
Dark chocolate cranberry almond granola, ⅓ cup	5
Peach apple walnut multigrain cereal, ¾ cup	9
Summer berry granola, ⅓ cup	4
Supergrains maple pecan raisin flavored oatmeal, 1 package (70 g)	10
Quaker Simply	
Cereal, granola, oats apples cranberries and almonds, ½ cup	7
Cereal, granola, oats honey and almonds, ½ cup	7
Cereal, granola, oats honey raisins and almonds, ½ cup	8
Raisin Bran	
Cereal, 1 cup	7
Cereal with cranberries, 1 ¼ cups	8
Cinnamon almond cereal, 1 ¼ cups dry	8

	SmartPoints™ value
Wheat bran flakes with raisins, 1 cup	7
Whole grain wheat and bran cereal with raisins, 1 cup	8
Raisin Bran Crunch	
Cereal, 1 container (80 g)	12
Toasted flakes, raisins and crunchy oat clusters cereal, 1 cup	8
Raisin Nut Bran	
Cereal, almonds, and covered raisins, ¾ cup	7
Slivered almonds and crisp bran flakes cereal, ¾ cup dry	7
Reese's Puffs	
Hershey's cocoa and Reese's peanut butter sweet and crunchy corn puffs, ¾ cup	5
Rice Krispies	
Cereal, toasted, with brown rice, gluten free, 1 ¼ cups	4
Multi grain shapes cereal, 1 cup	4
Rice Krispies Treats	
Crispy marshmallow squares, ¾ cup	5
Rocky Mountain Chocolate Factory Limited Edition	
Chocolatey almond cereal, 1 cup	9
Safeway Kitchens	
Cereal, bran flakes, ¾ cup	4
ShopRite	
Cereal, bran flakes, ¾ cup	3
Shredded Wheat	
Cereal, honey nut, spoon size, 1 cup dry	8
Cereal, lightly frosted, spoon size, 1 cup dry	7
Shredded Wheat Natural Advantage	
Cereal, original, spoon size, 1 cup dry	5
Cereal, wheat 'n bran, spoon size, 1 ¼ cups (dry)	5

Silver Palate Grain Berry

Cereal, whole grain, toasted oat, honey nut, 1 cup dry	4

Smart Start

Original antioxidants cereal, 1 cup	7

Smart Start Antioxidants

Cereal, 1 box (43 g)	6

Special K

Cereal, blueberry, ¾ cup	4
Cereal, chocolate almond, ⅔ cup	4
Cereal, chocolatey strawberry, ¾ cup	4
Cereal, fruit & yogurt, ¾ cup	5
Cereal, low fat, granola, touch of honey, ½ cup dry	6
Cereal, multigrain oats & honey, ⅔ cup	4
Cereal, oats & honey, ⅔ cup	4
Chocolatey delight cereal, ¾ cup	5
Chocolatey strawberry cereal, ¾ cup	4
Cinnamon pecan cereal, ¾ cup	4
Low fat granola cereal, ½ cup	6
Multigrain cereal, 1 cup	4
Oats and honey cereal, ⅔ cup	4
Original toasted rice cereal, 1 cup	4
Protein plus cereal, ¾ cup	4
Red berries cereal, 1 container (71 g)	10
Red berries cereal, 1 cup	4
Red berries waffles, 2 waffles (70 g)	5
Vanilla almond cereal, ¾ cup	4

Special K Gluten Free

Cereal with a touch of brown sugar, 1 cup	6

Special K Protein

Cereal, ¾ cup	4
Cinnamon brown sugar crunch cereal, ¾ cup	4

Stop & Shop

Cereal, shredded wheat, bite size, 1 ¼ cups	5

Sunbelt

Cereal, granola, fruit & nut, ⅔ cup dry	10

Sunbelt Bakery

Simple granola whole grain cereal, ½ cup	8

Sunbelt Snacks & Cereals

Granola cereal, banana nut, banana's & almonds, ⅔ cup dry	9

Trader Joe's

Bran flakes, ¾ cup	3
Country pumpkin spice granola cereal, ⅔ cup	10
Crunchy oats and honey granola bars, 2 bars (42 g)	7
Fruity O's multigrain cereal, 1 cup	4
Gluten free granola cranberry maple nut, ⅓ cup	5
Gluten free granola loaded fruit & nut, ⅓ cup	5
High fiber cereal, ⅔ cup	3
Honey nut o's, ¾ cup	5
Joe's o's, 1 cup	3
Just the clusters vanilla almond granola cereal, ⅔ cup	8
Low fat granola mixed berry, ¾ cup	8
Lowfat granola with almonds, ¾ cup	8
Multigrain o's cereal, 1 cup	4
Organic high fiber o's cereal, 1 ¼ cups	6
Pecan praline granola, ½ cup	7
Puffed wheat cereal, 1 cup	3
Raisin bran, 1 cup	7
Shredded bite size wheats, 1 cup	5
Toasted oatmeal flakes, ¾ cup	4

Breakfast

Breakfast

	SmartPoints™ value
Trader Joe's Organic	
Honey crunch 'n oats cereal, ¾ cup	4
Joe's o's cereal, 1 cup	3
Trix	
Cereal, reduced sugar, 1 cup	4
Cereal, wildberry red swirls, 1 cup	5
Udi's	
Granola, ¼ cup	4
Granola, cranberry, ¼ cup	4
Granola, natural artisan, au naturel, ¼ cup	4
Granola, natural artisan, vanilla, ¼ cup	4
Granola, original, ¼ cup	4
Granola, vanilla, ¼ cup	4
Uncle Sam	
Cereal, original, value size, ¾ cup	5
Van's	
Cereal, cinnamon heaven, ¾ cup	5
Cereal, honey nut crunch, ¾ cup	4
Cranberry almond granola clusters, ⅓ cup	5
Viki's Granola	
Original honey granola, ¼ cup	5
Weetabix Organic	
Cereal, whole grain biscuit, 2 biscuits	3
Wegman's	
Cereal, bite size shredded wheat, 1 ¼ cups	5
Cereal, crunchy raisin bran, 1 cup	8
Cereal, fiber essentials, ½ cup	2
Cereal, fruit hoops, organic, 1 cup	5
Cereal, natural granola, ½ cup	8
Cereal, oats & honey, with almonds, ¾ cup	4
Cereal, shredded wheat, frosted, bite-size, 1 cup	7

	SmartPoints™ value
Cereal, toasted oats, 1 cup	3
Honey and nut toasted oats cereal, 1 cup	4
Wegman's Food You Feel Good About	
Granola, organic, ancient grain, ¼ cup	4
Wegman's Organic Food You Feel Good About	
Ancient grain granola, ¼ cup	4
Blueberry and flax granola, ¼ cup	5
Cocoa and chia granola, ¼ cup	4
Vanilla and almonds granola, ¼ cup	5
Wheatena	
Cereal, toasted wheat, ⅓ cup	4
Wheaties	
Cereal, ¾ cup	3
Toasted whole wheat flakes, ¾ cup	3
Whole Foods 365 Everyday Value	
Bite size shredded wheat cereal, 1 cup	5
Bran flakes cereal, ¾ cup	3
Wild Harvest Natural	
Granola, crunchy vanilla almond, ⅔ cup	9
Wild Oats Marketplace Organic	
Instant maple & brown sugar oatmeal, 1 packet (40 g)	6

French Toast

Aunt Jemima	
French toast, cinnamon, 2 slices (118 g)	7
French toast, homestyle, 2 slices (118 g)	7
Eggo	
French toaster sticks, original, 2 pieces (90 g)	8

Jimmy Dean Jimmy D's

French toast griddlers, 1 sandwich (102 g)	7

Kroger

French toast, cinnamon swirl, 2 slices (118 g)	8

Krusteaz

French toast, cinnamon swirl, 2 slices (118 g)	8

Trader Joe's

French toast, 1 slice (57 g)	4

Pancakes & Pancake Mixes

Aunt Jemima

Blueberry pancakes, 3 pancakes (104 g)	9
Mini pancakes, 13 pieces (117.4 g)	8
Pancake & waffle mix, buttermilk, complete, three 4" pancakes	5
Pancake & waffle mix, original, 4 pancakes (48 g)	5
Pancake & waffle mix, original, complete, 2 pancakes (45 g)	5
Pancake and waffle mix, buttermilk, ¼ cup mix	3
Pancake, buttermilk, 3 pancakes (105 g)	9

Bisquick

Pancake & baking mix, original all-purpose, ⅓ cup	5
Pancake and baking mix, ⅓ cup	4
Pancake and baking mix, heart smart, ⅓ cup	4
Pancake mix, whole grain, 3 pancakes (62 g)	7

Bisquick Complete

Pancake & waffle mix, simply buttermilk with whole grain, ½ cup mix	7

Bisquick Shake 'N Pour

Pancake mix, buttermilk, 3 pancakes (58 g)	7

De Wafelbakkers

Pancakes, blueberry, 3 pancakes (117 g)	9
Pancakes, buttermilk, 3 pancakes (117 g)	9

Eggo

Pancakes, chocolate chip, 3 pancakes (105 g)	10
Pancakes, minis, 11 pancakes (110 g)	9

Eggo Bites

Chocolatey chip pancakes, 1 pouch (48 g)	5

Fiber One

Buttermilk complete pancake mix, ½ cup dry	5
Original complete pancake mix, ½ cup mix	5

Golden

Pancakes, sweet potato, 1 pancake (38 g)	3

Great Value

Blueberry pancakes, 3 pancakes (117 g)	9

Hodgson Mill

Pancake mix, whole wheat, buttermilk, ⅓ cup	4

Hungry Jack

Buttermilk pancake & waffle mix, ⅓ cup	5
Complete buttermilk pancake & waffle mix, three 4" pancakes	5
Complete extra light & fluffy pancaked & waffle mix, three 4" pancakes	5

Hungry Jack Complete

Belgian waffle mix, ⅔ cup mix	11
Chocolate chip pancake and waffle mix, ⅓ cup dry	6

Breakfast

SmartPoints™ value

Hungry Jack Complete Wheat Blends

Pancake & waffle mix, buttermilk, ⅓ cup	5

Jimmy Dean

Original pancake and sausage on a stick, 1 serving (71 g)	8

Kodiak Cakes

Frontier flapjack and waffle mix, buttermilk & honey, ⅓ cup	4
Frontier flapjack and waffle mix, whole wheat, oat & honey, ⅓ cup	4

Kodiak Cakes Power Cakes

Whole grain buttermilk flapJack and waffle mix, ½ cup	5

Kroger

Pancake & waffle mix, original, 3 pancakes (39 g)	5

Log Cabin

Pancake mix, all natural, ⅓ cup	5

Melissa's

French crepes, nine-inch, 1 crepe (14.2 g)	2

Mrs. Butterworth's

Pancake & waffle mix, buttermilk complete, ⅓ cup mix	6

Pillsbury Heat-N-Go!

Pancakes, mini blueberry, 1 pouch (80 g)	7
Pancakes, mini, maple burst'n, 1 pouch (80 g)	7

Simply Nature

Oatmeal pancake mix, 1 ¾ oz	5
Whole wheat pancake mix, 1 ¾ oz	5

Trader Joe's

Pumpkin pancake and waffle mix, ⅓ cup dry	6
Toasted coconut pancake mix, 1 oz	4

SmartPoints™ value

Van's

Pancakes, multigrain, all natural, 2 pancakes (88 g)	5
Pancakes, wheat gluten free, 2 pancakes (88 g)	6

Toaster Pastries

Glutino

Toaster pastry, gluten free, apple cinnamon flavored, 1 pastry (52 g)	7
Toaster pastry, gluten free, strawberry flavored, 1 pastry (52 g)	7

Kellogg's Limited Edition

Frosted red velvet pastry, 1 pastry (50 g)	8

Kellogg's Pop-Tarts

Birthday cake toaster pastry, 1 (50 g)	8
Frosted blueberry muffin toaster pastry, 1 pastry (50 g)	8
Frosted pumpkin pie toaster pastries, 1 pastry (50 g)	8
Oatmeal delights frosted strawberry toaster pastries, 1 pastry (50 g)	8
Strawberry flavor mini crisps, 1 pouch (14 g)	2
Toasted pastries, frosted chocolatey strawberry, 1 pastry (50 g)	8
Toasted pastries, low fat frosted strawberry, 1 pastry (50 g)	7
Toaster pastries, brown sugar cinnamon unfrosted, 1 pastry (50 g)	8
Toaster pastries, chocolate chip, 1 pastry (52 g)	9
Toaster pastries, frosted blueberry, 1 pastry (52 g)	8
Toaster pastries, frosted chocolate chip cookie dough, 1 pastry (50 g)	8

	SmartPoints™ value
Toaster pastries, frosted cinnamon roll, 1 pastry (50 g)	8
Toaster pastries, frosted confetti cupcake, 1 pastry (50 g)	8
Toaster pastries, frosted cookies & creme, 1 pastry (50 g)	8
Toaster pastries, frosted cookies & crème, 1 pastry (50 g)	8
Toaster pastries, frosted pumpkin pie, 1 (50 g)	8
Toaster pastries, frosted wild! berry, 1 pastry (54 g)	9
Toaster pastries, frosted, brown sugar cinnamon, 1 pastry (50 g)	9
Toaster pastries, frosted, cherry, 1 pastry (52 g)	8
Toaster pastries, frosted, chocolate fudge, 1 pastry (52 g)	8
Toaster pastries, frosted, raspberry, 1 pastry (52 g)	8
Toaster pastries, frosted, s'mores, 1 pastry (52 g)	8
Toaster pastries, frosted, strawberry, 1 pastry (52 g)	8
Toaster pastries, low fat frosted brown sugar cinnamon, 1 pastry (50 g)	7
Toaster pastries, strawberry, unfrosted, 1 pastry (52 g)	8
Toaster pastries, unfrosted blueberry, 1 pastry (52 g)	8
Wildlicious frosted wild cherry toaster pastries, 1 pastry (50 g)	8

Kellogg's Pop-Tarts Gone Nutty!

Chocolate peanut butter toaster pastries, 1 pastry (50 g)	9
Frosted pb and j strawberry toaster pastry, 1 pastry (50 g)	8
Peanut butter toaster pastries, 1 pastry (50 g)	8

Kellogg's Pop-Tarts Printed Fun

	SmartPoints™ value
Frosted sugar cookie toaster pastries, 1 pastry (50 g)	8
Frosted sugar cookie toaster pastry, 1 pastry (50 g)	8

Kellogg's Special K

Blueberry fruit crisps, 2 crisps (25 g)	4
Blueberry pastry crisps, 2 crisps (25 g)	4
Pastry crisps, brown sugar cinnamon, 2 crisps (25 g)	4
Pastry crisps, chocolatey delight, 2 crisps (25 g)	4
Pastry crisps, strawberry, 2 crisps (25 g)	4

Millville

Strawberry pastry crisps, 2 (25 g)	4

Millville 100 Calorie

Blueberry pastry crisps, 2 crisps (25 g)	4

Pillsbury Toaster Scrambles

Pastries, cheese sauce, egg & bacon, 1 pastry (47 g)	6
Pastry, apple with icing, 1 (54 g)	7

Pillsbury Toaster Strudel

Pastries, apple, 1 pastry (54 g)	7
Pastries, blueberry, 1 pastry (54 g)	7
Pastries, cherry, 1 pastry/icing (54 g)	8
Pastries, cinnamon roll, 1 pastry (54 g)	7
Pastries, cream cheese & strawberry, 1 pastry (54 g)	7
Pastries, Danish style cream cheese, 1 pastry (54 g)	8
Pastries, raspberry, 1 pastry (54 g)	7
Pastries, strawberry, 1 pastry (54 g)	7
Pastries, strawberry, value size, 1 pastry, icing (54 g)	7

Breakfast

Breakfast

	SmartPoints™ value
Pastries, sweet delights, Boston cream pie, 1 pastry, icing (54 g)	7
Pastries, wildberry, 1 pastry (54 g)	7
Toaster pastries, with icing packets, chocolate strawberry, 1 pastry (54 g)	7
Rhodes	
Cinnamon rolls, with cream cheese frosting, 1 roll (71 g)	7
Trader Joe's	
Organic cherry and pomegranate frosted toaster pastries, 1 pastry (52 g)	9

Waffles

	SmartPoints™ value
Aunt Jemima	
Waffles, blueberry, 2 waffles (70 g)	6
Waffles, buttermilk, 2 waffles (70 g)	6
Waffles, homestyle, 2 waffles (70 g)	5
Waffles, low fat, 2 waffles (70 g)	5
Eating Right For Gluten Free	
Waffles, gluten free, blueberry, 2 waffles (70 g)	8
Waffles, gluten free, homestyle, 2 waffles (70 g)	7
Eggo	
Chocolate chip waffles, 2 waffles (70 g)	7
Cinnamon toast waffles (3 sets of 4), 3 waffles (92 g)	11
Strawberry waffles, 2 waffles (70 g)	7
Waffles, blueberry, 2 waffles (70 ml)	7
Waffles, buttermilk, family pack, 2 waffles (70 g)	6
Waffles, French toast, 1 waffle (45 g)	5

	SmartPoints™ value
Waffles, homestyle, 2 waffles (70 g)	6
Waffles, homestyle, family pack, 2 waffles (70 g)	6
Waffles, homestyle, value pack, 2 waffles (70 g)	6
Waffles, minis, buttery maple syrup, 3 sets (93 g)	10
Waffles, nutri-grain honey oat, 2 waffles (140 g)	7
Waffles, special k, 2 waffles (70 ml)	5
Waffles, thick & fluffy, cinnamon brown sugar, 1 waffle (55 g)	6
Waffles, thick & fluffy, mixed berry, 1 waffle (55 g)	6
Waffles, thick & fluffy, original recipe, 1 waffle (55 g)	5
Eggo Bites	
Maple flavored waffle, 1 pouch (62 g)	7
Eggo FiberPlus	
Waffles, buttermilk, 2 waffles (70 g)	5
Waffles, chocolate chip, 2 waffles (70 g)	7
Eggo Gluten Free	
Cinnamon waffles, 2 waffles (70 g)	6
Original waffles, 2 waffles (70 g)	6
Eggo Nutri-Grain	
Low fat whole grain waffles, 2 waffles (70 g)	4
Whole wheat waffles, 2 waffles (70 g)	5
Eggo Seasons	
Waffles, pumpkin spice, 2 waffles (70 g)	7
Eggo Thick & Fluffy	
Waffles, original recipe, family pack, 1 waffle (55 g)	5

Eggo Wafflers

Waffle bars, chocolatey chip muffin, 2 waffles (76 g)	10

Fit & Active

Multigrain waffles, 2 waffles (70 g)	6

Giant

Waffles, low fat, homestyle, 2 waffles (70 g)	5
Waffles, multigrain, 2 waffles (70 g)	6

Kashi

Waffles, 7 grain, 2 waffles (72 g)	5
Waffles, blueberry, 2 waffles (72 g)	5

Kellogg's Eggo

Blueberry cobbler Belgian-style waffles, 1 (55 g)	6

Kroger

Waffles, blueberry, 2 waffles (70 g)	7
Waffles, chocolate chip, 2 waffles (70 g)	7
Waffles, cinnamon, 2 waffles (70 g)	7
Waffles, multigrain, 2 waffles (70 g)	6

Nature's Path

Pumpkin spice waffles, 2 waffles (70 g)	7

Nature's Path Organic

Waffles, buckwheat, wildberry, 2 waffles (70 g)	6
Waffles, chia plus, 2 waffles (70 g)	7

Publix

Waffles, whole wheat, 2 waffles (70 g)	6

Trader Joe's

Blueberry waffles, 2 waffles (78 g)	7
Multi grain toaster waffles, 2 waffles (78 g)	8
Toaster waffles (wheat free), 2 waffles (78 g)	8

Van's

Waffles, apple cinnamon, 2 waffles (85 g)	8
Waffles, blueberry, 2 waffles (85 g)	8
Waffles, buckwheat with berries, 2 waffles (85 g)	8
Waffles, lite, totally natural, 2 waffles (76 g)	4
Waffles, mini, homestyle, 8 mini waffles (23.3 ml)	4
Waffles, totally natural, 2 waffles (85 g)	8

Van's Love Your Heart

Totally natural waffle, 2 waffles (76 g)	4

Van's Natural Foods

Gluten free ancient grains waffles, 2 waffles (76 g)	7
Organic waffles, 2 waffles (76 g)	6

Van's Organics

Waffles, blueberry, 2 waffles (80 g)	7

Van's Whole Grains

Multigrain waffles, 2 waffles (76 g)	4

Whole Foods 365 Everyday Value

Multigrain waffles, 2 waffles (70 g)	5

Breakfast

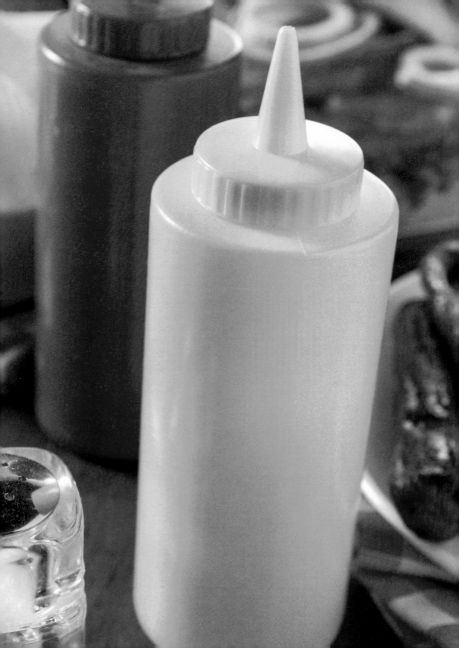

condiments

Sauces & Gravies

Asian Sauces & Condiments

A Taste of Thai

Peanut satay sauce, 2 Tbsp	4

Bennetts

Sweet and sour sauce, Oriental, 2 Tbsp	2

Bragg

Liquid aminos, ½ tsp	0

Campbell's

Skillet sauces, sweet & sour chicken, ¼ cup	2

Coconut Secret

Coconut aminos, raw, 1 tsp	0

Dynasty

Sesame seed oil, 1 Tbsp	4

Frontera

Skillet sauce, classic fajita, medium, 2 Tbsp	1
Skillet sauce, Texas original taco, mild, 2 Tbsp	1

House of Tsang

General tsao sauce, 1 Tbsp	2
Peanut sauce, bangkok padang, 1 Tbsp	2
Stir-fry sauce, classic, 1 Tbsp	1
Stir-fry sauce, szechuan spicy, 1 Tbsp	1

Iron Chef

Sauce & glaze, General Tso's, 2 Tbsp	4

Kikkoman

Orange sauce, 2 Tbsp	4
Ponzu, 1 Tbsp	0
Soy sauce, 1 Tbsp	0
Soy sauce, less sodium, 1 Tbsp	0
Stir-fry sauce, 1 Tbsp	1

Kikkoman Takumi Collection

Teriyaki, original, 1 Tbsp	2

La Choy

Soy sauce, lite, 1 tsp	1
Stir fry marinade sauce, orange ginger, 1 Tbsp	1

Stir fry marinade sauce, teriyaki, 1 Tbsp	0
Sweet & sour sauce, 2 Tbsp	3

Lee Kum Kee

Sriracha mayo, 1 Tbsp	3
Thai sweet chili sauce, 1 Tbsp	1

Lee Kum Kee Select

Hoisen sauce, 2 Tbsp	6

McCormick Skillet Sauce

Sesame chicken stir fry, ¼ cup	2

Panda Express

Sauce, Kung Pao, 2 Tbsp	1

Patak's Simmer Sauce

Medium tikka masala curry, ½ cup	5

Red Shell

Dressing, Japanese miso, 1 tsp	2

Seoul

Kim chi, original, 1 oz	0

Simply Asia

Stir-fry sauce, general tso, 2 Tbsp	4

Soy Vay

Veri veri teriyaki, 1 Tbsp	2

Stonewall Kitchen

Dressing, balsamic fig, 2 Tbsp	4

Sun Luck

Garlic sauce, black bean, Chinese style, 1 Tbsp	1

Terry Hos

Yum yum sauce, 2 Tbsp	6

Trader Joe's

Island soyaki sauce, 1 Tbsp	1
Thai red curry sauce, ¼ cup	4
Thai yellow curry sauce, ¼ cup	4

Trader Ming's

General tsao stir fry sauce, ¼ cup	7
Gyoza dipping sauce, 2 Tbsp	1
Soyaki sauce, 1 Tbsp	2

Wegman's

Thai peanut sauce, 2 Tbsp	2

World Classics

General Tso's sauce, 1 Tbsp	2

Yoshida's

Sauce, original marinade, 1 Tbsp	2

Barbecue & Grilling Sauces

Aunt Jenny's Barbeque Sauce

Barbeque sauce, 2 tsp	2

Bulls-Eye

Bbq sauce, original, 2 Tbsp	3

Campbell's Slow Cooker

Apple bourbon bbq sauce, ¼ cup	3

Famous Dave's

Bbq sauce, rich & sassy, original recipe, 2 Tbsp	3
Bbq sauce, sweet & zesty, 2 Tbsp	4

Head Country

Bar-B-Q sauce, original, 2 tsp	2

IGA

Barbeque sauce, original, 2 Tbsp	2

Jack Daniel's

Barbecue sauce, original no. 7 recipe, 2 Tbsp	2

Jim Beam Sauce

Bbq sauce, 2 Tbsp	1

KC Masterpiece

Barbecue sauce, classic blend, 2 Tbsp	0
Barbecue sauce, original, 2 Tbsp	3
Original barbecue sauce, 2 Tbsp	3

Kinder's

Bbq sauce, mild, 2 Tbsp	4

Kraft

Barbecue sauce, hickory smoke, 2 Tbsp	2
Barbecue sauce, honey hickory smoke, 2 Tbsp	4
Barbecue sauce, original, 2 Tbsp	3
Honey barbecue sauce, 2 Tbsp	3
Original barbecue sauce, 2 Tbsp	3
Slow simmered sweet honey barbecue sauce, 2 Tbsp	3

Montgomery Inn

Sauce, barbecue, 2 Tbsp	2

Muirhead

Barbeque sauce, 1 Tbsp	1

Open Pit

Bbq sauce, original, 2 Tbsp	2

Russell's Barbecue

Sauce, original, 2 Tbsp	1

Sticky Fingers

Barbecue sauce, Carolina sweet, 2 Tbsp	3

Stubb's

Bar-b-q sauce, original, 2 Tbsp	1
Bbq sauce, smokey mesquite, 2 Tbsp	2
Bbq sauce, spicy, 2 Tbsp	1

Sweet Baby Ray's

Barbecue sauce, 2 Tbsp	4
Barbecue sauce, honey, 2 Tbsp	4
Barbecue sauce, honey chipotle, 2 Tbsp	4
Barbecue sauce, sweet 'n spicy, 2 Tbsp	4
Barbecue sauce, sweet vidalia onion, 2 Tbsp	4
Dipping sauce, ray's signature sauce, 2 Tbsp	4
Gourmet sauces, hickory barbecue, 2 Tbsp	4
Hickory and brown sugar barbecue sauce, 2 Tbsp	4

Trader Joe's

All natural barbecue sauce, 2 Tbsp	2
Organic sriracha and roasted garlic bbq sauce, 2 Tbsp	3

Weber's Original

Real molasses bbq sauce, 2 Tbsp	2

Buffalo Wing Sauce

Frank's Red Hot

Wings sauce, buffalo, 1 Tbsp	0
Wings sauce, hot buffalo, 1 Tbsp	0

Condiments, Sauces & Gravies

	SmartPoints™ value
Ken's Steak House	
Marinade & sauce, buffalo wing sauce, 1 Tbsp	0
Moore's	
Buffalo wing sauce, medium, 1 Tbsp	0
Sweet Baby Ray's	
Marinade & sauce, buffalo wing sauce, 1 Tbsp	0
Texas Pete	
Buffalo style wing sauce, 2 Tbsp	1

Cheese Sauce

	SmartPoints™ value
Campbell's	
Skillet sauces, creamy parmesan chicken, ¼ cup	4
Rico's	
Cheddar cheese sauce, nacho, ¼ cup	3
Nacho cheese sauce, 1 cup	5
Velveeta	
Cheese sauce, ¼ cup	6

Chili Sauce

	SmartPoints™ value
A Taste of Thai	
Chili sauce, sweet, red, 1 tsp	1
Frank's Red Hot	
Chili sauce, sweet, 2 Tbsp	4
Heinz	
Sauce, chili, 1 Tbsp	1
Huy Fong	
Chili sauce, sriracha, hot, 1 tsp	0
Maggi	
Sweet chili sauce, mild, 1 Tbsp	2
Texas Pete	
Chili sauce, 1 Tbsp	0
Trader Joe's	
Sweet chili sauce, 1 Tbsp	1

Dessert Sauce

	SmartPoints™ value
Torani	
Sauce, caramel, 2 Tbsp	6
Sauce, chocolate, 2 Tbsp	5

Fruit Sauce

	SmartPoints™ value
GoGo Squeez	
Appleberry applesauce on the go, 1 pouch (90 g)	3
Ocean Spray	
Cranberry sauce, jellied, ¼ cup	6
Cranberry sauce, whole berry, ¼ cup	6
Panda Express	
Sauce, Mandarin, 2 Tbsp	4
Sauce, orange, 2 Tbsp	4

Gravy & Gravy Mixes

	SmartPoints™ value
Bob Evans	
Sausage gravy, 1 cup	10
Campbell's	
Gravy, beef, ¼ cup	1
Gravy, chicken, ¼ cup	2
Gravy, golden pork, ¼ cup	2
Gravy, mushroom, ¼ cup	1
Gravy, turkey, ¼ cup	1
Campbell's Oven Sauces	
Creamy garlic butter chicken sauce, ¼ cup	4
Heinz	
Gravy, fat free, classic chicken, ¼ cup	0
Gravy, fat free, savory beef, ¼ cup	1
Heinz HomeStyle	
Gravy, classic chicken, ¼ cup	1
Gravy, fat free, roasted turkey, ¼ cup	1
Gravy, pork, ¼ cup	1
Gravy, rich mushroom, ¼ cup	1
Gravy, roasted turkey, ¼ cup	1
Gravy, savory beef, ¼ cup	1
Libby's	
Gravy, country sausage, ¼ cup	3
McCormick	
Brown gravy mix, 30% less sodium, 1 Tbsp	1
Country gravy mix, peppered, ¼ cup	2

Gravy mix, brown, 1 Tbsp dry	1
Gravy mix, chicken, 1 Tbsp dry mix	1
Gravy mix, country, original, 1 ⅓ Tbsp dry mix	1
Gravy mix, pork, 1 tsp dry mix	1
Gravy mix, turkey, 2 tsp	1
Mix, brown gravy, 1 Tbsp dry mix	1
Omaha Steaks	
Country style white gravy, 2 oz	2
Pioneer	
Gravy mix, country, ¼ cup gravy	2
Gravy mix, country sausage flavor, ¼ cup gravy	2
Gravy mix, peppered, ¼ cup gravy	2

Hollandaise Sauce

Knorr	
Sauce mix, hollandaise, 1 tsp	0

Horseradish & Horseradish Sauce

Beano's	
Horse radish sauce, 1 Tbsp	1
Boar's Head	
Horseradish sauce, pub style (gluten free), 1 tsp	1
Heinz	
Sauce, horseradish, premium, 1 tsp	1
Inglehoffer	
Horseradish, cream style, 1 tsp	0
Kraft	
Horseradish sauce, creamy, 1 tsp	1
Woeber's Sandwich Pal	
Horseradish sauce, 1 tsp	1

Hot & Latin Sauce

Boar's Head	
Bold fiery chipotle gourmaise, 1 Tbsp	3
Cholula	
Hot sauce, chipotle, 1 tsp	0
Hot sauce, original, 1 tsp	0

Frank's Red Hot	
Cayenne pepper sauce, original, 1 tsp	0
Las Palmas	
Enchilada sauce, green chile, medium, ¼ cup	1
Louisiana	
Hot sauce, 1 tsp	0
Old El Paso	
Enchilada sauce, mild, ¼ cup	1
Ortega	
Taco sauce, hot, 1 Tbsp	0
Taco sauce, mild, 1 Tbsp	1
Taco sauce, original, medium, 1 Tbsp	0
Taco sauce, original, medium, thick & smooth, 1 Tbsp	0
Taco sauce, thick & smooth, original, mild, 1 Tbsp	0
Pace	
Mild original picante sauce, 2 Tbsp	1
Picante sauce, hot, 2 Tbsp	0
Picante sauce, medium, 2 Tbsp	1
Picante sauce, mild, 2 Tbsp	1
The original medium picante sauce, 2 Tbsp	0
Robert Rothschild Farm Gourmet Sauce	
Roasted pineapple and habanero sauce, 2 Tbsp	4
Tabasco	
Pepper sauce, chipotle, 1 tsp	0
Pepper sauce, original flavor, 1 tsp	0
Taco Bell	
Fire sauce, 1 tsp	0
Hot sauce, 1 tsp	0
Mild taco sauce, 1 Tbsp	0
Taco Bell Home Originals	
Bold & creamy sauce, chipotle, 2 Tbsp	4
Tapatio	
Hot sauce, 1 tsp	0

Condiments, Sauces & Gravies

Ketchup

Annie's

Ketchup, 1 Tbsp	1

Heinz

Ketchup, tomato, 1 Tbsp	1
Ketchup, tomato, jalapeño, 1 Tbsp	1
Ketchup, tomato, organic, 1 Tbsp	1
Ketchup, tomato, reduced sugar, 1 Tbsp	0

Heinz Simply Heinz

Ketchup, tomato (no high fructose corn syrup), 1 Tbsp	1

Hunt's

Ketchup, tomatoes, perfect squeeze, 1 Tbsp	1
Tomato ketchup, 1 Tbsp	1

SnowFloss

Tomato catsup, 1 Tbsp	1

Springfield

Tomato catsup, 1 Tbsp	1

Marinades

Bernstein's Light Fantastic

Dressing & marinade, cheese fantastico, 2 Tbsp	1

Garlic Expressions

Salad dressing & marinade, classic vinaigrette, 1 Tbsp	2

Gazebo Room

Salad dressing & marinade, Greek, 1 Tbsp	3
Salad dressing & marinade, Greek, lite, 1 Tbsp	1

Greek Goddess

Salad dressing & marinade, 2 Tbsp	5

KC Masterpiece

Marinade, honey teriyaki with sesame, 1 Tbsp	2

Kikkoman

Marinade & sauce, teriyaki, less sodium, 1 Tbsp	1
Teriyaki marinade & sauce, 1 Tbsp	1

Lawry's

Marinade, Hawaiian, 1 Tbsp	1
Marinade, sesame ginger, 1 Tbsp	2

Lawry's 30 Minute

Marinade, teriyaki with pineapple juice, 1 Tbsp	1

Olde Cape Cod

Vinaigrette & marinade dressing, toasted sesame soy & ginger, fat free, 2 Tbsp	2
Vinaigrette & marinade dressing, wasabi soy & ginger, fat free, 2 Tbsp	2
Vinaigrette & marinade, fat free, toasted sesame soy & ginger, 2 Tbsp	2

Soy Vay

Marinade & sauce, hoisin garlic, 1 Tbsp	3
Marinade & sauce, veri veri teriyaki, 1 Tbsp	2

Mayonnaise

Bama

Mayonnaise, real, 1 Tbsp	3

Best Foods

Dijonnaise, 1 tsp	0
Mayonnaise, low fat, 1 Tbsp	1
Mayonnaise, with canola oil, 1 Tbsp	3

Best Foods Easy Out!

Mayonnaise, light, 1 Tbsp	1

Blue Plate

Light mayonnaise, 1 Tbsp	2
Real mayonnaise, 1 Tbsp	3

Blue Plate Light

Mayonnaise, 1 Tbsp	2

Burman's

Real mayonnaise, 1 Tbsp	3

Cains

Mayonnaise, 1 Tbsp	3
Reduced calorie mayonnaise, light, 1 Tbsp	2

Condiments, Sauces & Gravies

Duke's

Mayonnaise, light, 1 Tbsp	2
Mayonnaise, light, with olive oil, 1 Tbsp	2
Mayonnaise, real, 1 Tbsp	3
Mayonnaise, real, sugar-free, 1 Tbsp	3
Real mayonnaise, smooth & creamy, 1 Tbsp	3

Duke's Light

Mayonnaise, 1 Tbsp	2
Mayonnaise with olive oil, 1 Tbsp	2

Earth Balance Mindful Mayo

Dressing and sandwich spread made with olive oil, 1 Tbsp	3

Essential Everyday

Mayonnaise dressing, with olive oil, 1 Tbsp	2

Gefen

Mayo, lite, 1 Tbsp	2

Gefen Lite

Mayonnaise, 1 Tbsp	2

Hampton Creek

Mayo, 1 Tbsp	3

Heinz

Mayonnaise, real, 1 Tbsp	3

Hellmann's

Aioli, real, classic, 1 Tbsp	2
Dressing, mayonnaise, creamy balsamic, 1 Tbsp	2
Dressing, mayonnaise, low fat, 1 Tbsp	1
Dressing, mayonnaise, with olive oil, 1 Tbsp	2
Mayonnaise, canola, 1 Tbsp	1
Mayonnaise, light, 1 Tbsp	1
Mayonnaise, real, 1 Tbsp	3

Kirkland Signature

Real mayonnaise, 1 Tbsp	3

Kraft

Light mayo, 1 Tbsp	1
Mayo, fat free, 1 Tbsp	0

Mayo, homestyle, 1 Tbsp	3
Mayo, light, 1 Tbsp	1
Mayo, reduced fat, chipotle, 1 Tbsp	1
Mayo, reduced fat, ranch, 1 Tbsp	1
Mayo, reduced fat, with olive oil, 1 Tbsp	1
Mayonnaise, reduced fat, with olive oil, cracked pepper, 1 Tbsp	1
Reduced fat mayo with olive oil, 1 Tbsp	1

Kraft Mayo

Mayonnaise, reduced fat, light, 1 Tbsp	2

Kraft Sandwich Shop

Mayo, hot & spicy, 1 Tbsp	3
Mayo, reduced fat, horseradish-Dijon, 1 Tbsp	1

Kroger

Classic mayo, 1 Tbsp	3
Lite mayo, 1 Tbsp	2
Mayo, classic, 1 Tbsp	3
Mayonnaise, real, classic mayo, 1 Tbsp	3

Market Basket

Mayonnaise, light, reduced calorie, 1 Tbsp	2
Light mayonnaise, 1 Tbsp	1

McCormick

Mayonnaise, with lime juice, 1 Tbsp	4

Meijer

Mayonnaise, lite, 1 Tbsp	1

Safeway

Mayo, canola, 1 Tbsp	2
Mayo, with extra virgin olive oil, 1 Tbsp	2
Mayonnaise, light, 1 Tbsp	1

ShopRite

Mayonnaise, light, 1 Tbsp	1

Smart Balance

Light mayonnaise, 1 Tbsp	2
Light mayonnaise dressing, non-hydrogenated, 1 Tbsp	2

Condiments, Sauces & Gravies

Mayonnaise (cont'd)

Spectrum
Mayonnaise, organic, 1 Tbsp	3

Spectrum Naturals
Light canola mayo, eggless, vegan, 1 Tbsp	1

Trader Joe's
Organic mayonnaise, 1 Tbsp	3
Reduced fat mayonnaise, 1 Tbsp	1
Wasabi mayonnaise, 1 Tbsp	3

Walden Farms
Miracle mayo, 1 Tbsp	0

Wegman's
Mayonnaise, light, 1 Tbsp	2

Wildwood
Mayo alternative, aioli, zesty garlic, 1 Tbsp	3

Woebers Mayo Gourmet
Mayonnaise, roasted chipotle, 1 Tbsp	3

Olives

Alma
Calamata olives, 7 olives	1
Calamata olives, pitted, 7 olives	1

Giuliano
Olives, kalamata, pitted, 4 olives	1

Krinos
Kalamata olives, in vinegar brine, 3 olives	2

Kroger
Olives, kalamata, pitted, 4 olives	1
Olives, ripe, sliced, 2 Tbsp	1

Lindsay
Olives, extra large, pitted, 3 each (14 g)	1
Olives, manzanilla, pimento stuffed, 5 olives	1
Olives, pitted, California ripe, large, 4 olives	1
Olives, sliced, 2 Tbsp	1

Mario
Manzanilla olives, 3 olives	1
Olives, black, sliced, 2 Tbsp	1

Sliced black olives, 2 Tbsp	1
Spanish green olives stuffed with minced pimiento, 2 pieces (16 g)	1

Mezzetta
Blue cheese stuffed olives, 2 olives	1
Greek olives, imported, calamata, 4 olives	1
Olives, calamata, 4 olives	1
Olives, garlic stuffed, 1 olive	0
Olives, jalapeño stuffed, 1 olive	0
Olives, kalamata, sliced Greek, 9 pieces (15 g)	1
Olives, pitted Greek kalamata, 4 olives	1
Olives, stuffed, bleu cheese, 1 olive	0
Olives, whole, green, Italian castelvetrano, 2 olives	1
Stuffed olives, garlic, 1 ½ olives	1

Paesana
Kalamata olives, 2 olives	1

Pearl's
Olives, black California ripe, sliced, 2 Tbsp	1
Olives, black pitted California ripe, large, 4 olives	1
Olives, black pitted California ripe, medium, black, 5 olives	1
Olives, black pitted California ripe, small, 6 olives	1
Olives, black ripe, sliced, 2 Tbsp	1

Pearl's Olives To Go!
Kalamata pitted Greek olives, 5 olives	2
Olives, black ripe, pitted, California, large, 4 olives	0
Olives, pimiento stuffed Spanish green, 3 olives	1

Pearl's Specialties
Olives, Greek, pitted Kalamata, 5 olives	2

ShopRite
Kalamata olives, whole olives, 4 olives	1

Tasso's

Olives, super mammoth, double stuffed jalapeño garlic, 2 olives	1

Trader Joe's

Sliced black olives, 2 Tbsp	1

Tuscan Garden Classics

Stuffed Spanish olives, 5 olives	1

Wegman's

Kalamata olives, pitted, 5 olives	1

Lindsay Recloseables

California sliced ripe olives, 2 Tbsp	1

Pasta Sauce

Artisan Fresh

Pesto, 2 Tbsp	4

Barilla

Pasta sauce, chunky, traditional, ½ cup	3
Pasta sauce, flavored with meat, ½ Cup	3
Pasta sauce, roasted garlic, /2 cup	3
Pasta sauce, tomato and basil, ½ cup	3
Sauce, traditional, ½ cup	3

Bertolli

Alfredo sauce, light, ¼ cup	2
Arrabbiata spicy tomato and red pepper sauce, ½ cup	2
Four cheese rosa sauce, ¼ cup	4
Garlic Alfredo sauce, light, ¼ cup	2
Portobello mushroom with merlot sauce, ½ cup	4

Buitoni

Alfredo sauce, ¼ cup	6
Alfredo sauce, light, ¼ cup	4
Marinara sauce, ½ cup	3
Pesto with basil, ¼ cup	9

Classico

Pasta sauce, parmesan & romano, ½ cup	3
Pasta sauce, traditional, ½ cup	3

Classico Organic

Pasta sauce, tomato, herbs & spices, ½ cup	3

Classico Seasonal Selections

Creamy spinach and parmesan pasta sauce, ½ cup	4

Classico Signature Recipes

Pasta sauce, asiago romano Alfredo, light, ¼ cup	3
Sauce & spread, sun-dried tomato pesto, ¼ cup	4

Classico Traditional Favorites

Pasta sauce, tomato & basil, ½ cup	2
Pasta sauce, traditional sweet basil, value size, ½ cup	3
Tomato and basil pasta sauce, ½ cup	2

Contadina

Sauce, ¼ cup	1

Del Monte Garden Quality

Traditional pasta sauce, ½ cup	3

Hunt's

Pasta sauce (no added sugar), ½ cup	1

Hunt's Pasta Sauce

Chunky vegetable sauce, ½ cup	3

Hunt's Premium

Pasta sauce, cheese & garlic, ½ cup	2
Pasta sauce, Italian sausage flavored, ½ cup	3
Pasta sauce, mushroom, ½ cup	2

Knorr

Pesto sauce mix, 2 tsp	1

Kroger

Homestyle, tomato and basil pasta sauce, ½ cup	4
Traditional pasta sauce, ½ cup	4

Market Pantry

Tomato, basil and garlic pasta sauce, ½ cup	3

Condiments, Sauces & Gravies

Condiments, Sauces & Gravies

	SmartPoints™ value
Mids	
Pasta sauce, homestyle, garlic & onion, ½ cup	3
Pasta sauce, tomato, basil, mushroom, homestyle, ½ cup	2
Newman's Own	
Marinara pasta sauce, ½ cup	3
Newman's Own Organic	
Marinara pasta sauce, ½ cup	3
Prego	
Sauce, Alfredo, basil pesto, ¼ cup	3
Sauce, Alfredo, roasted garlic parmesan, ¼ cup	3
Sauce, creamy cheddar, ¼ cup	3
Sauce, homestyle Alfredo, ¼ cup	3
Sauce, Italian, creamy sundried tomato, ½ cup	5
Sauce, Italian, creamy vodka, ½ cup	7
Sauce, Italian, flavored with meat, ½ cup	4
Sauce, Italian, Florentine spinach and cheese, ½ cup	4
Sauce, Italian, marinara, ½ cup	3
Sauce, Italian, merlot marinara, ½ cup	3
Sauce, Italian, roasted garlic & herb, ½ cup	4
Sauce, Italian, spicy sausage, ½ cup	4
Sauce, Italian, traditional, ½ cup	3
Sauce, meat, Italian sausage & garlic, ½ cup	4
Sauce, meat, mini-meatball, ½ cup	4
Sauce, pasta, savory bacon Alfredo, ½ cup	3
Sauce, pesto, marinara Italian sauce, ½ cup	4
Prego Alfredo Sauce	
Artisan three cheese, ¼ cup	3

	SmartPoints™ value
Prego Chunky Garden	
Italian sauce combo, ½ cup	3
Italian sauce mushroom and green pepper, ½ cup	4
Italian sauce, tomato, onion & garlic, ½ cup	4
Prego Heart Smart	
Italian sauce roasted red pepper and garlic, ½ cup	3
Mushroom Italian sauce, ½ cup	3
Traditional Italian sauce, ½ cup	3
Prego Italian Sauce	
Fontina and asiago cheese, ½ cup	4
Prego Light	
Homestyle Alfredo sauce, ¼ cup	2
Prego Traditional	
Italian sauce fresh mushroom, ½ cup	3
Italian sauce three cheese, ½ cup	4
Italian sauce tomato basil garlic, ½ cup	3
Private Selection	
Authentic restaurant style salsa, 2 Tbsp	0
Sauce, basil pesto, 2 Tbsp	4
Progresso	
Sauce, white clam with garlic and herb, ½ cup	3
Ragu	
Sauce, old world style traditional, ½ cup	3
Sauce, organic, cheese, ½ cup	3
Ragu Carb Options	
Alfredo sauce, ¼ cup	4
Garden style sauce, ½ cup	3
Ragu Cheese Creations	
Sauce, creamy tomato, ¼ cup	3
Sauce, four cheese, ¼ cup	3
Ragu Meat Creations	
Grilled steak flavored sauce, ½ cup	3

Rana

Sauce, pesto basil, ¼ cup	10

Rao's Homemade

Marinara sauce, sensitive formula, ½ cup	3

Rico's

Cheese sauce, restaurant style, white queso, ¼ cup	4

Trader Giotto's

Organic tomato basil marinara sauce, ½ cup	2
Roasted garlic marinara sauce, ½ cup	3
Tomato basil marinara sauce, ½ cup	4
Traditional marinara sauce, ½ cup	2

Trader Joe's

Marinara sauce, ½ cup	2
Organic vodka sauce, ½ cup	4
Pesto and quinoa, 2 Tbsp	4

Victoria

Marinara sauce, family size, ½ cup	2

Pickles

Ba-Tampte

Dill pickles, garlic, 1 oz	0

Best Maid

Pickles, hamburger slices, 15 slices (28 g)	0

Boar's Head

Pickle spears, kosher dill, 1 spear	0

Bubbies

Pickles, bread & butter chips, 1 oz	2

Claussen

Kosher dill pickle spears, 1 spear	0
Kosher dill, halves, ½ pickle half	0
Kosher dill, mini, 1 pickle	0
Kosher dill, sandwich slices, 2 slices (34 g)	0
Kosher dill, wholes, ⅓ pickle	0

Pickles, kosher dill, deli style, halves, ½ pickle half	0
Pickles, kosher dill, deli style, spears, 1 spear	0
Sandwich slices, bread 'n butter, 2 slices (34 g)	1
Sandwich slices, hearty garlic, deli style, 2 slices (34 g)	0

Claussen Deli Style

Dill halves, kosher, ½ pickle half	0
Dill spears, kosher, 1 spear	0

Famous Dave's

Spicy pickle spears (serves 17), 1 serving (28 g)	1

Famous Dave's Signature Spicy

Spicy pickle chips, 4 slices (28 g)	2

Gedney

Pickles, dill, babies, 3 pickles	0

Great Gherkins

Baby dills, kosher, fresh pack, 1 pickle	0

Grillo's Pickles

Bread and butter chips, 3 pieces (24 g)	1

Kroger

Pickles chips, dill, 11 slices (59 g)	0
Pickles, chips, bread & butter, 5 slices (28 g)	2
Pickles, chips, hamburger dill, 5 slices (28 g)	0
Pickles, spears, kosher dill, 1 spear	0
Pickles, whole, dill, ⅓ pickle	0

Mt. Olive

Baby dills, kosher, fresh pack, 1 pickle	0
Bread & butter chips, old fashioned sweet, fresh pack, 6 chips (28 g)	1
Bread & butter chips, old-fashioned sweet, fresh pack, 6 chips (28 g)	1
Deli style kosher dill relish made with sea salt, 1 Tbsp	0
Dill petites, kosher, pickle pak, 1 pak (51 g)	0

Condiments, Sauces & Gravies

Condiments, Sauces & Gravies

	SmartPoints™ value
Dill spears, kosher, fresh pack, 1 spear	0
Dills, kosher, fresh pack, ½ pickle	0
Gherkins, sweet, 2 pickles (28 g)	2
Hamburger dill chips, 2 chips	0
Kosher spears, zesty garlic, fresh pack, ¾ spear (28 g)	0
Salad cubes, sweet, 1 Tbsp	1
Sandwich stuffers, bread & butter, old fashioned sweet, fresh pack, 1 ½ slices (28 g)	1
Sandwich stuffers, kosher dill, fresh pack, 1 slice (28 g)	0
Snack crunchers, petite, kosher dill, fresh pack, 3 pickles	0
Snack crunchers, sweet petite, 6 pickles (28 g)	2
Spears, kosher dill, fresh pack, ¾ spear (28 g)	0
Safeway	
Pickle spears, kosher dill, 1 oz	0
ShopRite	
Pickles, half sours, whole, deli style, 1 oz	0
Tree of Life Organic	
Pickles, sweet bread and butter chips, 4 slices (47 ml)	2
Vlasic	
Baby wholes, kosher dill, 1 pickle	0
Bread & butter chips, 3 slices (28 g)	1
Bread & butter chips, zesty, 3 chips (28 g)	2
Bread & butter spears, ⅔ spear (28 g)	1
Dill relish, 1 Tbsp	0
Dill spears, kosher, 1 spear	0
Hamburger dill chips, ovals, 2 ¼ slices (28 g)	0
Kosher dill baby wholes, 1 ¼ pickles	0
Kosher dill gherkins, 3 pickles	0
Kosher dill, wholes, fresh pack, ¼ pickle	0

	SmartPoints™ value
Kosher dills, ½ pickle	0
Pickles, kosher dill, 1 oz	0
Reduced sodium kosher dill spears, ⅔ spear (48 ml)	0
Stackers, bread & butter, 1 ½ slices (28 g)	1
Stackers, kosher dill, 1 ½ slices (28 g)	0
Sweet gherkins, 3 pickles (28 g)	2
Sweet midgets, 3 pickles (28 g)	2
Sweet relish, 1 Tbsp	1
Vlasic Farmer's Garden	
Chips, bread & butter, 3 chips (28 g)	1
Spears, kosher dill, 1 spear	0
Vlasic Great For Sandwiches!	
Pickles, stackers zesty dill, 1 oz	0
Vlasic Snak'mms	
Kosher dill, 3 pickles	0
Wickles	
Pickles, a wickedly delicious, original, 3 slices (28 g)	2

Pizza Sauce

	SmartPoints™ value
Classico Signature Recipes	
Pizza sauce, fire roasted, ¼ cup	1
Pizza sauce, traditional, ¼ cup	2
Essential Everyday	
Pizza sauce, homemade style, ¼ cup	1
Prego	
Sauce, pizza, ¼ cup	2
Sauce, pizzeria style pizza, ¼ cup	2
Trader Giotto's	
Fat free pizza sauce, ¼ cup	1

Relish

	SmartPoints™ value
Claussen	
Pickle relish, sweet, 1 Tbsp	1
Heinz	
Dill relish, 1 Tbsp	0
Relish, dill, 1 Tbsp	0
Relish, sweet, 1 Tbsp	1

Kroger

Relish, dill, 1 Tbsp	0
Sweet relish, 1 Tbsp	1

Mt. Olive

Relish, dill, 1 Tbsp	0
Relish, sweet, 1 Tbsp	1
Relish, sweet, squeeze, 1 Tbsp	1

Safeway

Pickle relish, dill, 1 Tbsp	0

Vlasic

Home style relish, dill relish, squeezable, 1 Tbsp	0
Relish, sweet, 1 Tbsp	1
Squeezable home style relish, sweet relish, 1 Tbsp	1

Wickles

Relish, hoagie sub sandwich, spicy, 1 Tbsp	0
Relish, original, 1 Tbsp	1

Seafood Sauce

Frisch's

Tartar sauce, original, 2 Tbsp	7

Heinz

Sauce, cocktail, original, ¼ cup	3
Tartar sauce, premium, 2 Tbsp	4

Hellmann's

Sauce, tartar, 2 Tbsp	3

Kraft

Tartar sauce, 2 Tbsp	2

Kroger

Tarter sauce, squeezable, 2 Tbsp	4

McCormick

Original cocktail sauce for seafood, ¼ cup	5
Sauce for seafood, tartar, fat free, 2 Tbsp	2

McCormick Golden Dipt

Tartar sauce, original, 2 Tbsp	5

Shur Fine

Tarter sauce, 2 Tbsp	2

Sloppy Joe Sauce

Del Monte

Sloppy Joe sauce, original, ¼ cup	3

Heinz

Sloppy Joe sauce, classic recipe, ¼ cup	2

Hormel Not-So-Sloppy-Joe

Sauce, sloppy Joe, ¼ cup	3

Hunt's Manwich

Original sloppy joe, ¼ cup	3
Sloppy Joe sauce, ¼ cup	2
Sloppy Joe sauce, thick & chunky, ¼ cup	2

Manwich

Sloppy Joe sauce, barbecue, ¼ cup	3
Sloppy Joe sauce, bold, ¼ cup	3
Sloppy Joe sauce, original, ¼ cup	2

Steak & Meat Sauce

A1

Steak sauce, 1 Tbsp	1
Steak sauce, thick & hearty, 1 Tbsp	1

Campbell's Slow Cooker

Tavern style pot roast sauce, ¼ cup	2
Hawaiian luau, ¼ cup	5
Sweet Korean bbq sauce, ¼ cup	6

Peter Luger

Sauce, steak house, old fashioned, 1 Tbsp	2

Worcestershire Sauce

Lea & Perrin's

Worcestershire sauce, the original, 1 tsp	0

Condiments, Sauces & Gravies

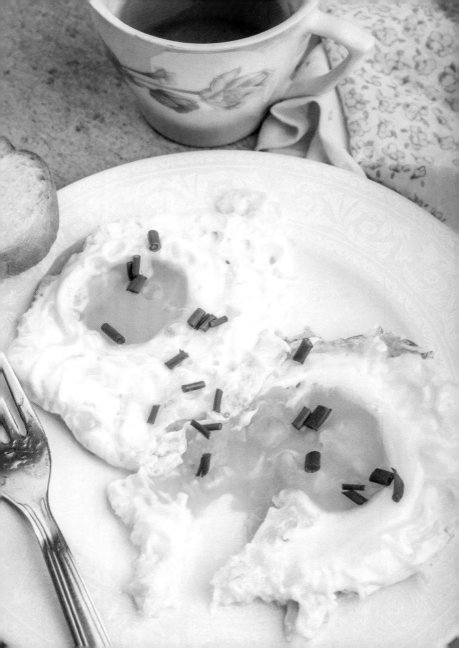

dairy
& Eggs

Dairy & Eggs

Butter & Butter Substitutes

Balade

Light butter, 1 Tbsp	2

Breakstone's

Whipped butter, salted, 1 Tbsp	3

Breakstone's Organic

Whipped butter, salted, 1 Tbsp	3

Butter Buds

Butter flavor granules, 1 tsp	1

Canola Harvest

Buttery spread, original, 1 Tbsp	3

Challenge

Butter, light, 1 Tbsp	2
Butter, salted, 1 Tbsp	5
Butter, spreadable, with canola oil, 1 Tbsp	4
Butter, whipped, salted, 1 Tbsp	3
Spreadable butter, lite, 1 Tbsp	2

Country Crock

Original spreadable butter with canola oil, 1 Tbsp	4

Country Crock Simply Delicious

Shedd's spread, 1 Tbsp	4

Countryside Creamery

Salted sweet cream butter, 1 Tbsp	5

Daily Chef

Salted sweet cream butter, 1 Tbsp	5

Darigold

Butter, natural, salted, 1 Tbsp	5

Earth Balance

Buttery spread, natural, original, 1 Tbsp	4
Natural buttery spread, 1 Tbsp	3
Natural soy free buttery spread, 1 Tbsp	4

Essential Everyday

Salted sweet cream butter, 1 Tbsp	5

Kroger

Butter spread, with canola oil, 1 Tbsp	4
Butter, unsalted, 1 Tbsp	5
Salted butter, 1 Tbsp	5

Land O' Lakes

Butter spread, cinnamon sugar, 1 Tbsp	3
Butter spread, honey, 1 Tbsp	3
Butter spread, light, with canola oil, 1 Tbsp	2
Butter spread, with canola oil, 1 Tbsp	4
Butter spread, with olive oil, 1 Tbsp	4
Butter with canola oil, 1 Tbsp	4
Butter, honey, 1 Tbsp	4
Butter, light, 1 Tbsp	2
Butter, light, whipped, 1 Tbsp	2
Butter, salted, 1 Tbsp	5
Butter, unsalted sweet, 1 Tbsp	5
Butter, unsalted, sweet, half sticks, 1 Tbsp	5
Butter, whipped, 1 Tbsp	2
Butter, with olive oil & sea salt, half sticks, 1 Tbsp	5

Land O' Lakes Saute Express

Butter & olive oil saute starter, seasoned, garlic & herb, ½ oz	3
Butter & olive oil saute starter, seasoned, Italian herb, ½ oz	4

Lucerne

Butter, spreadable, light, 1 Tbsp	2
Butter, spreadable, with canola oil, 1 Tbsp	4
Spreadable butter, light, with canola oil, 1 Tbsp	2

Molly McButter

Natural butter flavor sprinkles, fat free, 1 tsp	0

Olivio

Spreadable butter, with canola & olive oil, 1 Tbsp	4

Olivio Organic

Premium coconut spread, 1 Tbsp	3

Organic Valley

Butter, organic, cultured, unsalted, 1 Tbsp	5
Butter, organic, salted, 1 Tbsp	5

Purity Farms Ghee

Clarified butter, 1 tsp	2

Shedd's Spread Country Crock

Original spreadable butter with canola oil, 1 Tbsp	4

ShopRite

Butter, whipped, salted, 1 Tbsp	3

Smart Balance

Butter & canola oil blend, light, spreadable, 1 Tbsp	2
Butter and canola oil spreadable blend, 1 Tbsp	4
Butter blend, 50/50, 1 Tbsp	4
Butter blend, 50/50, original, 1 Tbsp	4
Butter, & canola and extra virgin olive oil blend, 1 Tbsp	4
Buttery spread, 1 Tbsp	3
Buttery spread, light, original, 1 Tbsp	2
Buttery spread, low sodium, lightly salted, 1 Tbsp	3
Buttery spread, made with extra virgin olive oil, 1 Tbsp	2
Buttery spread, non-hydrogenated, 1 Tbsp	3
Buttery spread, original, 1 Tbsp	3
Buttery spread, original, with flax, 1 Tbsp	3
Non gmo original buttery spread, 1 Tbsp	3

Smart Balance Heart Right

Buttery spread, light, 1 Tbsp	2

Smart Balance Omega

Buttery spread, light, 1 Tbsp	2
Butter, spread, whipped, 1 Tbsp	3

Tillamook

Butter, sweet cream, salted, 1 Tbsp	5

Trader Joe's

Clarified butter (ghee), 1 tsp	2

Wegman's

Butter, sweet cream, salted, 1 Tbsp	5

Cheese

4C

Grated cheese, homestyle parmesan, 1 Tbsp	1

Adams Reserve

Cheese, New York extra sharp cheddar, ¾ oz	3

Albertson's

Cottage cheese, lowfat, 4 oz	2
Cottage cheese, small curd, fat free, ½ cup	1
Cottage cheese, small curd, low fat, ½ cup	2

Alouette

Creme de brie, original, 2 Tbsp	4
Crumbled cheese, blue, ¼ cup	4
Crumbled cheese, feta, ¼ cup	3
Crumbled cheese, goat, ¼ cup	3
Crumbled cheese, gorgonzola, ¼ cup	4
Soft spreadable cheese, spinach artichoke, 2 Tbsp	3

Alouette Light

Soft spreadable cheese, garlic and herb, 2 Tbsp	2

Alpenhaus Le Gruyere

Cheese, gruyere, 1 oz	4

Dairy & Eggs

	SmartPoints™ value
Alpine Lace	
Cheese, deli thin, reduced fat cheddar, 1 slice (23 g)	2
Cheese, deli thin, reduced fat provolone, 1 slice (23 g)	2
Cheese, deli thin, reduced fat Swiss, 1 slice (23 g)	2
American Heritage	
Fancy shredded Mexican blend cheese, ⅓ cup	4
American Heritage	
Shredded mild cheddar cheese, ¼ cup	4
AMPI	
Fancy shredded cheddar cheese, ¼ cup	4
Apple Smoked Cheese	
Cheese, smoked cheddar, 1 oz	4
Applegate	
Cheese slices, Monterey Jack, 1 slice (19 g)	3
Cheese, aged cheddar, New York extra sharp, 1 slice (28 g)	4
Cheese, American, 1 slice (21 g)	3
Cheese, cheddar, medium, 1 slice (19 g)	3
Cheese, Swiss, emmentaler, 1 slice (19 g)	3
Applegate Naturals	
Cheese slices, havarti, 1 ½ slice (43 g)	8
Cheese, muenster, 1 slice (21 g)	3
Argitoni	
Parmesan cheese, 1 Tbsp	1
ARZ	
Kefir cheese, labne, 2 Tbsp	3
Athenos	
Cheese chunk, feta, 1" cube	3
Cheese chunk, feta, reduced fat, 1 oz	2
Cheese, fat free, feta, 1" cube	0

	SmartPoints™ value
Crumbled cheese, blue, 3 Tbsp	4
Crumbled cheese, feta with tomato & basil, ¼ cup	3
Crumbled cheese, feta, garlic & herb, ¼ cup	3
Crumbled cheese, feta, traditional, ¼ cup	3
Crumbled cheese, feta, traditional, ¼ cup	3
Crumbled cheese, feta, traditional, fat free, ¼ cup	0
Crumbled cheese, feta, traditional, reduced fat, ¼ cup	2
Axelrod Easy-Dieter	
Cottage cheese, lowfat, 1% milkfat, ½ cup	2
Cottage cheese, nonfat, ½ cup	2
Cottage cheese, nonfat, with added pineapple, ½ cup	2
Baker	
String cheese, 1 piece (28 g)	2
String cheese, light, 1 stick (24 g)	1
String cheese, part-skim, mozzarella, 1 piece (28 g)	2
String cheese, smoked, 1 piece (28 g)	2
Bakers & Chefs	
Natural shredded cheddar cheese, ⅓ cup	4
BelGioioso	
Asiago cheese, freshly shredded, 1 Tbsp	1
Cheese shreds, four cheese, 1 Tbsp	1
Gorgonzola cheese, crumbly, Italian blue, 2 Tbsp	4
Mozzarella cheese, fresh, 1 oz	2
Mozzarella cheese, fresh, burrata, 1 oz	3
Mozzarella cheese, fresh, ciliegine, 1 oz	2

Dairy & Eggs

	SmartPoints™ value
Mozzarella cheese, fresh, snacking cheese, 1 oz	2
Parmesan cheese, freshly shaved, 1 Tbsp	1
Provolone cheese, mild, sliced, 1 oz	4
Salad blend cheese, freshly shaved, 1 Tbsp	1
Belmont	
100% feta cheese fat free, 1 oz	0
Best Choice	
Cheese food, American, 2% milk singles, 1 slice (21 g)	2
Cheese product, American, fat free singles, 1 slice (21 g)	1
Cheese, deluxe, sliced American, 1 slice (21 g)	3
Shredded cheese, fat free, mild cheddar, ⅓ cup	1
Boar's Head	
25% lower fat, 25% lower sodium American cheese (gluten free), 1 oz	3
44% lower sodium provolone cheese (gluten free), 2 slices (28 g)	4
Baby Swiss cheese (gluten free), 1 oz	4
Bold 3 pepper colby Jack cheese (gluten free), 1 oz	4
Bold horseradish cheddar cheese (gluten free), 1 oz	4
Cheese, American (gluten free), 1 oz	4
Cheese, chipotle gouda, medium, 1 oz	4
Cheese, colby Jack (gluten free), 1 oz	4
Cheese, cream havarti (gluten free), 1 oz	5
Cheese, extra aged yellow cheddar, 1 oz	4

	SmartPoints™ value
Cheese, longhorn colby (gluten free), 1 oz	4
Cheese, muenster (gluten free), 1 oz	4
Cheese, vermont cheddar (gluten free), 1 oz	4
Feta cheese (crumbled), ¼ cup	2
Lacey Swiss cheese, 1 oz	3
Low sodium muenster cheese (gluten free), 1 oz	4
Monterey Jack cheese (gluten free), 1 oz	4
Pepper Jack cheese (gluten free), 1 oz	4
Picante provolone cheese (gluten free), 1 oz	4
Sharp Wisconsin cheddar cheese (gluten free), 1 oz	4
Smoked gouda, pasteurized process gouda and cheddar cheese (gluten free), 1 oz	4
Whole milk low moisture mozzarella cheese (gluten free), 1 oz	3
Boar's Head Master Cheesemaker's Selections	
Cheese, cream havarti with dill (gluten free), 1 oz	5
Cheese, imported Swiss, 1 oz	4
Cheese, Monterey Jack with jalapeño, 1 oz	4
Boar's Head Old World Delicacies	
Cheese, gouda (gluten free), 1 oz	4
Borden	
2% milk reduced fat singles, American, 1 each (21 g)	2
Cheddar and Monterey Jack finely shredded cheese, ¼ cup	4
Cheese product slices, American, 2% milk, reduced fat, 1 slice (19 g)	2
Cheese product, lactose free singles, American, 1 slice (19 g)	2

Dairy & Eggs

	SmartPoints™ value
Cheese product, pasteurized prepared, 2% milk reduced fat, sharp, 1 slice (19 g)	2
Cheese product, pasteurized prepared, 2% milk reduced fat, singles, sharp, 1 slice (21 g)	2
Cheese product, pasteurized prepared, fat free, singles, American, 1 slice (21 g)	1
Cheese product, pasteurized prepared, fat free, singles, sharp, 1 slice (21 g)	1
Cheese product, singles, white American, 1 slice (21 g)	3
Cheese, American, family pack, singles, 1 slice (19 g)	2
Cheese, colby & Monterey Jack, 2 oz	8
Cheese, extra sharp cheddar, 1 oz	4
Cheese, pasteurized prepared, American, 1 slice (19 g)	2
Cheese, sharp cheddar, 1 oz	4
Cheese, sharp cheddar, slices, 2 slices (32 g)	5
Finely shredded cheese, four cheese Mexican, ¼ cup	4
Natural mild cheddar cheese slices, 1 slice (17 g)	3
Sharp cheddar finely shredded cheese, ¼ cup	4
String cheese, mozzarella cheese, 1 stick (24 g)	2
Borden Dairy	
Cheese product, grilled cheese melts, 1 slice (21 g)	2
Cheese product, singles, American, 1 slice (21 g)	3
Borden Dairy Fat Free	
Pepper Jack singles, 1 slice (21 g)	1
Borden Dairy Singles Sensations	
Cheese product, southwest pepperjack, 1 slice (23 g)	3

	SmartPoints™ value
Borden Double Twist	
String cheese, 1 (24 g)	2
Borden Natural	
Finely shredded cheese, cheddar & Monterey Jack cheese, reduced fat, ¼ cup	3
Borden Singles	
Cheese product, pastuerized prepared, American, 1 slice (21 g)	3
Boursin	
Cheese, gournay, shallot & chive, 2 Tbsp	6
Spreadable cheese, gourmet, garlic & herbs, 2 Tbsp	3
Spreadable cheese, gourmet, light, garlic & herbs, 2 Tbsp	2
Breakstone's	
2% lowfat small curd cottage cheese snack size, 1 container (113 g)	3
2% milkfat lowfat 30% less sodium cottage cheese, ½ cup	3
2% milkfat lowfat large curd cottage cheese, ½ cup	3
4% milkfat small curd cottage cheese, ½ cup	4
4% milkfat smooth and creamy small curd cottage cheese snack size, 1 container (113 g)	4
Fat free small curd cottage cheese, ½ cup	2
Fat free small curd cottage cheese snack size, 1 container (113 g)	2
Breakstone's 100 Calorie Cottage Doubles	
2% milkfat lowfat small curd cottage cheese with pineapple, 1 container (113 g)	4
2% milkfat lowfat cottage cheese & pineapple topping, 1 container (110 g)	4
Cottage cheese, 2% milkfat, lowfat, mango topping, 1 container (110 g)	4

Cottage doubles, apple cinnamon, 1 container (110 g)	4
Cottage doubles, blueberry, 1 container (110 g)	4
Cottage doubles, peach, 1 container (110 g)	4
Cottage cheese, raspberry, 1 container (110 g)	4
2% milkfat lowfat cottage cheese & strawberry topping, 1 container (110 g)	4
Cottage cheese, lowfat, & raspberry topping, 1 container (156 g)	5
Cottage cheese, lowfat, blueberry topping, 1 container (156 g)	5
Cottage cheese, lowfat, peach topping, 1 container (156 g)	5
Cottage cheese, lowfat, pineapple topping, 1 container (156 g)	5
Cottage cheese, lowfat, strawberry topping, 1 container (156 g)	5

Breakstone's LiveActive

2% milkfat lowfat cottage cheese, 1 container (113 g)	2

Brunckhorst's Boar's Head

Gold label switzerland Swiss cheese (gluten free), 2 slices (28 g)	4

Buitoni

Cheese, parmesan, freshly shredded, 1 Tbsp	1

Buttermilk Blue

Blue cheese crumbles, 1 oz	4

Cabot

75% reduce fat cheddar cheese, 1" cube	1
Cheddar cheese, classic vermont sharp, 1 cube (28 g)	4
Cheddar cheese, sharp, 1 cube (28 g)	4
Cheese, cheddar, 50% reduced fat, 1 oz	2

Cheese, cheddar, extra sharp, 1 oz	4
Cheese, cheddar, horseradish, 1 oz	4
Cheese, cheddar, seriously sharp, 1"cube	4
Cheese, extra sharp aged cheddar, 1 oz	4
Cheese, jalapeño cheddar, 50% reduced fat, 1 oz	2
Cheese, Monterey Jack, 1 oz	4
Cheese, New York extra sharp cheddar, 1 oz	4
Cheese, pepper Jack, 1 oz	4
Cheese, premium naturally aged cheddar, seriously sharp, 1 oz	4
Cheese, sharp cheddar, 50% reduced fat, 1 oz	2
Cheese, sharp cheddar, 75% reduced fat, 1 oz	1
Natural vermont cheddar cheese seriously sharp snack packs, 1 bar (21 g)	3
No fat cottage cheese, ½ cup	1
No fat vermont style cottage cheese, ½ cup	1
Sharp cheddar cheese slice, 1 slice (28 g)	4

Cabot Serious Snacking

Cheese, sharp cheddar, 50% reduced fat, 1 bar (21 g)	2
Sharp cheddar cheese, 1 bar (21 g)	3

Cabot Vermont Snack Packs

50% light cheddar cheese, 1 snack bar (21 g)	2

Cacique

Cheese, panela, 1 oz	3
Queso fresco, 1 oz	3

Cacique Ranchero

Cheese, part skim milk, 1 oz	3

Calabro

Fat free ricotta, ¼ cup	1

Dairy & Eggs

Cheese (cont'd)

SmartPoints™ value

Castle Wood Reserve

Light Swiss cheese, 1 slice (21 g)	1

Castle Wood Reserve Heart Healthy

Baby Swiss cheese, 1 slice (18 g)	3

Challenge

Cream cheese spread, whipped, 2 Tbsp	3

Chavrie

Cheese, goat's milk, 2 Tbsp	2

Cheez Whiz

Cheese spread, pasteurized process, 2 Tbsp	4

Chuck E. Cheese's

Mozzarella string cheese, 1 (24 g)	2

Cracker Barrel

Asiago cheese slice, 1 slice (18 g)	3
Baby Swiss cheese, 1" cube	4
Cheese bars, extra sharp cheddar, 1 bar (21 g)	2
Cheese bars, jalapeño cheddar, 1 bar (21 g)	3
Cheese bars, sharp cheddar, 1 bar (21 g)	3
Cheese slices, extra sharp white cheddar, 1 slice (18 g)	3
Cheese sticks, extra sharp cheddar, 1 stick (28 g)	5
Cheese, cheddar, extra sharp, 1 oz	4
Cheese, cheddar, extra sharp, aged reserve, 1 oz	4
Cheese, cracker cuts, sharp-white cheddar, 3 slices (28 g)	4
Cheese, extra sharp cheddar, 1 oz	5
Cheese, extra sharp cheddar, natural reduced fat, 1 oz	3
Cheese, extra sharp cheddar, reduced fat, 1" cube	3
Cheese, extra sharp-white cheddar, 1" cube	4
Cheese, natural sharp cheddar, vermont sharp-white, 1" cube	4

Cheese, natural, sharp cheddar, slices, 1 slice (20 g)	3
Cheese, reduced fat, extra sharp, 1 oz	3
Cheese, sharp cheddar, 1 oz	4
Cracker barrel sharp white cheddar cheese, 1" cube	5
Cracker cuts, sharp white cheddar, 4 slices (33 g)	5
Extra sharp cheddar cracker cuts, 4 slices (33 g)	5
Extra sharp white cheddar cheese bars, 1 bar (21 g)	3
Havarti cheese slices, 1 slice (20 g)	3
Jalapeño cheddar cracker cuts, 4 slices (33 g)	5
Reduced fat extra sharp white cheddar cheese, 1" cube	3
Shreds, cheddar cheese, extra sharp, ¼ cup	4
Shreds, vermont white, cheddar cheese, sharp, ¼ cup	4

Cracker Barrel Cracker Cuts

Cheese, extra sharp cheddar, 3 slices (28 g)	5

Cracker Barrel Vermont Sharp White

Reduced fat sharp cheddar cheese, 1" cube	3

Crowley

Nonfat cottage cheese, ½ cup	2

Crystal Farms

Cheese food, singles, American, 1 slice (21 g)	2
Cheese product, pasteurized processed, light, creamy Swiss, 1 wedge (19 g)	1
Cheese product, pasteurized processed, light, garlic & herb, 1 wedge (19 g)	1
Cheese product, pasteurized processed, light, jalapeño pepper, 1 wedge (19 g)	1

Dairy & Eggs

230

Cheese slices, pepper Jack, med, 1 slice (23 g)	3
Cheese, 4 cheese blend, Mexican style, ¼ cup	4
Cheese, cheddar, ¼ cup	4
Cheese, mozzarella, low moisture part-skim, ⅓ cup	4
Cheese, Wisconsin sharp cheddar, ¼ cup	4
Finely shredded cheese, taco cheese blend, Mexican style, ¼ cup	4
Marble Jack cheese slice, 1 slice (23 g)	4
Provolone cheese slice, 1 slice (23 g)	3
Shaved parmesan cheese, ¼ cup	4
Shredded cheese, Mexican style 3 cheese blend, ¼ cup	4
Swiss cheese slices, 1 slice (20 g)	2
Wisconsin marble Jack cheese stick, 1 piece (28 g)	4
Wisconsin sharp cheddar cheese, ¼ cup	4
Wisconsin sharp cheddar cheese slices, 1 slice (23 g)	4
Wisconsin string cheese, 1 stick (24 g)	2

Crystal Farms Cheezoids

Reduced fat mozzarella string cheese, 1 stick (24 g)	2

Crystal Farms Cheezoids Spirals

Mozzarella cheese snacks, 1 piece (24 g)	2

Crystal Farms Light

Wisconsin string cheese, 1 piece (24 g)	1

Daily Chef

2% low fat small curd cottage cheese, ½ cup	2
Sharp cheddar cheese, 1 oz	4

Daisy

2% milkfat small curd low fat cottage cheese, ½ cup	2
Cottage cheese, small curd, ½ cup	3
Low fat cottage cheese, ½ cup	2

Daiya

Cheddar style slices, deliciously dairy free, 1 slice (20 g)	2
Plain cream cheese style spread, 2 Tbsp	4
Provolone style slices, deliciously dairy free, 1 slice (20 g)	3
Shreds, pepperjack style, ¼ cup	3

Darigold

Cottage cheese, trim, ½ cup	3

Dean's

4% milkfat minimum small curd cottage cheese, ½ cup	3
Cottage cheese, small curd, fat free, ½ cup	2
Cottage cheese, small curd, low fat, ½ cup	2
Fat free small curd cottage cheese, ½ cup	2
Lowfat small curd cottage cheese, ½ cup	2

Deli Deluxe

Cheese product, pasteurized process, American slices, 1 slice (21 g)	3
Cheese product, pasteurized process, white American slices, 1 slice (19 g)	3
Cheese, colby Jack, slices, 1 each (23 g)	3

Denmark's Finest

Havarti dill cheese, 1 oz	4

Dietz & Watson

Cheese, meunster, ¾ oz	3
Cheese, white American, ¾ oz	3

Dairy & Eggs

	SmartPoints™ value
DiGiorno	
Shaved cheese, parmesan, ¼ cup	4
Dofino	
Creamy havarti deli slices, 1 oz	4
Easy Cheese	
Easy cheese, American, 2 Tbsp	3
Easy cheese, cheddar, 2 Tbsp	3
Easy cheese, sharp cheddar, 2 Tbsp	3
Eating Right For Calorie Counting	
Cheese wedge, light spreadable, garlic & herb, 1 wedge (19 g)	1
Cheese wedge, light spreadable, white cheddar, 1 wedge (19 g)	1
El Mexicano	
Cheese, cotija, 1 oz	4
Essential Everyday	
Cheese product, pasteurized process, non fat, singles, American, 1 slice (19 g)	0
Cheese product, pasteurized process, non fat, singles, white American, 1 slice (19 g)	0
Cheese product, pasteurized process, reduced fat, singles, American, 1 slice (19 g)	2
Cheese, colby Jack, deli style, 1 slice (23 g)	3
Cheese, mild cheddar, deli style, 1 slice (22 g)	4
Cheese, mozzarella, deli style, 1 slice (23 g)	2
Cheese, muenster, deli style, 1 slice (22 g)	3
Cheese, pepper Jack, deli style, 1 slice (22 g)	3
Cheese, provolone, deli style, 1 slice (23 g)	3
Cheese, reduced fat, sharp cheddar, 1 oz	3
Cheese, sharp cheddar, deli style, 1 slice (22 g)	4

	SmartPoints™ value
Cottage cheese, small curd, 1% milkfat, low fat, ½ cup	2
Cottage cheese, small curd, fat free, ½ cup	2
Cream cheese, fat free, 2 Tbsp	1
Cream cheese, reduced fat, 2 Tbsp	3
Fancy shredded sharp cheddar cheese, ⅓ cup	4
Jalapeño string cheese, 1 piece (24 g)	2
Low fat cottage cheese, ½ cup	3
Neufchatel cheese, 2 Tbsp	3
Reduced fat 2% milk Mexican style four cheese blend, ¼ cup	3
Shredded cheese, fancy, colby Jack, ¼ cup	4
Shredded cheese, fancy, colby Jack, reduced fat, ¼ cup	3
Shredded cheese, fancy, Italian style, parmesan, ⅓ cup	3
Shredded cheese, fancy, Mexican style, cheddar Jack, ¼ cup	4
Shredded cheese, fancy, mild cheddar, ¼ cup	4
Shredded cheese, fancy, mild cheddar, reduced fat, ¼ cup	3
Shredded cheese, fancy, mozzarella, ¼ cup	3
Shredded cheese, fancy, mozzarella, reduced fat, ⅓ cup	2
Shredded cheese, fancy, sharp cheddar, reduced fat, ¼ cup	3
Shredded cheese, fat free, mozzarella, ¼ cup	0
Shredded cheese, four cheese blend, Mexican style, ⅓ cup	4
Shredded cheese, low-moisture part-skim mozzarella, ¼ cup	3
Shredded cheese, Mexican style cheddar Jack, ⅓ cup	4

Dairy & Eggs

Shredded cheese, Mexican style four cheese blend, ¼ cup	4
Shredded cheese, Mexican style, four cheese blend, ⅓ cup	4
Shredded cheese, Mexican style, taco blend, ⅓ cup	4
Shredded cheese, mild cheddar, ¼ cup	4
Shredded cheese, mild cheddar, fat free, ¼ cup	1
Shredded cheese, pizza blend, ¼ cup	4
Shredded cheese, sharp cheddar, fancy, ¼ cup	4
Shredded cheese, six cheese blend, Italian style, ¼ cup	3
String cheese twists, low-moisture part-skim mozzarella & cheddar, 1 piece (24 g)	2
String cheese, light low-moisture part-skim mozzarella, 1 piece (28 g)	2
String cheese, low-moisture part-skim mozzarella, 1 piece (28 g)	3

Essential Everyday Deli Style

Natural Swiss cheese, 1 slice (23 g)	3

FairPlay Packaging

Mild cheddar string cheese, 1 stick (23.6 g)	4

FarmRich

Mozzarella bites, 4 pieces (48 g)	5

Fiber One

Lowfat cottage cheese with fiber, ½ cup	2

Fit & Active

2% milk Mexican shredded cheese blend, ¼ cup	3
Neufchatel cheese, 1 oz	3
Reduce fat provolone cheese deli slices, 1 slice (19 g)	2
Reduced fat colby Jack cheese deli slices, 1 slice (19 g)	2

Food Club

Cheese product, nonfat pasteurized process, American, fat free, singles, 1 slice (21 g)	1
Cheese, natural, baby Swiss, deli-style sliced, 1 slice (21 g)	3
Colby Jack cheese, 1 oz	4
Finely shredded cheese blend, natural, Mexican style, reduced fat, ¼ cup	3
Light string cheese, 1 stick (24 g)	1

Fred Meyer

Cottage cheese, lowfat, ½ cup	2
Fat free cottage cheese, ½ cup	1

Friendly Farms

Low fat small curd cottage cheese, ½ cup	2

Friendship

0% milkfat small curd cottage cheese with pineapple, ½ cup	2
1% milkfat whipped cottage cheese, ½ cup	2
Cottage cheese, 1% milkfat, no salt added, small curd, ½ cup	2
Cottage cheese, 1% milkfat, small curd, ½ cup	2
Cottage cheese, 1% milkfat, small curd, with pineapple, ½ cup	4
Cottage cheese, 2% milkfat, large curd, pot style, ½ cup	2
Cottage cheese, 4% milkfat minimum, small curd, California style, ½ cup	3

Frigo

Cheese, Italian, shredded, parmesan, asiago & romano, ¼ cup	3
Cheese, parmesan, shaved, ¼ cup	3
Crumbled blue cheese, ¼ cup	4

Dairy & Eggs

	SmartPoints™ value
Frigo Cheese Heads	
Cheese sticks, reduced fat, colby Jack, 1 piece (24 g)	2
Light string mozzarella cheese, 1 piece (24 g)	1
Sharp cheddar & beef sticks, 1 beef stick (21 g)	3
String cheese & meat sticks, pepperoni flavored, 1 stick (22 g)	3
String cheese, 100% natural, light, mozzarella, 1 oz	1
String cheese, 100% natural, mozzarella, 1 package (28 g)	3
String cheese, mozzarella, 1 piece (28 g)	3
String cheese, natural, light swirls, 1 oz	1
String cheese, natural, swirls, 1 oz	3
String cheese, pepper Jack string, 12 pack, 1 piece (24 g)	3
Frigo Cheese Heads Premium Snacking	
Cheese stick, natural, chipotle cheddar, 1 piece (24 g)	3
Cheese stick, natural, garlic & herb white cheddar, 1 piece (24 g)	4
Cheese stick, natural, Wisconsin sharp cheddar, 1 piece (24 g)	4
Wisconsin colby Jack cheese sticks, 1 piece (24 g)	3
Frigo Cheese Heads String	
100% natural string cheese, 1 stick (28 g)	3
Frigo Cheese Heads Superstring	
Natural string cheese, 1 piece (24 g)	2
String cheese, natural, 1 oz	3
Frigo Cheese Heads Swirls	
String cheese, natural, double cheese swirl, 1 each (28 g)	3
String cheese, natural, light, 1 oz	1

	SmartPoints™ value
Galbani Sticksters	
Cheddar cheese snacks, 1 stick (24 g)	4
Genuine Locatelli	
Grated cheese, pecorino romano, 1 Tbsp	1
Giant	
Cheese, medium cheddar, slices, 1 slice (21 g)	3
Cheese, mozzarella, slices, 1 slice (21 g)	2
Cheese, muenster, orange rind style, slices, 1 slice (21 g)	3
Cheese, provolone, slices, 1 slice (21 g)	3
Cheese, Swiss, slices, 1 slice (21 g)	3
Colby Jack, colby & Monterey Jack cheese, 1 oz	4
Cottage cheese, lowfat, ½ cup	2
Cottage cheese, small curd, 1% milkfat, lowfat, ½ cup	2
Cottage cheese, small curd, fat free, ½ cup	1
Shredded cheese, mild cheddar, ¼ cup	4
Shredded cheese, mozzarella, ¼ cup	3
Shredded cheese, reduced fat, mild cheddar, ¼ cup	3
Shredded cheese, reduced fat, mozzarella, ¼ cup	2
String cheese, mozzarella cheese, reduced fat, 1 stick (28 g)	2
Giant Fancy	
Cheese, nacho taco blend, ¼ cup	4
Shredded cheese, Italian blend, ¼ cup	3
Shredded cheese, Mexican blend, ¼ cup	4
Shredded cheese, sharp cheddar, ¼ cup	4

Dairy & Eggs

Giant/Stop & Shop

Fat free cottage cheese with pineapple, ½ cup	4
Finely shredded reduced fat sharp cheddar, ¼ cup	3
Reduced fat mozzarella string cheese, 1 stick (28 g)	1
String cheese mozzarella, 1 stick (28 g)	3

Giant/Stop & Shop Cracker Cuts

Extra sharp cheddar cheese slices, 4 slices (32 g)	5

Gordo's

Cheese dip, original, 2 Tbsp	3

Great Lakes Cheese

American cheese singles, 1 slice (19 g)	2
Cheese, slices, pepper Jack, 1 slice (21 g)	3
Cheese, slices, provolone, 1 slice (21 g)	3
Fat free American cheese singles, 1 slice (21 g)	1
Muenster shingle slice, 1 slice (19 g)	3
Provalone shingle slice, 1 slice (19 g)	3

Great Value

100% parmesan grated cheese, 1 Tbsp	1
American cheese singles, 1 slice (21 g)	3
Brown sugar and cinnamon cream cheese spread, 2 Tbsp	5
Cheese food, pasteurized process, reduced fat, singles, American, 1 slice (19 g)	2
Cheese product, pasteurized prepared, singles, American, 1 slice (21 g)	3
Cheese product, pasteurized prepared, singles, white American, 1 slice (19 g)	2

Cheese, finely shredded, colby & Monterey Jack, ⅓ cup	4
Cheese, finely shredded, fiesta blend, ⅓ cup	4
Cheese, finely shredded, Italian style, ⅓ cup	3
Cheese, finely shredded, mild, cheddar, ⅓ cup	3
Cheese, finely shredded, mozzarella, ⅓ cup	3
Cheese, finely shredded, parmesan, ⅓ cup	3
Cheese, finely shredded, pizza blend, ⅓ cup	3
Cheese, finely shredded, sharp, cheddar, ⅓ cup	4
Cheese, finely shredded, taco blend, ⅓ cup	4
Cheese, pasteurized process, deluxe, American, 1 slice (19 g)	3
Cheese, pasteurized process, fat free, singles, 1 slice (21 g)	1
Cheese, shredded, mozzarella, ¼ cup	3
Cottage cheese, low fat, ½ cup	2
Cottage cheese, low fat, small curd, ½ cup	2
Cottage cheese, small curd, ½ cup	4
Cottage cheese, small curd, fat free, ½ cup	2
Deli style sliced colby and Monterey Jack cheese, 1 slice (19 g)	3
Deli style sliced provolone cheese, 1 slice (19 g)	2
Fat free cream cheese, 1 oz	1
Finely shredded cheese, fiesta blend, reduced fat, ⅓ cup	3
Pasteurized prepared cheese product, singles, American, 1 slice (19 g)	2
Shredded cheese, mild cheddar, ¼ cup	4

Dairy & Eggs

Dairy & Eggs

	SmartPoints™ value
Green Mountain Farms	
Greek cream cheese, 2 Tbsp	2
Greek cream cheese whipped yogurt, 2 Tbsp	2
Happy Farms	
Cheese wedges, spreadable, light, 1 wedge (19 g)	1
Cheese, provolone, sliced, 1 slice (21 g)	3
Cheese, string mozzarella, low-moisture, part-skim, 1 piece (24 g)	2
Happy Farms Light	
Cheese wedges, spreadable, jalapeño pepper, 1 wedge (19 g)	1
Heluva Good!	
Cheese, colby-Jack, 1 oz	4
Cheese, natural, sharp cheddar cheese, 1 oz	4
Hoffman's	
Cheese, cheddar, mild, deli style slices, 1 slice (19 g)	3
Cheese, colby-Jack, 1 slice (23 g)	3
Cheese, cubes, cheddar, 4 cubes (29 g)	5
Cheese, muenster, 1 slice (23 g)	3
Cheese, slices, hot pepper, 1 slice (23 g)	3
Cheese, super-sharp cheddar, 1 slice (23 g)	4
Home Made Brand	
Spread, cheese, pimento, 2 Tbsp	4
Hood	
Cottage cheese (4%) with pineapple, ½ cup	5
Cottage cheese with chive, ½ cup	4
Cottage cheese with pineapple, 1 container (170 g)	8
Cottage cheese, fat free, ½ cup	2
Cottage cheese, low fat, ½ cup	2

	SmartPoints™ value
Cottage cheese, low fat, small curd, with chive & toasted onion, ½ cup	2
Cottage cheese, lowfat, small curd, ½ cup	2
Cottage cheese, small curd, 1% milkfat, low fat, with pineapple & cherry, ½ cup	4
Cottage cheese, small curd, fat free, ½ cup	2
Cottage cheese, with pineapple, fat free, ½ cup	4
Hood Country Style	
Cottage cheese, small curd, 4% milkfat, ½ cup	3
Hood Low Fat	
Small curd cottage cheese, 1 container (170 g)	3
Horizon	
Cottage cheese, lowfat, organic, small curd, ½ cup	3
Horizon Organic	
American cheese singles, 1 slice (19 g)	3
Hy-Vee	
Cheese product, pasteurized prepared, reduced fat, singles, American, 1 slice (21 g)	2
Cheese product, pasteurized process, fat free, singles, American, 1 slice (21 g)	1
Cheese product, pasteurized process, fat free, singles, Swiss flavored, 1 slice (21 g)	1
Cheese, natural, colby Jack, sliced, 1 slice (21 g)	3
Cheese, natural, Mexican, ¼ cup	5
Cheese, natural, Swiss, sliced, 1 slice (21 g)	3
Cheese, provolone, sliced, 1 slice (21 g)	3

Finely shredded cheese,
cheddar Jack, ¼ cup — 4

Finely shredded cheese,
natural, mild cheddar, ¼ cup — 4

Shredded cheese, natural,
colby Jack, ¼ cup — 4

Hy-Vee Lil' Hunk

Cheese strings, mozzarella,
1 piece (28 g) — 3

String cheese, natural, light,
mozzarella, 1 piece (28 g) — 1

Ile de France

Cheese, soft ripened, brie bites,
1 mini cheese (25 g) — 3

Imo's

Shredded cheese, provel, ¼ cup — 4

Jarlsberg

Cheese dip, with red onion,
original, 1 oz — 4

Cheese slices, reduced fat,
lite, Swiss, ¾ oz — 2

Cheese, semi soft, part skim, 1 oz — 4

Cheese, Swiss, 1 oz — 4

Minis 100% all natural
cheese snack, 1 piece (20 g) — 2

Jarlsberg Lite

Reduced fat Swiss cheese
slices, 1 slice (21 g) — 1

Karoun Kefir Cheese Labne

Yogurt cheese, spreadable,
mediterranean style, 2 Tbsp — 3

Kaukauna

Spreadable cheese,
port wine, 2 Tbsp — 4

Kemps

1% lowfat cottage cheese, ½ cup — 2

2% lowfat cottage cheese, ½ cup — 2

Kemps Free

Fat free cottage cheese, ½ cup — 2

Kemps Singles

1%, lowfat cottage cheese,
1 container (160 g) — 3

Kirkland Signature

Mexican style shredded cheese,
⅓ cup — 4

Shredded parmigiano reggiano,
1 Tbsp — 1

Kitchen Table Bakers

Parmesan crisps, aged,
3 crisps (15 g) — 3

Knudsen

Cottage cheese, lowfat,
with pineapple, ½ cup — 4

Cottage cheese, small curd,
½ cup — 4

Lowfat 2% milk fat small curd
cottage cheese, ½ cup — 3

Knudsen Cottage Doubles 100 Calorie

Cottage doubles, blueberry,
1 container (110 g) — 4

2% milkfat, lowfat cottage cheese
with raspberry topping,
1 container (110 g) — 4

Cottage cheese, 2% milkfat lowfat,
and pineapple topping,
1 container (110 g) — 4

Cottage cheese, 2% milkfat,
lowfat, and peach topping,
1 container (110 g) — 4

Cottage cheese, 2% milkfat,
lowfat, and strawberry topping,
1 container (110 g) — 4

Cottage cheese, 2% milkfat,
lowfat, mango topping,
1 container (110 g) — 4

Knudsen Free

Nonfat cottage cheese, ½ cup — 2

Knudsen On the Go!

Cottage cheese, lowfat,
1 container (113 g) — 3

Dairy & Eggs

SmartPoints™ value

Kraft

100% grated parmesan cheese, 2 tsp	1
Cheese crumbles, blue cheese, 3 Tbsp	4
Cheese crumbles, feta, ¼ cup	3
Cheese cubes, made with 2% milk, cheddar & Monterey Jack, 7 pieces (30 g)	3
Cheese slices, big slice, American, 1 slice (23 g)	3
Cheese slices, colby Jack, with a touch of Philadelphia, 1 slice (20 g)	3
Cheese slices, pepper Jack, with a touch of Philadelphia, 1 slice (20 g)	3
Cheese twists, made with 2% milk, mozzarella & cheddar, 1 stick (21 g)	1
Cheese twists, mozzarella & cheddar, 1 stick (21 g)	2
Cheese, shredded parmesan, ¼ cup	2
Cheese, shredded, with a touch of Philadelphia, Mexican style, four cheese, ¼ cup	4
Cheese, shredded, with a touch of Philadelphia, mozzarella, ¼ cup	3
Cheese, Swiss, deli thin slices, 1 slice (19 g)	3
Finely shredded cheese, Mexican style taco, ¼ cup	4
Finely shredded cheese, sharp cheddar, reduced fat, ¼ cup	3
Finely shredded sharp cheddar cheese, ¼ cup	4
Grated cheeses, natural, parmesan & romano, 2 tsp	1
Grated parmesan cheese, 2 tsp	0
Parmesan style grated topping, reduced fat, 2 tsp	1

SmartPoints™ value

Season grated parmesan cheese, 2 tsp	1
Shaved cheese, parmesan, ¼ cup	4
Shredded cheese, American & cheddar Jack, ¼ cup	3
Shredded cheese, classic, American & cheddar, ¼ cup	3
Shredded cheese, four cheese blend, ¼ cup	3
Shredded cheese, Italian five cheese, ¼ cup	3
Shredded cheese, Italian five cheese, with a touch of Philadelphia, ¼ cup	3
Shredded cheese, Monterey Jack, ¼ cup	4
Shredded cheese, mozzarella, ¼ cup	3
Shredded cheese, mozzarella, fat free, ¼ cup	0
Shredded cheese, parmesan, romano and asiago, ¼ cup	4
Shredded cheese, pepper Jack, with a touch of Philadelphia, ¼ cup	4
Shredded cheese, three cheese, with a touch of Philadelphia, ¼ cup	4
Shredded cheese, triple cheddar, with a touch of Philadelphia, ¼ cup	4
Shredded Mexican style four cheese, ¼ cup	4
String cheese, cracked black pepper, 1 stick (24 g)	2
String cheese, jalapeño, 1 stick (24 g)	2
String cheese, low-moisture part-skim, mozzarella, 1 stick (28 g)	3
String cheese, made with 2% milk, mozzarella, 1 stick (24 g)	2

Dairy & Eggs

	SmartPoints™ value
String cheese, tomato basil, 1 stick (24 g)	2
Three cheese blend, 100% grated, 2 tsp	1
Velveeta, made with 2% milk, ¼" slice	2

Kraft Combo

Cheese slices, combo pack (mild cheddar), 2 slices (23 g)	4

Kraft Deli Deluxe

American pasteurized process cheese (19 gm slices), 1 slice (19 g)	3
Cheese slices, pasteurized process, American, family size!, 2 slices (25 g)	4
Cheese slices, pasteurized process, white American, 1 slice (21 g)	3
Cheese slices, reduced fat pasteurized process, American, 1 slice (19 g)	2
Pasteurized process cheese, sharp cheddar, slices, 1 slice (19 g)	3

Kraft Free

Shredded cheese, cheddar, ¼ cup	0

Kraft Natural

Big cheese slices, aged Swiss, 1 slice (23 g)	3
Big cheese slices, colby Jack, 1 slice (23 g)	3
Big cheese slices, jalapeño cheddar, 1 slice (21 g)	3
Big cheese slices, mild cheddar, 1 slice (23 g)	4
Big cheese slices, pepper Jack, medium heat, 1 slice (23 g)	3
Big cheese slices, sharp cheddar, 1 slice (23 g)	4
Big cheese slices, smoky chipotle, 1 slice (21 g)	3

	SmartPoints™ value
Big cheese slices, Swiss, 1 slice (23 g)	3
Cheese crumbles, three cheese, ¼ cup	4
Cheese cubes, cheddar & Monterey Jack, 7 pieces (30 g)	5
Cheese cubes, marbled colby & Monterey Jack, 7 pieces (30 g)	4
Cheese cubes, mild cheddar, 7 pieces (30 g)	5
Cheese cubes, sharp cheddar, 7 pieces (30 g)	5
Cheese slices, combo pack (sharp cheddar), 2 slices (23 g)	4
Cheese slices, extra thin, extra sharp white cheddar, slim cut, 3 slices (35 g)	4
Cheese slices, extra thin, Swiss, 1 slice (16 g)	2
Cheese slices, havarti, 1 slice (20 g)	3
Cheese slices, hot habanero, extra hot, big slice, 1 slice (21 g)	3
Cheese slices, low-moisture part-skim, mozzarella, 1 slice (19 g)	2
Cheese slices, made with 2% milk, sharp cheddar, 1 slice (20 g)	2
Cheese slices, marbled colby and Monterey Jack, 1 slice (19 g)	3
Cheese slices, mozzarella, slim cut, 3 slices (33 g)	3
Cheese slices, Swiss, made with 2% milk, 1 slice (18 g)	2
Cheese sticks, extra sharp cheddar cheese, 1 stick (28 g)	5
Cheese sticks, snacks, reduced fat, sharp cheddar, 1 stick (28 g)	3
Cheese, extra sharp cheddar, ⅛ package (28 g)	5
Cheese, jalapeño white cheddar, 1" cube	4

Dairy & Eggs

	SmartPoints™ value
Cheese, made with 2% milk, colby & Monterey Jack, 1/7 package (28 g)	3
Cheese, made with 2% milk, sharp cheddar, 1 oz	3
Cheese, marbled colby & Monterey Jack, high moisture, 1/8 package (28 g)	4
Cheese, medium cheddar, 1/8 package (28 g)	5
Cheese, mild cheddar, 1 oz	5
Cheese, mild cheddar, made with 2% milk, 1 oz	3
Cheese, Monterey Jack, 1/8 package (28 g)	4
Cheese, Monterey Jack, mild cheddar & colby, reduced fat, 1 oz	3
Cheese, mozzarella, low moisture, part-skim, 1/8 package (28 g)	3
Cheese, provolone, 1 slice (19 g)	2
Cheese, sharp cheddar, 1/8 package (28 g)	5
Cheese, Swiss, slices, 1 slice (23 g)	3
Extra hot habanero string cheese snack, 1 stick (24 g)	2
Finely shredded cheese, aged Wisconsin sharp cheddar, ¼ cup	4
Finely shredded cheese, authentic Mexican style, ¼ cup	3
Finely shredded cheese, cheddar pepper Jack, Mexican style, ¼ cup	4
Finely shredded cheese, colby & Monterey Jack, ¼ cup	4
Finely shredded cheese, made with 2% milk, Mexican style cheddar Jack, ¼ cup	3
Finely shredded cheese, made with 2% milk, Mexican style four cheese, ¼ cup	3
Finely shredded cheese, Mexican style cheddar Jack, ¼ cup	4

	SmartPoints™ value
Finely shredded cheese, mild cheddar, ¼ cup	4
Finely shredded cheese, mild cheddar, reduced fat, ¼ cup	3
Finely shredded cheese, mozzarella, ¼ cup	3
Finely shredded cheese, parmesan, ¼ cup	4
Finely shredded cheese, triple cheddar, ¼ cup	4
Mexican style taco shredded cheese made with 2% milk, ¼ cup	3
Mozzarella string cheese, 1 stick (28 g)	3
Sharp cheddar aged Wisconsin shredded cheese, ¼ cup	4
Shredded cheese, colby & Monterey Jack, reduced fat, ¼ cup	3
Shredded cheese, made with 2% milk, mozzarella, ¼ cup	2
Shredded cheese, mild cheddar, ¼ cup	4
Shredded cheese, mild cheddar & Monterey Jack, ¼ cup	4
Shredded cheese, mozzarella, fat free, ¼ cup	0
Shredded cheese, pepper Jack, medium, ¼ cup	4
Shredded cheese, pizza, mozzarella cheddar, ¼ cup	3
Shredded cheese, reduced fat, mild cheddar, ¼ cup	3
Shredded cheese, sharp cheddar, reduced fat, ¼ cup	3
Shredded cheese, sharp white cheddar, ¼ cup	4
Shredded cheese, Swiss, ¼ cup	4
Shredded colby and Monterey Jack cheeses, ¼ cup	4

Dairy & Eggs

	SmartPoints™ value
Slim cut cheese slices, reduced fat, Swiss, 3 slices (33 g)	4
Slim cut cheese, reduced fat, colby Jack, 1 slice (35 g)	4
Slim cut cheese, reduced fat, sharp cheddar, 3 slices (35 g)	4
Kraft Simply	
Cottage cheese, large curd, 4% milkfat minimum, ½ cup	4
Cottage cheese, small curd, 2% milkfat, low fat, ½ cup	3
Cottage cheese, small curd, 4% milkfat minimum, ½ cup	4
Cottage cheese, small curd, fat free, ½ cup	2
Kraft Singles	
American cheese pasteurized cheese product, 1 slice (19 g)	2
American cheese pasteurized prepared cheese product (19 gm slices), 1 slice (19 g)	2
American cheese pasteurized prepared cheese product (21 gm slices), 1 slice (21 g)	3
Cheese product slices, made with skim milk, sharp cheddar, 1 slice (19 g)	0
Cheese product slices, sharp cheddar, 1 slice (21 g)	2
Cheese product, made with 2% milk, Swiss, 1 slice (19 g)	2
Cheese product, made with skim milk, Swiss, 1 slice (19 g)	0
Cheese product, pasteurized prepared, made with 2% milk, sharp cheddar, 1 slice (19 g)	2
Cheese product, pasteurized prepared, made with 2% milk, white American, 1 slice (19 g)	2
Cheese product, pasteurized prepared, made with skim milk, American, 1 slice (19 g)	0

	SmartPoints™ value
Cheese product, pasteurized prepared, reduced fat 2%, American, 1 slice (19 g)	2
Cheese product, pasteurized prepared, reduced fat, 2% milk, American, 1 slice (21 g)	2
Cheese product, pasteurized prepared, white American, 1 slice (21 g)	3
Cheese product, pasteurized, Swiss, 1 slice (21 g)	2
Cheese product, pepperjack, made with 2% milk, 1 slice (19 g)	1
Kroger	
2% milk reduced fat American cheese product singles, 1 slice (21 g)	2
Cheese cubes, mild cheddar Jack, 6 pieces (28 g)	4
Cheese food, hot pepper, 1" cube	3
Cheese food, singles, Swiss style, 1 slice (21 g)	2
Cheese product, fat free singles, Swiss, 1 slice (21 g)	1
Cheese product, pasteurized process, nice'n cheesy slices, 1 slice (21 g)	3
Cheese product, singles, 3 cheese blend, 1 slice (21 g)	2
Cheese product, singles, American, 1 slice (19 g)	2
Cheese product, singles, pepper Jack, 1 slice (21 g)	2
Cheese product, Swiss flavored, pasteurized process, 1 wedge (19 g)	1
Cheese slices, aged sharp white cheddar, 1 slice (21 g)	3
Cheese slices, colby, 1 slice (21 g)	3
Cheese slices, havarti, 1 slice (21 g)	4
Cheese slices, mild cheddar, 1 slice (21 g)	3

Dairy & Eggs

	SmartPoints™ value
Cheese slices, mozzarella, 1 slice (21 g)	2
Cheese slices, orange rind muenster, 1 slice (21 g)	3
Cheese slices, pepper Jack, 1 slice (21 g)	3
Cheese spread, lite, pimento, 1 Tbsp	1
Cheese spread, pimento, 1 Tbsp	3
Cheese, colby Monterey Jack, 1" cube	4
Cheese, colby, finely shredded, ¼ cup	4
Cheese, deli thin slices, aged Swiss, 1 slice (21 g)	3
Cheese, deli thin slices, medium cheddar, 1 slice (21 g)	3
Cheese, deli thin slices, smoke flavored provolone, 1 slice (21 g)	3
Cheese, extra sharp cheddar, 1" cube	4
Cheese, finely shredded, 4 cheese Mexican blend, reduced fat, ¼ cup	3
Cheese, marble cheddar, shredded, ¼ cup	4
Cheese, medium cheddar, 1" cube	4
Cheese, Mexican style, finely shredded, ¼ cup	4
Cheese, Mexican style, shredded, ¼ cup	4
Cheese, mild cheddar, 1" cube	4
Cheese, mild cheddar, finely shredded, ¼ cup	4
Cheese, Monterey Jack, 1" cube	4
Cheese, mozzarella, finely shredded, ¼ cup	2
Cheese, nacho & taco, finely shredded, ¼ cup	4
Cheese, natural, colby Monterey Jack, 1" cube	4

	SmartPoints™ value
Cheese, natural, extra sharp cheddar, 1" cube	4
Cheese, natural, medium cheddar, 1 oz	4
Cheese, natural, mozzarella, low moisture part skim, 1 oz	2
Cheese, natural, sharp cheddar, 1" cube	4
Cheese, pizza, shredded, ¼ cup	3
Cheese, reduced fat, mild cheddar, 2% milk, 1" cube	3
Cheese, reduced fat, mild cheddar, finely shredded, ¼ cup	3
Cheese, sharp cheddar, 1" cube	4
Cheese, sharp cheddar, shredded, ¼ cup	4
Cheese, sliced, Swiss, 1 slice (38 g)	5
Cheese, slices, colby Jack, 1 slice (21 g)	3
Cheese, string, low moisture part skim mozzarella, twists, 1 piece (24 g)	2
Cheese, Swiss, reduced fat, slices, 1 slice (28 g)	2
Cottage cheese, large curd, ½ cup	3
Cottage cheese, low fat, with pineapple, ½ cup	3
Cream cheese spread, whipped, 2 Tbsp	3
Cream cheese, fat free, 2 Tbsp	1
Cream cheese, light, 2 Tbsp	2
Cream cheese, original, 2 Tbsp	5
Cream cheese, soft, 2 Tbsp	5
Fat free American cheese singles, 1 slice (21 g)	1
Fat free cottage cheese, ½ cup	1
Fat-free cottage cheese, ½ cup	1
Finely shredded cheese, colby Jack, ¼ cup	4

Dairy & Eggs

Finely shredded cheese, Italian blend, ¼ cup	3
Finely shredded cheese, mild cheddar, ¼ cup	4
Finely shredded cheese, mild cheddar Jack, ¼ cup	4
Finely shredded cheese, natural, colby Jack, ¼ cup	4
Finely shredded cheese, sharp cheddar, ¼ cup	4
Finely shredded cheese, sharp cheddar, reduced fat, ¼ cup	3
Large curd cottage cheese, ½ cup	3
Light mozzarella string cheese, 1 stick (28 g)	2
Lowfat cottage cheese, ½ cup	3
Neufchatel cheese, 2 Tbsp	3
Shredded cheese, Mexican style, ¼ cup	4
Shredded cheese, mild cheddar, ¼ cup	4
Shredded cheese, mild cheddar & Monterey Jack, ¼ cup	4
Shredded cheese, Monterey Jack, ¼ cup	4
Shredded cheese, mozzarella style, fat free, ¼ cup	1
Shredded cheese, mozzarella, low moisture part skim, ¼ cup	2
Shredded cheese, sharp cheddar, ¼ cup	4
Smoke flavor string cheese, 1 stick (24 g)	2

Kroger CowPals

Cheese, snack, colby Jack, 1 piece (28 g)	3
Cheese, string, mozzarella, low moisture part skim, 1 piece (28 g)	3
Snack cheese, 1 piece (21 g)	3
Snack cheese, colby Jack, 1 piece (21 g)	3

Snack cheese, mild cheddar, 1 piece (21 g)	3
String cheese, mozzarella, 1 piece (28 g)	3

Kroger Deluxe

Cheese, pasteurized process, American, 1 slice (21 g)	3

La Bonne Vie

Goat cheese crumbles, 1 oz	3

Lactaid

Cottage cheese, lowfat, ½ cup	2

Land O' Lakes

American singles, white, 1 each (21 g)	3
Cheese, 30% less sodium, American, 1 oz	5
Cheese, deli, thin, American, 1 slice (23 g)	3
Cheese, muenster, 1 slice (23 g)	3
Cheese, pasteurized process, American, 1 slice (23 g)	4
Cheese, provolone, 1 slice (23 g)	3
Cheese, reduced fat, 2% milk, American, 1 oz	3
Cheese, thin, baby Swiss, 1 slice (21 g)	3
Cheese, thin, pepper Jack, 1 slice (23 g)	3
Cottage cheese, 1% lowfat, small curd, ½ cup	2
Cottage cheese, 2% lowfat, small curd, ½ cup	2
Deli cheese, American, slices, 1 slice (19 g)	3
Deli cheese, American, white, 1 slice (23 g)	4
Deli cheese, American, yellow, 1 slice (23 g)	4
Deli cheese, white American, 1 slice (19 g)	3
Deli cheese, yellow American, 1 slice (19 g)	3

Dairy & Eggs

Dairy & Eggs

	SmartPoints™ value
Fat free small curd cottage cheese, ½ cup	2
Low fat 1% milkfat small curd cottage cheese, ½ cup	2
Reduced fat cheddar cheese, 1 portion (19 g)	2
Land O' Lakes Snack 'N Cheese To-Go!	
Cheese, natural, co-Jack, 1 bar (21 g)	3
Cheese, natural, mild cheddar, 1 bar (21 g)	3
Laughing Cow	
Creamy spicy pepper Jack spreadable cheese wedges, 1 wedge (21 g)	1
Spreadable cheese wedges, creamy mozzarella sun-dried tomato & basil, 1 wedge (21 g)	1
Spreadable cheese wedges, creamy queso fresco chipotle, 1 wedge (21 g)	1
Spreadable cheese wedges, creamy Swiss French onion, 1 wedge (21 g)	1
Spreadable cheese wedges, creamy Swiss, light, 1 wedge (21 g)	1
Spreadable cheese wedges, creamy Swiss, original, 1 wedge (21 g)	2
Spreadable cheese wedges, white cheddar flavor, creamy, 1 wedge (21 g)	1
Laughing Cow Light	
Garlic and herb spreadable cheese wedge, 1 wedge (21 g)	1
Laughing Cow Mini Babybel	
Semi-soft cheese, gouda, 1 piece (21 g)	3
Semisoft cheese, mozzarella style, reduced fat, 1 piece (21 g)	2
Semisoft cheeses, cheddar variety, 1 piece (21 g)	2

	SmartPoints™ value
Semisoft cheeses, original, 1 piece (21 g)	3
Semisoft cheeses, sharp original, 1 piece (20 g)	2
Semisoft cheeses, white cheddar variety, 1 piece (20 g)	3
Lorraine Cheese	
Deli sliced cheese, lorraine, original, 1 slice (28 g)	4
Deli sliced cheese, lorraine, reduced fat, 1 slice (28 g)	4
Lucerne	
Cheese product, 2% milk American slices, 1 slice (21 g)	2
Cheese sticks, sharp cheddar, reduced fat 2% milk, 1 stick (28 g)	3
Cheese, American, fat free slices, 1 slice (21 g)	1
Cheese, American, reduced fat, slices, 1 slice (19 g)	2
Cheese, colby Jack, reduced fat, 1 oz	3
Cheese, havarti, sliced, 1 slice (22 g)	4
Cheese, medium cheddar, sliced, 1 slice (22 g)	3
Cheese, muenster, sliced, 1 slice (21 g)	3
Cheese, natural, 2% milk, reduced fat, sliced, provolone, 1 slice (21 g)	2
Cheese, natural, medium cheddar, 2% reduced fat, 1 oz	3
Cheese, natural, reduced fat, sliced, medium, ¾ oz	2
Cheese, natural, reduced fat, sliced, Swiss, 1 slice (21 g)	2
Cheese, natural, sliced, aged Swiss, ¾ oz	3
Cheese, natural, sliced, colby Jack, 1 slice (21 g)	3
Cheese, natural, sliced, mozzarella, ¾ oz	2

	SmartPoints™ value
Cheese, natural, sliced, pepper Jack, 1 slice (21 g)	3
Cheese, pepper Jack, colby Jack, sliced, Jack pack, 1 slice (22 g)	3
Cheese, sliced, havarti, 1 slice (21 g)	4
Cheese, sliced, Monterey Jack, 1 slice (21 g)	3
Cheese, sliced, sharp cheddar, 1 slice (21 g)	3
Cheese, smoked gouda, sliced, 1 slice (21 g)	3
Cottage cheese, 1% milkfat min., no salt added, ½ cup	2
Cottage cheese, 2% milkfat, lowfat, ½ cup	2
Cottage cheese, fat free, ½ cup	2
Cottage cheese, lowfat, 1% milkfat min., ½ cup	2
Cream cheese spread, whipped, 2 Tbsp	3
Cream cheese spread, whipped, with chives, 2 Tbsp	3
Cream cheese, light, 2 Tbsp	3
Cream cheese, with garden vegetables, 2 Tbsp	4
Crumbled cheese, reduced fat, feta, ¼ cup	2
Deluxe American cheese slices, 1 slice (19 g)	3
Fat free cottage cheese, ½ cup	2
Finely shredded cheese, cheddar Jack, ¼ cup	4
Finely shredded cheese, Mexican, ¼ cup	4
Light string cheese, 1 stick (24 g)	1
Low fat 1% milkfat min cottage cheese, ½ cup	2
Mozzarella fat free shredded cheese, ¼ cup	0
Shredded cheese, fat free cheddar, ¼ cup	0

	SmartPoints™ value
Shredded cheese, medium cheddar, ¼ cup	4
Shredded cheese, mozzarella, ¼ cup	2
Shredded cheese, sharp cheddar, ¼ cup	4
String cheese, 1 piece (28 g)	3
String cheese, light, 1 piece (24 g)	1
Swiss cheese, jarlsberg lite, reduced fat, 1 slice (21 g)	1
Lucerne Dairy Farms	
Low moisture part skim mozzarella string cheese, 1 stick (24 g)	2
Lucerne Thin Slices	
Natural medium cheddar cheese slices, 3 slices (32 g)	5
Natural Swiss cheese slices, 3 slices (32 g)	4
Lynn	
Cheese, munster, 1" cube	4
Market Pantry	
100% grated parmesan cheese, 1 Tbsp	1
Cheese bars, colby Jack, 1 bar (21 g)	3
Cheese bars, mild cheddar, 1 bar (21 g)	3
Cheese food, American, singles, 1 slice (21 g)	3
Cheese product, American, reduced fat, singles, 1 slice (21 g)	2
Cheese slices, deli-style, colby Jack, 1 slice (19 g)	3
Cheese slices, deli-style, colby Jack, reduced fat, 2% milk, 1 slice (19 g)	2
Cheese slices, deli-style, mild cheddar, 1 slice (19 g)	3
Cheese slices, deli-style, mild cheddar, reduced fat, 2% milk, 1 slice (19 g)	2
Cheese slices, deli-style, mozzarella, 1 slice (19 g)	2

Dairy & Eggs

Dairy & Eggs

	SmartPoints™ value
Cheese slices, deli-style, muenster, 1 slice (12 g)	3
Cheese slices, deli-style, provolone, 1 slice (19 g)	2
Cheese slices, deli-style, sharp cheddar, 1 slice (19 g)	3
Cheese slices, deli-style, Swiss, reduced fat, 2% milk, 1 slice (19 g)	2
Cheese sticks, colby Jack, 1 stick (28 g)	4
Cheese sticks, colby Jack, reduced fat, 1 piece (28 g)	3
Cheese sticks, mild cheddar, 1 stick (28 g)	4
Cheese sticks, pepper Jack, 1 stick (28 g)	4
Cheese, deluxe American, slices, 1 slice (19 g)	2
Cheese, natural, sharp cheddar, reduced fat, 2% milk, ⅛ package (28 g)	3
Colby Jack ultra thin cheese slices, 2 slices (25 g)	3
Fat free cottage cheese, ½ cup	2
Finely shredded cheese, cheddar Jack, ¼ cup	4
Finely shredded cheese, Mexican style taco blend, ¼ cup	4
Finely shredded cheese, mild cheddar, ¼ cup	4
Finely shredded cheese, mozzarella, ⅓ cup	4
Mild cheddar ultra-thin cheese slices, 2 slices (25 g)	4
Pepper Jack ultra thin cheese slices, 2 slices (25 g)	3
Provolone ultra thin cheese slices, 2 slices (25 g)	3
Reduced fat deli style provolone cheese slice, 1 slice (19 g)	2

	SmartPoints™ value
Shredded cheese, cheddar Jack, ¼ cup	4
Shredded cheese, colby Jack, ¼ cup	4
Shredded cheese, colby Jack, reduced fat, 2% milk, ¼ cup	3
Shredded cheese, Mexican style four cheese blend, ¼ cup	4
Shredded cheese, Mexican style four-cheese blend, reduced fat, 2% milk, ¼ cup	3
Shredded cheese, mozzarella, ¼ cup	3
Shredded cheese, mozzarella, reduced fat, ¼ cup	2
Sliced cheese, deli-style, pepper Jack, 1 slice (19 g)	3
Small curd cottage cheese, ½ cup	2
String cheese, light, mozzarella, 1 piece (28 g)	2
String cheese, mozzarella, 1 piece (28 g)	3
String cheese, mozzarella double twist, 1 piece (24 g)	2
Merkts	
Cheese spread, cold pack, port wine, 2 Tbsp	4
Mexica	
Queso fresco, semi-soft white cheese, 1 oz	3
Michigan	
Small curd cottage cheese, ½ cup	3
Miller's Cheese	
Cheese, natural, muenster, 1 oz	4
Mini Babybel	
Light semisoft cheese, 1 piece (21 g)	1
Mozzarella Fresca	
Fresh mozzarella, 1 oz	2

My Essentials 2% Milk

Fancy shredded Mexican blend cheese, ¼ cup	3
Fancy shredded sharp cheddar cheese, ¼ cup	3

My Essentials Cheese Twisters

Part skim mozzarella string cheese, 1 (28 g)	3

Nancy's

Cottage cheese, cultured lowfat, ½ cup	2
Cottage cheese, organic, cultured lowfat, ½ cup	2

Nordica

Cottage cheese, lowfat, 1% milkfat min, ½ cup	2

O Organics

Light mozzarella low moisture part skim string cheese, 1 stick (28 g)	2

Odyssey

Crumbled cheese, feta, Greek style, crumbled, fat free, 2 Tbsp	1

Old Home

Cottage cheese, small curd, ¼ cup	4

Organic Valley

Cheese, American singles, high-moisture colby-style, 1 slice (19 g)	3
Cheese, fancy shredded, mozzarella, organic, ¼ cup	3
Cottage cheese, lowfat, organic small curd, ½ cup	2
Cream cheese, organic, 2 Tbsp	5
Fancy shredded cheese, organic, Mexican blend, ¼ cup	4
Neufchatel cheese, organic, 2 Tbsp	3

Our Family

Cheese product, American, 2% milk, singles, 1 slice (21 g)	2

Palmetto

Cheese spread, 2 Tbsp	5
Palmetto cheese spread with jalapeños, 2 Tbsp	5

Paneer

Cheese, paneer, 1 oz	4

Pauly

Swiss cheese slices, 1 slice (18 g)	3

Philadelphia

Cream cheese spread, ⅓ less fat, 2 Tbsp	3
Cream cheese spread, ⅓ less fat, chive and onion, 2 Tbsp	3
Cream cheese spread, ⅓ less fat, garden vegetable, 2 Tbsp	3
Cream cheese spread, ⅓ less fat, strawberry, 2 Tbsp	3
Cream cheese spread, bacon flavor, 2 Tbsp	3
Cream cheese spread, blueberry, 2 Tbsp	3
Cream cheese spread, brown sugar and cinnamon, 2 Tbsp	4
Cream cheese spread, chipotle, 2 Tbsp	3
Cream cheese spread, chive & onion, 2 Tbsp	4
Cream cheese spread, fat free, 2 Tbsp	1
Cream cheese spread, garden vegetable, 2 Tbsp	3
Cream cheese spread, honey pecan, 2 Tbsp	4
Cream cheese spread, light, 1 Tbsp	2
Cream cheese spread, milk chocolate, 2 Tbsp	6
Cream cheese spread, original, 2 Tbsp	4
Cream cheese spread, pineapple, 2 Tbsp	3

Dairy & Eggs

	SmartPoints™ value
Cream cheese spread, pumpkin spice, 2 Tbsp	4
Cream cheese spread, regular, brown sugar & cinnamon, 2 Tbsp	4
Cream cheese spread, regular, honey nut flavor, 2 Tbsp	4
Cream cheese spread, regular, salmon, 2 Tbsp	4
Cream cheese spread, smoked salmon, 2 Tbsp	3
Cream cheese spread, spicy jalapeño, 2 Tbsp	3
Cream cheese spread, strawberry, 2 Tbsp	4
Cream cheese, reduced fat (individual pouch), 1 pouch (28 g)	3
Philadelphia 2x Protein	
Cream cheese spread, 2 Tbsp	2
Philadelphia Cream Swirls	
Cream cheese spread, brown sugar 'n cinnamon spice, 2 Tbsp	4
Philadelphia Deli Style	
Cream cheese, 2 Tbsp	4
Philadelphia Fat Free	
Cream cheese spread, strawberry, 2 Tbsp	2
Philadelphia Whipped	
Cream cheese spread, chive, 2 Tbsp	2
Cream cheese spread, mixed berry, 2 Tbsp	3
Cream cheese spread, original, 2 Tbsp	2
Polly-O	
Cheese, fresh mozzarella, 1 oz	3
Cheese, mozzarella, fat free, 1 oz	0
Cheese, mozzarella, part skim, 1 oz	2
Cheese, part skim mozzarella, 1 serving (28 g)	2
String cheese, jalapeño, 1 stick (24 g)	2

	SmartPoints™ value
String cheese, mozzarella, natural reduced fat, 1 stick (28 g)	2
String cheese, mozzarella, reduced fat, 1 stick (24 g)	2
String cheese, mozzarella, reduced fat, family size, 1 stick (24 g)	2
Twists, mozzarella & cheddar cheeses, 1 stick (21 g)	2
Polly-O Snackables Twists	
Cheese, cheddar & mozzarella, 1 stick (21 g)	2
Polly-O String	
Mozzarella cheese, 1 stick (28 g)	3
Prairie Farms	
Cottage cheese, fat free, ½ cup	2
Cottage cheese, low fat, ½ cup	2
Cottage cheese, low fat, snack cups, ½ cup	2
Cottage cheese, small curd, ½ cup	4
Precious	
Cheese, mozzarella, 1 oz	3
Cheese, ricotta part skim, ¼ cup	3
Cheese, ricotta, fat free, ¼ cup	1
Cheese, ricotta, low fat, ¼ cup	2
Precious Sticksters	
Cheese stick, colby Jack, 1 stick (24 g)	3
Cheese stick, pepper-Jack, 1 stick (24 g)	3
Cheese sticks, pepper-Jack, 1 stick (24 g)	3
Precious Stringsters	
String cheese, 1 string (28 g)	3
String cheese, reduced fat, 1 string (28 g)	2
String cheese, reduced fat mozzarella, 1 stick (28 g)	2
String cheese, riddles, 1 stick (28 g)	3

Dairy & Eggs

President

Cheese, fat free, crumbled, mediterranean herbs, 1 oz	1
Cheese, feta, chunks, 1 oz	3
Cheese, feta, crumbled, herb, 1 oz	0
Cheese, feta, fat free, chunks, 1 oz	0

President Pub Cheese

Cheese, spreadable, cheddar & horseradish, 2 Tbsp	4

Primo Taglio

Goat cheese, crumbles, 1 oz	3

Private Selection

Cheese, blue, reduced fat, crumbled, ¼ cup	3
Cheese, creamy, small eye, baby Swiss, 1 slice (22 g)	3
Cheese, extra sharp, New York white cheddar, 3 slices (28 g)	4
Cheese, feta, crumbled, traditional, ¼ cup	3
Cheese, feta, reduced fat, crumbled, traditional, ¼ cup	3
Cheese, hand crafted provolone, sliced, 1 slice (22 g)	3
Cheese, hand marbled, Colby Jack, sliced, 1 slice (22 g)	3
Cheese, havarti, sliced, 1 slice (22 g)	4
Cheese, mild cheddar, sliced, 1 slice (22 g)	3
Cheese, natural, vermont extra sharp white cheddar, 1 piece (28 g)	4
Cheese, parmesan, shaved, ¼ cup	3
Cheese, pepper Jack, sliced, 1 slice (22 g)	4
Cheese, sliced mild Wisconsin muenster, 1 slice (22 g)	3
Cheese, sliced, Colby, 1 slice (22 g)	3
Cheese, smoked gouda, sliced, 1 slice (22 g)	3

Pub Cheese

Cheese, spreadable, Sharp cheddar gourmet, 2 Tbsp	4

Publix

Cheese, cream spread, regular soft, 2 Tbsp	5
Cheese, sharp American, singles, 1 slice (21 g)	3
Cottage cheese, fat free, small curd, ½ cup	1
Cottage cheese, small curd, lowfat, ½ cup	2
Cottage cheese, with pineapple, low fat, 1% milkfat, small curd, ½ cup	4
Cream cheese spread, whipped, 2 Tbsp	3

Publix Singles

American pasteurized process cheese singles, 1 slice (19 g)	2

Rosenborg

Cheese, Danish blue, crumbled, traditional, 1 oz	4

Roth

Gouda cheese, sliced, Van Gogh natural smoked, 1 slice (21 g)	3

Roundy's

String cheese, reduced fat, 1 piece (24 g)	2

Saladena

Goat cheese crumbles, ¼ cup	3

Salemville

Cheese crumbles, Amish gorgonzola, 2 Tbsp	4
Cheese crumbles, blue, Amish, 2 Tbsp	4

Sandwich Mate

Cheese food, pasteurized, imitation, singles, American flavor, 1 slice (19 g)	2

Saputo Frigo Cheese Heads

String cheese, light, 1 piece (24 g)	1

Dairy & Eggs

Dairy & Eggs

	SmartPoints™ value
Saputo Frigo Cheese Heads Swirls	
Natural string cheese, 1 piece (24 g)	2
Sara Lee Premium Deli	
Baby Swiss natural cheese custom slices, 3 slices (34 g)	5
Colby and Monterey Jack natural cheese custom thin slices, 3 slices (34 g)	5
Mild cheddar cheese custom thin slices, 3 slices (34 g)	5
Smoked provolone natural cheese, 1 slice (23 g)	3
Sargento	
Cheese slices, reduced fat, colby Jack, 1 slice (19 g)	2
Cheese slices, reduced fat, medium cheddar, 1 slice (19 g)	2
Cheese sticks, Colby Jack, 1 piece (21 g)	3
Cheese sticks, pepper Jack, 1 piece (21 g)	3
Cheese sticks, reduced fat, colby Jack, 1 piece (21 g)	2
Cheese sticks, reduced fat, mild cheddar, 1 piece (21 g)	2
Cheese sticks, reduced fat, natural mild cheddar, 1 piece (21 g)	2
Cheese sticks, reduced fat, sharp cheddar, 1 piece (21 g)	2
Cheese, light ricotta, ¼ cup	2
Cheese, natural Monterey Jack, deli style, slices, 1 slice (21 g)	3
Cheese, natural Swiss baby cheese, ultra thin slices, 3 slices (30 g)	4
Cheese, natural, extra sharp cheddar, 1 slice (20 g)	3
Cheese, reduced fat, 4 cheese Italian, shredded, ¼ cup	2

	SmartPoints™ value
Cheese, reduced fat, 4 cheese Mexican, shredded, ¼ cup	3
Cheese, reduced fat, cheddar Jack, shredded, ¼ cup	3
Cheese, reduced fat, Colby Jack, shredded, ¼ cup	3
Cheese, reduced fat, mild cheddar, shredded, ¼ cup	3
Cheese, reduced fat, mozzarella, shredded, ¼ cup	2
Cheese, reduced fat, pepper Jack, 1 slice (19 g)	2
Cheese, reduced fat, provolone cheese, slices, 1 slice (19 g)	2
Cheese, reduced fat, sharp cheddar, shredded, ¼ cup	3
Cheese, reduced fat, Swiss cheese, slices, 1 slice (21 g)	2
Cheese, reduced sodium, pepper Jack, slices, 1 slice (19 g)	3
Natural deli style sliced baby Swiss cheese, 1 slice (18 g)	3
Natural deli style sliced chipotle cheddar cheese, 1 slice (21 g)	3
Natural deli style sliced Colby Jack cheese, 1 slice (19 g)	3
Natural deli style sliced gouda cheese, 1 slice (20 g)	3
Natural deli style sliced medium cheddar cheese, 1 slice (21 g)	3
Natural deli style sliced muenster cheese, 1 slice (21 g)	3
Natural deli style sliced provolone cheese, 1 slice (19 g)	2
Natural deli style sliced Swiss cheese, 1 slice (18 g)	2
Natural deli style sliced Vermont sharp white cheddar cheese, 1 slice (20 g)	3
String cheese, light mozzarella, 1 piece (21 g)	1

Sargento Artisan Blends

Authentic Mexican shredded cheese, ¼ cup	4
Mozzarella and provolone shredded cheese, ¼ cup	3
Shredded cheese, whole milk mozzarella, ¼ cup	3
Shredded parmesan cheese, 2 tsp	1
Shredded parmesan cheese (stand up pouch), 2 tsp	1

Sargento Chef Blends

4 cheese pizzeria shredded cheese, ¼ cup	3
4 state cheddar, ¼ cup	4
4 state cheddar shredded cheese, ¼ cup	4
6 cheese Italian shredded cheese, ¼ cup	3
Nacho and taco flavor shredded cheese, ¼ cup	4
Taco flavor shredded cheese, ¼ cup	4

Sargento Classic

4 cheese Mexican, ¼ cup	4
Traditional cut shredded mozzarella cheese (16 oz bag), ¼ cup	3

Sargento Deli Style

Natural deli style sliced sharp cheddar cheese, 1 slice (21 g)	3

Sargento Natural Blends

Cheddar mozzarella cheese sticks, 1 piece (21 g)	3
Cheddar-mozzarella cheese slices, 1 slice (19 g)	3
Cheddar-mozzarella cheese snacks, 1 stick (21 g)	3
Colby-pepper Jack cheese slices, 1 slice (19 g)	3
Double cheddar cheese slices, 1 slice (19 g)	3

Double cheddar cheese sticks, 1 piece (21 g)	3
Provolone-mozzarella cheese slices, 1 slice (19 g)	2
Sharp cheddar-Jack cheese slices, 1 slice (19 g)	3
Sharp cheddar-Jack cheese snacks, 1 piece (21 g)	3

Sargento Off the Block

4 cheese Mexican fine cut cheese, ¼ cup	4
Fine cut 4 cheese Mexican shredded cheese (16 oz bag), ¼ cup	4
Fine cut shredded 4 cheese Mexican blend, ¼ cup	4
Fine cut shredded cheddar Jack cheese (8 oz bag), ¼ cup	4
Fine cut shredded colby Jack cheese, ¼ cup	4
Fine cut shredded mild cheddar cheese, ¼ cup	4
Fine cut shredded sharp cheddar cheese (16 oz bag), ¼ cup	4
Fine cut shredded sharp cheddar cheese (8 oz bag), ¼ cup	4
Sharp cheddar traditional cut shredded cheese, ¼ cup	4
Shredded cheese, sharp cheddar, traditional cut, ¼ cup	4
Traditional cut 4 cheese Mexican shredded cheese, ¼ cup	4
Traditional cut extra sharp cheddar shredded cheese, ¼ cup	4
Traditional cut shredded mozzarella cheese (8 oz bag), ¼ cup	3

Sargento Snacks

Cheese sticks, natural, extra sharp cheddar, 1 piece (21 g)	3
Cheese, Colby Jack, cubes, 7 cubes (30 g)	4

Dairy & Eggs

	SmartPoints™ value
Mozzarella string cheese, 1 piece (21 g)	2
Sharp cheddar cheese stick, 1 piece (21 g)	3
Sargento Ultra Thin	
Baby Swiss cheese slices, 3 slices (32 g)	4
Cheddar Jack cheese slices, 3 slices (32 g)	5
Colby-Jack cheese slices, 3 slices (31 g)	5
Longhorn colby cheese slices, 3 slices (32 g)	5
Mild cheddar cheese slices, 3 slices (32 g)	5
Provolone cheese slices, 3 slices (31 g)	4
Sharp cheddar cheese slices, 3 slices (32 g)	5
Sartori Reserve	
Cheese, merlot bellavitano, 1 oz	4
Shamrock Farms	
Cottage cheese, low fat, ½ cup	3
ShopRite	
Cheese slices, American, white, 1 slice (21 g)	3
Cheese slices, Swiss, 1 slice (21 g)	3
Cheese, ricotta, fat free, ¼ cup	1
Cottage cheese, small curd, 1% milkfat, lowfat, ½ cup	2
Cottage cheese, small curd, fat free, ½ cup	2
Cream cheese, soft, light, 2 Tbsp	3
Finely shredded cheese, natural, cheddar Jack, ¼ cup	4
Finely shredded cheese, natural, Mexican blend, ¼ cup	4
Finely shredded cheese, natural, mild cheddar, ¼ cup	4
Shredded cheese, mozzarella, part-skim, ¼ cup	3

	SmartPoints™ value
Shredded cheese, mozzarella, whole milk, ¼ cup	3
Shredded cheese, natural, sharp yellow cheddar, ¼ cup	4
Shredded cheese, sharp yellow, ¼ cup	4
Shredded cheese, taco blend, ¼ cup	4
Singles, 2% milk, white, 1 slice (21 g)	2
Singles, 2% milk, yellow, 1 slice (21 g)	2
String cheese, mozzarella, 1 stick (28 g)	3
ShopRite Singles	
Cheese product, non-fat white, 1 slice (21 g)	1
Cheese product, non-fat yellow, 1 slice (21 g)	1
Skinny Cheese	
Cheese, fat free, sharp cheddar, 1" cube	1
Skyline	
Cheese, finely shredded. mild cheddar, ¼ cup	4
Sonoma Jack's	
Hot pepper Jack cheese, 1 slice (28 g)	4
Sonoma Jack's Sonoma Cheese	
Cheese wedges, gourmet, garlic & herb, 1 wedge (19 g)	2
Cheese wedges, gourmet, light, garlic & herb, 1 wedge (19 g)	1
Cheese wedges, gourmet, light, pepper Jack, 1 wedge (19 g)	1
Cheese wedges, gourmet, light, smoked gouda, 1 wedge (19 g)	1
Cheese wedges, gourmet, light, white cheddar, 1 wedge (19 g)	1

Dairy & Eggs

Sorrento

Cheese, mozzarella, part skim, 1 oz	3
Ricotta cheese, low fat, ¼ cup	2
Ricotta cheese, part skim, deli style, ¼ cup	4

Sorrento Sticksters

Cheese sticks, cheddar, 1 stick (28 g)	4
Cheese sticks, colby Jack, 1 stick (24 g)	3
Cheese sticks, pepperjack, 1 stick (24 g)	3
Cheese, reduced fat, cheddar, 1 stick (24 g)	2
Cheese, reduced fat, colby Jack, 1 stick (24 g)	2
Stick cheese, reduced fat, colby Jack, 1 stick (24 g)	2

Sorrento Stringsters

String cheese, 100% natural, reduced fat mozzarella, 1 stick (28 g)	2
String cheese, mozzarella, low moisture, part skim, 1 oz	3
String cheese, reduced fat, 1 oz	2
String cheese, reduced fat, mozzarella, 1 oz	2

Specially Selected

Crumbled blue cheese, 2 Tbsp	4
Crumbled feta cheese, 1 oz	2

Stella

Blue cheese freshly crumbled, ¼ cup	4
Finely shredded cheese, 3 cheese Italian, ¼ cup	3

Stella Reduced Fat

Crumbled blue cheese, ¼ cup	3

Stilton

Cheese, blue stilton, 1" slice	4

Supremo

Chihuahua, familiar fam-pack, ¼ cup	4

Supremo Chihuahua

Melting cheese, quesadilla, Mexican style, ¼ cup	4

Temp Tee

Cream cheese, 2 Tbsp	4
Cream cheese, whipped, 2 Tbsp	4

Tillamook

Cheese shred, Mexican, ¼ cup	4
Cheese, colby Jack, 1 oz	5
Cheese, extra sharp natural cheddar, special reserve, 1 oz	5
Cheese, medium cheddar, 1 oz	4
Cheese, medium cheddar, baby loaf, 1 oz	4
Cheese, Monterey Jack, 1 oz	4
Cheese, reduced fat cheddar, 1 slice (23 g)	2
Cheese, sharp cheddar, 1 oz	4
Cheese, sharp cheddar, vintage white extra, 1" cube	4
Cheese, sliced pepper Jack, 1 oz	3
Cheese, sliced sharp cheddar, 1 oz	4
Cheese, sliced Swiss, 1 oz	4
Cheese, sliced, Colby Jack, 1 slice (28 g)	5
Cheese, sliced, medium cheddar, 1 slice (28 g)	4
Cheese, smoked cheddar, 1 oz	4
Cheese, vintage white extra sharp cheddar, 1 oz	4
Deli sliced cheese, cheddar cheese, reduced fat, 1 slice (21 g)	2
Deli sliced cheese, Colby Jack, 1 slice (21 g)	3
Deli sliced cheese, medium cheddar, 1 slice (21 g)	3

Dairy & Eggs

Dairy & Eggs

	SmartPoints™ value
Deli sliced cheese, pepper Jack, 1 slice (21 g)	3
Deli sliced cheese, sharp cheddar, 1 slice (21 g)	3
Deli sliced cheese, Swiss cheese, 1 slice (21 g)	3
Finely shredded cheese, Mexican 2 cheese, ¼ cup	4
Shredded cheese, 4 cheese blend, Mexican, ¼ cup	4
Sliced cheese, combo pack, 1 slice (21 g)	3
Sliced cheese, medium cheddar, 1 oz	4
Sliced cheese, Monterey Jack cheese, 1 slice (28 g)	4
Tillamook Pack-it-Pals Tilla-Moos	
Cheese, colby Jack, 1 piece (21 g)	3
Cheese, medium cheddar, 1 piece (21 g)	3
Tillamook Special Reserve	
Cheese, cheddar, extra sharp, 1 oz	4
Tillamook Vintage White	
Cheese, extra sharp cheddar, 1 oz	4
Cheese, medium cheddar, 1 oz	4
Trader Giotto's	
Fat free ricotta cheese, ¼ cup	1
Trader Joe's	
Cottage cheese (fat free), 1 oz	0
Crumbled blue cheese, 1 oz	4
Fancy shredded lite Mexican blend, ¼ cup	2
Fancy shredded Mexican cheese blend, ¼ cup	4
Fat free crumbled feta, 1 oz	0
Fresh goat cheese medallions, 1 oz	3
Fresh mozzarella cheese sticks, 1 stick (28 g)	2

	SmartPoints™ value
Goat's milk creamy cheese, 1 oz	2
Light whipped cream cheese, 2 Tbsp	3
Lite havarti cheese, 1 slice (28 g)	2
Lite mild cheddar cheese snack sticks, 1 stick (24 g)	1
Lite shredded 3 cheese blend with mozzarella, Monterey Jack, & cheddar, ¼ cup	2
Lite shredded mozzarella cheese, 1 oz	1
Mild cheddar cheese snack sticks, 1 stick (24 g)	3
Mini brie bites, 1 piece (25 g)	3
Monterey Jack cheese snack sticks, 1 stick (24 g)	3
Sliced lite cheddar cheese, 1 slice (28 g)	2
Sliced lite provolone cheese, 1 slice (28 g)	2
Sliced muenster, 1 slice (28 g)	4
Sliced sharp cheddar, 1 slice (28 g)	4
Sliced smoked gouda cheese, 1 slice (28 g)	4
String cheese, low moisture part-skim mozzarella, 1 stick (28.35 g)	2
String cheese, low moisture part-skim mozzarella lite, 1 stick (28.35 g)	2
Unexpected cheddar cheese, 1 oz	4
Trader Joe's Organic	
Light string cheese, 1 stick (28 g)	2
Light whipped cream cheese, 2 Tbsp	3
String cheese, 1 stick (28 g)	2
Trader Jose's	
Fancy shredded Mexican cheeses blend, ¼ cup	4

Treasure Cave

Crumbled cheese, gorgonzola, ¼ cup	4
Crumbled cheese, reduced fat, blue, ¼ cup	3

Velveeta

Cheese food, pasteurized process, slices, 1 slice (19 g)	2
Cheese product, pasteurized prepared, made with 2% milk, ¼" slice	2
Cheese, Mexican, mild, 1 oz	3
Original cheese, ¼" slice	3
Original flavor cheese product slices, 1 slice (21 g)	1

Velveeta Shreds

Cheese product, original flavor, shredded, ¼ cup	3
Shredded cheese product, cheddar flavor, ¼ cup	2
Shredded cheese product, Mexican style cheddar blend, ¼ cup	2
Shredded cheese product, mozzarella flavor, ¼ cup	2

Velveeta Slices

3 cheese blend pasteurized prepared cheese product, 1 slice (21 g)	2
Cheese product, jalapeño, 1 slice (21 g)	2
Cheese product, pasteurized prepared, Swiss, 1 slice (21 g)	2
Cheese product, sharp cheddar, 1 slice (21 g)	2
Original cheese, 1 slice (19 g)	1
Queso blanco, 1 slice (21 g)	1

Wegman's

2% slices, Swiss, 1 slice (21 g)	2
Cheese food, reduced fat pasteurized process, American, white slices, 1 slice (21 g)	2

Cheese food, reduced fat pasteurized process, American, yellow slices, 1 slice (21 g)	2
Cheese product, non fat pasteurized process, sharp cheddar, yellow slices, 1 slice (21 g)	1
Cheese product, non fat pasteurized process, white American, 1 slice (21 g)	1
Cheese sticks, mozzarella, 1 stick (28 g)	3
Cheese, muenster, 1 slice (21 g)	3
Cheese, sharp cheddar, 1 oz	4
Cheese, thin sliced, sharp cheddar, 1 slice (23 g)	3
Cottage cheese, 1% milkfat, ½ cup	2
Cottage cheese, small curd, 1% milkfat, lowfat, ½ cup	2
Cream cheese, fat free, 2 Tbsp	1
Singles, American cheese, white, 1 slice (21 g)	3
Thin sliced cheese, provolone, 1 slice (23 g)	3
Thin sliced cheese, provolone, 2% milk, 1 slice (21 g)	2
Thin sliced cheese, Swiss, 2% milk, 1 slice (21 g)	1
Thin sliced pepper Jack cheese, 1 slice (21 g)	3
Traditional fat free crumbled feta cheese, ¼ cup	1

Wegman's Delicatessen

Cheese, American, sliced, ¾ oz	3
Cheese, Swiss, light, ¾ oz	1

Wegman's Food You Feel Good About

Cottage cheese, small curd, fat free, ½ cup	2

Westminster

Cheese, sharp English cheddar cheese, 1 oz	5

Dairy & Eggs

	SmartPoints™ value
Whole Foods 365 Everyday Value	
Colby Jack stick cheese, 1 piece (28 g)	4
Shredded parmesan cheese, 1 Tbsp	1
Whole Foods 365 Organic	
Mild cheddar shredded cheese, ¼ cup	4
World Classics	
Cheese, American, slices, 1 slice (19 g)	3

Coffee Creamers

	SmartPoints™ value
Albertson's	
Coffee creamer, French vanilla, 1 Tbsp	3
Coffee creamer, hazelnut, 1 Tbsp	3
Baileys Non-Alcoholic	
Coffee creamer, caramel, 1 Tbsp	2
Coffee creamer, chocolate, 1 Tbsp	2
Coffee creamer, chocolatini, 1 Tbsp	2
Coffee creamer, cinnamon dolce, 1 Tbsp	2
Coffee creamer, creme brulee, 1 Tbsp	2
Coffee creamer, fat free, French vanilla, 1 Tbsp	1
Coffee creamer, fat free, original, 1 Tbsp	1
Coffee creamer, French vanilla, 1 Tbsp	2
Coffee creamer, mudslide, 1 Tbsp	2
Coffee creamer, the original Irish cream, 1 Tbsp	2
Coffee creamer, toffee almond cream, 1 Tbsp	2
Coffee creamer, vanilla brown sugar, 1 Tbsp	2
Coffee creamer, white chocolate raspberry swirl, 1 Tbsp	2

	SmartPoints™ value
Califia Farms	
Hazelnut almondmilk creamer, 1 Tbsp	1
Vanilla almondmilk creamer, 1 Tbsp	1
Coffee House Inspirations	
Coffee creamer, chai latte, 1 Tbsp	2
Coffee-Mate	
Classic vanilla liquid coffee creamer, 1 Tbsp	2
Coffee creamer, amaretto, 1 Tbsp	2
Coffee creamer, caramel apple, 1 Tbsp	2
Coffee creamer, chocolate raspberry, 1 Tbsp	2
Coffee creamer, creamy chocolate, 4 tsp	3
Coffee creamer, creme brulee, 1 Tbsp	2
Coffee creamer, eggnog latte, 1 Tbsp	2
Coffee creamer, fat free, cinnamon/ vanilla creme, 1 Tbsp	1
Coffee creamer, fat free, French vanilla, 4 tsp	2
Coffee creamer, French vanilla, single serve, 1 tub (11 ml)	2
Coffee creamer, French vanilla, sugar free, 1 Tbsp	1
Coffee creamer, gingerbread, 4 tsp	3
Coffee creamer, gingerbread latte, 1 Tbsp	2
Coffee creamer, Girl Scouts, caramel & coconut, 1 Tbsp	2
Coffee creamer, Girl Scouts, thin mints, 1 Tbsp	2
Coffee creamer, hazelnut, 1 Tbsp	2
Coffee creamer, hazelnut, fat free, 1 Tbsp	1
Coffee creamer, hazelnut, pantry pack, 1 Tbsp	2

	SmartPoints™ value
Coffee creamer, hazelnut, single serve, 1 tub (11 ml)	2
Coffee creamer, hazelnut, sugar free, liquid, 1 Tbsp	0
Coffee creamer, lite, the original, 1 tsp	0
Coffee creamer, low fat, 1 Tbsp	0
Coffee creamer, original, 1 Tbsp	1
Coffee creamer, original, 1 Tbsp	1
Coffee creamer, original, lite, 1 tsp	0
Coffee creamer, peppermint mocha, 1 Tbsp	2
Coffee creamer, pumpkin spice, 1 Tbsp	2
Coffee creamer, sugar free, hazelnut, 1 Tbsp	1
Coffee creamer, sugar free, peppermint mocha, 1 Tbsp	0
Coffee creamer, sugar free, vanilla caramel, 1 Tbsp	1
Coffee creamer, sweetened original, 2 tsp	2
Coffee creamer, the original, 1 tsp	0
Coffee creamer, the original, single serve, 1 tub (11 ml)	1
French vanilla liquid coffee creamer, 1 Tbsp	2
French vanilla pantry pack coffee creamer, 1 Tbsp	2
Non dairy creamer, hazelnut, 4 tsp	2
Non-dairy creamer, cinnamon vanilla creme, 1 Tbsp	2
Original sweetened coffee creamer, 4 tsp	3
Sugar free vanilla caramel powder coffee creamer, 1 Tbsp	1
The original fat free liquid coffee creamer, 1 Tbsp	0
The original fat free powder coffee creamer, 1 tsp	0

	SmartPoints™ value
Vanilla caramel powder coffee creamer, 4 tsp	3
White chocolate caramel latte liquid coffee creamer, 1 Tbsp	2
Coffee-Mate 2Go	
French vanilla concentrated coffee creamer, 1 tsp	1
Hazelnut concentrated coffee creamer, 1 tsp	1
Coffee-Mate Cafe Collection	
Coffee creamer, cafe latte, 1 Tbsp	1
Coffee creamer, caramel macchiato, 1 Tbsp	2
Coffee creamer, white chocolate caramel latte, 1 Tbsp	2
Sugar free caramel macchiato liquid coffee creamer, 1 Tbsp	0
Coffee-Mate Italian Series	
Italian sweet creme liquid coffee creamer, 1 Tbsp	2
Sugar free Italian sweet creme liquid coffee creamer, 1 Tbsp	0
Coffee-Mate Natural Bliss	
Cinnamon cream all-natural coffee creamer, 1 Tbsp	2
Coffee creamer, caramel flavor, 1 Tbsp	2
Coffee creamer, sweet cream, 1 Tbsp	2
Vanilla flavor liquid coffee creamer, 1 Tbsp	2
Coffee-Mate Powder	
Original coffee creamer, 1 tsp	0
Coffee-Mate Special Edition	
Coffee creamer, cinnamon bun, 1 Tbsp	2
Coffee-Mate Sugar Free	
French vanilla powder coffee creamer, 1 Tbsp	1

Dairy & Eggs

257

	SmartPoints™ value
Coffee-Mate World Cafe Collection	
Coffee creamer, Italian sweet creme, 1 Tbsp	2
Community	
Creamer, 1 tsp	0
Daily Chef	
Rich and creamy non-dairy creamer, 1 tsp	0
Darigold	
Creamer, fat free, French vanilla, 1 Tbsp	1
Creamer, French vanilla, 1 Tbsp	2
Creamer, hazelnut, 1 Tbsp	2
Dunkin' Donuts	
Extra extra lquid coffee creamer, 1 Tbsp	2
Fat free coffee creamer, 1 Tbsp	1
Original liquid coffee creamer, 1 Tbsp	1
Unsweetened original coffee creamer, 1 Tbsp	1
Vanilla non dairy liquid coffee creamer, 1 Tbsp	2
Essential Everyday	
Coffee creamer, French vanilla, 1 Tbsp	2
Coffee creamer, original, fat free, 1 tsp	0
Coffee creamer, sugar free, French vanilla, liquid, 1 Tbsp	0
Friendly Farms	
Vanilla caramel creamer, 1 Tbsp	2
Giant/Stop & Shop	
Fat free French vanilla coffee creamer, 1 Tbsp	1
Great Value	
Fat free powder creamer, 1 tsp	0
French vanilla liquid coffee creamer, 1 Tbsp	2
French vanilla powder creamer, 1 Tbsp	3

	SmartPoints™ value
Hazelnut liquid coffee creamer, 1 Tbsp	2
Irish cream liquid coffee creamer, 1 Tbsp	2
Non dairy extra rich powder coffee creamer, 1 tsp	0
Non dairy powder creamer, 1 tsp	0
Non-dairy powder coffee creamer, 1 tsp	0
Original liquid coffee creamer, 1 Tbsp	0
Sugar free French vanilla powder creamer, 1 Tbsp	1
Vanilla caramel liquid coffee creamer, 1 Tbsp	2
Hood Country Creamer	
Fat free liquid coffee creamer, 1 Tbsp	0
International Delight	
Coffee creamer singles, heath, 1 creamer (13 ml)	2
Coffee creamer, almond joy, 1 Tbsp	2
Coffee creamer, amaretto, fat free, 1 Tbsp	2
Coffee creamer, chocolate cream, 1 Tbsp	2
Coffee creamer, cinnabon, 1 Tbsp	2
Coffee creamer, cinnamon hazelnut, 1 Tbsp	2
Coffee creamer, cinnamon hazelnut, fat free, 1 Tbsp	2
Coffee creamer, gourmet, caramel macchiato, 1 Tbsp	2
Coffee creamer, gourmet, cinnabon, 1 Tbsp	2
Coffee creamer, gourmet, cold stone creamery sweet cream, 1 Tbsp	2
Coffee creamer, gourmet, fat free, caramel macchiato, 1 Tbsp	2
Coffee creamer, gourmet, fat free, French vanilla, 1 Tbsp	2

Dairy & Eggs

	SmartPoints™ value
Coffee creamer, gourmet, fat free, white chocolate mocha, 1 Tbsp	2
Coffee creamer, gourmet, heath, 1 Tbsp	2
Coffee creamer, gourmet, salted caramel mocha, seasonal edition, 1 Tbsp	2
Coffee creamer, gourmet, sugar free caramel macchiato, 1 Tbsp	1
Coffee creamer, gourmet, vanilla caramel creme, 1 Tbsp	2
Coffee creamer, gourmet, white chocolate mocha, 1 tbsp	2
Coffee creamer, gourmet, york, 1 Tbsp	2
Coffee creamer, singles, almond joy, 1 creamer (13 ml)	2
Coffee creamer, singles, pumpkin pie spice, 1 creamer (13 ml)	2
Coffee creamer, vanilla hazelnut, 1 Tbsp	2
Creamer singles, liquid, hazelnut, 1 creamer (13 ml)	2
Creamer singles, liquid, Irish creme, 1 creamer (13 ml)	2
French vanilla flavored non dairy creamer, 1 container (13 ml)	2
French vanilla gourmet coffee creamer, 1 Tbsp	2
French vanilla sugar free single serve liquid coffee creamer, 1 creamer (13 ml)	1
Frosted sugar cookie gourmet liquid coffee creamer, 1 Tbsp	2
Gingerbread latte liquid coffee creamer, 1 Tbsp	2
Gourmet coffee creamer, cold stone creamery sweet cream, 1 Tbsp	2
Gourmet coffee creamer, york, 1 Tbsp	2

	SmartPoints™ value
Hazelnut coffee creamer, 1 Tbsp	2
Hazelnut liquid gourmet coffee creamer, 1 Tbsp	2
Heath gourmet coffee creamer, 1 Tbsp	2
Hershey's chocolate caramel gourmet coffee creamer, 1 Tbsp	2
Irish creme gourmet coffee creamer, 1 Tbsp	2
Peppermint chocolate truffle gourmet liquid coffee creamer, 1 Tbsp	2
Peppermint mocha creamer, 1 Tbsp	2
White chocolate and raspberry flavored gourmet coffee creamer, 1 Tbsp	2
White chocolate macadamia gourmet coffee creamer, 1 Tbsp	2
International Delight Coffee House Inspirations	
Coffee creamer, dark chocolate cream, 1 Tbsp	2
Coffee creamer, hazelnut cream, 1 Tbsp	2
Coffee creamer, skinny vanilla latte, fat free, 1 Tbsp	2
Coffee creamer, vanilla caramel cream, 1 Tbsp	2
Coffee creamer, vanilla latte, 1 Tbsp	2
Creamer singles, caramel macchiato, 1 creamer (11 ml)	2
Creamer singles, white chocolate mocha, 1 creamer (11 ml)	2
Peppermint mocha coffee creamer, 1 Tbsp	2
Vanilla caramel coffee creamer, 1 Tbsp	2

Dairy & Eggs

Coffee Creamers (cont'd)

SmartPoints™ value

International Delight Cold Stone Creamery

Churro caramel gourmet coffee creamer, 1 Tbsp	2
Coffee creamer, gourmet, brownie sundae, 1 Tbsp	2
Hot for cookie sundae coffee creamer, 1 Tbsp	2
Sweet cream single serve non dairy creamer, 1 container (13 ml)	2

International Delight Fat Free & Sugar Free

Caramel creme gourmet coffee creamer, 1 Tbsp	0
Caramel marshmallow gourmet coffee creamer, 1 Tbsp	0
Chocolate almond biscotti gourmet coffee creamer, 1 Tbsp	0
Gourmet toasted hazelnut coffee creamer, 1 Tbsp	0
Pumpkin pie spice liquid coffee creamer, 1 Tbsp	0
Toasted hazelnut gourmet coffee creamer, 1 Tbsp	0

International Delight Mini I.D.'s

Coffee creamer, Hershey's chocolate caramel, single serve, 1 creamer (13 ml)	2
French vanilla single serve coffee creamer, 1 creamer (13 ml)	2

International Delight Seasonal Celebrations

Coffee creamer, chocolate mint truffle, 1 Tbsp	2
Coffee creamer, white chocolate raspberry, 1 Tbsp	2

International Delight Seasonal Edition

Pumpkin pie spice creamer, 1 Tbsp	2
Pumpkin pie spice gourmet coffee creamer, 1 Tbsp	2
Salted caramel mocha gourmet coffee creamer, 1 Tbsp	2

SmartPoints™ value

International Delight Vanilla Heat

Flavored gourmet coffee creamer, 1 Tbsp	2

Kroger

Cinnamon creme powder coffee creamer, 4 tsp	3
Coffee creamer, lactose free, original, powder, 4 tsp	3
Creamer, non-dairy, 4 tsp	3
Creamer, non-dairy, fat free, powder, 4 tsp	3
Creamer, non-dairy, French vanilla, 4 tsp	3
Creamer, non-dairy, hazelnut, 4 tsp	3
Creme brulee liquid coffee creamer, 1 Tbsp	2
Fat free French vanilla lactose free liquid coffee creamer, 1 Tbsp	2
French vanilla liquid coffee creamer, 1 Tbsp	2
Hazelnut liquid coffee creamer, 1 Tbsp	2
Lactose free French vanilla powder coffee creamer, 4 tsp	3
Limited edition liquid coffee creamer, 1 Tbsp	2
Original powder coffee creamer, 4 tsp	0
Sugar free hazelnut flavored coffee creamer, 1 Tbsp	0
Sugar free hazelnut liquid coffee creamer, 1 Tbsp	0
Vanilla caramel powder coffee creamer, 4 tsp	3

Kroger Sugar Free

French vanilla liquid coffee creamer, 2 Tbsp	1

Land O' Lakes

Coffee creamer, sweetened with sugar, sweet valley creams, 2 Tbsp	3

Land O Lakes Mini Moo's

Half and half liquid single serve creamer, 1 each (9 ml)	0
Dairy creamers, 1 creamer (9 ml)	0

Lucerne

Coffee creamer, Belgian chocolate toffee, 1 Tbsp	2
Coffee creamer, caramel macchiato, 1 Tbsp	2
Coffee creamer, cinnamon vanilla, 1 Tbsp	2
Coffee creamer, creme brulee, 1 Tbsp	2
Coffee creamer, French vanilla, 1 Tbsp	1
Coffee creamer, hazelnut, 1 Tbsp	2
Coffee creamer, Mexican cinnamon chocolate, 1 Tbsp	2
Coffee creamer, peppermint white chocolate, 1 Tbsp	2
Coffee creamer, salted caramel, 1 Tbsp	2
Coffee creamer, sugar free, French vanilla, 1 Tbsp	0
Coffee creamer, sugar free, hazelnut, 1 Tbsp	0
Coffee creamer, vanilla caramel, 1 Tbsp	2
Coffee creamer, white chocolate mocha, 1 Tbsp	2

Market Pantry

Coffee creamer, original, 1 tsp	0

Meijer Organics

Creamer, French vanilla, 1 Tbsp	2
Creamer, hazelnut, 1 Tbsp	2

Mocha Mix

Coffee creamer, non-dairy, original flavor, 1 Tbsp	1
Non-dairy coffee creamer, original flavor, 1 Tbsp	1

Nestlé

Sugar free pumpkin spice coffee creamer, 1 Tbsp	0

Nestlé Coffee-Mate

Butter toffee coffee creamer, 1 Tbsp	2
Cafe mocha coffee creamer, 1 Tbsp	2
Chocolate chip cookie coffee creamer, 1 Tbsp	2
Coffee creamer, sugar free, creamy chocolate, 2 tsp	2
Coffee creamer, sugar free, peppermint mocha, 1 Tbsp	0
Coffee creamer, sugar free, pumpkin spice, 1 Tbsp	0
Dulce de leche coffee creamer, 1 Tbsp	2
Mexican chocolate style coffee creamer, 1 Tbsp	2
Natural bliss hazelnut flavor all-natural coffee creamer, 1 Tbsp	2
Snickerdoodle coffee creamer, 1 Tbsp	2
Spiced rum cake coffee creamer, 1 Tbsp	2

Nestlé Coffee-Mate Cafe Collection

Vanilla latte non-dairy powdered coffee creamer, 4 tsp	3

Nestlé Coffee-Mate The Original

Single serve portion creamer, 1 container (11 ml)	1

N'Joy

Coffee creamer, 1 tsp	0

Open Nature

Creamer, dairy, sweet cream, 1 Tbsp	2
Vanilla dairy creamer, 1 Tbsp	2

Organic Valley

Soy creamer, French vanilla, 1 Tbsp	1
Soy creamer, original, 1 Tbsp	1

Dairy & Eggs

SmartPoints™ value

Publix

Coffee creamer, French vanilla, non-dairy, 4 tsp	3
Coffee creamer, lite, non-dairy, 1 tsp	0
Coffee creamer, rich & creamy, non-dairy, 1 tsp	0

Rich's Coffee Rich

Non-dairy creamer, 1 Tbsp	1

Safeway

Creamer, non-dairy, French vanilla, 1 Tbsp	1

ShopRite

Coffee creamer, sugar free, French vanilla, 1 Tbsp	0
Coffee creamer, sugar free, hazelnut, 1 Tbsp	0

Silk

Almond creamer, vanilla, 1 Tbsp	1
Creamer, French vanilla, 1 Tbsp	1
Creamer, hazelnut, 1 Tbsp	1
Creamer, original, 1 Tbsp	1
French vanilla soy creamer, 1 Tbsp	1

So Delicious

Coconut milk, hazelnut creamer, 1 Tbsp	1
Creamer, coconut milk, French vanilla, 1 Tbsp	1
Creamer, coconut milk, original, 1 Tbsp	0
Creamer, original, coconut milk, 1 Tbsp	0
Original almond milk creamer, 1 Tbsp	0

So Delicious Dairy Free

Creamer, coconut milk, French vanilla, barista style, 1 Tbsp	0
Creamer, coconut milk, original, barista style, 1 Tbsp	0
French vanilla almond milk creamer, 1 Tbsp	1

SmartPoints™ value

Tassimo

Creamer, cappuccino, foaming milk, 1 disc (370 ml)	2

Trader Joe's

Original flavor coffee creamer, 1 Tbsp	1
Soy milk creamer, 1 Tbsp	1

Wide Awake Coffee Co.

Coffee creamer, non-dairy, fat free, French vanilla, 1 Tbsp	1

Cream

Cabot

Whipped cream, sweetened, light, 2 Tbsp	1

Classic Cream

Whipped cream, real light, 2 Tbsp	1
Whipped cream, real light, sweetened, 2 Tbsp	1

Creamland

Heavy cream, 1 Tbsp	3

Garelick Farms

Light cream, 1 Tbsp	1

Great Value

Whipping cream, heavy, 1 Tbsp	2

Hood

Light liquid cream, 1 Tbsp	1

Horizon Organic

Heavy whipping cream, 1 Tbsp	2

Land O' Lakes

Heavy cream, whipped, extra creamy, 2 Tbsp	1
Whipped light cream, 2 Tbsp	1

Land O' Lakes Zero Carbs

Ultra pasteurized whipped heavy cream, 1 Tbsp	1

Reddi Wip

Whipped light cream, original, 2 Tbsp	1

Dairy & Eggs

Egg & Egg Substitutes

4Grain
Eggs, large, omega 3, 1 egg	2

Abbotsford Farms
100% liquid egg whites, 3 Tbsp	0

AllWhites
100% liquid egg whites, 3 Tbsp	0

Almark Foods
Eggs, hard-boiled, 1 egg	2

Better'n Eggs
Liquid egg whites, 3 Tbsp	0
Healthier real egg product, 3 Tbsp	0

Better'n Eggs Plus
Pasteurized real egg product, 3 Tbsp	0

Daily Chef Gourmet Foods
100% liquid egg whites, 3 Tbsp	0

Dutch Farms
Eggs, large, 1 egg	2

Egg Beaters
100% egg whites, liquid, 3 Tbsp	0
Egg product, ham cheese, ¼ cup	1
Egg product, with yolk, ¼ cup	1
Frozen egg product, pasteurized, ¼ cup	0
Liquid egg product, garden vegetable, with yolk, ¼ cup	1
Original liquid egg, ¼ cup	0
Real egg product, cheese & chive, ¼ cup	1
Real egg product, original, 3 Tbsp	0
Southwestern flavored egg whites, ¼ cup	0
Southwestern style made of real eggs, 3 Tbsp	0
Three cheese flavored egg whites, 3 Tbsp	0

Egg Beaters All Natural
Florentine egg whites, 3 Tbsp	1

Egg Beaters SmartCups
All natural 100% egg whites, 1 container (113 g)	0

Egg-Land's Best
100% liquid egg whites, 3 Tbsp	0
Eggs, brown, organic, large, 1 egg	2
Eggs, grade A, extra large, 1 egg	2
Eggs, grade A, large, 1 egg	2
Extra large grade A eggs, 1 egg	2
Hard cooked peeled medium egg, 1 egg	2
Jumbo grade A egg, 1 egg	2
Large egg, 1 egg	2

Essential Everyday
Large egg, 1 egg	2
The amazing egg liquid egg product, 3 Tbsp	0
The amazing egg whites, 3 Tbsp	0

Essential Everyday The Amazing Egg
Pasteurized liquid egg white, 3 Tbsp	0

Farm Fresh
Grade A large eggs, 1 egg	2

Farmers Harvest Fresh Eggs
Large brown egg, 1 egg	2

Fit & Active
Egg substitute, ¼ cup	0
Liquid egg whites, 3 Tbsp	0

Giant
Egg whites, ¼ cup	0
Egg whites, liquid, ¼ cup	0
Eggs, large, grade A, 1 egg	2

Giant Eggs Made Simple
99% egg product, ¼ cup	0

Giroux's
Eggs, 2 ½ dozen, grade A, small, 1 egg	2

Great Day Foods
Farmers market large farm fresh egg, 1 egg	2
Hard boiled eggs, 1 egg	2

Dairy & Eggs

	SmartPoints™ value
Great Day Foods Farmers Market	
Large grade A farm fresh egg, 1 egg	2
Great Value	
Original liquid eggs, ¼ cup	0
Hannaford	
Egg mates, ¼ cup	0
Happy Egg	
Egg, brown, large, free range, 1 egg	2
Harris Teeter	
Eggs, large, white, 1 egg	2
H-E-B	
Egg whites, real, ¼ cup	0
Horizon Organic	
Eggs, brown, grade A, large, 1 egg	2
IGA	
Eggs, large, 1 egg	2
Kirkland Signature	
100% liquid egg whites, 3 Tbsp	0
Kirkland Signature Organic	
Large brown eggs, 1 egg	2
Kroger	
Grade A jumbo eggs, 1 egg	2
Real egg product, break-free, ¼ cup	0
Kroger Break Free	
100% liquid egg whites, 3 Tbsp	0
Real egg product, ¼ cup	0
Land O' Lakes	
All natural extra large brown eggs, 1 egg	2
Eggs, brown, cage free, large, 1 egg	2
Large brown eggs, 1 egg	2
Lucerne Best of the Egg	
Original pasteurized real egg product, 3 Tbsp	0
Lucerne Best of the Egg Whites	
100% liquid egg whites, 3 Tbsp	0

	SmartPoints™ value
Market Pantry	
Egg substitute, original, ¼ cup	0
Meijer	
Eggs, large, 1 egg	2
Nature's Harmony	
Grade A large eggs, 1 large	2
Nearby Eggs	
Grade A extra large eggs, 1 egg	2
Nellie's Nest	
Eggs, grade A large, fresh brown, 1 each (57 g)	2
NestFresh	
Large eggs, 1 egg	2
Nulaid ReddiEgg	
Real egg product, ¼ cup	0
O Organics	
Eggs, brown, large, organic, 1 egg	2
Open Nature	
Cage free 100% liquid egg whites, 3 Tbsp	0
Large, grade AA cage free eggs, 1 egg	2
Organic Valley	
Egg whites, organic, ¼ cup	0
Eggs, large brown, omega-3, organic, 1 egg	2
Eggs, large brown, organic, 1 egg	2
Penrose	
Pickled eggs, 1 egg	1
Pickled eggs, beet flavored, 1 egg	2
Pete And Gerry's	
Eggs, organic, grade A large brown, 1 egg	2
Publix	
Eggs, extra large, 1 egg	2
Eggs, jumbo, 1 egg	2
Eggs, large, 1 egg	2
Eggstirs, ¼ cup	0

Dairy & Eggs

S&S Brands, Inc.

Egg, Large, grade A, 1 egg	2

Sauder's Quality Eggs

Fresh hard-cooked peeled eggs, 1 egg	2

ShopRite

Egg whites, ¼ cup	0
Eggs, large, white, 1 egg	2
Large white eggs, 1 egg	2

ShopRite The Great Eggscape

99% real egg product, ¼ cup	0

Simple Truth

Natural cage free grain fed large brown egg, 1 egg	2

Simple Truth Natural

Cage-free grain-fed large brown eggs, 1 egg	2

Sunny Meadow

Large grade A farm fresh eggs, 1 egg	2

Trader Joe's

Cage free 100% liquid egg whites, 3 Tbsp	0
Cage free fresh hard-cooked peeled eggs, 1 egg	2

Wegman's Food You Feel Good About

Egg busters, ¼ cup	0
Egg whites, liquid, ¼ cup	0
Eggs, organic, brown, large, 1 egg	2

Whole Foods 365 Organic

Egg whites, 3 Tbsp	0

Winter Gardens

Eggs, red beet, 1 egg	3

Half & Half

Barber's

Half & half, 2 Tbsp	2

Berkeley Farms

Half & half, 2 Tbsp	2

Borden

Half & half, 2 Tbsp	2
Half & half, fat free, 2 Tbsp	1

C.F. Burger Creamery

Half & half, ultra-pasteurized, 2 Tbsp	2
Half & half, 2 Tbsp	2

Clover

Half and half, 2 Tbsp	2

Creamland

Half & half, 2 Tbsp	2

Darigold

Fat free half and half, 2 Tbsp	1
Half & half, 2 Tbsp	2

Farmland

Half and half liquid creamer, 2 Tbsp	2

Farmland Special Request

Fat free half and half skim plus liquid coffee creamer, 2 Tbsp	1

Garelick Farms

Half & half, 2 Tbsp	2
Half & half, fat free, 2 Tbsp	1

Great Value

Half & half, 2 Tbsp	2
Half & half, fat free, 2 Tbsp	1

Hood

Half and half liquid coffee creamer, 2 Tbsp	2

Horizon Organic

Half & half, 2 Tbsp	2
Half & half, ultra-pasteurized, 2 Tbsp	2

Dairy & Eggs

Dairy & Eggs

	SmartPoints™ value
Knudsen	
Half and half, 2 Tbsp	2
Kroger	
Half & half, 2 Tbsp	2
Land O' Lakes	
Fat free half and half, 2 Tbsp	1
Fat free half and half liquid creamer, 2 Tbsp	1
Half & half, 2 Tbsp	2
Half & half, ultra-pasteurized, 2 Tbsp	2
Low fat half and half, 2 Tbsp	1
Lehigh Valley	
Half & half, 2 Tbsp	2
O Organics	
Half & half, organic, 2 Tbsp	2
Organic Valley	
Half & half, organic, 2 Tbsp	2
Publix	
Half and half cream, 2 Tbsp	2
Shamrock Farms	
Half and half, fat free, 2 Tbsp	1
ShopRite	
Half and half, 2 Tbsp	2
Half and half, fat free, 2 Tbsp	1
Half and half, ultra pasteurized, 2 Tbsp	2
Simple Truth Organic	
Half and half cream, 2 Tbsp	2
Snapple Diet	
Half 'n half, 12 fl oz	0
Sunnyside Farms	
Half & half, fat free, 2 Tbsp	1
Swiss Dairy	
Half & half, 2 Tbsp	2
Trader Joe's Organic	
Ultra pasteurized half and half, 2 Tbsp	2

	SmartPoints™ value
Tuscan	
Half & half, fat free, 2 Tbsp	1
Upstate Farms	
Half & half, fat free, 2 Tbsp	1
Half and half, ultra-pasteurized, 2 Tbsp	2
Wegman's	
Half & half, 2 Tbsp	2

Milk & Milk Based Drinks

	SmartPoints™ value
AE	
Milk, fat free, chocolate, skim, 1 cup	3
Alta Dena	
Milk, 1% low fat, 1 cup	5
America's Choice	
Fat free skim milk, 1 cup	3
Milk, fat free, 1 cup	3
Bayview Farms	
Milk, fat free, 1 cup	3
Milk, light, 1% milkfat, 1 cup	5
Milk, fat free, 1 cup	3
Borden	
1% lowfat milk, 1 cup	4
2% reduced fat milk, 1 cup	5
Condensed milk, fat free, sweetened, 2 Tbsp	6
Milk, Dutch chocolate, 1 cup	10
Milk, reduced fat, 2% milkfat, 1 cup	5
Milk, skim, fat free, 1 cup	3
Milk, sweetened condensed, 2 Tbsp	7
Milk, vitamin D, 1 cup	7
Borden Plus	
Lite line skim milk, 1 cup	3
Borden Viva	
Fat free milk, 1 cup	3
Milk, 1% lowfat milk, 1 cup	4

Carnation

Evaporated milk, fat free, 2 Tbsp	1
Milk, evaporated, 2 Tbsp	2
Milk, evaporated, lowfat 2%, 2 Tbsp	1
Milk, sweetened condensed, 2 Tbsp	7

Centrella

Fat free milk, 1 cup	3

Clear Value

Milk, skim, fat free, 1 cup	3

Core Power

Milk shake, high protein, chocolate, 11 ½ oz	4
Milk shake, high protein, strawberry banana, 11 ½ fl oz	4
Milk shake, protein, vanilla, 11 ½ fl oz	8

Country Fresh

Milk, ½% lowfat, 1 cup	4

Creamland

Fat free milk, 1 cup	3
Milk, 2% reduced fat, 2% milkfat, 1 cup	5

Cub

Fat free milk, 1 cup	3

Daily Chef

1% lowfat milk, 1 cup	4
2% reduced fat milk, 1 cup	5
Fat free skim milk, 1 cup	3

Darigold

Milk, creamy, fat free, 1 cup	4
Milk, fat free, 1 cup	3
Milk, lowfat, 1% milk fat, 1 cup	4
Milk, lowfat, 1% milkfat, 1 cup	4
Milk, reduced fat, 2% milk fat, 1 cup	5
Milk, reduced fat, 2% milkfat, 1 cup	5

Dean's

Fat free milk, 1 cup	3
Milk, fat free, 1 cup	3
Milk, reduced fat, 2% milkfat, 1 cup	5

Dean's Easy

Milk, fat free, 1 cup	3

Deans Milk Chug

Milk, fat free, skim, 1 cup	3

Dean's TruMoo

Lowfat 1% chocolate milk, 1 cup	6

Edaleen

Milk, low fat, 1% milk fat, 1 cup	4

Essential Everyday

Milk, fat free, lactose free, 1 cup	3

Fairlife

2% lactose free chocolate milk, 1 cup	5
2% low fat chocolate milk, 11 ½ fl oz	7
Lactose free 2% milk, 1 cup	4
Lactose free skim milk, 1 cup	2

Farmland Special Request

Milk, skim plus, 1 cup	4
Milk, skim plus, 100% lactose free, 1 cup	4
Milk, skim plus, fat free, 1 cup	4

Fit & Active

Milk chocolate flavored weight loss shake, 1 bottle (325 ml)	7

Friendly Farms

1% lowfat milk, 1 cup	4
2% reduced fat milk, 1 cup	5

Garelick Farms

Milk, 1% lowfat, 1% milkfat, 1 cup	4
Milk, fat free skim, 1 container (236 ml)	3

Garelick Farms Dairy Pure

Milk, lowfat, 1% milkfat, 1 cup	4

Dairy & Eggs

Dairy & Eggs

SmartPoints™ value

Giant	
Milk, 2% reduced fat, lactose free, 2% milkfat, 1 cup	5
Milk, fat free, lactose free, 1 cup	3
Good Karma	
Flax milk, original, 1 cup	2
Flax milk, unsweetened, 1 cup	1
Flax milk, vanilla, 1 cup	3
Great Value	
Milk, 1% low fat, 1% milkfat, 1 cup	4
Milk, 2% reduced fat, 2% milkfat, 1 cup	5
Milk, fat free, 0% milkfat, 1 cup	3
Milk, fat free, lactose free, 1 cup	3
Milk, fat free, organic, 1 cup	3
Milk, lactose free, 1 cup	7
Milk, low fat, chocolate, 1% milkfat, 1 cup	8
Milk, reduced fat, lactose free, 2% milkfat, 1 cup	5
Milk, reduced fat, organic, 2% milkfat, 1 cup	5
Milk, vitamin D, 1 cup	6
Green Valley Organics	
Kefir, lactose free, plain, 1 cup	3
Harris Teeter	
Milk, low fat, 1% milkfat, 1 cup	4
Milk, skim, non-fat, 1 cup	3
Harris Teeter Naturals	
Milk, fat free, organic, 1 cup	3
H-E-B	
Milk, reduced fat, 8 fl oz	5
Helios	
Kefir, nonfat, with fos, organic, original, 1 cup	3
Heritage	
Milk, fat free, organic, 1 cup	3
Highland Crest	
Milk, reduced fat, 2% milk, 1 cup	5
Milk, skim, fat free, 1 cup	3

SmartPoints™ value

Hiland	
Milk, lowfat, 1%, 1 cup	4
Milk, reduced fat, 2%, 1 cup	5
Milk, skim, fat free, 1 cup	3
Hills Bros.	
Drink mix, cappuccino, white chocolate caramel, 3 Tbsp	6
Hood	
Milk, fat free, 8 fl oz	3
Milk, fat free, skim, 1 cup	3
Milk, fat free, skim, vitamins A, C & D, 1 cup	3
Milk, lowfat, 1% milkfat, 8 fl oz	4
Milk, reduced fat, 2% milkfat, 1 cup	5
Hood Carb Countdown	
Dairy beverage, 2% reduced fat, 1 cup	3
Dairy beverage, fat free, 1 cup	1
Hood Simply Smart	
Fat free half and liquid coffee creamer, 2 Tbsp	1
Milk, 1% lowfat, 1 cup	5
Milk, fat free, 1 cup	3
Horizon	
Milk, chocolate, lowfat, organic, 1 container (236 ml)	7
Milk, dha omega-3, fat-free, 1 cup	4
Milk, fat-free, 1 cup	3
Milk, reduced fat, 2%, 1 cup	5
Milk, whole, 1 cup	7
Horizon Organic	
2% organic reduced fat milk, 1 cup	5
Dha omega-3, 2% organic reduced fat milk, 1 cup	5
Fat free milk, 1 cup	3
Milk, 2% reduced fat, 1 cup	5
Milk, dha omega-3 vitamin D organic whole milk, 1 cup	6
Milk, fat-free, 1 cup	3

Milk, lowfat, chocolate, 1% milkfat, 1 cup	8
Milk, lowfat, organic, 1 container (236 ml)	4
Milk, organic, 100% lactose-free, reduced fat, 2%, 1 cup	5
Milk, organic, fat-free, 1 cup	3
Whole milk with vitamin D, 1 cup	6
Hunter Farms	
Milk, skim, less than ½% milkfat, 1 cup	3
Jewel	
Fat free skim milk, 1 cup	3
Kirkland Signature	
Fat free milk, 1 cup	3
Milk, reduced fat, 2% milkfat, 1 cup	5
Kirkland Signature Organic	
1% lowfat milk, 1 cup	4
Kroger	
1% lowfat milk, 8 fl oz	4
2% reduced fat milk, 8 fl oz	5
Condensed milk, sweetened, 2 Tbsp	6
Low fat chocolate milk, 8 fl oz	9
Milk, lowfat, chocolate, 8 fl oz	9
Milk, vitamin D, 8 fl oz	6
Vanilla carbmaster nonfat reduced sugar milk, 8 fl oz	1
Kroger Value CARBmaster	
Nonfat reduced sugar milk, 8 fl oz	1
Lactaid	
Fat free milk, 1 cup	3
Milk, fat free, 1 cup	3
Milk, fat free, 100% lactose free, calcium enriched, 1 cup	3
Milk, lowfat, 1% milkfat, 1 cup	4
Milk, lowfat, 1% milkfat, 100% lactose free, calcium enriched, 1 cup	4

Milk, lowfat, 1% milkfat, chocolate, 1 cup	7
Milk, lowfat, 100% lactose free, 1% milkfat, 1 cup	4
Milk, reduced fat, 2% milkfat, 1 cup	5
Milk, whole, 1 cup	7
Milk, whole, 100% lactose free, 1 cup	7
Land O' Lakes	
Milk, 1% lowfat, 1 cup	4
Milk, fat free, skim, 1 cup	4
Land O' Lakes Dairy Ease	
Fat free milk, 1 cup	3
Land O' Lakes Original	
Milk, skim, fat free, 1 cup	3
Lehigh Valley	
Milk, fat free, 1 cup	3
Milk, lowfat, 1% milkfat, 1 cup	4
Milk, reduced fat, 2% milkfat, 1 cup	5
Lifeway	
Kefir cultured milk, nonfat, Greek style, strawberry, 1 cup	7
Kefir cultured milk, nonfat, plain, unsweetened, 1 cup	3
Lifeway Organic	
Kefir, lowfat, plain unsweetened, 1 cup	4
Magnolia	
Condensed milk, sweetened, 2 Tbsp	7
Market Pantry	
Lactose-free skim milk, 1 cup	3
Milk, lowfat, 1% milkfat, 1 cup	4
Milk, reduced fat, 2% milkfat, 1 cup	5
Milk, skim, 1 cup	3
Milk, whole, 1 cup	6

Dairy & Eggs

Dairy & Eggs

	SmartPoints™ value
Mayfield	
Milk, 2% reduced fat, 2% milkfat, 1 cup	5
Milk, fat free skim, 1 cup	3
Milk, reduced fat, 2% milkfat, 1 cup	5
Mayfield Nurture	
Milk, lowfat, 1% milkfat, 1 cup	4
Meadow Gold TruMoo	
Milk, fat free, chocolate (0.5 pt), 1 container (236 ml)	6
Meijer	
Milk, 1% lowfat, 1 cup	4
Milk, ½% lowfat, 1 cup	4
Milk, fat free, 1 cup	3
Milk, lowfat, 1% milkfat, 1 cup	4
Milk, lowfat, ½% milkfat, 1 cup	4
Milk, reduced fat, 2% milkfat, 1 cup	5
Meijer Organics	
Milk, fat free, 1 cup	3
Midwest Country Fare	
Milk, fat free skim, 1 cup	3
My Essentials	
1% lowfat milk, 1 cup	4
Nature's Promise Organics	
Milk, fat free, organic, 1 cup	3
Milk, lowfat, organic 1%, 8 fl oz	4
Organic fat free milk, 8 fl oz	3
Nestlé Nesquik	
Lowfat chocolate milk, 1 bottle (236 ml)	8
Milk, fat free, chocolate, 1 cup	7
Milk, low fat, chocolate, 1 bottle (236 ml)	7
No Frills Fresh	
Milk, fat free, skim, 1 cup	3

	SmartPoints™ value
O Organics	
Milk, organic, fat free, 1 cup	3
Milk, organic, lowfat, 1% milkfa, 1 cup	4
Organic fat free milk, 1 cup	3
Oak Farms	
Milk, reduced fat, 2% milkfat, 1 cup	5
Oberweis	
Milk, fat free, 1 cup	3
Organic Valley	
Milk, fat free, lactose free, 1 cup	4
Milk, fat free, organic, 1 cup	3
Milk, lowfat, 1% milkfat, organic, 1 cup	4
Milk, lowfat, organic, 1% milkfat, 1 cup	4
Milk, organic, fat free, 0% milkfat, 1 cup	3
Milk, organic, reduced fat, 2% milkfat, 1 cup	5
Milk, reduced fat, 2% milkfat, organic, 1 cup	5
Milk, reduced fat, organic, 2% milkfat, 1 cup	5
Milk, reduced fat, organic, lactose free, 2% milkfat, 1 cup	5
Milk, whole, organic, 1 cup	6
Organic lowfat milk, lactose free, 1 cup	5
Over The Moon	
Fat free milk, 1 cup	5
Milk, fat free, 1 cup	4
Pantry Essentials	
Milk, fat free, 1 cup	3
Milk, lowfat, 1% milkfat, 1 cup	5
Milk, reduced fat, 2% milkfat, 1 cup	6

Piggly Wiggly

Milk, fat free skim, 1 cup	3

Prairie Farms

Milk, lowfat, 1% milkfat, 1 cup	4
Milk, lowfat, chocolate, 1% milkfat, 1 cup	8
Milk, reduced fat, 2%, 1 cup	5
Milk, skim, fat free, 1 cup	3

Price First

Milk, 2% reduced fat, 1 cup	5
Milk, fat free, 1 cup	3
Milk, whole, with vitamin D, 1 cup	6

Publix

Milk, fat free, all natural grade A, 1 cup	3

ShopRite

Milk, fat free, 1 cup	3
Milk, low fat, 1% milkfat, 1 cup	4
Milk, reduced fat, 2% milkfat, 1 cup	5

ShopRite Certified Organic

Milk, fat free, 1 cup	3
Milk, low fat, organic, 1% milkfat, 1 cup	4

Simple Truth Organic

2% reduced fat milk, 8 fl oz	5

Simply Balanced

Fat free organic skim milk, 1 cup	3
Milk, organic, low fat, 1% milk fat, 1 cup	4
Milk, fat free, and omega-3s, 1 cup	4
Milk, lactose free, fat free, 1 cup	4

Springdale

2% reduced fat milk, 8 fl oz	5

Starbucks Verismo

Milk pods, 1 pod (10 g)	2

Stonyfield Farm Organic

Fat free milk, 1 cup	3
Lowfat milk, 1% milkfat, 1 cup	4
Milk, reduced fat, 2% milkfat, 1 cup	5
Whole milk, 1 cup	7

Sunnyside Farms

Milk, fat free, 1 cup	3

Swiss Premium TruMoo

1% lowfat chocolate milk, 1 cup	6

Trader Joe's

Fat free milk, 1 cup	3
Low fat kefir, 8 fl oz	3

Trader Joe's Organic

Fat free milk, 1 cup	3

TruMoo

Milk, lowfat, chocolate, 1% milkfat, 1 cup	7

Tuscan

Milk, fat free, 1 cup	3
Milk, reduced fat, 2% milkfat, 1 cup	5

Valu Time

Milk, lowfat, 1% milkfat, 1 cup	4
Milk, lowfat, 2% milkfat, 1 cup	5

Viva

Milk, 2% reduced fat, 2% milkfat, 1 cup	5
Milk, fat free, 1 cup	3

Wal-Mart

1% low fat milk, 1 cup	4

Wegman's

Milk, lactose free, fat free, 1 cup	3
Milk, lactose free, reduced fat, 2% milkfat, 1 cup	5
Milk, low fat, 1% milkfat, 1 cup	4
Milk, reduced fat, 2% milkfat, 1 cup	5

Dairy & Eggs

	SmartPoints™ value
Wegman's Food You Feel Good About	
Milk, 1% low fat, 1 cup	4
Milk, fat free, 1 cup	3
Milk, fat free, skim rich, 1 cup	3
Whole Foods 365 Organic	
Skim fat free milk, 1 cup	3

Sour Cream

	SmartPoints™ value
Axelrod	
Sour cream, 2 Tbsp	3
Axelrod Easy-Dieter	
Sour cream, light, 2 Tbsp	2
Breakstone's	
All natural sour cream, 2 Tbsp	3
Reduced fat sour cream, 2 Tbsp	1
Sour cream, 2 Tbsp	3
Sour cream, fat free, 2 Tbsp	1
Cabot	
Light sour cream, 2 Tbsp	1
Sour cream, 2 Tbsp	2
Country Fresh	
Sour cream, low fat, 2 Tbsp	1
Daisy	
Light sour cream, 2 Tbsp	2
Sour cream, 2 Tbsp	3
Essential Everyday	
Light sour cream, 2 Tbsp	2
Sour cream, fat free, 2 Tbsp	1
Friendly Farms	
Light sour cream, 2 Tbsp	1
Friendship	
Sour cream, 2 Tbsp	3
Sour cream, light, 2 Tbsp	2
Giant	
Sour cream, fat free, 2 Tbsp	1
Hood	
Sour cream, all natural, 2 Tbsp	3
Sour cream, low fat, 2 Tbsp	1

	SmartPoints™ value
Hood Light	
Sour cream, 2 Tbsp	2
Horizon Organic	
Lowfat sour cream, 2 Tbsp	1
Kemps	
Smooth and creamy fat free sour cream, 2 Tbsp	1
Smooth and creamy light sour cream, 2 Tbsp	2
Knudsen	
Sour cream, fat free, 2 Tbsp	1
Kraft Simply	
Sour cream, 2 Tbsp	3
Sour cream, light, 2 Tbsp	2
Kroger	
Original sour cream, 2 Tbsp	3
Sour cream, 2 Tbsp	3
Sour cream, original, 2 Tbsp	3
Sour cream, reduced fat, 2 Tbsp	2
Lakeview Farms	
Lite sour cream, 2 Tbsp	1
Lowe's Foods Lite	
Sour cream, 2 Tbsp	2
Lucerne	
Sour cream, light, 2 Tbsp	2
Meijer	
Sour cream, fat free, 2 Tbsp	1
Sour cream, light, 2 Tbsp	1
Mid-America Farms Top The Tater	
Chive-onion sour cream, 2 Tbsp	3
Naturally Yours	
Fat free sour cream, 2 Tbsp	1
Organic Valley	
Sour cream, organic, 2 Tbsp	3
Prairie Farms	
Sour cream, lite, 2 Tbsp	2

Dairy & Eggs

Publix

Sour cream, fat free, 2 Tbsp	1
Sour cream, light, 2 Tbsp	2
Sour cream, regular, 2 Tbsp	3

ShopRite

Sour cream, light, 2 Tbsp	2

Spartan

Sour cream, low fat, 2 Tbsp	2

Tillamook

Sour cream, fat free, 2 Tbsp	1
Sour cream, light, 2 Tbsp	2
Sour cream, natural, 2 Tbsp	3
Sour cream, premium, 2 Tbsp	3

Tofutti

Sour cream, imitation, milk free, 2 Tbsp	3

Tofutti Sour Supreme

Sour cream, non-dairy, 2 Tbsp	2

Wegman's Food You Feel Good About

Sour cream, light, 2 Tbsp	2

Whole Foods 365 Organic

Low fat sour cream, 2 Tbsp	2

Yogurt & Yogurt Drinks

Activia

Black cherry flavored lowfat ogurt, 1 container (113 g)	5
Blueberry flavored light yogurt, 1 container (113 g)	2
Blueberry flavored lowfat yogurt, 1 container (113 g)	6
Mixed berry flavored lowfat yogurt, 1 container (113 g)	5
Peach flavored lowfat yogurt, 1 container (113 g)	5
Prune lowfat yogurt, 1 container (113 g)	5
Strawberry banana flavored lowfat yogurt, 1 container (113 g)	5
Strawberry flavored lowfat yogurt, 1 container (113 g)	5
Vanilla flavored lowfat yogurt, 1 container (113 g)	5

Activia Fiber

Peach and cereal lowfat yogurt, 1 container (113 g)	5
Strawberry and cereal lowfat yogurt, 1 container (113 g)	5
Vanilla and cereal lowfat yogurt, 1 container (113 g)	5

Activia Fruit on the Bottom

Black cherry nonfat Greek yogurt, 1 container (150 g)	6

Activia Greek

Banana cream blended yogurt, 1 container (150 g)	5
Garden blueberry fruit on the bottom nonfat yogurt, 1 container (150 g)	5
Orchard peach fruit on the bottom nonfat yogurt, 1 container (150 g)	5
Strawberry patch fruit on the bottom nonfat yogurt, 1 container (150 g)	5
Toasted coconut vanilla flavor blended yogurt, 1 container (150 g)	5
Tropical fruit on the bottom nonfat yogurt, 1 container (150 g)	5
Vanilla flavored nonfat yogurt, 1 container (150 g)	6

Activia Light

Blueberry fruit on the bottom nonfat Greek yogurt, 1 container (150 g)	2
Cherry on the bottom nonfat Greek yogurt, 1 container (150 g)	2
Peach favored yogurt, 1 container (113 g)	2
Raspberry flavored nonfat yogurt, 1 container (113 g)	2
Strawberry banana flavored nonfat yogurt, 1 container (113 g)	2

SmartPoints™ value

	SmartPoints™ value
Strawberry flavored nonfat yogurt, 1 container (113 g)	2
Strawberry fruit on the bottom non fat Greek yogurt, 1 container (150 g)	2
Vanilla flavored nonfat yogurt, 1 container (113 g)	2
Almond Dream	
Coconut flavored non dairy low fat yogurt, 1 container (170 g)	5
Mixed berry low fat almond non dairy yogurt, 1 container (170 g)	7
Strawberry low fat almond non dairy yogurt, 1 container (170 g)	7
Yogurt, almond non-dairy, low fat, vanilla, 1 container (170 g)	7
Axelrod	
Yogurt, fat free, vanilla, 1 container (170 g)	4
Brown Cow	
Cherry vanilla cherry on the bottom cream top yogurt, 1 container (170 g)	9
Yogurt, cream top, maple, 1 container (170 g)	8
Yogurt, cream top, plain, 1 cup	7
Yogurt, cream top, smooth & creamy vanilla, 1 container (170 g)	8
Yogurt, cream top, vanilla, 1 cup	10
Yogurt, nonfat, Greek, plain, 1 container (150 g)	2
Yogurt, nonfat, Greek, strawberry on the bottom, 1 container (150 g)	5
Yogurt, nonfat, Greek, vanilla, 1 container (150 g)	3
Cabot	
Yogurt, Greek-style, plain, 1 cup	12
Yogurt, lowfat, Greek-style, plain, 1 cup	5
Yogurt, lowfat, Greek-style, vanilla, 1 cup	9

	SmartPoints™ value
Chobani	
Black cherry non fat Greek yogurt, 1 container (150 g)	5
Indulgent banana & dark chocolate Greek yogurt, 1 container (99 g)	6
Indulgent mint & dark chocolate Greek yogurt, 1 container (99 g)	6
Key lime blended low fat Greek yogurt, 1 container (150 g)	6
Peach non fat Greek yogurt, 1 container (150 g)	4
Pineapple low fat Greek yogurt, 1 container (150 g)	6
Plain Greek non fat yogurt, 1 cup	3
Chobani Flip	
Almond coco loco Greek low fat yogurt, 1 container (150 g)	10
Blueberry power Greek non fat yogurt, 1 container (150 g)	6
Chocolate haze craze flavored Greek yogurt, 1 container (150 g)	10
Clover honey Greek low fat yogurt, 1 container (150 g)	6
Key lime crumble Greek low fat yogurt, 1 container (150 g)	8
Nutty for 'nana Greek low fat yogurt, 1 container (150 g)	8
Peachy pistachio Greek low fat yogurt, 1 container (150 g)	8
Salted caramel crunch flavored Greek yogurt, 1 container (150 g)	7
Strawberry sunrise non fat Greek yogurt, 1 container (150 g)	6
Tropical escape Greek low fat yogurt, 1 container (150 g)	9
Vanilla golden crunch Greek non fat yogurt, 1 container (150 g)	7
Chobani Fruit On The Bottom	
Apple cinnamon Greek non fat yogurt, 1 Container (150 g)	4
Apricot Greek low fat yogurt, 1 container (150 g)	6

Dairy & Eggs

	SmartPoints™ value
Black cherry Greek non fat yogurt, 1 container (150 g)	5
Blackberry Greek non fat yogurt, 1 oz	4
Blood orange Greek non fat yogurt, 1 container (150 g)	4
Blueberry Greek non fat yogurt, 1 container (150 g)	5
Mango Greek low fat yogurt, 1 container (150 g)	6
Passion fruit Greek low fat yogurt, 1 container (150 g)	6
Peach flavored non-fat yogurt (variety pack), 1 container (170 g)	5
Peach Greek non fat yogurt, 1 container (150 g)	4
Pineapple Greek low fat yogurt, 5 oz	6
Pomegranate Greek non fat yogurt, 1 container (150 g)	4
Raspberry Greek non fat yogurt, 1 container (150 g)	5
Strawberry banana Greek low fat yogurt, 1 container (150 g)	6
Strawberry Greek non fat yogurt, 1 container (150 g)	4

Chobani Indulgent

Banana and dark chocolate Greek yogurt, 1 container (99 g)	6
Dulce de leche caramel and dark chocolate Greek yogurt, 1 container (99 g)	6
Mint and dark chocolate Greek yogurt, 1 container (99 g)	6
Raspberry and dark chocolate Greek yogurt, 1 container (99 g)	6

Chobani Kids

Banana flavored Greek low fat yogurt, 1 tube (57 g)	2
Chocolate dust flavored low fat Greek yogurt, 1 tube (57 g)	2

	SmartPoints™ value
Chocolate dust Greek yogurt, 1 tube (57 g)	2
Strawberry flavored low fat Greek yogurt, 1 tube (57 g)	2
Watermelon and grape flavored Greek low fat yogurt, 1 tube (57 g)	2

Chobani Oats

Apple cinnamon with steel cut oats low fat Greek yogurt, 1 container (150 g)	6
Apricot ancient grain blend low fat Greek yogurt, 1 container (150 g)	7
Banana maple low fat Greek yogurt, 1 container (150 g)	6
Blueberry low fat Greek yogurt, 1 container (150 g)	6
Cranberry low fat Greek yogurt, 1 container (150 g)	6
Mixed berry ancient grain blend Greek yogurt, 1 container (150 g)	7

Chobani Simply 100

Black cherry on the bottom Greek non fat yogurt, 1 container (150 g)	3
Blueberry on the bottom Greek non fat yogurt, 1 container (150 g)	3
Key lime blended Greek non fat yogurt, 1 container (150 g)	3
Peach on the bottom Greek non fat yogurt, 1 container (150 g)	3
Pineapple coconut blended Greek non fat yogurt, 1 container (150 g)	3
Pineapple on the bottom Greek non fat yogurt, 1 container (150 g)	3
Raspberry lemon blended Greek non fat yogurt, 1 container (150 g)	3
Strawberry on the bottom Greek non fat yogurt, 1 container (150 g)	3
Tropical citrus blended Greek yogurt, 1 container (150 g)	3
Vanilla blended Greek non fat yogurt, 1 container (150 g)	3

Dairy & Eggs

Dairy & Eggs

	SmartPoints™ value
DanActive	
Light strawberry flavored probiotic dairy drink, 1 bottle (93 ml)	1
Strawberry flavored probiotic drink, 1 bottle (93 ml)	4
Vanilla flavored probiotic dairy drink, 1 bottle (93 ml)	3
Dannon All Natural	
Plain lowfat yogurt, 1 cup	6
Plain nonfat yogurt, 1 cup	4
Plain yogurt, 1 cup	6
Vanilla flavored lowfat yogurt, 1 container (170 g)	8
Dannon Classics	
Coffee lowfat yogurt, 1 container (170 g)	8
Dannon Fruit on the Bottom	
Blueberry flavored lowfat yogurt, 1 container (170 g)	7
Cherry flavored lowfat yogurt, 1 container (170 g)	7
Mixed berry flavored lowfat yogurt, 1 container (170 g)	7
Peach flavored lowfat yogurt, 1 container (170 g)	7
Raspberry flavored lowfat yogurt, 1 container (170 g)	7
Strawberry banana flavored lowfat yogurt, 1 container (170 g)	7
Strawberry flavored lowfat yogurt, 1 container (170 g)	7
Dannon Greek	
Yogurt, nonfat, plain, 1 container (150 g)	2
Dannon Light & Fit	
Banana flavored nonfat yogurt, 1 container (170 g)	3
Banana protein shake, 1 bottle (296 ml)	5
Blueberry flavored nonfat yogurt, 1 container (170 g)	3

	SmartPoints™ value
Cherry flavored nonfat yogurt, 1 container (170 g)	3
Cherry vanilla flavored nonfat yogurt, 1 container (170 g)	3
Key lime flavored nonfat yogurt, 1 container (170 g)	3
Mixed berry protein shake, 1 bottle (296 ml)	5
Peach flavored nonfat Greek yogurt, 1 container (150 g)	2
Peach flavored nonfat yogurt, 1 container (170 g)	3
Pineapple coconut flavored nonfat yogurt, 1 container (170 g)	3
Raspberry flavored nonfat yogurt, 1 container (170 g)	3
Strawberry banana flavored nonfat yogurt, 1 container (170 g)	3
Strawberry cheesecake flavored nonfat yogurt, 1 container (170 g)	3
Strawberry cheesecake Greek nonfat yogurt, 1 container (150 g)	2
Strawberry flavored nonfat yogurt, 1 container (170 g)	3
Strawberry protein shake, 1 bottle (296 ml)	5
Vanilla flavored nonfat yogurt, 1 container (170 g)	3
Vanilla flavored nonfat yogurt, 1 cup	4
Vanilla protein shake, 1 bottle (296 ml)	5
Dannon Light & Fit 50 Calorie Packs	
Strawberry flavored nonfat yogurt, 1 container (113 g)	2
Dannon Light & Fit Carb & Sugar Control	
Strawberries and cream flavored cultured dairy snack, 1 container (113 g)	1
Vanilla cream flavored cultured dairy snack, 1 container (113 g)	1

Dannon Light & Fit Greek

Banana cream flavored nonfat yogurt, 1 Container (150 g)	2
Blackberry flavored nonfat yogurt, 1 container (150 g)	2
Blueberry flavored nonfat yogurt, 1 container (150 g)	2
Boston cream pie nonfat yogurt, 1 container (150 g)	2
Cherry chocolate flavored nonfat yogurt, 1 container (150 g)	2
Cherry flavored nonfat yogurt, 1 container (150 g)	2
Key lime flavored nonfat yogurt, 1 container (150 g)	2
Mango lemonade flavored nonfat yogurt, 1 container (150 g)	2
Peach flavored nonfat yogurt, 1 container (150 g)	2
Peach flavored nonfat yogurt, 1 container (150 g)	2
Pineapple flavored nonfat yogurt, 1 container (150 g)	2
Pomegranate berry flavored nonfat yogurt, 1 container (150 g)	2
Raspberry flavored nonfat yogurt, 1 container (150 g)	2
Strawberry banana flavored nonfat yogurt, 1 container (150 g)	2
Strawberry banana flavored nonfat yogurt, 1 container (150 g)	2
Strawberry cheesecake nonfat yogurt, 1 container (150 g)	2
Strawberry flavored nonfat yogurt, 1 container (150 g)	2
Strawberry fruit on the bottom yogurt, 1 container (150 g)	2
Toasted coconut flavored nonfat yogurt, 1 container (150 g)	2
Toasted coconut vanilla flavored nonfat yogurt, 1 container (150 g)	2
Vanilla flavored nonfat yogurt, 1 container (150 g)	2

Dannon Light & Fit Greek Blends

Caramel macchiato flavored nonfat yogurt, 1 container (150 g)	2
Caramel macchiato nonfat yogurt, 1 container (150 g)	2
Cherry chocolate non fat yogurt, 1 container (150 g)	2
Orange cream flavored nonfat yogurt, 1 container (150 g)	2
Raspberry chocolate nonfat yogurt, 1 container (150 g)	2
Strawberry cheesecake flavored nonfat yogurt (variety pack), 1 container (150 g)	2

Dannon Oikos

Triple zero banana creme nonfat yogurt, 1 container (150 g)	3

Dannon Superstars

Strawberry slide flavored Greek lowfat yogurt, 1 container (113 g)	4

Elli

Creamy german style strawberry quark, 1 container (170 g)	2

Essential Everyday

Plain Greek nonfat yogurt, 1 cup	3
Plain nonfat yogurt, 1 cup	5
Yogurt, fat free, strawberry, 1 container (170 g)	4
Yogurt, nonfat, Greek, vanilla, 1 cup	6

Fage

All natural strawberry goji nonfat Greek strained yogurt, 1 container (150 g)	4
Peach Greek yogurt, 1 container (170 g)	5
Yogurt, Greek strained, lowfat, total 2%, with peach, 1 container (150 g)	5
Yogurt, Greek strained, total, with honey, 1 container (150 g)	13

Dairy & Eggs

SmartPoints™ value

Fage Fruyo

	SmartPoints™ value
Yogurt, Greek, nonfat strained, blended with blueberry, 1 container (170 g)	6
Yogurt, Greek, nonfat strained, blended with cherry, 1 container (170 g)	7
Yogurt, Greek, nonfat strained, blended with pineapple, 1 container (170 g)	7
Yogurt, Greek, nonfat strained, blended with raspberry, 1 container (170 g)	7
Yogurt, Greek, nonfat strained, blended with strawberry, 1 container (170 g)	6
Yogurt, Greek, nonfat strained, blended with vanilla, 1 container (170 g)	7

Fage Fruyo Classic

Yogurt, Greek, strained, blended with coconut, 1 container (170 g)	9
Yogurt, Greek, strained, blended with coffee, 1 container (170 g)	8

Fage Total

Yogurt, Greek, strained, with peach, 1 container (150 g)	7
Yogurt, Greek, strained, 1 cup	8

Fage Total 0%

Greek strained cherry yogurt, 1 container (150 g)	4
Greek strained nonfat yogurt with orange cinnamon, 1 container (150 g)	5
Nonfat Greek strained yogurt, 1 cup	3
Nonfat Greek strained yogurt with blueberry acai, 1 container (150 g)	4
Nonfat Greek strained yogurt with cherry pomegranate, 1 container (150 g)	4
Nonfat Greek strained yogurt with honey, 1 container (150 g)	7
Nonfat Greek strained yogurt with mango guanabana, 1 container (150 g)	4
Nonfat Greek strained yogurt with strawberry goji, 1 container (150 g)	4
Nonfat Greek yogurt with peach, 1 container (150 g)	4
Yogurt, Greek strained, with blueberry, 1 container (150 g)	4
Yogurt, Greek strained, with raspberry, 1 container (150 g)	4
Yogurt, Greek strained, with strawberry, 1 container (150 g)	4
Yogurt, Greek, nonfat, strained, with apple cranberry, 1 container (150 g)	4
Yogurt, nonfat Greek strained, with apple cinnamon raisins, 1 container (150 g)	4

Fage Total 2%

Greek strained lowfat yogurt, 1 cup	5
Lowfat Greek strained yogurt, 1 cup	5
Lowfat Greek strained yogurt with blueberry, 1 container (150 g)	5
Lowfat Greek strained yogurt with honey, 1 container (150 g)	9
Lowfat Greek strained yogurt with strawberry, 1 container (150 g)	5
Nonfat Greek strained yogurt with cherry, 1 container (150 g)	5
Yogurt, Greek, lowfat, strained, with blood orange, 1 container (150 g)	5
Yogurt, Greek, lowfat, strained, with key lime, 1 container (150 g)	5
Yogurt, Greek, lowfat, strained, with mixed berries, 1 container (150 g)	6

Dairy & Eggs

Fit & Active

Black cherry Greek strained nonfat yogurt, 1 container (150 g)	3
Boston cream pie nonfat yogurt, 1 container (170 g)	5
Coconut cream flavored nonfat yogurt, 1 container (170 g)	4
Pineapple upside down cake flavoured nonfat yogurt, 1 container (170 g)	4
Pumpkin pie nonfat yogurt, 1 container (170 g)	4
Vanilla nonfat yogurt, 1 cup	5
Yogurt, nonfat, cherries jubilee, 1 container (170 g)	4
Yogurt, nonfat, key lime pie, 1 container (170 g)	4
Yogurt, nonfat, strawberry cheesecake, 1 container (170 g)	4

Friendly Farms

Blood orange Greek strained nonfat yogurt, 1 container (170 g)	4
Greek peach nonfat strained yogurt, 1 container (170 g)	5
Greek strawberry yogurt, 1 container (170 g)	5

Friendly Farms 100 Calories

Mixed berries Greek nonfat strained yogurt, 1 container (150 g)	3
Tropical fruit Greek nonfat strained yogurt, 1 container (150 g)	3

Giant

Nonfat yogurt, plain, 1 cup	5
Yogurt, nonfat, vanilla, 1 cup	9

Giant/Stop & Shop

Vanilla Greek 100 calorie nonfat yogurt, 1 container (150 g)	4

Great Value

Black cherry Greek nonfat yogurt, 1 container (170 g)	5
Light peach flavor Greek nonfat yogurt, 1 container (150 g)	2
Plain nonfat yogurt, 1 cup	4
Strawberry Greek nonfat yogurt, 1 container (170 g)	5
Vanilla Greek nonfat yogurt, 1 cup	7
Yogurt, light, banana cream pie, 6 oz	3
Yogurt, lowfat, blueberry, 6 oz	7
Yogurt, lowfat, cherry, 6 oz	7
Yogurt, lowfat, key lime pie, 6 oz	7
Yogurt, lowfat, peach, 6 oz	7
Yogurt, lowfat, strawberry, 1 cup	10
Yogurt, lowfat, vanilla, 1 cup	9
Yogurt, lowfat, vanilla (6 oz), 1 container (170 g)	7
Yogurt, nonfat, light, banana cream pie, 6 oz	3
Yogurt, nonfat, light, blueberry, 6 oz	3
Yogurt, nonfat, light, blueberry, 1 unit (170 g)	3
Yogurt, nonfat, light, cherry, 6 oz	3
Yogurt, nonfat, light, key lime pie, 6 oz	3
Yogurt, nonfat, light, orange creme pie, 6 oz	3
Yogurt, nonfat, light, peach, 6 oz	3
Yogurt, nonfat, light, raspberry, 6 oz	3
Yogurt, nonfat, light, raspberry, 1 unit (170 g)	3
Yogurt, nonfat, light, strawberry, 6 oz	3
Yogurt, nonfat, light, strawberry banana, 6 oz	3
Yogurt, nonfat, light, vanilla, 6 oz	3

Dairy & Eggs

	SmartPoints™ value
Great Value Light	
Pina colada flavored nonfat yogurt, 1 container (170 g)	3
Greek Gods	
Yogurt, Greek style, honey salted caramel, 1 cup	14
Yogurt, Greek style, traditional, honey flavored, 4 oz	8
Yogurt, Greek, honey & strawberry flavored, 1 cup	15
Yogurt, Greek, nonfat, plain, 4 oz	2
Yogurt, Greek, vanilla honey, 1 cup	14
Green Mountain Farms	
Whipped Greek cream cheese and Greek yogurt, 2 Tbsp	2
Green Valley Organics	
Yogurt, low fat, lactose free, plain, 1 container (170 g)	3
Yogurt, low fat, lactose free, vanilla, 1 container (170 g)	5
Healthy Choice	
Frozen yogurt, Greek, blueberry, 1 container (71 g)	4
Frozen yogurt, Greek, strawberry, 1 container (71 g)	4
Frozen yogurt, Greek, vanilla bean, 1 container (67 g)	4
Kirkland Signature	
Plain nonfat Greek yogurt, 1 cup	3
Kroger	
Peach Greek yogurt, 1 container (170 g)	4
Plain Greek nonfat yogurt, 1 container (170 g)	2
Vanilla Greek yogurt, 1 container (170 g)	3
Yogurt, lite, blackberry pomegranate, 1 container (170 g)	3

	SmartPoints™ value
Yogurt, lite, vanilla cranberry, 1 container (170 g)	3
Yogurt, nonfat, lite, blueberry, 1 container (170 g)	3
Yogurt, nonfat, lite, cherry cheesecake, 1 container (170 g)	3
Yogurt, nonfat, lite, cherry vanilla, 1 container (170 g)	3
Yogurt, nonfat, lite, strawberry, 1 container (170 g)	3
Yogurt, nonfat, lite, strawberry banana, 1 container (170 g)	3
Kroger CARBmaster	
Banana cream pie cultured dairy blend yogurt, 1 container (170 g)	2
Black forest cake flavored cultured dairy blend, 1 container (170 g)	2
Blackberry cultured dairy blend, 1 container (170 g)	2
Caramel spice cake cultured dairy blend, 1 container (170 g)	2
Cherry cultured dairy blend, 1 container (170 g)	2
Cinnamon roll cultured dairy blend, 1 container (170 g)	2
Key lime cultured dairy blend, 1 container (170 g)	2
Peach cultured dairy blend, 1 container (170 g)	2
Raspberry cultured dairy blend, 1 container (170 g)	2
Raspberry yumberry cultured lowfat dairy blend, 1 container (170 g)	2
Strawberry banana cultured dairy blend, 1 container (170 g)	2
Strawberry pomegranate cultured low fat dairy blend, 1 container (170 g)	2
Strawberry yogurt, 1 container (170 g)	2

Dairy & Eggs

Tropical fruit cultured dairy blend, 1 container (170 g) — 2

Vanilla cultured dairy blend yogurt, 1 container (170 g) — 2

White chocolate flavored raspberry cultured dairy blend, 1 container (170 g) — 2

Kroger Greek

Blended vanilla nonfat yogurt, 1 container (150 g) — 2

Lite blueberry nonfat yogurt, 1 container (150 g) — 2

Lite peach nonfat yogurt, 1 container (150 g) — 2

Lite raspberry nonfat yogurt, 1 container (150 g) — 2

Lite strawberry nonfat yogurt, 1 container (150 g) — 2

Lite vanilla nonfat yogurt, 1 container (150 g) — 2

Original plain nonfat yogurt, 1 container (150 g) — 2

Kroger Lite

Lemon flavoured yogurt, 1 container (170 g) — 3

La Yogurt

Light nonfat strawberry yogurt, 1 container (170 g) — 3

La Yogurt Probiotic

Blended nonfat yogurt, blueberry, light, 1 container (170 g) — 4

Yogurt, nonfat, blended, strawberry banana, 1 container (170 g) — 4

Blended nonfat yogurt, vanilla, 1 container (170 g) — 3

Liberte Mediterranee

Lemon flavored yogurt, 1 container (170 g) — 12

Rich and creamy coconut flavored yogurt, 1 container (170 g) — 12

Strawberry flavored yogurt, 1 container (170 g) — 11

Yogurt, French vanilla, 1 container (170 g) — 13

Lucerne

Black cherry light nonfat yogurt, 6 oz — 4

Blueberry light nonfat yogurt, 6 oz — 4

Plain Greek nonfat yogurt, 8 oz — 3

Vanilla light nonfat yogurt, 6 oz — 4

Yogurt, Greek 100 calorie, nonfat, strawberry flavor, 6 oz — 3

Yogurt, nonfat, Greek, vanilla, 6 oz — 5

Lucerne Greek 100 Calorie

Black cherry nonfat yogurt, 1 container (170 g) — 3

Vanilla nonfat yogurt, 1 container (170 g) — 3

Yoplain nonfat yogurt, 6 oz — 3

Mountain High

Yoghurt, all natural, fat free, plain, 1 cup — 4

Yoghurt, all natural, fat free, vanilla, 1 cup — 7

Yoghurt, all natural, lowfat, plain, 1 cup — 6

Yoghurt, all natural, lowfat, vanilla, 1 cup — 8

Yoghurt, all natural, original style, 1 cup — 8

Yoghurt, all natural, original style, vanilla, 1 cup — 10

Muller

Yogurt, raspberry chocolate chip, 1 container (150 g) — 10

Muller Corner

Chocolate coconut crunch Greek lowfat yogurt, 1 container (150 g) — 7

Lowfat yogurt with crispy crunch, 1 container (150 g) — 9

Lowfat yogurt with dark chocolate shavings and raspberry, 1 container (150 g) — 8

Yogurt, lowfat vanilla, with crunchy granola, 1 container (150 g) — 9

Yogurt, lowfat, dark chocolate & cherry, 1 container (150 g) — 8

Dairy & Eggs

SmartPoints™ value

Yogurt, lowfat, with choco balls, 1 container (150 g)	10
Yogurt, lowfat, with strawberry, 1 container (150 g)	7
Muller Fruit Up	
Yogurt, lowfat, with fruit mousse, luscious lemon, 1 container (150 g)	7
Yogurt, lowfat, with fruit mousse, splendid strawberry, 1 container (150 g)	7
Muller Greek 100	
Nonfat yogurt with black cherry and pomegranate, 1 container (150 g)	4
Nonfat yogurt with blackberry and raspberry, 1 container (150 g)	4
Nonfat yogurt with strawberry, 1 container (150 g)	4
Muller Greek Corner	
Lowfat strawberry Greek yogurt, 1 container (150 g)	7
Lowfat yogurt with blackberry and raspberry, 1 container (150 g)	6
Lowfat yogurt with caramelized almonds, 1 container (150 g)	8
Lowfat yogurt with mango, 1 container (150 g)	6
Lowfat yogurt with strawberry, 1 container (150 g)	7
Yogurt, Greek style, lowfat, with blueberry, 1 container (150 g)	6
Nancy's	
Yogurt, nonfat, plain, 1 cup	5
Nancy's Organic	
Yogurt, nonfat, plain, 1 cup	5
Noosa	
Blueberry aussie style yogurt, 1 container (113 g)	6
Blueberry yoghurt, 8 oz	12
Tart cherry aussie style yogurt, 1 container (113 g)	6
Yoghurt, finest, coconut, 8 oz	13
Yoghurt, finest, pineapple, 8 oz	12

SmartPoints™ value

Yoghurt, finest, plain, 8 oz	10
Yoghurt, finest, strawberry rhubarb, 8 oz	13
Yoghurt, finest, tart cherry, 8 oz	13
Yoghurt, lemon, 4 oz	8
Yoghurt, mango, 4 oz	5
Yoghurt, passion fruit, 4 oz	7
Yoghurt, peach, 4 oz	7
Yoghurt, raspberry, 4 oz	5
Yoghurt, strawberry rhubarb, 4 oz	5
Nostimo	
Greek nonfat yogurt blueberry fruit on the bottom, 1 container (150 g)	5
Plain nonfat Greek yogurt, 1 container (150 g)	2
Oikos	
Apricot mango flavored Greek nonfat yogurt, 1 container (150 g)	6
Black cherry fruit on the bottom Greek nonfat yogurt, 1 container (150 g)	5
Black cherry fruit on the bottom Greek nonfat yogurt, 1 container (150 g)	5
Blueberry flavored Greek nonfat yogurt (variety pack), 1 container (150 g)	5
Blueberry fruit on the bottom Greek nonfat yogurt, 1 container (150 g)	5
Blueberry fruit on the bottom organic Greek nonfat yogurt, 1 container (133 g)	3
Caramel macchiato flavored Greek yogurt with caramel on top, 1 container (150 g)	10
Caramel on top bananas foster Greek yogurt, 1 container (150 g)	10
Key lime traditional Greek yogurt, 1 container (150 g)	7
Pineapple fruit on the bottom Greek nonfat yogurt, 1 container (150 g)	5

Dairy & Eggs

Plain nonfat Greek yogurt, 1 cup	3
Pumpkin pie flavored Greek yogurt, 1 container (150 g)	7
Strawberry flavored Greek nonfat yogurt (variety pack), 1 container (150 g)	5
Strawberry fruit on the bottom Greek nonfat yogurt, 1 container (150 g)	5
Strawberry fruit on the bottom organic Greek nonfat yogurt, 1 container (133 g)	3
Traditional toasted coconut vanilla flavor blended yogurt, 1 container (150 g)	7
Vanilla flavored Greek nonfat yogurt, 1 container (150 g)	5
Vanilla flavored Greek nonfat yogurt, 1 container (150 g)	5
Yogurt, nonfat, Greek, pomegranate, 1 container (150 g)	5

Oikos Fruit on the Bottom

Blackberry Greek nonfat yogurt, 1 container (150 g)	5
Blueberry Greek nonfat yogurt, 1 container (150 g)	5
Peach Greek nonfat yogurt, 1 container (150 g)	5
Strawberry banana Greek nonfat yogurt, 1 container (150 g)	5
Strawberry Greek nonfat yogurt, 1 container (150 g)	5

Oikos Greek

Strawberry fruit on the bottom nonfat yogurt, 1 container (150 g)	5

Oikos Traditional

Apple pie flavored Greek yogurt, 1 container (150 g)	7
Banana cream flavor Greek yogurt, 1 container (150 g)	7
Cafe latte flavored Greek yogurt, 1 container (150 g)	7

Caramel macchiato Greek yogurt, 1 container (150 g)	7
Chocolate covered strawberry Greek yogurt, 1 container (150 g)	10
Key lime flavored Greek yogurt, 1 container (150 g)	7
Key lime Greek yogurt, 1 container (150 g)	7
Lemon meringue flavored Greek yogurt, 1 container (150 g)	7
Orange cream flavored Greek yogurt, 1 container (150 g)	7
Raspberry flavored Greek yogurt, 1 container (150 g)	7
Raspberry Greek yogurt, 1 container (150 g)	7
Strawberry flavored Greek yogurt, 1 container (150 g)	7

Oikos Triple Zero

Vanilla flavored blended Greek nonfat yogurt, 1 cup	5
Yogurt, Greek, nonfat, blended, coconut creme flavor, 1 container (150 g)	3
Yogurt, Greek, nonfat, blended, mixed berry flavor, 1 container (150 g)	3
Yogurt, Greek, nonfat, blended, strawberry flavor, 1 container (150 g)	3
Yogurt, Greek, nonfat, blended, vanilla, 1 container (150 g)	3

Open Nature

Greek nonfat strained vanilla yogurt, 6 oz	4
Yogurt, Greek, nonfat strained, strawberry on the bottom, 6 oz	5
Yogurt, Greek, nonfat, peach, 1 container (170 g)	6
Yogurt, Greek, nonfat, strained, blueberry on the bottom, 6 oz	5
Yogurt, Greek, nonfat, strained, lemon, 6 oz	4

Dairy & Eggs

Dairy & Eggs

	SmartPoints™ value
Yogurt, Greek, nonfat, strained, plain, 1 container (170 g)	2
Yogurt, nonfat, strained, Greek, honey, 1 container (170 g)	5
Open Nature Greek	
Nonfat plain yogurt, 8 oz	2
Nonfat yogurt strained black cherry on the bottom, 1 container (170 g)	5
Private Selection Organic	
Yogurt, lowfat, vanilla, 1 cup	10
Publix	
Yogurt, fat free, light, blueberry, 1 cup	5
Yogurt, fat free, light, strawberry, 1 cup	6
Yogurt, fat free, light, vanilla, 1 cup	5
ShopRite	
Yogurt, fat free, light, blueberry, 1 container (170 g)	4
Yogurt, fat free, light, vanilla, 1 container (170 g)	3
Siggi's	
Acai and mixed berries icelandic style skyr strained non-fat yogurt, 1 container (150 g)	3
Blueberry icelandic style skyr strained non-fat yogurt, 1 container (150 g)	3
Blueberry icelandic style strained skyr low-fat yogurt tube, 1 tube (57 g)	2
Coconut icelandic style skyr strained low-fat yogurt, 1 container (150 g)	6
Orange and ginger icelandic style skyr strained non-fat yogurt, 1 container (150 g)	3
Peach icelandic style skyr strained non-fat yogurt, 1 container (150 g)	3
Plain icelandic style skyr strained on-fat yogurt, 1 cup	2

	SmartPoints™ value
Pomegranate and passion fruit icelandic style skyr strained non-fat yogurt, 1 container (150 g)	3
Pumpkin and spice icelandic style cream skyr low fat strained yogurt, 1 container (150 g)	4
Raspberry non fat strained yogurt, 1 container (150 g)	3
Strawberry flavored icelandic style skyr strained non fat yogurt, 1 container (150 g)	3
Strawberry icelandic style skyr strained low-fat yogurt tube, 1 tube (57 g)	2
Vanilla icelandic style skyr strained non-fat yogurt, 1 container (150 g)	3
Silk Fruity and Creamy	
Peach mango dairy-free yogurt alternative, 1 container (150 g)	6
Simply Balanced	
Vanilla flavoured Greek yogurt, ¼ container (227 g)	5
Simply Balanced Fruit on the Bottom	
Black cherry Greek yogurt, 1 container (150 g)	4
Blueberry Greek yogurt, 1 container (150 g)	4
Raspberry Greek yogurt, 1 container (150 g)	4
Strawberry Greek yogurt, 1 container (150 g)	4
Stonyfield Farm	
Blueberry on the bottom organic nonfat Greek yogurt, 1 container (150 g)	4
Plain organic nonfat Greek yogurt, 1 container (150 g)	2
Strawberry on the bottom nonfat organic Greek yogurt, 1 container (150 g)	5

	SmartPoints™ value
Vanilla organic nonfat Greek yogurt, 1 container (150 g)	5
Yogurt, whole milk, French vanilla, 1 cup	11

Stonyfield Farm Oh My Yog!

Madagascar vanilla bean organic trilayer yogurt, 1 container (170 g)	9

Stonyfield Farm Oikos

Organic super fruits on the bottom Greek nonfat yogurt, 1 container (150 g)	5
Plain organic nonfat Greek yogurt, 1 container (113 g)	2
Strawberry organic Greek nonfat yogurt, 1 container (113 g)	3

Stonyfield Farm Organic

Belle blueberry petite low fat creme, 1 container (150 g)	5
Black cherry on the bottom nonfat Greek yogurt, 1 container (150 g)	4
Blood orange Greek nonfat yogurt & chia seeds, 1 container (150 g)	5
Chocolate flavor Greek nonfat yogurt, 1 container (150 g)	6
Greek blueberry nonfat yogurt & chia seeds, 1 container (150 g)	5
Greek strawberry raspberry cranberry nonfat yogurt & chia seeds, 1 container (150 g)	5
La vie en strawberry petite low fat crème, 1 container (150 g)	5
Nonfat yogurt, plain, 1 container (170 g)	3
Smooth and creamy plain nonfat yogurt, 1 cup	4
Strawberry fruit on the bottom low fat Greek yogurt, 1 container (150 g)	5
Super fruits on the bottom nonfat Greek yogurt, 1 container (150 g)	3
Vanilla nonfat Greek yogurt, 1 cup	8

	SmartPoints™ value
Vive la vanilla petite low fat creme, 1 container (150 g)	6
Yogurt, Greek, nonfat, peach mango on the bottom, 1 container (150 g)	5
Yogurt, low fat, French vanilla, 1 container (170 g)	6
Yogurt, lowfat, banilla, 1 cup	10
Yogurt, lowfat, plain, 1 container (170 g)	4
Yogurt, nonfat, Greek, plain, 1 cup	3
Yogurt, nonfat, Greek, vanilla, 1 container (113 g)	2
Yogurt, nonfat, organic, Greek, caramel on the bottom, 1 container (150 g)	6
Yogurt, plain, 1 cup	7

Stonyfield Farm Organic Oikos

Vanilla smooth and creamy organic Greek nonfat yogurt, 1 cup	5

Stonyfield Farm Organic O'Soy

Soy yogurt, strawberry, 1 container (170 g)	8

Stonyfield Farm Organic YoKids

Yogurt, lowfat, organic, squeezers, assorted, 1 tube (56 g)	3

Stonyfield Farm Smooth & Creamy

French vanilla fat free organic yogurt, 1 cup	7

Stonyfield Farm YoBaby

Yogurt, vanilla, 1 container (113 g)	3

Stonyfield Farm YoKids

Yogurt, organic lowfat, blueberry, strawberry vanilla, 1 container (113 g)	4

Stonyfield Organic Greek

Nonfat yogurt with lemon on the bottom, 1 container (150 g)	5

Taste of Inspirations

Vanilla flavored Greek non fat yogurt, 1 cup	5

Dairy & Eggs

SmartPoints™ value

SmartPoints™ value

The Greek Gods

Honey and strawberry flavored Greek yogurt, 1 cup	15
Yogurt, Greek style, traditional plain, 4 oz	6

Tillamook

Yogurt, lowfat, 1.5% milkfat, key lime, 6 oz	10
Yogurt, lowfat, dark cherry, 6 oz	9
Yogurt, lowfat, vanilla bean, 8 oz	14

Tillamook Farmstyle Greek

Old fashioned vanilla flavored strained yogurt, 1 container (150 g)	5
Oregon marionberry strained yogurt, 1 container (150 g)	4
Oregon strawberry flavored strained yogurt, 1 container (150 g)	5
Pacific northwest honey strained yogurt, 1 container (150 g)	5
Washington raspberry flavored strained yogurt, 1 container (150 g)	5

Trader Joe's

European style organic plain nonfat yogurt, 1 cup	3
Greek style nonfat plain yogurt, 1 oz	0
Greek style nonfat vanilla bean yogurt, 1 container (150 g)	5
Greek style nonfat yogurt, 1 container (150 g)	3
Low fat vanilla yogurt with almonds, 1 container (130 g)	7
Organic Greek style nonfat yogurt - plain, 1 container (150 g)	2
Organic Greek style vanilla nonfat yogurt, 1 container (150 g)	5
Strawberry kefir, 1 cup	7

Trader Joe's Organic

Greek style honey nonfat yogurt, 1 container (150 g)	5

Voskos

Yogurt, Greek, blended Greek honey, 1 container (150 g)	5
Yogurt, Greek, blended wild blueberry, 1 container (150 g)	4
Yogurt, Greek, blended wild strawberry, 1 container (150 g)	4
Yogurt, Greek, honey vanilla bean, 1 container (150 g)	5

Wallaby Organic

Greek nonfat yogurt with mixed berries, 1 container (150 g)	4
Greek plain nonfat yogurt, 1 container (170 g)	2
Yogurt, Greek, lowfat, plain, 2% milkfat, 1 container (170 g)	3
Yogurt, Greek, lowfat, with blueberries, 1 container (150 g)	5
Yogurt, Greek, lowfat, with cherries, 1 container (150 g)	5
Yogurt, Greek, lowfat, with strawberries, 1 container (150 g)	5
Yogurt, lowfat, Greek, plain, 1 cup	4
Yogurt, lowfat, vanilla, 1 cup	9

Wegman's

Yogurt, blended, nonfat, light, blueberry, 6 oz	4
Yogurt, blended, nonfat, light, raspberry, 6 oz	4
Yogurt, blended, nonfat, light, strawberry, 6 oz	4
Yogurt, blended, nonfat, light, vanilla, 6 oz	4
Yogurt, nonfat, light, blackberry, 6 oz	4

Wegman's Food You Feel Good About

Yogurt, Greek, nonfat, raspberry, 6 oz	5
Yogurt, Greek, pineapple, 6 oz	5
Yogurt, Greek, plain, 1 cup	3

Dairy & Eggs

	SmartPoints™ value
Yogurt, Greek, vanilla flavored, 1 cup	5
Yogurt, lowfat, organic, super pre- & probiotic, vanilla, 6 oz	7
Blueberry Greek yogurt, 1 container (150 g)	4

Yakult

Probiotic drink, nonfat, 1 bottle (80 ml)	3

Yasso

Frozen Greek yogurt bar, mango, 1 bar (70 g)	3
Frozen Greek yogurt bar, vanilla bean, 1 bar (70 g)	3

YoCrunch

Lemon flavored Greek nonfat yogurt with shortbread cookie pieces, 1 container (150 g)	4
Lowfat strawberry yogurt, 1 container (170 g)	8
Yogurt, lowfat, cookies n' cream, 1 container (113 g)	6
Yogurt, lowfat, vanilla, 1 container (113 g)	7
Yogurt, lowfat, vanilla, with snickers pieces, 1 container (113 g)	4
Yogurt, lowfat, vanilla, with twix pieces, 1 container (113 g)	4

YoCrunch Cereal Bowl

Vanilla lowfat yogurt with Kellogg's frosted flakes, 1 container (133 g)	4
Vanilla lowfat yogurt, with Kellogg's fruit loops, 1 container (133 g)	7

YoCrunch Fruit Parfait

Vanilla non fat yogurt with strawberries and lowfat granola, 1 container (113 g)	9

YoCrunch M&Ms

Vanilla nonfat yogurt with milk chocolate candies, 1 container (170 g)	15

YoCrunch Oreo

	SmartPoints™ value
Cookies and cream low fat yogurt with oreo cookie pieces, 1 container (170 g)	14

YoCrunch Yopa!

Yogurt, Greek nonfat, key lime, graham cracker pieces, 1 container (150 g)	4
Yogurt, Greek, nonfat, blueberries, includes 9 whole grain granola, 1 container (150 g)	6
Yogurt, Greek, nonfat, strawberries, includes 9 whole grain granola, 1 container (150 g)	7
Yogurt, Greek, nonfat, toasted almonds vanilla, includes toppings, 1 container (150 g)	7

Yopa YoCrunch

Vanilla flavor and dove® dark chocolate pieces Greek nonfat yogurt, 1 container (150 g)	8

Yoplait

All natural plain nonfat yogurt, 8 oz	5
Cafe mocha Greek yogurt with 2% milkfat, 1 container (150 g)	6
Caramel flavored original low fat yogurt, 1 container (170 g)	8
Cookies 'n cream original low fat yogurt, 1 container (170 g)	8
Harvest peach original low fat yogurt, 1 container (170 g)	8
Key lime 2% fat Greek yogurt, 1 container (150 g)	6
Orange crème original low fat yogurt, 1 container (170 g)	8
Peaches 'n cream 2% fat Greek yogurt, 1 container (150 g)	6
Strawberry original low fat yogurt, 1 container (170 g)	8

Yoplait 100 Calorie

Apple pie blended Greek fat free yogurt, 1 container (150 g)	3
Blended blueberry fat free Greek yogurt, 1 container (150 g)	3

Dairy & Eggs

	SmartPoints™ value

Yoplait Blended

Blueberry fat free Greek yogurt, 1 container (150 g)	5
Cherry fat free Greek yogurt, 1 container (150 g)	5
Coconut low fat Greek yogurt, 1 container (150 g)	6
Pineapple fat free Greek yogurt, 1 container (150 g)	5
Raspberry fat free Greek yogurt, 1 container (150 g)	5
Strawberry fat free Greek yogurt, 1 container (150 g)	5
Strawberry raspberry fat free Greek yogurt, 1 container (150 g)	5
Tangerine fat free Greek yogurt, 1 container (150 g)	5

Yoplait Fruitful

Yogurt with blueberries, 1 container (170 g)	8
Yogurt with peaches, 1 container (170 g)	7
Yogurt with strawberries, 1 container (170 g)	6

Yoplait Fruitplait

Strawberry yogurt, 1 container (113 g)	5

Yoplait Go-Gurt

Berry blue blast flavored portable low fat yogurt, 1 tube (64 g)	3
Burstin melon berry low fat portable yogurt, 1 tube (64 g)	3
Perry cherry flavored portable low fat yogurt, 1 tube (64 g)	3
Strawberry banana burst low fat portable yogurt, 1 tube (64 g)	3
Strawberry riptide low fat potable yogurt, 1 tube (64 g)	3
Strawberry splash spongebob squarepants portable low fat yogurt, 1 tube (64 g)	3

Yoplait Go-Gurt Simply

Mixed berry flavored portable low fat yogurt, 1 tube (64 g)	3
Strawberry flavored portable low fat yogurt, 1 tube (64 g)	3

Yoplait Greek

Caramel flavored yogurt with 2% milk fat, 1 container (150 g)	6
Cinnamon roll 2% fat yogurt, 1 container (150 g)	6
Honey flavored lowfat yogurt with 2% milk fat, 1 container (150 g)	6
Lemon meringue lowfat yogurt, 1 container (150 g)	6
Piña colada lowfat Greek yogurt, 1 container (150 g)	6
Vanilla fat free yogurt, 1 container (150 g)	5

Yoplait Greek 100

Banana caramel fat free yogurt, 1 container (150 g)	3
Black cherry fat free yogurt, 1 container (150 g)	3
Blackberry pie fat free yogurt, 1 container (150 g)	3
Blended blueberry fat free yogurt, 1 container (150 g)	3
Blended blueberry fat free yogurt, 1 container (150 g)	3
Blended strawberry banana fat free yogurt, 1 container (150 g)	3
Blended strawberry cheesecake fat free yogurt, 1 container (150 g)	3
Boston cream pie fat free yogurt, 1 container (150 g)	3
Caramel apple flavored nonfat yogurt, 1 container (150 g)	3
Caramel macchiato fat free yogurt, 1 container (150 g)	3
Coconut flavor fat free yogurt, 1 container (150 g)	3
Fat free yogurt, blended strawberry banana, 1 container (150 g)	3

Dairy & Eggs

Key lime fat free yogurt, 1 container (150 g)	3
Lemon fat free yogurt, 1 container (150 g)	3
Mango fat free yogurt, 1 container (150 g)	3
Mixed berry fat free yogurt, 1 container (150 g)	3
Mixed berry fat free yogurt fruit on the bottom, 1 container (150 g)	3
Orange creme fat free yogurt, 1 container (150 g)	3
Peach fat free yogurt, 1 container (150 g)	3
Pineapple fat free yogurt, 1 container (150 g)	3
Plain nonfat yogurt, 1 cup	3
Raspberry fat free yogurt, 1 container (150 g)	3
Strawberry banana blended fat free yogurt, 1 container (150 g)	3
Strawberry fat free yogurt, 1 container (150 g)	3
Tropical fruit fat free yogurt, 1 container (150 g)	3
Vanilla fat free yogurt, 1 cup	4
Yogurt, fat free, apple pie, 1 container (150 g)	3
Yoplait Greek 100 Whips!	
Blackberry fat free yogurt mousse, 1 container (113 g)	4
Blueberry fat free yogurt mousse, 1 container (113 g)	4
Lemon meringue fat free yogurt, 1 container (113 g)	4
Raspberry fat free yogurt mousse, 1 container (113 g)	4
Strawberry cheesecake fat free yogurt mousse, 1 container (113 g)	4
Strawberry fat free yogurt, 1 container (113 g)	4
Tropical fat free yogurt mousse, 1 container (113 g)	4

Vanilla cupcake fat free yogurt mousse, 1 container (113 g)	4
Yoplait Lactose Free	
Cherry low fat yogurt, 1 container (170 g)	8
French vanilla low fat yogurt, 1 container (170 g)	8
Strawberry low fat yogurt, 1 container (170 g)	8
Yoplait Light	
Apple fritter flavored fat free yogurt, 1 container (170 g)	3
Apricot mango flavored fat free yogurt, 1 container (170 g)	3
Apricot mango sorbet flavored fat free yogurt, 1 container (170 g)	3
Banana cream pie flavored fat free yogurt, 1 container (170 g)	3
Blackberry flavored fat free yogurt, 1 container (170 g)	3
Blackberry pomegranate flavored fat free yogurt, 1 container (150 g)	3
Blackberry pomegranate flavored fat free yogurt, 1 container (170 g)	3
Blueberry flavored yogurt with nature valley granola, 1 container (170 g)	8
Blueberry patch fat free yogurt, 1 container (170 g)	3
Blueberry patch or blackberry pomegranate fat free yogurt (variety pack), 1 container (170 g)	3
Boston cream pie flavored fat free yogurt, 1 container (170 g)	3
Chocolate cherry cupcake flavored fat free yogurt, 1 container (170 g)	3
Chocolate mint fat free yogurt, 1 container (170 g)	3
Harvest peach flavored fat free yogurt, 1 container (170 g)	3
Harvest peach or watermelon flavored fat free yogurt (variety pack), 1 container (170 g)	3

Dairy & Eggs

Dairy & Eggs

	SmartPoints™ value
Key lime pie fat free yogurt, 1 container (170 g)	3
Key lime pie flavored fat free yogurt, 1 container (170 g)	3
Key lime pie or very vanilla flavored fat free yogurt, 6 oz	3
Lemon cream pie flavored fat free yogurt, 1 container (170 g)	3
Orange creme flavored fat free yogurt, 1 container (170 g)	3
Orange creme non fat yogurt, 1 container (170 g)	3
Pineapple upside down cake flavored fat free yogurt, 1 container (170 g)	3
Pumpkin pie flavored fat free yogurt, 1 container (170 g)	3
Pumpkin pie flavored fat free yogurt, 1 container (170 g)	3
Raspberry cheesecake flavored fat free yogurt, 1 container (170 g)	3
Raspberry sorbet fat free yogurt, 1 container (170 g)	3
Red raspberry flavored fat free yogurt, 1 container (170 g)	3
Red velvet cupcake non fat yogurt, 1 container (170 g)	3
Strawberries 'n bananas fat free yogurt, 1 container (170 g)	3
Strawberries n bananas non fat yogurt, 1 container (170 g)	3
Strawberries'n bananas flavored fat free yogurt, 1 container (170 g)	3
Strawberry flavored yogurt with nature valley granola, 1 container (170 g)	8
Strawberry or blueberry patch flavored fat free yogurt, 1 container (170 g)	3
Strawberry orange sunrise flavored fat free yogurt, 1 container (170 g)	3

	SmartPoints™ value
Strawberry shortcake fat free yogurt, 1 container (170 g)	3
Strawberry shortcake or Boston cream pie flavored fat free yogurt (variety pack), 1 container (170 g)	3
Triple berry torte flavored fat free yogurt, 1 container (170 g)	3
Vanilla cherry flavored fat free yogurt, 1 container (170 g)	3
Very cherry flavored fat free yogurt, 1 container (170 g)	3
Very vanilla flavored fat free yogurt, 1 container (170 g)	3
White chocolate strawberry flavored fat free yogurt, 1 container (170 g)	3
Yoplait Light Thick & Creamy	
Key lime pie flavored fat free yogurt, 1 container (170 g)	4
Strawberry fat free yogurt, 1 container (170 g)	4
Yoplait Original	
Blackberry harvest low fat yogurt, 1 container (170 g)	8
Cherry orchard low fat yogurt, 1 container (170 g)	8
French vanilla low fat yogurt, 1 container (170 g)	8
Harvest peach low fat yogurt, 1 container (170 g)	8
Key lime pie flavored low fat yogurt, 1 container (170 g)	8
Lemon burst low fat yogurt, 1 container (170 g)	8
Mixed berry low fat yogurt, 1 container (170 g)	8
Mountain blueberry low fat yogurt, 1 container (170 g)	8
Orange creme flavored low fat yogurt, 1 container (170 g)	8
Pina colada low fat yogurt, 1 container (170 g)	8

Red raspberry low fat yogurt, 1 container (170 g)	8
Strawberry & strawberry banana flavored low fat yogurt family pack, 1 container (170 g)	8
Strawberry banana low fat yogurt, 1 container (170 g)	8
Strawberry cheesecake low fat yogurt, 1 container (170 g)	8
Strawberry flavored low fat yogurt, 1 container (170 g)	8
Strawberry kiwi low fat yogurt, 1 container (170 g)	8
Strawberry mango low fat yogurt, 1 container (170 g)	8
Tropical low fat yogurt, 1 container (170 g)	8
Tropical peach low fat yogurt, 1 container (170 g)	8

Yoplait Protein

Blueberry nonfat yogurt, 1 container (113 g)	4

Yoplait Thick & Creamy

Vanilla low fat yogurt, 1 container (170 g)	9

Yoplait Trix

Strawberry banana bash low fat yogurt, 1 container (113 g)	4

Yoplait Whips!

Cherry cheesecake flavored low fat yogurt mousse, 1 container (113 g)	7
Chocolate raspberry chocolate mousse style yogurt mousse, 1 container (113 g)	8
Chocolate yogurt mousse, 1 container (113 g)	8
Key lime pie flavored low fat yogurt mousse, 1 container (113 g)	7
Lemon burst flavored low fat yogurt mousse, 1 container (113 g)	7

Orange creme flavored low fat yogurt mousse, 1 container (113 g)	7
Raspberry mousse flavored low fat yogurt mousse, 1 container (113 g)	7
Strawberry mist low fat mousse yogurt, 1 container (113 g)	7
Vanilla creme flavored low fat yogurt mousse, 1 container (113 g)	8

Yulu

Vanilla bean aussie style yogurt, 1 container (150 g)	7

Zoi

Yogurt, Greek, nonfat, honey, 8 oz	9
Yogurt, Greek, nonfat, plain, 8 oz	4
Yogurt, Greek, nonfat, vanilla, 8 oz	8
Yogurt, Greek, traditional style, honey, 8 oz	15
Yogurt, Greek, traditional style, plain, 8 oz	10
Yogurt, Greek, vanilla, 8 oz	10

Dairy & Eggs

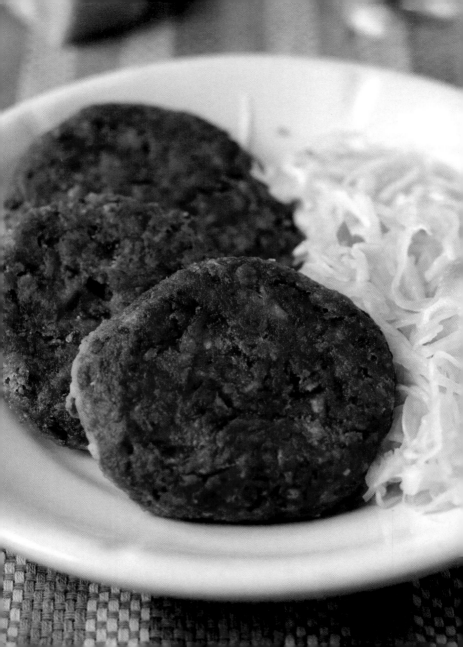

Dairy *substitutes* & Meat Substitutes

Dairy Substitutes & Meat Substitutes

Bacon Substitutes

Betty Crocker Bac-Os

Bacon flavor chips, 1 ½ Tbsp	1

Lightlife

Organic smoky tempeh strips, fakin' bacon, 3 slices (57 g)	2

Lightlife Smart Bacon

Veggie protein strips, bacon style, 1 slice (10 g)	0

McCormick

Bac'n pieces, chips, 1 Tbsp	1
Bits bac'n pieces, 1 Tbsp	1

Turtle Island Foods

Smoky maple bacon marinated tempeh, 7 slices (99 g)	3

Beef Substitutes

Beyond Meat

Beefy beef free crumble, ½ cup	2

Gardein

Beefless tips, home style, 3 ½ oz	2

Lightlife Smart Ground

Veggie protein crumbles, Mexican style, ⅓ cup	1
Veggie protein crumbles, original, ⅓ cup	1

Quorn

Grounds, meatless and soy-free, ⅔ cup	2

Bologna Substitutes

Lightlife Smart Deli

Veggie protein slices, bologna style, 4 slices (57 g)	1

Yves

Veggie bologna, 4 slices (62 g)	1

Cheese, Non-Dairy

4C

Grated cheese, homestyle, parmesan - romano, 1 Tbsp	1

Daiya

Shreds, cheddar style, ¼ cup	3
Shreds, mozzarella style, ¼ cup	3

Follow Your Heart Vegan Gourmet

Cheese alternative, mozzarella, 1 oz	2

Galaxy

Veggie shreds, cheddar flavor, ¼ cup	2
Veggie shreds, mozzarella flavor, ¼ cup	2
Veggie slices, American flavor, 1 slice (17 g)	1
Veggie slices, cheddar flavor, 1 slice (17 g)	1
Veggie slices, pepper Jack flavor, 1 slice (17 g)	1

Galaxy Nutritional Foods Veggie Slices

Cheese food alternative, pasteurized process, cheddar flavor with jalapeños, 1 slice (17 g)	1
Cheese food alternative, provolone, 1 ½ slices (30 g)	1

Go Veggie

Cream cheese alternative, classic plain, 2 Tbsp	4
Shreds, mozzarella style, ⅓ cup	3

Smart Beat

Healthy fat free non-dairy slices, American flavor, 1 slice (19 g)	0

Tofutti Better Than Cream Cheese

Imitation cream cheese, plain, 2 Tbsp	2

Chicken Substitutes

Beyond Meat

Beyond chicken grilled strips, 6 strips (85 g)	2

Morningstar Farms

Buffalo chik patties, 1 patty (71 g)	5
Italian herb chik patties, 1 patty (71 g)	4

Fish Substitutes

Gardein

Golden fishless filet, 2 pieces (96 g)	5

Frankfurter Substitutes

Lightlife Smart Dogs

Veggie protein links, 1 link (42 g)	1
Veggie protein links, jumbo, 1 link (76 g)	1

Morningstar Farms

Veggie dogs, 1 link (40 g)	1

Ham Substitutes

Lightlife Smart Deli

Veggie protein slices, baked ham style, 4 slices (52 g)	1

Sausage Substitutes

Boca

Veggie breakfast links, 2 links (45 g)	2

El Burrito

Soyrizo, 2 oz	3

Frieda's

Soy chorizo, meatless, 4 Tbsp	3

Lightlife Gimme Lean

Veggie protein, ground sausage style, 2 oz	1

Lightlife Smart Sausages

Veggie protein sausages, Italian style, 1 link (85 g)	3

Morningstar Farms

Sausage patties, veggie, breakfast, original, value pack, 1 patty (38 g)	2

Soy Yogurt

Silk

Blueberry dairy-free yogurt alternative, 1 container (150 g)	6
Strawberry dairy-free yogurt alternative, 1 container (150 g)	5
Vanilla dairy-free yogurt alternative, 1 container (150 g)	6

Tofu

House Foods

Tofu, shirataki, angel hair, 4 oz	1
Tofu, shirataki, fettuccine, 4 oz	1
Tofu, shirataki, spaghetti, 4 oz	1

House Foods Organic

Tofu, firm, 1" slice	1

Nasoya

Tofu, extra firm, 1 serving (79 g)	2
Tofu, firm, 1 serving (79 g)	1
Tofu, lite, 1 serving (79 g)	1
Tofu, super firm, cubed, ⅓ package (79 g)	2

Trader Joe's

Extra firm organic tofu, ¼ block (84 g)	2

Trader Joe's Organic

Teriyaki flavored baked tofu, 1 piece (100 g)	4

Turkey Substitutes

Lightlife Smart Deli

Veggie protein slices, roast turkey style, 4 slices (52 g)	2

Dairy Substitutes & Meat Substitutes

Dairy Substitutes & Meat Substitutes

Veggie Burgers

Amy's

Black bean veggie burger, 1 burger (71 g)	4
California garden vegetables veggie burger, 1 burger (71 g)	4
Veggie burger, all American, 1 burger (71 g)	3
Veggie burger, California, 1 burger (71 g)	3
Veggie burgers, 1 burger (71 g)	4

Boca

All American classic veggie burger, 1 burger (71 g)	1
All American flame grilled veggie burger, 1 burger (71 g)	3
Spicy chik'n veggie patty, 1 patty (71 g)	3
Vegan veggie burger, 1 burger (71 g)	1
Veggie burgers, grilled vegetable, 1 burger (71 g)	1
Veggie ground crumbles, ½ cup	1
Veggie patties, bruschetta tomato basil parmesan, 1 patty (71 g)	2

Dominex

Eggplant burgers, 1 burger (78 g)	2

Don Lee Farms

Veggie patty, 1 patty (85 g)	5

Dr. Praeger's Sensible Foods

Kale veggie burgers, 1 burger (71 g)	4

Franklin Farms

Veggiburger, fresh, original recipe, 1 patty (71 g)	2
Veggiburger, fresh, portabella, 1 patty (71 g)	2

Gardein

Beefless burger, the ultimate, 1 burger (85 g)	2

Gardenburger

Burgers, garden vegan, 1 patty (71 g)	2
Burgers, veggie medley, 1 patty (71 g)	2
Original veggie burgers, 1 patty (29 g)	4

Lightlife

Veggie protein patties, veggie burgers, 1 patty (71 g)	4

Morningstar Farms

Mediterranean chickpea veggie burger, 1 burger (67 g)	3
Veggie burgers, grillers original, 1 burger (64 g)	3
Veggie burgers, roasted garlic & quinoa, 1 burger (67 g)	4

Qrunch

Burger, quinoa, veggie gluten free, 1 burger (91 g)	6

Trader Joe's

Pizza veggie burgers with tomato basil and mozzarella cheese, 1 patty (67 g)	4

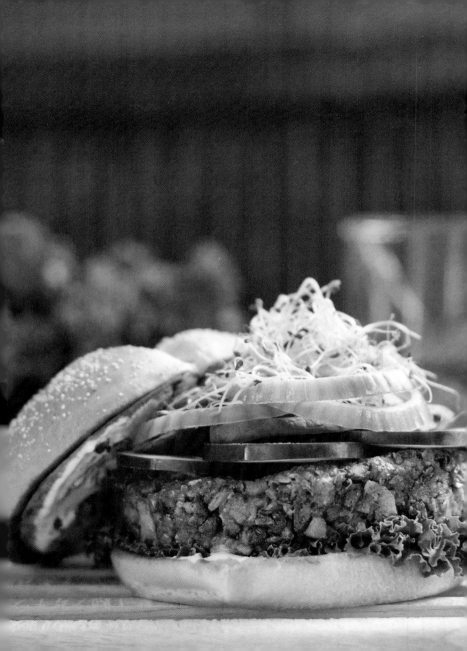

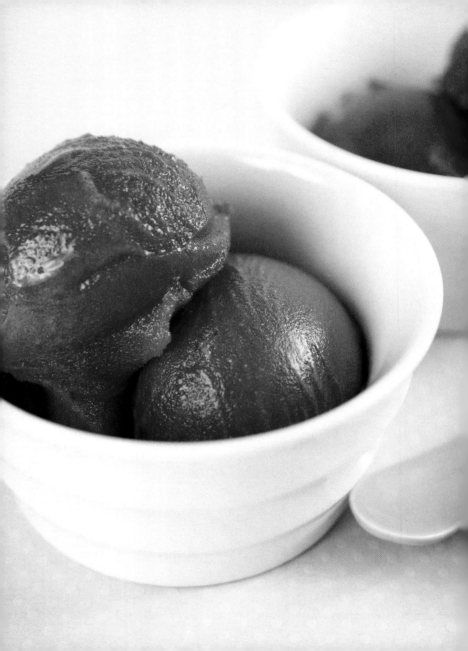

desserts
Cakes, Candy & Cookies

Brownie & Brownie Mixes

Betty Crocker

Brownie mix, fudge brownies, unprepared, 1 serving (26 g)	5
Brownie mix, fudge, dark chocolate, unprepared, 1 serving (28 g)	5
Brownie mix, low fat, unprepared, 1 serving (32 g)	6
Brownie mix, premium, with Hershey's, ultimate fudge, 1 serving (32 g)	6
Brownie mix, traditional, milk chocolate, unprepared, 1 serving (29 g)	5

Breads From Anna

Brownie mix, black bean, ⅔ oz	3

Duncan Hines

Premium brownie mix, family-style, milk chocolate, unprepared, 1 serving (29 g)	6

Fiber One 90 Calorie Brownie

Chocolate chip cookie, 1 brownie (25 g)	4
Chocolate fudge, 1 brownie (25 g)	4

Ghirardelli Brownie Mix

Triple fudge, 3 Tbsp dry	7

Homestyle

Brownies, two-bite, 2 brownies (39.88 g)	8

Kellogg's Special K

Blondie brownie bites, 1 package (21 g)	4
Divine fudge brownies, 1 brownie (20 g)	3
Fudge brownie bites, 1 package (21 g)	4
Heavenly caramel brownies, 1 brownie (20 g)	3

Kroger

High fiber brownie chocolate chip cookie, 1 (25 g)	4

Little Debbie

Brownies, 1 (48 g)	9
Cosmic brownie, 1 brownie (113 g)	22
Little brownies, 1 pouch (47 g)	8

Pillsbury

Brownie bites, fudgy, 2 brownie bites (48 g)	9
Brownie mix, milk chocolate, family size (serves 20), 1 serving (26 g)	5
Brownies, traditional chocolate fudge, ready made dough, 1 serving (38.9 g)	7
Chocolate fudge brownie mix family size (serves 20), 1 serving (26 g)	5

Pillsbury Brownie Minis

Brownie mix, chocolate fudge, ⅓ tray (33 g)	7
Brownie mix, milk chocolate, ⅓ tray (33 g)	7

Safeway Select

Brownie bites, petite, 1 brownie (28 g)	6

Sara Lee

Cake, brownie chocolate chip, 1 cake (50 g)	10

Toll House

Brownie bites, mini, 4 mini brownies (45 g)	10
Brownie dough, fudgy brownies, 1 brownie (34 g)	7

Trader Joe's

Reduced guilt brownie mix - fat free (1/12 box), 1 serving (1 g)	6

Udi's

Gluten free dark chocolate brownie bites, 2 brownies (44 g)	7

Vitalicious VitaBrownie 100 Calories

Deep velvety chocolate, 1 brownie (55 g)	4

Whole Foods

Brownies, two-bite, Belgian chocolate, 2 brownies (38 g)	8

Cake & Cake Mixes

1-2-3 Gluten Free

Cake mix, deliriously delicious, devil's food chocolate, 1 serving (23 g)	2

Baker's Treat Swiss Rolls

Chocolate cream filled cakes, 2 cakes (62 g)	11

Bakery Fresh

Angel food cake, classic white, 1 slice (57 g)	6

BBC

Angel food cake, fat-free, 1 serving (50 g)	7

Benson's Bakery

Fruit cake, premium, 1 piece (76 g)	13

Betty Crocker

Cake mix, angel food, 1 package mix (38 g)	7

Betty Crocker Super Moist

Cake mix, butter recipe, chocolate (serves 10), 1 serving (43 g)	7
Cake mix, butter recipe, yellow (serves 10), 1 serving (43 g)	7
Cake mix, devil's food (serves 10), 1 serving (43 g)	7
Cake mix, strawberry (serves 10), 1 serving (43 g)	7
Cake mix, white unprepared (serves 10), 1 serving (46 g)	8

Betty Crocker Warm Delights Minis

Cake mix, molten chocolate cake, 1 bowl (35 g)	7

Drake's

Coffee cakes, 2 cakes (70 g)	12
Devil dogs, 1 cake (49 g)	9
Ring dings, 2 cakes (80 g)	18
Yodels, 2 cakes (67 g)	15

Duncan Hines

Cake & frosting mix, decadent, red velvet cake, unprepared, cake only, 1 serving (28 g)	9

Duncan Hines Decadent

German chocolate cake mix (serves 12), 1 serving (50 g)	10

Duncan Hines Holiday Velvets

Cake mixes, red velvet, green velvet, limited edition, 1 serving (42 g)	8

Duncan Hines Signature

Cake mix, French vanilla (unprepared), 1 serving (39 g)	7

Entenmann's

Loaf cake, cinnamon crunch, 1 serving (61 g)	12
Loaf cake, lemon, 1 serving (54 g)	9

Entenmann's Little Bites

Creme filled chocolate cupcake, 2 pouches (64 g)	12
Creme filled golden cupcakes, 2 pouches (64 g)	13

Giant/Stop & Shop

Sponge cake dessert shells, 1 shell (24 g)	3

Hill & Valley

Angel food cake, sugar free, 1 slice (43 g)	2

Homestyle

Cupcakes, red velvet, 3 cakes (71 g)	14

Desserts, Cakes, Candy & Cookies

Desserts, Cakes, Candy & Cookies

	SmartPoints™ value
Hostess	
Cinnamon streusel coffee cakes, 2 cakes (82 g)	14
Coffee cakes, cinnamon streusel, 1 cake (41 g)	7
Ding dongs, 2 cakes (72 g)	17
Ho hos, 3 cakes (85 g)	19
Twinkies, 1 cake (42 g)	7
Twinkies, chocodile, fun size, 1 cake (41 g)	9
Zingers, iced vanilla, 2 cakes (72 g)	14
Hostess CupCakes	
Cup cakes, 1 cake (45 g)	8
Frosted orange flavored cake with creamy filling, 1 cupcake	9
Frosted red velvet cake with creamy filling, 1 cake (45 g)	8
Hostess Snack Classics	
Cupcakes, chocolate, 2 cakes (90 g)	16
Sno balls coconut and marshmallow covered chocolate cake with creamy filling, 2 cakes (99 g)	18
Twinkies, 2 cakes (77 g)	14
LaBree's	
Carrot cake, with cream cheese icing, 1 serving (76 g)	13
Little Debbie	
Be my valentine red velvet cakes, 2 cakes (62 g)	15
Butterfly cakes, 2 cakes (61 g)	14
Cinnamon streusel cakes, 1 cake (46 g)	7
Cloud cakes, 1 cake (43 g)	7
Cocoa cremes, 1 cake (40 g)	8
Fall tree cakes, 1 cake (42 g)	9
Snacks, oatmeal creme pie, double decker, 1 cookie (112 g)	21
Swiss rolls, 2 cakes (95 g)	20

	SmartPoints™ value
Little Debbie Christmas Tree Cakes	
Red velvet (5-count), 1 (28 g)	10
Mam Papaul's	
Cake mix, mardi gras king, 3 ½ oz	14
Marie Callender's	
Red velvet cake, 1 mini bag (82 g)	13
Meijer Fresh	
Pound cake, sliced lemon, 1 slice (45 g)	6
Mila's European Bakery	
Birthday cake, 5" yellow, white buttercream, 2 oz	8
Mrs. Freshley's	
Chocolate cupcake, 1 cupcake	10
Mrs. Smith's Homestyle Cakes	
Carrot cake, 1 serving (49 g)	13
Nice!	
Butter cake, gooey, st. louis style, 2 oz	8
Pepperidge Farm	
Cake, 3 layer, chocolate fudge, ⅛ cake (69 g)	11
Cake, 3 layer, coconut, ⅛ cake (69 g)	11
Cake, 3 layer, german chocolate, ⅛ cake (69 g)	11
Cake, 3 layer, lemon, ⅛ cake (69 g)	11
Cake, 3 layer, red velvet, ⅛ cake (67 g)	11
Pillsbury Funfetti	
Cake & cupcake mix, premium, with candy bits, happy birthday!, unprepared, 1 serving (43 g)	8
Cake mix holiday with candy bits, 1 ½ oz	7
Cake pop kit (serves 12), 1 serving (26 g)	6

Pillsbury Moist Supreme

Cake mix, premium, classic white (makes 10 servings), 1 serving (43 g)	7
Cake mix, premium, classic yellow, unprepared, 1 serving (43 g)	7
Cake mix, premium, devil's food, unprepared, 1 serving (43 g)	7

Sara Lee

Cake, angel food cake (serves 12), 1 serving (52 g)	6
Cake, banana (serves 5), 1 serving (78 g)	13
Cake, crumb, 1 cake (57 g)	11
Cake, double chocolate pound slices, 1 slice (51 g)	8
Cake, pound slice, 1 slice (45 g)	7

Tastykake

Krimpets, cream filled, butterscotch, family pack, 2 cakes (67 g)	13
Red velvet mini donuts, 4 (57 g)	9

Tastykake Kandy Kakes

Snack cakes, coconut, 2 cakes (38 g)	9

Tortuga

Original caribbean rum cake, 4 oz	17

Trader Joe's

Chocolate lava cakes, 1 cake (108 g)	17
Flourless chocolate cake (serves 6), 1 serving (76 g)	19

VitaCake

Cake, mini fudgy chocolate, 1 (35 g)	2
Vitacakes, 1 (32 g)	2

Vitalicious Energy Loaf

Apple cinnamon crumb, 1 loaf (54 g)	4

Whole Foods

Cakes, itty bitty bundt, 1 cake (28 g)	5

YoGo

Cakes, Greek yogurt, tuxedo, 1 cake (43 g)	3

Candy, Chocolate

100 Grand

Caramel, milk chocolate and crispy crunchies bar, 2 bars (43 g)	10

3 Musketeers

Candy bar, fun size, 3 bars (45 g)	10

3 Musketeers Minis

Dark chocolate candy with strawberry marshmallow, 7 pieces (41 g)	10
Milk chocolate candy with marshmallow, 7 pieces (41 g)	10

3 Musketeers Unwrapped Bites

Candy bars, sharing size, ½ cup	10

After Eight

Dark chocolate thin mints, 5 pieces (40 g)	9

Almond Joy

Candy bar, king size, 2 pieces (46 g)	12

Andes

Mocha mint indulgence, 4 pieces (34.43 g)	9
Peppermint crunch thins, 8 pieces (38 g)	12

Atkins Snack

Bar, caramel chocolate peanut nougat, 1 bar (44 g)	6

Atkins Treat

Endulge chocolate candies, 1 package (28 g)	4
Endulge chocolate covered almonds, 1 pack (28 g)	5
Endulge chocolate peanut candies, 1 package (34 g)	5

Desserts, Cakes, Candy & Cookies

	SmartPoints™ value
Endulge milk chocolate caramel squares, 3 pieces (35 g)	6
Endulge peanut butter cups, 2 pieces (34 g)	7
Endulge pecan caramel clusters, 1 pack (28 g)	5
Baby Ruth	
Chocolate caramel peanut bar, 2 bars (37 g)	9
Fun size chocolate caramel peanut bar, 2 bars (37 g)	9
Baci	
Chocolates, finest Italian, 3 pieces (43 g)	10
Bark Thins	
Dark chocolate almond with sea salt snacking chocolate, 1 ½ oz	9
Dark chocolate mint snacking chocolate, 1 ½ oz	11
Dark chocolate pretzel with sea salt snacking chocolate, 1 ½ oz	9
Blue Diamond	
Almonds, sea salt dark chocolate flavored, 24 nuts (28 g)	5
Boyer	
Mallo cup, 2 pieces (45.3 g)	11
Brookside	
Acai and blueberry flavored dark chocolate, 16 pieces (40 g)	9
Acai and blueberry flavors dark chocolate, 16 pieces (40 g)	9
Dark chocolate acai and blueberry, 16 pieces (40 g)	9
Dark chocolate almonds, 10 pieces (41 g)	10
Dark chocolate berry medley flavor crunchy clusters, 22 pieces (40 g)	10
Dark chocolate goji and raspberry, ¼ cup	9
Dark chocolate goji raspberry, ¼ cup	9

	SmartPoints™ value
Dark chocolate pomegranate snack, 16 pieces (40 g)	9
Goji and raspberry flavored dark chocolate, 16 pieces (40 g)	9
Pomegranate flavor dark chocolate, 16 pieces (40 g)	9
Brown & Haley	
Dark roca, 3 pieces (36 g)	10
Butterfinger	
Bar, miniatures, 4 pieces (40.94 g)	9
Bars, mini's, 1 bar (9.8 g)	2
Candy bar, 1 bar (60 g)	13
Candy bar, king size, 1 piece (52 g)	11
Candy bar, miniatures, 4 bars (38.9 g)	9
Candy bar, minis, 4 bars (40 g)	9
Chocolate bars, 2 bars (37 g)	8
Chocolates, bell shaped jingles, 5 pieces (42.51 g)	10
Crispety crunchety peanut buttery candy bar, 1 bar (54 g)	12
Fun size crunchy peanut bars, 2 bars (37 g)	8
Peanut butter cups, 1 pack (42 g)	12
Butterfinger Bites	
Bite-sized butterfinger candy, 8 pieces (40 g)	9
Butterfinger candy, 8 pieces (40 g)	9
Butterfinger Minis	
Unwrapped peanut butter cups, 9 pieces (41 g)	11
Cadbury	
Caramel egg, 1 egg	8
Chocolate creme egg, 1 piece (34 g)	9
Creme egg, 1 egg	8
Dark chocolate, royal dark, 10 blocks (42 g)	11

	SmartPoints™ value
Fine milk chocolate, 7 blocks (39.6 g)	10
Milk chocolate, fruit and nut bar, 10 blocks (42 g)	10
Milk chocolate, roast almond, 7 blocks (39 g)	10
Cadbury Caramello	
Milk chocolate, & creamy caramel, 6 blocks (43 g)	10
Cadbury Crunchie	
Candy bar, 1 bar (40 g)	5
Cadbury Fruit & Nut	
Milk chocolate, with raisins & almonds, 7 blocks (42 g)	9
Cadbury Mini Eggs	
Creme egg, caramel, 4 pieces (36 g)	9
Creme eggs, 3 pieces (34 g)	8
Creme eggs, 4 pieces (36 g)	9
Milk chocolate, 12 pieces (40.43 g)	10
Milk chocolate, solid, with a crisp sugar shell, 12 pieces (40 g)	11
Original, 12 pieces (39.23 g)	10
Royal dark, 12 pieces (38.88 g)	10
Solid milk chocolate with a crisp sugar shell, 12 pieces (40 g)	10
White candy with a crisp sugar shell, 12 pieces (40 g)	10
Cadbury Royal Dark	
Dark chocolate, indulgent, semi-sweet, 10 blocks (42 g)	11
Caramello	
Candy bar, 1 bar (45 g)	11
Candy bar, king size, 1 bar (76 g)	18
Cella's	
Cherries, dark chocolate covered, 2 pieces (28 g)	7
Charleston Chews	
Nougat, chewy, vanilla flavored, mini, 13 pieces (45.2 g)	9

	SmartPoints™ value
Chocolite	
Chocolate, pecan cluster, 1 piece (12 g)	1
Chocolove	
Dark chocolate, almonds & sea salt, 1 bar (37 g)	10
Dark chocolate, almonds & sea salt, 55% cocoa, ⅓ bar (30 g)	7
Dark chocolate, ginger crystallized, ⅓ bar (30 g)	8
Dark chocolate, orange peel, ⅓ bar (30 g)	8
Crunch	
Candy bar, 1 bar (43.9 g)	11
Chocolate bars, 3 bars (38 g)	9
Daily Chef	
Milk chocolate covered almonds, 9 pieces (40 g)	10
Divine	
Dark chocolate, 85%, 10 blocks (42 g)	11
Dole	
Dark chocolate banana dippers, 4 slices (44 g)	5
Dole Dippers	
Strawberry halves coated in dark chocolate, 4 pieces (35 g)	3
Dove	
Blueberries, whole, dipped in dark chocolate, 1 ½ oz	11
Chocolate assortment, 5 pieces (38.75 g)	10
Chocolate hearts, silky smooth, dark chocolate, 5 hearts (40 g)	11
Chocolate hearts, silky smooth, milk chocolate, 5 hearts (40 g)	11
Chocolate promises, dark, peppermint bark, 5 pieces (40.17 g)	11
Chocolate, assortment, 5 pieces (41.48 g)	11
Chocolates, select, 4 pieces (43 g)	12

Desserts, Cakes, Candy & Cookies

SmartPoints™
value

SmartPoints™
value

Desserts, Cakes, Candy & Cookies

Dark chocolate, 1 bar (36.9 g)	10
Dark chocolate & cherry swirl, heart promises, 6 hearts (42 g)	12
Dark chocolate bars, 1 bar (36.9 g)	10
Dark chocolate hearts, silky smooth, almond, 6 pieces (40.17 g)	11
Dark chocolate promises, silky smooth, 5 pieces (38.47 g)	11
Dark chocolate promises, silky smooth, family size, 5 pieces (39.69 g)	11
Dark chocolate, eggs, silky smooth, 6 eggs (43 g)	11
Dark chocolate, extra dark, 63% cacao, 5 pieces (38 g)	11
Dark chocolate, hearts, 6 hearts (44.6 g)	11
Dark chocolate, silky smooth, 71% cacoa, 9 pieces (47 g)	12
Eggs, dark chocolate, 6 eggs (44.6 g)	12
Eggs, milk chocolate, 6 eggs (44.6 g)	12
Milk chocolate bars, 1 bar (36.9 g)	10
Milk chocolate promises, 5 pieces (38.99 g)	11
Milk chocolate promises, silky smooth, caramel, 5 pieces (44.88 g)	10
Milk chocolate, eggs, silky smooth, 6 eggs (43 g)	12
Milk chocolate, hearts, 6 hearts (44.6 g)	12
Milk chocolate, smooth with caramel, 5 pieces (39.13 g)	10
Milk chocolate, smooth, with almonds, 5 pieces (40.17 g)	10
Peppermint bark promises, dark chocolate, let it snow, 5 pieces (40.29 g)	11

Whole cherries dipped in dark chocolate, ¼ cup	10
Whole cranberries dipped in dark chocolate, ¼ cup	11
Dove Beautiful	
Milk chocolate, smooth, 11 sections (40.04 g)	11
Dove Collection	
Dark chocolate, silky smooth, 3 pieces (40.27 g)	11
Dove Moments	
Chocolate, thank you, silky smooth milk & dark promises, 5 pieces (42.53 g)	11
Chocolates, with love. silky smooth milk & dark, 5 pieces (42.53 g)	11
Dove Promises	
Dark chocolate, 5 pieces (40 g)	11
Dark chocolate, silky smooth, 6 hearts (42 g)	11
Milk chocolate, 5 pieces (40.29 g)	11
Milk chocolate and red velvet swirl heart shaped chocolates, 6 pieces (42 g)	12
Milk chocolate strawberry creme swirl, silky smooth, 5 hearts (42 g)	12
Milk chocolate, hearts, 6 hearts (42 g)	12
White chocolate with creamy center silky smooth, 5 pieces (40 g)	12
Dove Silky Smooth	
Coconut creme milk chocolate eggs, 3 eggs (37 g)	11
Dark chocolate promises, 5 pieces (35.22 g)	11
Milk chocolate eggs, 6 eggs (43 g)	12
Milk chocolate promises, 5 pieces (39.13 g)	9
Dove Silky Smooth Promises	
Chocolate candies, mint & dark chocolate swirl, 5 pieces (40 g)	11
Dark chocolate, sea salt caramel, 5 pieces (40 g)	10

Emily's

Almonds, dark chocolate covered, 10 pieces (42.5 g)	9
Espresso beans, dark chocolate covered, 26 pieces (40 g)	9

Endangered

Dark chocolate, extreme, ½ bar (43 g)	10
Dark chocolate, supreme, ½ bar (43 g)	10
Dark chocolate, with cranberries & almonds, 72% cocoa, ½ bar (43 g)	10
Dark chocolate, with deep forest mint, 72% cocoa, ½ bar (43 g)	10

Endangered Species

Dark chocolate, with sea salt & almonds, 72% cocoa, ½ bar (43 g)	11

Essential Everyday

Peanut clusters, chocolate covered, milk chocolate, 3 pieces (42 g)	10

Fannie May

Chocolates, assorted, 3 pieces (37.67 g)	10
Mint meltaways, 5 pieces (40.89 g)	11

Ferrero

Chocolates, fine hazelnut, 3 pieces (38 g)	10

Ferrero Rocher

Fine hazelnut chocolates, 3 pieces (38 g)	10

Ferrero Rocher Collection

Confections, fine assorted, 4 pieces (40 g)	11

Flipz

Pretzels, chocolate mint covered, 7 pieces (28 g)	7

Goldenberg's

Peanut chews, milk chocolatey, 6 pieces (56 g)	12

Goobers

Peanuts, milk chocolate covered, ¼ cup	9

Green & Black's Organic

Dark chocolate, 70% cocoa, 12 pieces (40 g)	10
Dark chocolate, 85% cocoa, 12 pieces (40 g)	12
Dark chocolate, mint, 12 pieces (40 g)	11

GuyLian

Chocolates, artisanal belgium, 4 pieces (45 g)	12

HannahMax Baking

Cookie chips, chocolate chip, crunchy, 5 cookies (28 g)	6

Hawaiian Host

Macadamia nuts, chocolate covered, 4 pieces (40 g)	11

Heath

Candy bar, snack size, 3 pieces (43 g)	12
Candy bars, 1 bar (39 g)	10
English toffee bar, milk chocolate, 1 bar (39 g)	11

Hershey's

Bar, almond joy, 1 bar (45 g)	11
Bars, friendship exchange, kit kat, 1 bars (15.9 g)	4
Bars, special dark, snack size, 3 pieces (38 g)	9
Bell candy, peppermint bark, 4 pieces (38 g)	10
Candy bar, cookies 'n' creme, 1 bar (43 g)	11
Candy bar, cookies 'n' creme, king size, 1 (73 g)	18
Candy bar, take 5, 1 package (42 g)	9
Chocolate bar, dark, sugar free, 5 pieces (40 g)	7
Chocolate bar, extra dark, 3 blocks (37 g)	8

	SmartPoints™ value
Chocolate bar, sugar free, 5 pieces (40 g)	7
Chocolate bar, xoxo, ⅓ bar (38 g)	10
Chocolate kisses, pumpkin spice, 9 pieces (41 g)	11
Eggs, chocolate, cookies'n'creme, 6 pieces (42 g)	11
Eggs, marshmallow, milk chocolate covered, 1 piece (26 g)	5
Eggs, milk chocolate, candy coated, 8 pieces (38 g)	9
Hugs, kisses hugged by white chocolate, 9 pieces (37.78 g)	11
Kisses, milk chocolates, filled with caramel, 9 pieces (42 g)	10
Milk chocolate, 1 bar (43 g)	11
Milk chocolate bar, special holiday design, ⅓ package (33 g)	9
Milk chocolate bar, with almonds, giant bar, 3 blocks (36 g)	9
Milk chocolate, bars, snack size, 3 pieces (42 g)	11
Milk chocolate, bells, extra creamy solid, 5 pieces (40.43 g)	10
Milk chocolate, bunnies, mini, 4 pieces (36.71 g)	9
Milk chocolate, extra creamy, hearts, 5 pieces (40.43 g)	11
Milk chocolate, large bars, 7 blocks (42 g)	12
Milk chocolate, santa, 1 each (34 g)	9
Milk chocolate, with almonds, 1 bar (41 g)	10
Miniatures, 5 pieces (43 g)	11
Nuggets, chocolates, with raisins and almonds, 4 pieces (39 g)	10
Nuggets, chocolates, with toffee and almonds, 4 pieces (38 g)	10
Nuggets, dark chocolate with almonds, 4 pieces (41.2 g)	10
Nuggets, milk chocolate with almonds, 4 pieces (41.2 g)	10

	SmartPoints™ value
Peanut butter cups, Reese's, 1 piece (15 g)	4
Peanut butter cups, Reese's, minatures, 4 pieces (44 g)	10
Whoppers, 6 tubes (41 g)	10
York peppermint patties, sugar free, 3 pieces (36 g)	5
Hershey's Bliss	
Candy, dark chocolate, 6 pieces (41.5 g)	11
Candy, milk chocolate, 6 pieces (43 g)	11
Candy, white chocolate, 6 pieces (40.5 g)	12
Hershey's Drops	
Candies, milk chocolate, 15 pieces (41 g)	10
Hershey's Eggs	
Milk chocolate, 7 pieces (40 g)	10
Milk chocolate, special dark, mildly sweet chocolate, 7 pieces (39 g)	10
Hershey's Factory Favorites	
Whoppers, snack size (variety pack candy), 6 packets (41 g)	11
Hershey's Kisses	
Candy cane, 9 pieces (42 g)	11
Chocolate, mildly sweet, 9 pieces (42.5 g)	12
Chocolate, truffles, 5 truffles (36 ml)	10
Dark chocolate, filled with mint truffle, 9 pieces (40.43 g)	11
Dark chocolate, truffle, 9 pieces (42 g)	11
Mildly sweet chocolate, special dark, 9 pieces (40 g)	10
Milk chocolate, 9 pieces (41 g)	10
Milk chocolate, Easter, 9 pieces (38.88 g)	10
Milk chocolate, filled with caramel, 9 pieces (42 g)	10

Desserts, Cakes, Candy & Cookies

Milk chocolate, with almonds, 9 pieces (40 g)	10
Milk chocolates, filled with cherry cordial crème, 9 pieces (42 g)	10

Hershey's Pot of Gold

Chocolates, assorted milk and dark, caramels collection, 4 pieces (41 g)	10
Chocolates, premium collection, 4 pieces (41 g)	10
Clusters, pecan caramel, 4 pieces (41 g)	10

Hershey's Special Dark

Candy bar, 1 bar (41 g)	10
Candy bar, giant bar, 3 blocks (36 g)	9
Chocolate bar, 100 calorie, mildly sweet chocolate, 1 bar (17 g)	5
Chocolate bar, mildly sweet, 5 blocks (38 g)	9
Chocolate bar, with almonds, 1 serving (43 g)	10
Chocolate bars, king size, 1 bar (73 g)	18
Miniatures, 5 pieces (40 g)	11

Hershey's Symphony

Milk chocolate bar, giant, 3 blocks (36 g)	9
Milk chocolate bar, with almonds & toffee chips, giant, 3 blocks (36 g)	9

Joyva

Ring jells, chocolate covered, 3 pieces (42 g)	9

Junior Mints

Creamy mints, 16 pieces (37.67 g)	10
Creamy mints, big box size!, 16 pieces (40 g)	10
Creamy mints, in pure chocolate, xl, 16 pieces (38.29 g)	10
Junior mint chews, 26 piece (49.5 g)	5
Junior mints, king size, 1 ½ oz	9

Kinder

Chocolate, 1 piece (12.5 g)	4

Kirkland Signature

Chocolate covered raisins, 20 pieces (40 g)	10
Dark chocolate super fruits, ¼ cup	9
Macadamia clusters, 2 pieces (39 g)	10
Milk chocolate almonds, 11 pieces (30 g)	7
Semi-sweet chocolate chips, 30 pieces (15 g)	4

Kirkland Signature Truffettes de France

Chocolate truffles, 4 pieces (32 g)	10

Kit Kat

Bar, 1 four-piece bar (42 g)	12
Bar, big kat, 1 bar (55 g)	15
Candy bar, crisp wafers, in milk chocolate, 1 bar (42 g)	11
Candy bar, dark, 1 bar (42 g)	11
Candy bar, king size, 1 bar (42 g)	11
Candy bar, white, 1 four-piece bar (42 g)	11
Candy bars, minis, 5 pieces (40.43 g)	11
Crisp wafers in milk chocolate (42gm bars), 3 two-piece bars (42 g)	11
Crisp wafers in milk chocolate, valentine exchange, 3 (42 g)	11
Crisp wafers, assorted, snack size pieces, 3 bars (42 g)	11
Crisp wafers, in milk chocolate, miniatures, 5 pieces (43 g)	11
Crisp wafers, in milk chocolate, minis, 9 pieces (42 g)	11
Crisp wafers, in milk chocolate, minis, king size, 1 package (62 g)	16
Crisp wafers, in milk chocolate, snack size, 3 (42 g)	11

Desserts, Cakes, Candy & Cookies

Desserts, Cakes, Candy & Cookies

	SmartPoints™ value
Kit Kat Extra Crispy	
Crisp wafers, in milk chocolate, 1 bar (45 g)	11
Kit Kat Miniatures	
Crisp wafers in milk chocolate, 5 pieces (43 g)	11
Milk chocolate crisp wafers, 5 pieces (43 g)	11
Kit Kat To Go	
Bites, kit kat, 1 package (77 g)	20
Klondike	
Kandy bars, cookies & cream, 1 bar (58 g)	10
Krackel	
Milk chocolate with crisped rice candy bar, 1 bar (43 g)	11
Kroger	
Chocolate peanut clusters, 3 pieces (40 g)	10
Lake Champlain Chocolates	
Chocolate, dark, 4 blocks (43 g)	11
Lily's	
Dark chocolate, original, 55% cocoa, ½ bar (40 g)	7
Lindt	
Chocolate, minis, assorted, 4 pieces (40 g)	11
Lindor truffles, assorted chocolates with a smooth filling, 3 balls (36 ml)	12
Lindor truffles, assorted milk, dark and white chocolates, 3 balls (36 g)	12
Lindor truffles, milk chocolate, 3 balls (36 g)	11
Lindor truffles, white chocolates with a smooth filling, 3 balls (36 g)	12
Milk chocolate eggs, lindor truffles, 2 eggs (32 g)	10
Milk chocolate hollow mini bear figure, 4 (40 g)	12

	SmartPoints™ value
Truffles, gourmet, 3 balls (47 g)	15
Truffles, lindor, peanut butter, 3 balls (36 g)	10
Lindt Classic Recipe	
Hazelnut milk chocolate, 1 square (4 g)	11
Milk chocolate, 10 squares (42 g)	11
White chocolate, 10 squares (42 g)	12
Lindt Excellence	
70% cocoa smooth dark chocolate, 4 squares (40 g)	12
85% cocoa extra dark chocolate, 4 squares (40 g)	9
90% cocoa supreme dark chocolate, 4 squares (40 g)	11
Assortment dark chocolates, 4 squares (40 g)	11
Caramel with a touch of sea salt dark chocolate, 4 squares (40 g)	10
Chili dark chocolate, 4 squares (40 g)	10
Coconut dark chocolate, 4 squares (40 g)	11
Intense mint dark chocolate, 4 squares (40 g)	10
Intense orange dark chocolate, 4 squares (40 g)	9
Touch of sea salt dark chocolate, 4 squares (40 g)	10
Lindt Hello My Name Is	
Caramel brownie chocolate stick, 1 stick (39 g)	11
Lindt Lindor	
Milk chocolate tablet, 1 bar (38 g)	13
Lindt Lindor Truffles	
60% extra dark chocolate, 3 (36 g)	12
Assorted chocolate, 3 pieces (36 g)	12
Assorted dark and white milk chocolates, 3 (36 g)	12

Caramel milk chocolate, 3 (36 g)	12
Chocolate, 3 pieces (36 g)	12
Coconut milk chocolate, 3 pieces (36 g)	12
Dark chocolate, 3 balls (36 g)	8
Dark chocolate with mint filling, 3 (36 g)	12
Extra dark chocolate, 3 balls (36 g)	12
Hazelnut milk chocolate, 3 (36 g)	11
Milk and white milk chocolate, 3 balls (36 g)	12
Milk chocolate, 3 pieces (36 g)	11
Milk chocolate with peanut butter and chocolate smooth filling, 1 (12 g)	3
Milk chocolate with smooth filling, 3 pieces (36 g)	11
Sea salt milk chocolate, 3 pieces (36 g)	11
White chocolate, 3 (36 g)	12
White chocolate with smooth filling, 3 (36 g)	12

M&M's

Chocolate bar, milk chocolate, 1 bar (42.5 g)	11
Chocolate candies, almond, ½ pack (40 g)	9
Chocolate candies, cherry, 1 ½ oz	11
Chocolate candies, dark chocolate, peanut, ¼ cup	10
Chocolate candies, eggs!, coconut, ¼ cup	11
Chocolate candies, fun size gift mix, milk chocolate, 2 packs (36 g)	9
Chocolate candies, milk chocolate peanut, ¼ cup	10
Chocolate candies, milk chocolate, fun size, 2 packs (36 g)	8
Chocolate candies, milk chocolate, minis, 2 packs (33 g)	8

Chocolate candies, milk chocolate, speck-tacular eggs!, ¼ cup	11
Chocolate candies, minis, milk chocolate, 1 tube (50 g)	13
Chocolate candies, mint, made with dark chocolate, 1 pack (42 g)	11
Dark chocolate chocolate candies, 1 ½ oz	11
Milk chocolate covered almonds, ¼ cup	10
Milk chocolate, fun size, 3 packs (45 g)	12
Peanut chocolate candies, ¼ cup	10
Peanut filled chocolate candy, ¼ cup	10
Peanut milk chocolate candies, ¼ cup	10
Peppermint white chocolate candies, ¼ cup	12
Storybook and puzzles milk chocolate candies, 3 packs (45 g)	11
White chocolate candies, ¼ cup	12

M&M's Birthday Cake

Chocolate candies, 1 pack (39.7 g)	10

M&M's Bunny Mix

Chocolate candies, milk chocolate, 1 ½ oz	11

M&M's Fun Size

Milk chocolate candies, 3 packs (45 g)	12
Peanut butter chocolate candies, 2 packs (34 g)	9
Peanut chocolate candies, 2 packs (36 g)	8

M&M's Happy Holidays

Peanut chocolate candies mix, ¼ cup	10

Desserts, Cakes, Candy & Cookies

Desserts, Cakes, Candy & Cookies

	SmartPoints™ value
M&M's Mega	
Chocolate candies, milk chocolate, 1 pack (42 g)	11
Milk chocolate covered candies, 15 pieces (41 g)	10
Peanut chocolate covered candies, ¼ cup	10
M&M's Premiums	
Chocolate candies, almond, ¼ cup	10
Chocolate candies, dark chocolate, 1 ½ oz	11
M&M's Speck-Tacular Eggs!	
Chocolate candies, crispy, ⅓ cup	10
Chocolate candies, milk chocolate, peanut butter, ¼ cup	11
Madelaine Duets	
Milk chocolate truffles, double-filled, milk truffle & white truffle, 1 duet (14 g)	4
Mauna Loa	
Macadamia nuts covered in milk chocolate, 4 pieces (40.29 g)	11
Mighty Malts	
Malted milk balls, 16 pieces (39 g)	9
Milk Duds	
Candy, 13 pieces (39 g)	8
Milka	
Milk chocolate confection, alpine milk, 10 sections (40 g)	11
Milky Way	
Candy bar, 1 bar (52 g)	13
Candy bar, midnight dark, 1 bar (49.9 g)	12
Candy bar, midnight dark, 1 bar (49.9 g)	12
Candy bar, simply caramel, 1 bar (54.1 g)	13
Candy bars, fun size, 2 bars (34 g)	9
Candy bars, miniatures, Christmas, 5 pieces (40.96 g)	10

	SmartPoints™ value
Candy bars, minis, 5 pieces (44.11 g)	10
Candy bars, simply caramel, 1 bar (22 g)	5
Candy bars, simply caramel, fun size, 1 bar (22 g)	5
Chocolate minis, 5 pieces (43 g)	10
Milky Way Bites	
Candy bar, unwrapped, 8 pieces (38 g)	9
Candy bar, unwrapped, sharing size, ½ package (40 g)	10
Milky Way Fun Size	
Chocolate bars, 2 bars (34 g)	8
Milky Way Midnight	
Dark chocolate golden caramel vanilla nougat minis, 5 pieces (43 g)	10
Milky Way Minis	
Candy, 5 pieces (40.75 g)	10
Milky Way Simply Caramel	
Bunny bar, 1 (31 g)	8
Milky Way Unwrapped Bites	
Simply caramel candy, 7 pieces (37 g)	9
Mounds	
Bars, dark chocolate, snack size, 1 bar (17 g)	4
Candy bars, dark chocolate, 1 package (49 g)	12
Candy bars, king size, 2 pieces (49 g)	12
Dark chocolate, coconut filled, 1 package (49 g)	12
Mr. Goodbar	
Candy bar, 1 bar (49 g)	12
Candy, snack size, 3 pieces (38 g)	9
Nestlé	
Buncha crunch, movie pack, ⅓ cup	10
Crunch bar, 1 serving (40 g)	10

Crunch candy bars (variety pack 13 gm bars), 3 bars (38 g)	9
Crunch, fun size, 1 bar (9.8 g)	2
Nest eggs, crunch, 5 pieces (36.85 g)	9
Nestlé Butterfinger	
Nest eggs shaped chocolates, 5 pieces (43 g)	11
Peanut bar, 2 bars (37 g)	8
Peanut bar fun size, 2 bars (37 g)	8
Nestlé Crunch	
Fun size chocolate bar, 3 bars (38 g)	9
Nestlé Skinny Cow	
Divine filled chocolate caramel flavor candy (variety pack), 1 pouch (28 g)	7
Nestlé Sno-Caps	
Nonpareils, semi-sweet chocolate, ¼ cup	10
Nestlé Toll House	
Chocolate morsels, semi-sweet, with red & green colored morsels, 1 Tbsp	4
Semi sweet chocolate morsels, 1 Tbsp	4
Ocean Spray Craisins	
Dried cranberries, chocolate covered, ¼ cup	9
Milk chocolate covered dried cranberries, ¼ cup	7
Orchard Valley Harvest	
Dark chocolate covered almonds, 1 package (28 g)	7
Oreo 100 Calorie Packs	
Candy bites, oreo, 1 package (22 g)	5
Pearson's	
Original mint patties, 5 pieces (38 g)	8

Peeps	
Marshmallow, milk chocolate covered, 1 chick (28 g)	5
Planters	
Almonds, cocoa, dark chocolate flavor, 24 pieces (28 g)	5
Queen Anne	
Cordial cherries, dark chocolate, 2 pieces (37.4 g)	8
Raisinets	
California raisins, classic milk chocolate, ¼ cup	10
California raisins, dark chocolate, ¼ cup	10
Reese's	
Bunnies, mini reester, 4 pieces (40.43 g)	10
Candy bar, nutrageous milk chocolate, 1 bar (47 g)	11
Candy, lovers' assortment, 1 piece (18 g)	4
Milk chocolate, filled with Reese's peanut butter, 4 blocks (40 g)	10
Peanut butter bells, milk chocolate, 5 pieces (41 g)	10
Peanut butter cups, milk chocolate, 1 package (42 g)	10
Peanut butter cups, milk chocolate, king size, 1 package (79 g)	19
Peanut butter cups, milk chocolate, snack size, 1 piece (15 g)	4
Peanut butter cups, white, 1 package (42 g)	10
Peanut butter eggs, 3 pieces (34 g)	9
Peanut butter eggs, milk chocolate, 1 piece (17 g)	4
Peanut butter eggs, milk chocolate, mini eggs, 5 pieces (40 g)	10
Peanut butter eggs, white, 1 package (34 g)	8

Desserts, Cakes, Candy & Cookies

Desserts, Cakes, Candy & Cookies

	SmartPoints™ value
Peanut butter trees, 1 piece (34 g)	8
Peanut butter trees, milk chocolate, 1 piece (17 g)	4
peanut butter, hearts, 1 piece (34 g)	8
Peanut butter, hearts, snack size, 1 piece (17 g)	4
Pieces, 1 package (45 g)	10
Reese's sticks, 1 package (42 g)	9
Reese's Big Cup	
Candy, milk chocolate, 1 package (39 g)	9
Candy, milk chocolate, king size, 1 package (79 g)	18
Peanut butter cups, king size, 1 package (79 g)	18
Reese's Dark	
Peanut butter cups, dark chocolate, 1 package (42 g)	10
Reese's FastBreak	
Candy bar, 1 bar (56 g)	12
Candy bar, king size, ½ bar (50 g)	11
Reese's Hearts	
Peanut butter filled milk chocolate candy, 5 pieces (41 g)	10
Reese's Miniatures	
Milk chocolate peanut butter cups, 5 pieces (44 g)	10
Milk chocolate peanut butter cups, 5 pieces (44 g)	10
Peanut butter cups, 5 pieces (39 g)	10
Reese's Minis	
Milk chocolate peanut butter cups, 11 pieces (39 g)	10
Peanut butter cups snack size (17.5 gm), 2 packages (35 g)	9
Reese's Pieces	
Candy, 21 pieces (36 g)	9
Candy, peanut butter, 51 pieces (40 g)	10

	SmartPoints™ value
Candy, peanut butter, in a crunchy shell, 51 pieces (40 g)	10
Candy, peanut butter, pastel eggs, 12 pieces (39 g)	10
Candy, peanut butter, snack size treats, 3 pouches (42 g)	11
Peanut butter eggs, pastel, 12 pieces (37.78 g)	10
Peanut butter, candies, 1 package (43 g)	11
Reese's Sticks	
Candy bar, king size, ½ package (42 g)	10
Ritter Sport	
Alpine milk chocolate 30% cocoa, 6 pieces (38 g)	10
Dark chocolate with marzipan, 6 pieces (38 g)	9
Dark chocolate with whole hazelnuts, 6 pieces (38 g)	9
Milk chocolate with butter biscuit, 6 pieces (38 g)	10
Milk chocolate with whole hazelnuts, 6 pieces (38 g)	9
Rolo	
Chewy caramels in milk chocolate, 7 pieces (42 g)	10
Rolo Mini	
Chewy caramels, unwrapped, in milk chocolate, 11 pieces (39 g)	10
Russell Stover	
Assorted chocolates, the gift box, 3 pieces (46.6 g)	11
Candies, cake assortment, 4 pieces (57 g)	14
Candies, fine chocolate, assorted sugar free, 3 pieces (46.8 g)	7
Candies, peanut butter egg, 1 piece (28 g)	7
Caramel egg, 1 piece (28 g)	7
Caramel heart, 1 piece (35 g)	8
Caramel santa, 1 piece (35 g)	8

Caramel, in fine milk chocolate, 3 pieces (42 g)	10
Chocolate candies, fine, sugar free, pecan delights, 2 pieces (47 g)	9
Chocolate candy miniatures covered with chocolate candy, sugar free, 5 pieces (37.78 g)	8
Chocolate covered nuts, 3 pieces (40.57 g)	9
Chocolates, all milk, 2 pieces (33.08 g)	8
Chocolates, assorted creams, 3 pieces (47 g)	11
Chocolates, fine, nut, chewy & crisp centers, 2 pieces (33 g)	8
Chocolates, fine, pecan delight, 2 pieces (52 g)	13
Coconut dreams, sugar free, 2 pieces (28 g)	4
Coconut miniatures covered with chocolate candy, sugar free, 5 pieces (37.78 g)	8
Coconut nest, 1 piece (28 g)	9
Coconut, in fine dark chocolate, 3 pieces (43 g)	10
Cream egg, coconut, 1 piece (28 g)	6
Cream egg, maple, 1 piece (28 g)	6
Cream egg, strawberry, 1 piece (28 g)	5
Cream egg, vanilla, 1 piece (28 g)	6
Fine assorted chocolates, 2 pieces (33 g)	8
Fine chocolates, all dark, 2 pieces (33 g)	8
Fine chocolates, all milk, 2 pieces (33 g)	8
Marshmallow & caramel egg, 1 piece (28 g)	6
Marshmallow egg, dark chocolate, 1 piece (28 g)	5
Marshmallow egg, milk chocolate, 1 piece (28 g)	5

Marshmallow heart, dark chocolate, 1 piece (28 g)	5
Marshmallow heart, milk chocolate, 1 bar (28 g)	5
Mint patties, covered with chocolate candy, sugar free, 2 pieces (28 g)	5
Peanut butter cups, sugar free, 2 pieces (34 g)	6
Pecan delights, pecans & caramel covered in milk chocolate, 2 pieces (28 g)	5
Pecan delights, sugar free, 2 pieces (47.33 g)	8
Premium assortment fine chocolates, 3 pieces (47 g)	11
Truffle egg, 1 piece (28 g)	7
Truffles, 3 pieces (48.57 g)	12
Whip egg, raspberry, 1 piece (28 g)	6
Russell Stover Sugar Free	
Assorted candies, 3 pieces (39.6 g)	6
Pecan delights, 4 pieces (57 g)	10
Toffee squares, 2 pieces (28 g)	4
Safeway Select	
Walnuts, covered in dark chocolate, ¼ cup	9
Seattle Chocolates	
Truffles, dark chocolate, 4 pieces (40.57 g)	11
See's Candies	
Almond clusters, 3 pieces (37.83 g)	9
Chocolates, assorted, 2 pieces (32.73 g)	8
Nuts & chews, 3 pieces (44.43 g)	10
Sheila G's	
Brownie brittle, mint chocolate chip, 1 oz	6

Desserts, Cakes, Candy & Cookies

SmartPoints™ value

Simply Lite

Dark chocolate, 50% cacao, 1 serving (25 g)	4

Sixlets

Candy, 1 package (49 g)	13
Candy coated chocolate flavored candy, 1 tube (7 g)	2

Skinny Cow

Candy bar, heavenly crisp, milk chocolate flavor, 1 bar (22 g)	5
Candy bar, peanut butter flavor, heavenly crisp, 1 bar (22 g)	5
Candy, dreamy clusters, milk chocolate, 1 pouch (28.3 g)	6
Dark chocolate blissful truffle candy bar, 1 bar (22 g)	6
Dreamy clusters candy, milk chocolate, 1 pouch (28 g)	6
Milk chocolate blissful truffle candy bar, 1 bar (22 g)	7
Mochaccino candy bar, 1 bar (47 g)	7
Peanut butter and chocolate candy bar, 1 bar (22 g)	5

Skinny Cow Dreamy Clusters

Dark chocolate candy, 1 pouch (28 g)	6

Skinny Cow Heavenly Crisp

Chocolate raspberry crème candy bar, 1 bar (22 g)	5

Skor

Candy bar, 1 bar (39 g)	11

Snack Factory

Pretzel crisps, dark chocolate & peppermint, 4 crackers (28 g)	6

SnackWell's

Fudge pretzels, 1 pack (22 g)	5

Snak Club

Tootsie roll, midgees, snack size, 6 midgees (40 g)	7

SmartPoints™ value

Snickers

Bite size milk chocolate candy bars, ½ pack (40 g)	9
Candy bar, fun size, 2 bars (34 g)	7
Candy bars (2 to go), 1 bar (47 g)	10
Candy bars, almond, 1 bar (46 g)	10
Candy bars, miniatures, Christmas, 4 pieces (36.86 g)	8
Candy bars, peanut butter squared, 2 bars (50.5 g)	12
Chocolate egg, 1 egg	8
Minis, 4 pieces (36 g)	8
Minis (variety pack), 4 pieces (38 g)	9
Nutcracker, 1 bar (31.2 g)	8
Slice n' share, snickers bar, 1" slice	11
Variety mix, fun size, 1 bar (26 g)	6

Snickers 100 Calorie Bars

Chocolate bars, 1 bar (21 g)	5

Snickers Bites

Candy bar, sharing size, ½ pack (40 g)	9
Candy bar, unwrapped, 8 pieces (41 g)	9
Candy bar, unwrapped, sharing size, ½ package (40 g)	9

Snickers Minis

Caramel & peanut chocolates, 4 pieces (36 g)	8

Snickers Snack Time Pack

Fun size chocolate bars, 2 bars (32 g)	7

Specially Selected

Dark chocolate covered sea salt caramels, 2 pieces (38 g)	7

Streit's

Almonds, chocolate covered, 9 pieces (40 g)	10

Sun-Maid

Chocolate covered raisins, milk chocolate, 30 pieces (37.78 g)	9
Yogurt raisins, dark chocolate, ¼ cup	6

Sweet's

Orange sticks, 5 sticks (42 g)	8

Symphony

Milk chocolate, almonds & toffee chips, 5 blocks (38 g)	10

Take 5

Candy bar, 1 package (42 g)	9

Terry's

Dark chocolate orange, orange flavored, 5 pieces (43.75 g)	12
Milk chocolate orange, orange flavored, 5 pieces (43.75 g)	12

Theo

Dark chocolate, salted almond, ½ bar (42 g)	10

Theo Organic Fair Trade

Coconut 70 % dark chocolate, ½ bar (42 g)	10

Toblerone

Chocolates, assorted, 5 chocolates (44 g)	12
Dark chocolate, Swiss, with honey and almond nougat, ⅓ bar (33 g)	8
Milk chocolate, Swiss, crunchy salted almond, ⅓ bar (33 g)	9
Milk chocolate, Swiss, with honey and almond nougat, 1 bar (35 g)	9
Toblerone bars, 1 bar (35 g)	10

Tootsie Midgees

Candy, 6 pieces (40 g)	7

Tootsie Roll

Chocolate flavor candy, 1 piece (14 g)	2
Tootsie miniature pops, 3 (15 g)	3

Tootsie Roll Midgees

Chewy candies, 6 pieces (40 g)	7
Chocolate candy, 6 pieces (40 g)	7

Trader Joe's

100 calories 70% dark chocolate bars, 1 bar (18 g)	5
Chocolate coconut almonds, ⅓ cup	10
Chocolate covered sea salt butterscotch caramels, 11 pieces (40 g)	10
Chocolate fondue, 2 Tbsp	12
Crispy milk chocolate, 1 bar (40 g)	11
Dark chocolate almonds, ¼ cup	10
Dark chocolate bar, 1 bar (50 g)	14
Dark chocolate caramel wedges 70% cacao, 2 pieces (13 g)	3
Dark chocolate covered blueberries, ¼ cup	9
Dark chocolate covered caramels, 2 pieces (42 g)	9
Dark chocolate covered espresso beans, ¼ cup	8
Dark chocolate covered powerberries, ¼ cup	9
Dark chocolate honey mints, 3 pieces (33 g)	7
Dark chocolate peanut butter and salted caramel truffles, 3 pieces (36 g)	9
Dark chocolate peanut butter cups, 3 pieces (36 g)	9
Dark chocolate sea salt caramels, 3 pieces (45 g)	12
Dark chocolate speculoos cookie butter cups, 3 pieces (34 g)	9
Fireworks chocolate bar, ½ bar (40 g)	10
Milk chocolate jumbles, 3 pieces (36 g)	7

Desserts, Cakes, Candy & Cookies

SmartPoints™ value

	SmartPoints™ value
Moist chewy coconut bonbons, 2 pieces (32 g)	9
Organic dark chocolate bar, 12 squares (40 g)	11
Organic dark chocolate truffle, 5 sections (42 g)	12
Premium milk & dark chocolate covered almonds, ¼ cup	9
Sea salt & turbinado sugar dark chocolate almonds, 13 pieces (40 g)	9
The dark chocolate lover's chocolate bar, ⅔ bar (40 g)	11

Turin Bailey's

The original Irish cream chocolates, 3 pieces (30 g)	7

Twix

Caramel milk chocolate cookie bars, 2 cookies (51 g)	12
Cookie bars, caramel milk chocolate, gingerbread, 1 bar (16 g)	4
Cookie bars, fun size, 1 cookie (16 g)	4
Milk chocolate egg, 1 (30 g)	8

Twix 4 To Go

Caramel milk chocolate cookie bars, 1 cookie (22 g)	5

Twix Bites

Unwrapped chocolate covered cookie with caramel, ⅓ pack (27 g)	6
Unwrapped milk chocolate candy, 5 pieces (28 g)	7

Twix Minis

Caramel and milk chocolate cookie bars, 3 pieces (30 g)	7
Cookie bars, caramel, milk chocolate, 3 pieces (29.64 g)	8

Virginia Diner

Peanut butter buckeyes, gourmet, 2 pieces (35 g)	8
Pecans, chocolate covered, gourmet, 10 pieces (44.5 g)	9

Whatchamacallit

Candy bar, 1 bar (45 g)	12
Candy bar, king size, 1 bar (73 g)	19

Whitman's

Chocolate mousse dark chocolates, 3 pieces (40 g)	8

Whitman's Sampler

Assorted chocolates, 3 pieces (35 g)	8
Assorted sugar free candies, 3 pieces (43 g)	7

Whoppers

Malted milk balls, the original, 18 pieces (40.29 g)	11
Malted milk candy, robin eggs, 8 pieces (40.43 g)	10
Mini robin eggs, 24 pieces (37.78 g)	10

Whoppers Robin Eggs

Candy, malted milk, mini, 24 pieces (41 g)	11

York

Dark chocolate covered peppermint patties eggs, 3 pieces (41 g)	8
Peppermint patties hearts, dark chocolate covered, 3 patties (41 g)	8
Peppermint patties, dark chocolate covered, 3 patties (39 g)	8
Peppermint patties, pumpkin shaped, 3 pieces (41 g)	8
Peppermint patties, valentine, 3 pieces (37.7 g)	8

York Eggs

Dark chocolate peppermint patties, 3 pieces (41 g)	8

York Minis

Dark chocolate covered peppermint patties unwrapped, 10 pieces (40 g)	8
Dark chocolate covered unwrapped peppermint patties king size, 1 package (70 g)	14

Desserts, Cakes, Candy & Cookies

Zachary

Chocolate covered marshmallow eggs, 4 pieces (47 g)	9

Zachary

Thin mints, 5 pieces (39 g)	9

Candy, Non-Chocolate

Airheads

Candy, cherry, 1 bar (15.6 g)	3

Altoids

Curiously strong peppermints, 3 pieces (2 g)	1
Mints, cinnamon, 3 pieces (2 g)	1
Mints, peppermint, 3 pieces (2 g)	1
Mints, wintergreen, 3 pieces (2 g)	1

Bit O Honey

Taffy flavored candy bites with real honey, 6 pieces (40 g)	7

Bobs

Candy balls, peppermint, 3 pieces (14 g)	2
Candy canes, peppermint, 1 piece (14 g)	2

Bobs Sweet Stripes

Candy, mint, soft, 3 pieces (15 g)	4
Candy, peppermint, soft mint, 3 pieces (15 g)	4
Mint candy, soft, 3 pieces (15 g)	4
Soft mint candy, 3 pieces (15 g)	4

Brach's

Chicks & rabbits, 6 pieces (43 g)	7
Christmas nougats, peppermint, 5 pieces (44 g)	8
Conversation heart, small, treat packs, 1 packet (14.2 g)	4
Conversation hearts candy, small, 12 pieces (15 g)	4
Conversation hearts, large, 5 pieces (15.72 g)	4
Conversation hearts, small, 12 pieces (15 g)	4
Jelly beans, 1 each (51 g)	10

Jelly bird eggs, classic, 14 pieces (41 g)	8
Jordan almonds, 10 pieces (38.57 g)	9
Original peppermint candy canes, 1 piece (14 g)	3
Star brites, peppermint & spearmint, 3 pieces (15 g)	3
Star brites, peppermint, value bag, 3 pieces (15 g)	3

Brach's Classic

Jelly bird eggs, 14 pieces (41 g)	8

Brach's Milk Maid

Caramels, 4 pieces (36 g)	7

Brach's Orchard Fruit

Jelly beans, 25 pieces (40 g)	8

Brown & Haley

Almond roca, 3 pieces (36 g)	10
Almond roca, buttercrunch toffee, 3 pieces (36 g)	10

Buddy Bears

Gummy bears, 18 pieces (38 g)	6

Campfire Giant Roasters

Marshmallows, 1 piece (28 g)	4

Charms

Blow pop, bubble gum filled, black cherry, 1 pop (18 g)	3
Blow pop, bubble gum filled, what a melon, 1 pop (18 g)	3
Blow pop, flavor zone, 1 pop (16 g)	3
Blow pops, assorted flavors, 1 piece (18.4 g)	4

Clif Shot Bloks

Electrolyte chews, black cherry flavor, 3 pieces (30 g)	4

Coffee Rio

Coffee candy, premium, caramel caffe, 4 pieces (15 g)	3
Original roast premium caramel coffee candy, 4 pieces (15 g)	3

Desserts, Cakes, Candy & Cookies

	SmartPoints™ value
CVS	
Mini candy canes, peppermint flavor, 3 canes (11.76 g)	2
Dots	
Gumdrops, assorted fruit flavored, 11 dots (40 g)	6
Dum Dum	
Dum dum pops, 1 pop (5 g)	1
Everlasting Gobstopper	
Heartbreakers sweets, 8 pieces (15 g)	3
Fannie May	
Pixies, 2 pieces (40 g)	9
Ferrara Pan	
Candy, cinnamon flavored, 20 pieces (17 g)	4
Candy, lemon, 10 pieces (14 g)	3
Candy, red hots, 20 pieces (19 g)	3
Fireball, atomic, 1 piece (9 g)	2
Ferrara Pan Lemon-Head	
Candy, 10 pieces (14 g)	3
Ferrara Pan Lemon-Head & Friends	
Candy, chewy assorted flavors, 26 pieces (40 g)	8
Ferrara Pan Red Hots	
Candy, 18 pieces (15 g)	3
Fluff	
Marshmallow fluff, 2 Tbsp	2
Fun Dip	
Fun dip, 1 packet (14 g)	3
Ghirardelli Chocolate	
Chocolate, intense dark, sea salt soiree, 3 sections (38 g)	9
Gobstopper	
Everlasting jawbreaker, 9 pieces (15 g)	4
Jawbreakers, everlasting, 9 pieces (15 g)	4
Good & Plenty	
Candy, licorice, 1 box (51 g)	8
Licorice candy, 33 pieces (40 g)	7

	SmartPoints™ value
Great Value	
Mini marshmallows, ⅔ cup	5
Starlight mints, peppermint, 3 pieces (15 g)	3
Halls Advanced Vapor Action	
Cough supressant, cherry, 1 drop (5 g)	0
Haribo	
Gummi candy, peaches, 4 pieces (40 g)	6
Haribo Gold-Bears	
Gummi candy, juicy, 16 pieces (38 g)	6
Gummi candy, the original, minis, 4 minibags (40 g)	7
Hawaiian Host	
Caramacs, maui, the original, 3 pieces (42 g)	10
Hershey's	
Twizzlers twist, 4 packages (36 g)	5
Hershey's Payday	
Candy bar, peanut caramel, 1 bar (328 g)	4
Hickory Farms	
Mints, melt away, mini, 62 pieces (40 g)	12
Hot Tamales	
Candies, chewy, cinnamon flavored, 20 pieces (40 g)	7
Candies, flavored chewy, fierce cinnamon, 20 pieces (40 g)	7
Candy, hot tamales, chewy cinnamon flavored candies, 20 pieces (37.67 g)	7
Jelly Belly	
Gourmet jelly bean, 49 flavors, 35 pieces (39.43 g)	8
Gourmet jelly beans, 40 flavors, 35 pieces (39.33 g)	8
Jelly bean, 35 pieces (40 g)	8
Jelly beans, 10 individual flavors, 35 pieces (40 g)	8

Jelly beans, 20 assorted flavors, 35 pieces (36.8 g)	8
Jelly beans, jelly belly ice cream parlor mix, 1 package (42 g)	8
Jelly belly, 50 individual flavors, 35 pieces (39.67 g)	8
Sugar free assorted flavors jelly beans, 35 pieces (40 g)	3

Jolly Rancher

Awesome reds hard candy, 3 pieces (18 g)	3
Crunch 'n chew, original flavors, 3 pieces (15 g)	3
Hard candy, apple, 3 pieces (18 g)	3
Hard candy, assorted original, 3 pieces (45 g)	2
Hard candy, cherry, 3 pieces (18.83 g)	3
Hard candy, cinnamon fire, 3 pieces (17 g)	3
Hard candy, original flavors, family bag, 3 pieces (18 g)	3
Jelly beans, fruit smoothie flavors, 30 pieces (40 g)	7
Watermelon hard candy, 3 pieces (11.3 g)	4

Jolly Rancher Bites

Chewy candy, soft, watermelon & green apple, 15 pieces (41 g)	5

Jujubes

Candy, 52 pieces (40.89 g)	6

Jujyfruits

Chewy fruity candy, 15 pieces (40 g)	6

Just Born

Jelly beans, original fruit flavored, 23 pieces (40 g)	8

Kirkland Signature Jelly Belly

Gourmet jelly beans, 35 pieces (40 g)	8

Kraft

Caramels, traditional, 5 pieces (41 g)	8

Kraft Jet-Puffed

Mallow bits, vanilla, 2 Tbsp	1
Marshmallow creme, 2 Tbsp	2
Marshmallows, jumbo mallows, 1 piece (26 g)	5
Marshmallows, miniature, ⅔ cup	5
Marshmallows, peppermint mallows, peppermint mini, ⅔ cup	5
Miniature marshmallows, ⅔ cup	5

Kroger

Fruit snack mix, fruit gummies, 9 pieces (26 g)	5
Marshmallows, mini, ⅔ cup	5
Starlight mints, 3 pieces (15 g)	3

Laffy Taffy

Candy, assorted flavors, 5 pieces (43 g)	9
Laffy taffy, mystery swirl, 1 package (23.1 g)	4
Laffy taffy, sour apple, 1 rope (22.9 g)	4

Lancaster

Caramel, soft cremes, 7 pieces (42 g)	10
Soft cremes, vanilla and caramel, 7 pieces (42 g)	9
Soft cremes, vanilla and raspberry, 7 pieces (42 g)	9

Life Savers

Candy, 5 flavors, 10 pieces (40 g)	7
Candy, pepomint, 3 mints	1
Candy, wintogreen, 4 mints	4
Fruit slices candy, five flavor, 9 pieces (37.83 g)	7
Hard candy, 5 flavors, 2 pieces (5 g)	1
Hard candy, butter rum, 2 pieces (5 g)	1
Hard candy, sugar free, wint o green, 4 mints	1
Mints, orange, 4 pieces (15 g)	4
Mints, pep o mint, 3 mints	1

Desserts, Cakes, Candy & Cookies

Desserts, Cakes, Candy & Cookies

	SmartPoints™ value
Mints, spear o mint, 3 pieces (5 g)	1
Mints, sugar free, pep o mint, 4 pieces (15 g)	1
Mints, wint o green, 4 pieces (15 g)	4
Mints, wint o green, big value, 4 mints	4
Life Savers Gummies	
Candy, tangy fruits, 1 package (56 g)	9
Five flavours gums, 10 pieces (40 g)	7
Luden's	
Wild cherry throat drops, 1 piece (3.5 g)	1
Mamba	
Fruit chews, 6 pieces (25 g)	5
Mary Jane	
Candy, original with peanuts, 1 piece (8 g)	1
Mentos	
Chewy mint, 1 piece (3 g)	1
Chewy mint, strawberry, 1 piece (64 g)	1
Chewy mints, rainbow, 1 piece (3 g)	1
Mints, chewy, fruit, 1 piece (3 g)	1
Mike and Ike	
Candies, chewy, assorted fruit flavored, original fruits, 23 pieces (40 g)	7
Candies, chewy, berry flavored, berry blast, 23 pieces (40 g)	7
Necco	
Wafers, assorted, 1 roll (57 g)	13
Nerds	
Candy, 1 Tbsp	4
Candy & card kit, 1 box (13 g)	3
Candy, rainbow, 1 Tbsp	4
Rope candy, rainbow, 1 rope (26 g)	5

	SmartPoints™ value
Nips	
Hard candy, mocha, 2 pieces (14 g)	3
Hard candy, rich & creamy, butter rum, 2 pieces (14.16 g)	3
Hard candy, rich & creamy, caramel, sugar free, 2 pieces (14.16 g)	2
Hard candy, rich & creamy, chocolate parfait, 2 pieces (14.16 g)	3
Hard candy, rich & creamy, coffee, 2 pieces (14 g)	2
Hard candy, rich & creamy, peanut butter parfait, 2 pieces (14 g)	3
Rich and creamy caramel hard candy, 2 pieces (14 g)	3
Ocean Spray Craisins	
Greek yogurt dried cranberries, ¼ cup	8
Panda	
Licorice, raspberry, 15 pieces (40 g)	6
Licorice, soft, 15 pieces (40 g)	6
Peeps	
Marshmallow bunnies, pink, 4 bunnies (32 g)	6
Marshmallow bunnies, yellow, 4 bunnies (31.67 g)	7
Marshmallow hearts, 2 hearts (32 g)	6
Marshmallow minions, 3 pieces (32 g)	6
Marshmallow, purple bunnies, 4 bunnies (32 g)	6
Marshmallows, candy cane flavored chicks, 5 pieces (42 g)	8
Marshmallows, party cake flavored, 5 (42 g)	8

Red Vines

Black licorice twists, 4 vines (35.25 g)	6
Original red licorice twists, 6 twists (40 g)	6
Strawberry licorice, sugar free, 7 twists (40 g)	3

Reed's

Ginger candy, chews, 1 piece (6 g)	1

Ricola

Natural cherry-honey herb throat drops, 1 drop (1 g)	1

Riesen

Caramel, chewy, chocolate covered, 4 pieces (36 g)	8

Runts

Candy, 12 pieces (15 g)	3

Russell Stover

Jelly beans, pectin, 19 pieces (40 g)	8

Sanders

Sea salt caramels, 1 serving (40 g)	3

Sather's

Atomic fire ball, 3 pieces (17 g)	4
Candy, cherry sours, 12 pieces (40 g)	8
Candy, cinnamon discs, 3 pieces (18 g)	4
Candy, dum-dums, original pops, 2 pops (13 g)	3
Candy, orange slices, 3 pieces (46 g)	8
Candy, root beer barrels, 3 pieces (18 g)	3
Candy, tootsie roll midgees, 6 pieces (40 g)	7
Cinnamon bears, 4 pieces (36 g)	6

See's Candies

Chocolate butter eggs, 2 eggs	11
Lollypops, gourmet, assorted, 1 lollipop (20 g)	4
Cherry sour balls, 10 pieces (42.5 g)	8

Skinny Cow

Divine filled chocolates candy, caramel, 1 pouch (28.3 g)	7

Skinny Cow Divine Filled Chocolates

Caramel, 1 pouch (28 g)	7
Peanut butter creme, 1 pouch (28 g)	7

Skittles

Bite size candies, desserts, 2 oz package, 1 package (57 g)	13
Bite size candies, original, ¼ cup	10
Bite size candies, sour, ¼ cup	9
Wild berry bite size candies, ¼ cup	10

Skittles Desserts

Bite size candies, ¼ cup	9

Skittles Fun Size

Original skittles, 3 packages (46 g)	10

Skittles Original

Bite sized candies, ¼ cup	9
Original bite size candies, 1 package (45 g)	10

Smarties

Candy rolls, assorted flavors, 1 roll (7.5 g)	2

Sour Patch

Candy, soft & chewy, watermelon, 16 pieces (40 g)	8
Soft and chewy candy, 16 pieces (40 g)	8
Sour patch fruits, 16 pieces (37.83 g)	8

Sour Patch Kids

Candy, soft & chewy, 16 pieces (40 g)	7
Candy, soft & chewy, extreme sour, 1 bag (51 g)	10

Starburst

Favereds fruit chews, 8 pieces (40 g)	8
Fruit chews, 8 pieces (40 g)	8
Fruit chews, minis, original, ¼ cup	8

Desserts, Cakes, Candy & Cookies

Desserts, Cakes, Candy & Cookies

	SmartPoints™ value
Hard candy, original fruits, 3 pieces (14.34 g)	3
Hard candy, tropical fruits, 3 pieces (12.97 g)	3
Jellybeans, sour, ¼ cup	8
Red fruits jellybeans, ¼ cup	8
Starburst FaveReds	
Fruit chews, 8 pieces (40 g)	8
Starburst Minis	
Fruit chews, unwrapped!, favereds, ¼ cup	8
Sugar Babies	
Candy coated milk caramels, 30 pieces (42.5 g)	9
Sunkist	
Fruit gems soft fruit candy, 4 pieces (40 g)	7
Sun-Maid	
Yogurt raisins, mini-snacks, vanilla, 1 box (14 g)	3
Yogurt raisins, vanilla, 1 box (28 g)	7
Sun-Maid Mini-Snacks	
Vanilla yogurt raisins, 1 box (14 g)	4
Swedish Fish	
Candy, soft & chewy, red, 7 pieces (42 g)	8
SweeTarts	
Candy, hearts, 14 pieces (14.15 g)	3
Candy, tangy, 23 pieces (15 g)	3
Jelly beans, tart fruit flavors, 27 pieces (40 g)	8
Tangy candy, 8 pieces (15 g)	3
Tangy candy, chicks, ducks & bunnies, 4 pieces (14 g)	3
Sweethearts	
Confectionary candies, 1 box (28 g)	7
Sweethearts candies, 40 pieces (40 g)	9
Sweet's	
Salt water taffy, 7 pieces (42 g)	8

	SmartPoints™ value
The Ginger People	
Ginger chews, original, 2 pieces (12 g)	2
Gin-gins, double strength, 3 pieces (8.4 g)	2
The Ginger People Ginger Chews	
Sweet hot ginger candy, 2 pieces (12 g)	2
Theo	
Dark chocolate, orange, ½ bar (42 g)	10
Tic Tac	
Candy, orange mints, 1 piece (108 g)	0
Tootsie	
Fruit rolls, assorted fruity flavored, 6 pieces (40 g)	7
Tootsie Midgees	
Vanilla flavored candy, 6 pieces (40 g)	7
Tootsie Roll	
Candy, dots, 12 (43 g)	7
Frooties, 13 pieces (40 g)	7
Mini chews, 30 pieces (41 g)	8
Pops, assorted, 1 pop (17 g)	3
Tootsie fruit rolls, 6 pieces (40 g)	7
Tootsie pop lollipops assortment, 1 (17 g)	3
Tootsie Roll Midgees	
Limited edition vanilla candies, 6 pieces (40 g)	7
Trader Jacque's	
Fleur de sel caramels, 4 pieces (40 g)	8
Trader Joe's	
English toffee with nuts, 3 pieces (36 g)	10
Gummy bears, 19 pieces (42 g)	7
Salt water taffy, 7 pieces (42 g)	8

Trolli

Gummi candy, sour brite crawlers, 12 pieces (40 g)	6
Sour brite crawlers gummi candy, 12 pieces (40 g)	6

Twizzlers

Bites, cherry, 18 pieces (39.6 g)	6
Candy, pull 'n' peel, twizted strawberry blast, snack size, 3 pieces (37 g)	5
Nibs, cherry, 27 pieces (39.6 g)	6
Nibs, licorice bits, 29 pieces (39 g)	6
Strawberry twists, 6 pieces (42 g)	7
Twists, chocolate, 4 pieces (45 g)	7
Twists, licorice, 1 package (70 g)	10
Twizzlers pull-n-peel, wild berry, 1 piece (36.33 g)	5

Twizzlers Bites

Cherry bites, 17 pieces (40 g)	6
Filled fruit twists, strawberry, 22 pieces (40 g)	7
Mixed berry flavored candy, 18 pieces (40 g)	7

Twizzlers Pull 'n' Peel

Candy, cherry, big bag, 1 piece (33 g)	5
Candy, cherry, family bag, 1 piece (33 g)	5

Twizzlers To Go

Twizzlers, cherry bites, 1 package (77 g)	12

Vitafusion

Multivites gummy vitamins, 2 gummies (5 g)	1

Walgreen's

Hard candy, peppermint, 3 pieces (14 g)	1
Root beer barrels, 3 pieces (17 g)	3

Wegman's

Swedish fish, 19 pieces (38.64 g)	8

Werther's

Classic candy, 3 pieces (14.29 g)	3
Hard candies, caramel apple, sugar free, 5 pieces (16 g)	1
Hard candies, creamy caramel filled, 2 pieces (12 g)	3
Hard candies, minis, sugar free, 5 pieces (16 g)	1

Werther's Original

Hard candies, 3 pieces (16 g)	4
Hard candies, caramel coffee, 4 pieces (16 g)	4

Wonka

Bottle caps candy, 13 pieces (15 g)	3
Candy, chewy, sweetarts shockers, 9 pieces (16 g)	3
Candy, sweetarts, giant chewy, 1 piece (11 g)	2
Laffy taffy, cherry, 1 bar (42.5 g)	8

Wonka Laffy Taffy

Strawberry and banana flavored candy, 4 pieces (39 g)	7

Wonka Nerds

Bumpy jelly beans, 23 pieces (40 g)	8

Wonka SweeTarts

Mini chewy tangy candy, 23 pieces (15 g)	3
Tangy candy, 13 pieces (15 g)	3
Tangy candy hearts, 11 pieces (15 g)	3

York

Mints, 3 mints	1

Zero

Candy bar, 1 bar (52 g)	12

Desserts, Cakes, Candy & Cookies

Cheesecake

Desserts by David Glass

| Cheese cake, the ultimate New York, 1 serving (61 g) | 9 |

Duncan Hines Decadent

| Strawberry cheesecake cupcake cake and frosting mix, 1 serving (74 g) | 10 |

Great Value

| Cheesecake, chocolate, 1 slice (82 g) | 12 |

Jell-O

| Cheesecake snacks, original, strawberry cheesecake, 1 container (99 g) | 7 |

Jell-O No Bake

| Dessert, strawberry cheesecake, 1 serving (69 g) | 10 |

Jell-O Temptations

| Cheesecake snacks, strawberry cheesecake, 1 container (100 g) | 7 |

Sara Lee Classic

| Original cream cheesecake smooth and creamy, ¼ cheesecake (121 g) | 15 |
| Cream strawberry cheesecake, ¼ cheesecake (135 g) | 15 |

The Cheesecake Factory

| Original cheesecake, 1 piece (151 g) | 24 |

Cookie & Cookie Mixes

Annie's

| Bunny grahams, honey, 31 cookies (30 g) | 5 |

Annie's Gluten Free

| Bunny cookies, cocoa & vanilla, 27 cookies (30 g) | 5 |
| Snickerdoodle cinnamon sugar bunny cookies, 27 cookies (30 g) | 5 |

Annie's Organic

| Honey grahams, 2 sheets (31 g) | 5 |

Annie's Totally Natural

| Bunny grahams, chocolate, 28 cookies (30.43 g) | 5 |
| Bunny grahams, friends, 31 cookies (28 g) | 5 |

Archway Classics

Crispy windmill cookies, 2 cookies (42 g)	8
Frosty lemon soft cookie, 1 cookie (26 g)	5
Soft iced molasses cookies, 3 cookies (33 g)	5

Austin

| Animal crackers, 16 pieces (33 g) | 5 |

Back To Nature

Cookies, chocolate chunk, 2 cookies (26 g)	5
Cookies, classic creme, 2 cookies (26 g)	6
Cookies, fudge mint, 4 cookies (31 g)	7
Cookies, peanut butter creme, 2 cookies (26 g)	5

Bakery Fresh

| Cookies, oatmeal raisin, 1 cookie (25.2 g) | 4 |

Barbara's Snackimals

| Animal cookies, chocolate chip, 10 cookies (30 g) | 5 |

Barry's Bakery

| French twists, original, 2 twists (15 g) | 2 |

BelVita Bites

| Breakfast biscuits, mini, chocolate, 1 pack (50 g) | 8 |
| Breakfast biscuits, mini, mixed berry, 1 pack (50 g) | 8 |

Benton's Cookies

| Cinnamon graham crackers, 8 crackers (35 g) | 6 |
| Vanilla wafers, 9 cookies (32 g) | 6 |

Best Express Foods

Traditional aussie bites biscuits with omega-3, 1 cookie (27 g)	5

Betty Crocker

Cookie mix, chocolate chip, 3 Tbsp mix	7
Cookie mix, peanut butter, 4 Tbsp mix	6
Cookie mix, salted caramel, 3 Tbsp	5

Betty Lou's

Nut butter balls, peanut butter, 1 ball (48 g)	6

Carr's

English tea cookies, ginger lemon cremes, 2 pieces (28.57 g)	7

Chips Ahoy!

Chocolate chip cookies, 3 cookies (32.36 g)	8
Cookies, chewy, real chocolate chip, family size, 2 cookies (31 g)	6
Cookies, chocolate chip, 1 cookie (15.74 g)	3
Cookies, chocolate chip, original, 3 cookies (33 g)	7
Cookies, chocolate chip, original, 3 cookies (33.23 g)	7
Cookies, chunky, 1 cookie (16 g)	3
Cookies, mini, 1 package (28 g)	6
Cookies, real chocolate chip, 3 cookies (34 g)	7
Cookies, real chocolate chip, candy blasts, 1 cookie (17 g)	4
Cookies, real chocolate chip, made with Reese's peanut butter cups, 2 cookies (30 g)	7
Cookies, real chocolate chip, mini, go-paks!, 14 cookies (30 g)	6
Cookies, real chocolate chip, original, 3 cookies (33 g)	7
Cookies, real chocolate chip, original, family size, 3 cookies (33 g)	7

Cookies, real chocolate chunk, chunky, 1 cookie (16 g)	3
Cookies, reduced fat, real chocolate chip, 3 cookies (33 g)	6
Cookies, white fudge chunky, 1 cookie (16 g)	3

Chips Ahoy! 100 Calorie Packs

Cookies, double chocolate chip, chips ahoy!, 1 package (22 g)	4

Chips Ahoy! Chewy

Cookies, chocolate chip, 2 cookies (31 g)	6
Cookies, Reese's, 2 cookies (30 g)	6
Cookies, Reese's peanut butter cups chocolate, 2 cookies (30 g)	6
Cookies, soft, birthday frosting filled, 2 cookies (32 g)	7
Cookies, soft, brownie filled, 1 cookie (18 g)	4
Cookies, soft, oreo cream filled, 2 cookies (32 g)	7
Cookies, soft, fudge filled, choco-fudge, 2 cookies (31 g)	7

Chips Ahoy! Mini

Cookies, chocolate chip, 1 package (28 g)	6

Chips Ahoy! Reduced Fat

Cookies, real chocolate chip, 3 cookies (32.36 g)	6

Chips Deluxe 100 Calorie Right Bites

Cookies, 1 pouch (21 g)	4

Clear Value

Cookies, soft, snicker doodle, 1 cookie (25 g)	4

Creme de Pirouline Artisan Rolled Wafers

Chocolate hazelnut wafers, 2 cookies (28 g)	8

Cybeles

Cookies, vegan & gluten-free, chocolate chip, 2 cookies (28 g)	6

Desserts, Cakes, Candy & Cookies

Desserts, Cakes, Candy & Cookies

	SmartPoints™ value
E.L. Fudge	
Cookies, sandwich, butter, with fudge creme filling, double stuffed, 2 cookies (34 g)	8
Fudge sandwich cookies with fudge creme filling, 2 each (25 g)	5
Sandwich cookies, original, 1 cookie (17.71 g)	4
Emily's	
Graham crackers, milk chocolate covered, 1 cookie (28 g)	7
Enjoy Life	
Cookies, soft baked chew chocolate chip, 2 cookies (28.33 g)	6
Cookies, soft baked double chocolate brownie, 2 cookies (28.33 g)	5
Cookies, soft baked no-oats oatmeal, 2 cookies (28.33 g)	5
Cookies, soft baked snickerdoodle, 2 cookies (28.33 g)	6
Entenmann's	
Cookies, chocolate chip, 3 cookies (28.25 g)	6
Cookies, black & white, 1 cookie (31.2 g)	6
Famous Amos	
Bite size chocolate chip cookies (snack packs), 1 pouch (34 g)	7
Chocolate chip cookies, 4 each (30.2 g)	6
Cookies, bite size, chocolate chip, 4 cookies (29 g)	6
Cookies, chocolate chip cookies, 4 cookies (35.25 g)	6
Fiber One	
Chocolate chip crunchy cookies, 1 cookie (26 g)	5
Double chocolate soft-baked cookie, 1 cookie (31 g)	5
Oatmeal raisin soft baked cookie, 1 cookie (31 g)	5
Soft baked chocolate chunk cookie, 1 cookie (31 g)	5

	SmartPoints™ value
Fig Newtons	
Bars, fig, 1 bar (36.88 g)	6
Cookies, 2 cookies (30.46 g)	5
Cookies, fruit chewy, 2 cookies (32.29 g)	5
Fruit chewy cookies, 1 cookie (30 g)	4
Fit & Active	
Raisin apple fruit crisps, 3 crisps (44 g)	7
S'mores drizzled mini crisps, 1 package (21 g)	4
Fit & Active 100 Calorie	
Baked chocolate wafer snacks, 1 package (23 g)	4
Franz	
Cookies, molasses, 1 cookie (23.67 g)	4
Fudge Shoppe	
Creme wafers, fudge covered, original, 3 cookies (29 g)	8
Cookies, dark chocolate, 3 cookies (31 g)	7
Gamesa Marias	
Cookies, 8 cookies (29 g)	5
Cookies, 8 cookies (35 g)	5
Giant	
Honey grahams, low fat, honey, 2 whole crackers (26.47 g)	4
Ginger Snaps	
Cookies, 4 cookies (28 g)	5
Ginger snaps, old fashioned, 4 cookies (28.31 g)	5
Girl Scout Cookies	
Caramel delites®, 1 cookie (14 g)	3
Cranberry citrus crisps, 1 serving (34 g)	6
Do-si-dos®, 1 cookie (11.33 g)	2
Lemonades, 1 cookie (15.5 g)	3
Peanut butter patties®, 1 cookie (12.5 g)	3

	SmartPoints™ value
Peanut butter sandwich, 1 cookie (11.67 g)	2
Rah-rah raisins™, 1 serving (25 g)	5
Samoas®, 1 cookie (14.5 g)	3
Savannah smiles, 1 cookie (6 g)	1
Shortbread, 1 cookie (6.5 g)	1
Tagalongs®, 1 cookie (12.5 g)	3
Thanks-a-lot, 1 cookie (15.5 g)	4
Thin mints®, 2 cookies (16 g)	4
Toffee-tastic™ (gluten free), 1 serving (28 g)	6
Trefoils™, 1 cookie (6.4 g)	1
Trios (gluten free), 1 serving (34 g)	7

Glutino Gluten Free

Wafer cookies, lemon, 3 wafer (33.33 g)	7

Glutino Gluten Free Dream Cookies

Cookies, chocolate chip, 4 cookies (27.22 g)	6
Cookies, chocolate vanilla creme, 2 cookies (28.57 g)	6
Cookies, vanilla creme, 2 cookies (28.57 g)	6

Goldfish

Baked graham snacks, strawberry shortcake, 35 pieces (30 g)	5
Graham snacks, baked, s'mores adventures, 54 pieces (31.17 g)	5
S'mores baked graham snacks, 52 pieces (30 g)	6

Goldfish Flavor Blasted

Grahams, vanilla cupcake, 35 pieces (31.17 g)	5
Grahams, xtra chocolatey, 35 pieces (31.17 g)	6

Goldfish Grahams

Vanilla cupcake baked graham snacks, 35 pieces (30 g)	5

Gourmet Center Biscoff

Cookie, the airline, snack pack, 4 biscuits	6

Goya

	SmartPoints™ value
Maria cookies, 5 cookies (33 g)	5

Grandma's

Chocolate brownie cookie, 1 cookie (41 g)	8
Cookies, sandwich, mini, vanilla, 9 cookies (31 g)	6
Peanut butter cookies, 5 cookies (39 g)	8

Grandma's Homestyle

Chocolate chip cookie, 1 cookie (41 g)	8
Chocolate chip soft cookie, 1 cookie (35 g)	7
Oatmeal raisin cookies, 1 cookie (41 g)	8
Peanut butter cookies, 1 cookie (40 g)	7

Grandma's Mini

Vanilla sandwich creme cookies, 1 package (48 g)	10

Grasshopper

Cookies, fudge mint, 4 cookies (29 g)	7

Great Value

Cinnamon grahams, 2 whole crackers (31.38 g)	5
Cookie cakes, chocolate, devil's food, 1 cookie (15.92 g)	2
Ginger snaps cookies, 4 cookies (28 g)	5
Honey grahams, 2 crackers (31.38 g)	5

Handi Snacks

Snack packs, oreo, 1 package (28 g)	6

HannahMax Baking

Cookie chips, cinnamon sugar, crunchy, 5 cookies (28 g)	6
Cookie chips, dark chocolate chocolate chip, crunchy, 5 cookies (28 g)	6
Cookie chips, original, crunchy, 5 cookies (28 g)	6

Desserts, Cakes, Candy & Cookies

SmartPoints™ value

SmartPoints™ value

Desserts, Cakes, Candy & Cookies

H-E-B The Big Chip

Cookies, chocolate chip, 2 cookies (33 g)	8

Homestyle

Macaroons, coconut, two-bite, chocolate dipped, 2 macaroons (33 g)	9

Honey Bunches

Chocolate chip breakfast biscuits, 4 biscuits	9
Honey roasted breakfast biscuits, 4 biscuits	8

Honey Maid

Chocolate grahams, 8 crackers (31 g)	5
Cinnamon grahams, 8 crackers (31 g)	5
Crackers, grahamfuls, peanut butter & chocolate filled, 1 package (25 g)	5
Despicable me graham crackers, 1 pack (28 g)	4
Graham crackers, squares, 4 squares (27 g)	5
Graham squares, 4 squares (30 g)	5
Grahamfuls, s'mores, 1 pack (25 g)	5
Grahams, honey, 8 crackers (31 g)	5
Grahams, low fat, honey, 8 crackers (34 g)	5
Honey graham crackers, baked with 100% whole grain, 8 crackers (31.38 g)	5
Honey grahams, 8 crackers (31 g)	5
Honey grahams, family size, 8 crackers (31.38 g)	5
Low fat cinnamon grahams, 8 crackers (31 g)	5

Honey Maid Despicable Me

Graham crackers, 17 pieces (30 g)	5

Honey Maid Go Bites

Chocolate filled snacks, 1 pack (30 g)	5
Vanilla filled snacks, 26 pieces (30 g)	5

Horizon

Snack grahams, honey, 17 cookies (30 g)	5

Immaculate Baking Co.

Cookie dough, gluten free, chocolate chunk, 1 cookie (33 g)	7

Kashi

Cookies, soft-baked, chocolate almond butter, 1 cookie (30 g)	5

Kashi Cookies

Oatmeal dark chocolate, 1 cookie (30 g)	5

Kashi TLC

Chewy cookies, all natural, oatmeal raisin flax, 1 cookie (30 g)	5
Cookies, oatmeal dark chocolate, 1 cookie (30 g)	5

Kedem

Tea biscuits, 2 biscuits	1
Tea biscuits, chocolate flavor, 2 biscuits	1
Tea biscuits, vanilla flavor, 2 biscuits	1

Keebler

Animals cookies, frosted, 8 cookies (33.45 g)	8
Baked graham cracker sticks, scooby-doo!, cinnamon, 1 package (28 g)	5
Baked graham cracker sticks, scooby-doo!, honey, 9 crackers (31.2 g)	5
Cookies, fudge, caramel & coconut, 2 cookies (30 g)	7
Cookies, sandwich, chocolate creme filled, 2 cookies (32.36 g)	6
Crackers, grahams, original, 8 crackers (30.4 g)	5
Elfin crackers, 23 pieces (30 g)	5
Fudge covered coconut dreams cookies, 2 cookies (32 g)	8
Fudge grahams cookies, 17 cookies (31 g)	6

Graham crackers, fudge covered, 3 pieces (27 g)	7
Original mini fudge stripes cookies, 14 cookies (30 g)	7
Wafers, vanilla, 8 cookies (30.91 g)	6

Keebler 100 Calorie Right Bites Chips Deluxe

Cookies, soft 'n chewy, 1 pouch (21 g)	4

Keebler 100 Calorie Right Bites Fudge Shoppe

Cookies, mini fudge stripes, 1 pouch (21 g)	5
Cookies, mini, value 12 pack, 1 pouch (21 g)	5
Fudge grahams, 1 pouch (20 g)	4

Keebler Chips Deluxe

Chocolate lovers cookies, 2 cookies (32 g)	7
Coconut cookies, 2 cookies (30 g)	7
Cookies, rainbow, 2 cookies (31.62 g)	7
Original chocolate chip cookie, 2 cookies (30 g)	7
Rainbow chocolate chip cookies, 2 cookies (31 g)	7
Rainbow mini cookies, 1 pouch (28 g)	6
Triple chocolate cookies, 2 cookies (30 g)	6

Keebler Fudge Shoppe

Cookies, mini fudge stripes, snack size, 1 package (56 g)	13

Keebler Fudge Stripes

Cookies, original, 2 cookies (27 g)	6
Original mini cookies, 1 pouch (28 g)	6
Red velvet cookies, 2 cookies (27 g)	6

Keebler Right Bites

Fudge grahams 100 calorie portions (variety pack), 1 pouch (20 g)	4

Keebler Sandies

Pecan shortbread cookies, 2 cookies (31 g)	7
Simply shortbread cookies, 2 cookies (31 g)	7

Keebler Scooby-Doo!

Baked graham cracker sticks, cinnamon, 10 crackers (31.2 g)	5

Keebler Simply Made

Butter cookies, 2 cookies (27 g)	6
Chocolate chip cookies, 2 cookies (27 g)	6

Keebler Soft Batch

Chocolate chip cookies, 2 cookies (32 g)	7

Keebler Vienna Fingers

Cookies, sandwich, crème filled, reduced fat, 2 cookies (31 g)	6
Sandwich cookies, creme filled, 2 cookies (31 g)	6

Kellogg's 100 Calorie Right Bites

Sunshine cheez-it, 1 pouch (21 g)	4

Kellogg's Pop-Tarts

Mini crisps frosted blueberry bites, 1 pouch (14 g)	2

Kellogg's Special K

Chocolatey caramel pastry crisps, 2 crisps (25 g)	4
Cookies and creme pastry crisps, 2 crisps (25 g)	4

Kellogg's To Go

Oatmeal raisin morning biscuits, 1 pouch (44 g)	7
Oats and honey morning biscuits, 1 pouch (44 g)	7

Kinnikinnick

Graham style, smoreables, 1 cookie (12 g)	2

Kirkland Signature

European cookies with Belgian chocolate, 3 cookies (30 g)	7

Desserts, Cakes, Candy & Cookies

SmartPoints™ value

Desserts, Cakes, Candy & Cookies

Knott's Berry Farm

Cookies, shortbread, raspberry, 1 package (57 g)	9

Kroger

Cookies, devil's food, fat free, 1 cookie (16 g)	2
Crackers, whole wheat, baked weavers, 8 crackers (30 g)	4
Graham crackers, cinnamon, 2 cracker sheets (31.38 g)	5
Graham crackers, honey, 4 crackers (27 g)	4
Graham crackers, original, 4 crackers (26.65 g)	4
Graham crackers, wild animal, chocolate flavored, 11 cookies (28.33 g)	5
Honey graham sticks, 9 cookies (28 g)	5
Original vanilla wafers, 7 cookies (30 g)	6

Kroger ChipMates

Chunky chocolate chip cookies, 2 cookies (28 g)	5

Lance

Cookies, van-o lunch, 4 cookies (46.5 g)	6
Real peanut butter nekot cookies, 1 package (50 g)	9

Lance Nekot

Peanut butter cookies, 1 package (50 g)	9
Peanut butter cookies, 4 cookies (33 g)	6

Lance Van-O Lunch

Rich vanilla creme filled sandwich cookies, 1 package (47 g)	10

Lazzaroni

Original Italian cookies, 5 cookies (30 g)	7

Lehi Roller Mills

Cookie mix, pumpkin chocolate chip, 2 cookies (38 g)	5

SmartPoints™ value

Leibniz

Fine European butter biscuits, 6 cookies (30 g)	5

Lil Dutch Maid

Cookies, almond windmill, 4 cookies (35.38 g)	6

Little Debbie Nutty Bars

Wafers with extra peanut butter, 2 cookies (60 g)	14

LiveGfree

Snickerdoodle soft baked cookies, 2 cookies (28 g)	5

Loacker Quadratini

Wafer cookies, bite size, dark chocolate, 9 cookies (31.25 g)	7

Lofthouse

Cookies, sugar, frosted, 1 cookie (42.5 g)	8
Delicious cookies, frosted sugar cookies, 1 cookie (42.5 g)	6
Frosted sugar cookies, 1 cookie (38 g)	7

Lorna Doone

Cookies, mini shortbread, 1 package (28 g)	5
Cookies, shortbread, 1 package (42 g)	8

Love Grown Super Oats

Hot cereal blend, chia, nuts & seeds, ½ cup dry	4

LU Petit Ecolier

Biscuits, European, dark chocolate, 2 cookies (25 g)	6
Biscuits, European, extra-dark chocolate, 2 cookies (25 g)	6
Biscuits, European, milk chocolate, 2 cookies (25 g)	6

Lucy's

Chocolate chip cookies, 3 cookies (32 g)	6
Cinnamon thin cookies, 3 cookies (32 g)	6
Ginger snap cookies, 3 cookies (32 g)	5

M&M's

Cookies, bite size, 5 cookies (30.91 g)	7

Mallomars

Cookies, pure chocolate, 2 cookies (25.11 g)	6

Marketside

Ultimate oatmeal raisin cookies, 1 cookie (42 g)	9

McVitie's

Digestives, milk chocolate, 2 cookies (35.71 g)	7
Hobnobs, 2 cookies (29 g)	6

Metamucil

Cinnamon spice multigrain wafers, 2 wafers (22 g)	4

Mi-Del

Ginger snaps, 5 cookies (28.38 g)	6
Ginger snaps, Swedish-style, 5 cookies (28.4 g)	5

Milano

Pepperidge farm cookies Milano candy cane limited edition, 2 cookies (25 g)	6

Mini Fudge Stripes 100 Calorie Right Bites

Fudge striped shortbread cookies, 1 pouch (21 g)	5

Miss Meringue

Cookies, meringue, chocolate, 13 cookies (30.6 g)	6
Cookies, meringue, minis, chocolate, 12 cookies (30 g)	6

Miss Meringue Classiques

Cookies, meringue, vanilla, 4 cookies (28.4 g)	7
Meringues, chocolate chip, 4 cookies (28.4 g)	7

Moon Pie Minis

Chocolate flavored marshmallow sandwich pies, 1 (28 g)	5

Mother's

Circus animal cookies, the original, 6 cookies (28.35 g)	8
Cookies, English tea, 2 cookies (37.75 g)	7
Cookies, taffy, 2 cookies (37.75 g)	8
Cookies, the original, circus animal, 7 cookies (30 g)	8
Iced oatmeal cookies, 4 cookies (32 g)	6
Peanut butter cookies, 2 each (28.33 g)	6

Mrs. Fields

Cookie, snickerdoodle, 1 cookie (42 g)	8
White chunk macadamia cookies, 1 cookie (28 g)	6

Mrs. Thinster's

Brownie batter cookie thins, 5 cookies (28 g)	7
Cake batter cookie thins, 5 cookies (28 g)	7

Mrs. Thinster's Cookie Thins

Chocolate chip, 5 cookies (28 g)	6
Chocolate chip cookies, 5 cookies (28 g)	6

Murray

Cookies, ginger snaps, 5 cookies (30.2 g)	6
Cookies, sandwich, sugar free, 3 cookies (30.67 g)	4
Cookies, sandwich, sugar free, chocolate, 3 cookies (30.67 g)	5
Cookies, sugar free, chocolate chip, 3 cookies (31 g)	6
Cookies, sugar free, fudge dipped vanilla wafers, 4 cookies (31.2 g)	6
Cookies, sugar free, lemon, 3 cookies (30.67 g)	4
Cookies, sugar free, shortbread, 8 cookies (34 g)	4

Desserts, Cakes, Candy & Cookies

Desserts, Cakes, Candy & Cookies

	SmartPoints™ value
Murray Sugar Free	
Dark fudge wafers, 4 cookies (28 g)	4
Wafers, vanilla, 4 cookies (28.33 g)	5
Nabisco 100 Cal	
Cookie crisps, shortbread, Lorna Doone, 1 package (21 g)	4
Oreo thin crisps, 1 pack (23 g)	4
Thin crisps, chips ahoy!, 1 package (23 g)	4
Nabisco 100 Calorie Packs	
Cookie crisps, shortbread, Lorna Doone, 1 package (21 g)	4
Cookies, mini, 1 package (21 g)	4
Nabisco Chips Ahoy! Holiday	
Chocolate chip cookies with festive candy, 3 cookies (33 g)	7
Nabisco Classics	
Cookies, snickerdoodle, 1 cookie (18.87 g)	4
Nabisco Famous	
Wafers, chocolate, 5 cookies (31.88 g)	6
Nabisco Lorna Doone	
Shortbread cookies, 1 package (42 g)	8
Nabisco Newtons	
Fig chewy cookies single serve pack, 1 pack (56 g)	9
Nabisco Oreo	
Chocolate sandwich cookies, 3 cookies (34 g)	7
Nabisco Oreo Halloween	
Chocolate sandwich cookie, 2 cookies (29 g)	6
Nestlé	
Cookie shapes, pre-cut, chocolate chip, 1 cookie (42.5 g)	5
Nestlé Crunch Girl Scouts	
Thin mints dark chocolate cookie wafers, 2 bars (37 g)	11

	SmartPoints™ value
Nestlé Toll House	
Cookie dough, double chocolate chip, 1 cookie (28 g)	6
Cookie dough, peanut butter chocolate chip, 1 cookie (19 g)	3
White chip lemon cookie dough (prepared), 1 cookie (19 g)	4
Newtons	
Chewy cookies, 100% whole grain, triple berry, 2 cookies (29 g)	4
Chewy cookies, fig, whole grain, 2 cookies (30 g)	5
Chewy cookies, fruit, baked apple & cinnamon, 2 cookies (29 g)	4
Chewy cookies, strawberry, 2 cookies (29 g)	5
Cookies, chewy, fig, 1 pack (28 g)	4
Cookies, fig, fat free, 2 cookies (28.33 g)	4
Cookies, fruit chewy, original fig, 2 cookies (31 g)	5
Crispy cookies, fruit thins, fig and honey, 3 cookies (29.7 g)	5
Newtons Fruit Thins	
Cookies, cherry vanilla, 3 cookies (31 g)	5
Cookies, crispy, cranberry citrus oat, 3 cookies (29.7 g)	5
Cookies, crispy, lemon crisp, 3 cookies (31 g)	5
Cookies, sandwich, peanut butter, 3 cookies (30 g)	5
Toasted coconut with dark fudge, 3 cookies (31 g)	6
Nilla	
Mini wafers, 1 pack (28 g)	5
Nilla wafers, mini, 20 wafers (30 g)	6
Wafers, 8 wafers (30 g)	6
Wafers, mini, 1 package (28 g)	5
Wafers, mini, go-paks!, 14 cookies (30 g)	6
Wafers, reduced fat, 8 wafers (28.27 g)	5

Nilla Wafers

Wafers, nilla, mini, 1 package (33 g)	6

Nob Hill Trading Co.

Cookies, white chocolate chip, with macadamia nuts, 1 cookie (25.5 g)	6

Nonni's

Almond dark chocolate biscotti bites, 3 cookies (26 g)	5
Almond thins, cinnamon raisin, 1 package (21 g)	4
Almond thins, cranberry, 1 package (21 g)	4
Almond thins, pistachio, 1 package (21 g)	3
Biscotti bites, almond dark chocolate, 3 cookies (26 g)	5
Biscotti, cioccolati, 1 biscotti	5
Biscotti, decadence, 1 biscotti	4
Biscotti, limone, 1 biscotti	5
Biscotti, originali, 1 biscotti	4
Biscotti, salted caramel, 1 biscotti	5
Biscotti, toffee almond, 1 biscotti	5
Biscotti, triple milk chocolate without nuts, 1 biscotti	5
Biscotti, turtle pecan, 1 biscotti	5
Pumpkin spice biscotti, 1 cookie (24 g)	5

Nonni's THINaddictives

Almond thins, banana dark chocolate, 1 package (21 g)	4
Pistachio almond thins, 2 packages (23 g)	4

Nutter Butter

Cookies, peanut butter sandwich, bites, go-paks!, 10 cookies (30 g)	6
Cookies, sandwich, peanut butter, 2 cookies (24.5 g)	5
Creme patties, 5 patties (33 g)	6
Peanut butter sandwich cookies, 2 cookies (25 g)	5

Nutter Butter Bites

Cookies, sandwich, peanut butter, 1 package (49 g)	9
Peanut butter sandwich cookies, 10 cookies (31.44 g)	6

Nutter Butter Snak-Saks Bites

Cookies, sandwich, peanut butter, 10 cookies (28.25 g)	6

Oreo

Chocolate sandwich cookies, 3 cookies (34 g)	7
Chocolate sandwich cookies, milk chocolate covered, 1 each (17.67 g)	4
Chocolate sandwich cookies, reduced fat, 3 cookies (33.35 g)	6
Cookie pieces, medium, ¼ cup	6
Cookies, chocolate sandwich, chocolate creme, 2 cookies (30.86 g)	7
Cookies, chocolate sandwich, cool mint creme, 2 cookies (28.8 g)	6
Cookies, chocolate sandwich, mini, 1 package (28 g)	6
Cookies, chocolate sandwich, nascar, 2 cookies (29 g)	6
Cookies, chocolate sandwich, peanut butter creme, 2 cookies (30.86 g)	6
Cookies, chocolate sandwich, reduced fat, 3 cookies (33.77 g)	6
Cookies, chocolate sandwich, triple double, 1 cookie (20.61 g)	4
Cookies, chocolate sandwich, white fudge covered, 1 cookie (20.08 g)	5
Cookies, fudge cremes, mint, 3 cookies (35.56 g)	8
Cookies, sandwich, birthday cake flavor creme, 2 cookies (28 g)	6
Cookies, sandwich, chocolate, 3 cookies (34 g)	7
Cookies, sandwich, chocolate, berry burst ice cream, 2 cookies (30.86 g)	7

	SmartPoints™ value
Cookies, sandwich, chocolate, birthday cake flavor, 2 cookies (29 g)	6
Cookies, sandwich, chocolate, double stuf, 2 cookies (29 g)	6
Cookies, sandwich, chocolate, family size, 3 cookies (34 g)	7
Cookies, sandwich, chocolate, mega stuf, 2 cookies (36 g)	8
Cookies, sandwich, chocolate, winter edition, 2 cookies (29 g)	6
Cookies, sandwich, golden, 3 cookies (34 g)	7
Cookies, sandwich, golden chocolate creme, 3 cookies (34 g)	7
Cookies, sandwich, golden double stuff, king size, 2 cookies (29 g)	6
Cookies, sandwich, golden, double stuf, 2 cookies (30 g)	7
Cookies, sandwich, golden, mega stuf, 2 cookies (36 g)	8
Cookies, sandwich, golden, original, 3 cookies (35.44 g)	7
Cookies, sandwich, red velvet, 2 cookies (29 g)	6
Double stuf chocolate sandwich cookies, 2 cookies (29 g)	6
Golden sandwich cookies, 3 cookies (34 g)	7
Lemon twist flavor cream sandwich cookies, 2 cookies (29 g)	6
Oreos, peppermint creme, 2 cookies (28.8 g)	6
Reduced fat chocolate sandwich cookies, 3 cookies (34 g)	7
Reese peanut butter cup cookie, 2 cookies (29 g)	6

Oreo Double Stuf

Chocolate sandwich cookies, 2 cookies (29 g)	6
Cookies, chocolate sandwich, king size!, 2 cookies (29 g)	6
Cookies, sandwich, chocolate, 1 package (42 g)	9

	SmartPoints™ value
Cookies, sandwich, chocolate, family size, 2 cookies (29 g)	6
Cookies, sandwich, heads or tails, 2 cookies (28.8 g)	6

Oreo Mini

Chocolate sandwich cookie, 9 cookies (29 g)	6
Cookies, sandwich, chocolate, bite size, go-paks!, 9 cookies (29 g)	6
Cookies, sandwich, chocolate, candy cane creme, 9 cookies (29 g)	6
Cookies, sandwich, golden, bite size, snak-saks, 9 cookies (29 g)	6
Mint creme flavored chocolate sandwich cookies, 9 cookies (29 g)	6
Reese's chocolate cookie sandwich, 9 cookies (29 g)	5

Oreo Snak-Saks

Cookies, sandwich, mini, chocolate, 9 cookies (28.25 g)	6

Oreo Spring

Chocolate sandwich cookies filled with yellow cream, 2 cookies (29 g)	6

Otis Spunkmeyer

Bars, lemon, 1 serving (78 g)	11
Cookie dough, chocolate chip, 1 cookie (38 g)	8
Cookie dough, oatmeal raisin, 1 cookie (38 g)	7
Cookie dough, white chocolate macadamia nut, 1 cookie (38 g)	8

Pamela's Simplebites

Mini cookies, chocolate chip, 4 cookies (24.75 g)	6

Pepperidge Farm

Cookies, Bordeaux, 4 cookies (27.29 g)	6
Cookies, Brussels, 3 cookies (29.8 g)	7
Cookies, chessmen, 3 cookies (25.75 g)	5
Cookies, classic favorites, 3 cookies (28 g)	6

	SmartPoints value
Cookies, ginger family collection, 3 cookies (26 g)	5
Cookies, gingerman, 4 cookies (28.4 g)	6
Cookies, lemon, 4 cookies (34 g)	6
Cookies, Milano favorites, 4 cookies (34 g)	7
Cookies, Milano milk chocolate, 3 cookies (35.4 g)	8
Cookies, Milano mint, 2 cookies (24.75 g)	6
Cookies, Milano, dark chocolate, 3 cookies (34 g)	8
Cookies, Milano, double chocolate, 2 cookies (26.63 g)	6
Cookies, Milano, raspberry, 2 cookies (24.75 g)	6
Cookies, Sausalito, milk chocolate macadamia, 1 cookie (25.5 g)	6
Cookies, shortbread, 2 cookies (26 g)	6
Cookies, Verona, strawberry, 3 cookies (31.83 g)	6

Pepperidge Farm Chocolate Chunk

Cookies, crispy, Chesapeake dark chocolate pecan, 1 cookie (26 g)	6
Cookies, crispy, Maui, milk chocolate coconut almond, 1 cookie (26 g)	6
Cookies, crispy, Nantucket, 1 cookie (25.75 g)	6
Cookies, crispy, Tahoe, 1 cookie (25.75 g)	6

Pepperidge Farm Double Chocolate Chunk

Cookies, crispy, dark chocolate, 1 cookie (27.5 g)	6

Pepperidge Farm Milano

Cookies, 1 package (34 g)	8
Cookies, dark chocolate, 1 package (21 g)	5
Cookies, dulce de leche, 2 cookies (25 g)	6
Cookies, lemon flavored chocolate, 2 cookies (25 g)	6
Cookies, orange flavored chocolate, 2 cookies (24.75 g)	6

Pepperidge Farm Milano Melts

Cookies, chocolate dark classic creme, 2 cookies (27.17 g)	6

Pepperidge Farm Milano Slices

Cookies, crispy peppermint, 3 cookies (29 g)	7
Cookies, crispy, salted pretzel, 3 cookies (29 g)	6

Pepperidge Farm On The Go!

Cookies, Milano, dark chocolate, 1 package (21 g)	5

Pepperidge Farm Pirouette

Rolled wafers, creme filled, chocolate fudge, 2 wafers (25.47 g)	5
Rolled wafers, creme filled, chocolate hazelnut, 2 wafers (25.47 g)	6
Rolled wafers, creme filled, French vanilla, 2 wafers (25.47 g)	6

Pepperidge Farm Soft Baked

Cookies, Montauk, milk chocolate, 1 cookie (30.5 g)	7
Cookies, Santa Cruz, oatmeal raisin, 1 cookie (30.5 g)	6

Pillsbury

Cookie dough, chocolate chip, 1 rounded tsp	6
Cookie dough, gluten free chocolate chip, 1 Tbsp	5
Cookie dough, sugar cookies, ½" slice	5

Pillsbury Big Deluxe

Cookie dough, oatmeal raisin, 1 cookie (38 g)	7
Cookies, chocolate chip, 1 cookie (38 g)	8
Cookies, peanut butter cup, cookie (38 g)	8

Desserts, Cakes, Candy & Cookies

	SmartPoints™ value
Pillsbury Dessert Melts	
Cookies, s'more sensation ready to bake, 1 cookie (37 g)	7
Molten fudge cake ready to bake cookies, 1 cookie (37 g)	7
Pillsbury Mini	
Chocolate chip cookies, 4 cookies (31 g)	6
Cookies, soft baked snickerdoodle, 4 cookies (31 g)	6
Pillsbury Ready To Bake!	
Chocolate chip cookies, with Hershey's chocolate chips, 1 cookie (25.5 g)	5
Cookie dough, sugar, pink hearts, 2 cookies (26 g)	5
Cookies & chocolates, peanut butter blossoms, 1 cookie (29.5 g)	6
Cookies, chocolate chip, 2 cookies (38 g)	7
Cookies, chocolate chunk & chip, 2 cookies (38 g)	8
Cookies, sugar, bunny shape, 2 cookies (26 g)	5
Cookies, sugar, Easter shape, 2 cookies (26 g)	5
Pillsbury Simply	
Cookies, chocolate chip, 1 cookie (33 g)	7
Pinwheels	
Pinwheels, 1 cookie (30.91 g)	6
Pirouline	
Creme de pirouline, chocolate hazelnut, 2 cookies (18.4 g)	4
Creme de pirouline, dark chocolate, 2 cookies (18.4 g)	5
Pizelle	
Pizelle, Italian style cookies, anise, 6 cookies (30 g)	5
Pizelle, Italian style cookies, vanilla, 6 cookies (30 g)	5

	SmartPoints™ value
Pocky	
Biscuit sticks, chocolate cream covered, 1 oz	7
Power Crunch	
Protein energy bar, cookies and creme, 1 bar (40 g)	7
Protein energy bar, original, French vanilla creme, 1 bar (40 g)	7
Protein energy bar, triple chocolate, 1 bar (40 g)	7
Priano Pizzelle	
Pizzelle vanilla flavored Italian style cookies, 6 cookies (30 g)	5
Quaker	
Cookies, crispy, peanut butter oatmeal, 1 package (38 g)	7
Quaker Oat & Yogurt	
Vanilla sandwich biscuits, 1 package (38 g)	7
Vanilla sandwich cookies, 2 cookies (38 g)	7
Quaker Soft Baked	
Raisins oatmeal cookies, 1 cookie (42 g)	7
Reko	
Vanilla pizzelle, 1 oz	5
Reko Pizzelle	
Anise Italian waffle cookie, 6 cookies (30 g)	5
Right Bites 100 Calorie	
Sandies fudge dipped cookies, 1 package (21 g)	4
Royal Dansk	
Cookies, Danish butter, 4 cookies (34 g)	7
Safeway	
Frosted sugar cookies, red velvet, 1 cookie (38 g)	8
Ginger snaps, triple ginger, 4 cookies (28.31 g)	5

Safeway Kitchens

Fat free devil's food cookie cake, 1 cookie (16 g)	2

Safeway Select

Madeleines cookie, 1 cookie (28 g)	6

Sandies

Cookies, pecan shortbread, 1 cookie (16.18 g)	3

Schar

Cookies, shortbread, 4 cookies (28.57 g)	5

Sheila G's

Brownie brittle, chocolate chip, 1 oz	6
Brownie brittle, salted caramel, 1 oz	6
Brownie brittle, salted caramel, 1 oz	6
Brownie brittle, toffee crunch, 6 pieces (28 g)	6

Sinful

Cookies, white chocolate chunk and macadamia nut, 2 cookies (28.33 g)	7

SnackWell's

Cookies, creme sandwich, 2 cookies (24 g)	5
Devil's food cookie cakes, 1 cookie (16 g)	2

SnackWell's 100 Calorie Packs

Cookies, chocolate chip, fudge drizzled, 1 pack (22 g)	4

Social Tea

Biscuits, 7 cookies (31.82 g)	5

Stauffer's

Animal cookies, original, 16 crackers (30 g)	4
Animal crackers, chocolate, 16 crackers (29.36 g)	5

Steenstra's

Cookies, almond st. claus, 1 cookie (16 g)	3

Stella D'oro

Coffee treats, anisette sponge, 2 cookies (24.71 g)	4
Cookies, margherite, 2 cookies (28.33 g)	5
Cookies, margherite combination, 2 cookies (28.33 g)	5
Cookies, Swiss fudge, 3 cookies (32.29 g)	8

Stella D'oro Breakfast Treats

Cookies, original, 1 cookie (21.25 g)	4

Stella D'oro Coffee Treats

Anisette toast, 3 cookies (38.33 g)	5
Cookies, almond toast, 2 cookies (27 g)	4
Cookies, anisette toast, 3 cookies (32.4 g)	5

Tate's Bake Shop

Cookies, chocolate chip, 1 cookie (14 g)	4
Cookies, chocolate chip walnut, 1 cookie (15 g)	4
Cookies, gluten free, chocolate chip, 1 cookie (15 g)	4
Cookies, gluten free, double chocolate chip, 1 cookie (14 g)	3
Cookies, gluten free, ginger zinger, 1 cookie (14 g)	3
Cookies, white chocolate chip macadamia nut, 1 cookie (14 g)	4
Cookies, whole wheat, dark chocolate, 1 cookie (15 g)	4

Teddy Grahams

Graham snacks, 13 pieces (29.89 g)	5
Graham snacks, chocolate, 9 cookies (31.44 g)	5
Graham snacks, cinnamon, 11 each (31.44 g)	5

Desserts, Cakes, Candy & Cookies

Desserts, Cakes, Candy & Cookies

	SmartPoints™ value
Graham snacks, honey, go-packs!, 24 pieces (30 g)	5
Graham snacks, mini, chocolate, snak-saks, 47 cookies (28.25 g)	5
Teddy Grahams 100 Calorie Packs	
Graham snacks, mini, cinnamon cubs, 1 package (22 g)	3
Teddy Grahams Mini	
Graham snacks, chocolatey chip, 53 cookies (28.25 g)	5
Toll House	
Cookie dough, chocolate chip, 1 cookie (28 g)	6
Cookie dough, oatmeal scotchies, 2 cookies (39 g)	7
Cookie dough, triple chip, cookie of the year, 1 cookie (19 g)	4
Cookie kit, chocolate chip, 2 cookies (27 g)	4
Cookies, chocolate chip, 1 cookie (19.5 g)	5
Peanut butter chocolate chip cookie dough (makes 18 cookies), 1 cookie (28 g)	6
Toll House Mini	
Chocolate chip cookie dough prepared, 3 cookies (35 g)	7
Toll House Ultimates	
Cookie dough, chocolate chip lovers, 1 cookie (38 g)	8
Cookie dough, turtle, 1 cookie (38 g)	8
Cookie dough, white chip macadamia nut, 1 cookie (38 g)	8
Trader Joe's	
100 calorie packs of oatmeal chocolate chip cookies, 1 package (25 g)	4
Cats cookies, 15 cookies (30 g)	5
Chocolate almond horns, 1 piece (43 g)	7

	SmartPoints™ value
Chocolate cats cookies, 15 cookies (30 g)	5
Chocolate chip cookie dunkers, 2 cookies (32 g)	7
Chocolate chip cookies, 1 cookie (21 g)	4
Cookie butter sandwich cookies, 2 cookies (32 g)	8
Cookie thins - meyer lemon, 9 cookies (28 g)	7
Cookie thins - triple ginger, 9 cookies (28 g)	6
Crispy cookies filled with Belgian chocolate, 1 oz	7
Dark chocolate covered peppermint Joe joe's, 1 cookie (27 g)	7
Dress circle crispy crunchy chocolate chip cookies, 12 cookies (30 g)	7
Gluten free chocolate chocolate chip cookies, 1 cookie (26 g)	5
Joe-joe's chocolate sandwich creme cookies, 2 cookies (27 g)	6
Oatmeal cranberry dunkers cookies, 2 cookies (38 g)	7
Organic animal crackers, 17 cookies (30 g)	4
Pfeffernusse german spice cookies, 2 cookies (40 g)	7
Speculoos cookies, 4 cookies (32 g)	6
Triple ginger snaps, 6 cookies (30 g)	6
Ultimate vanilla wafers, 5 cookies (28 g)	5
Vanilla meringues, 4 cookies (30 g)	7
Twin Dragon	
Fortune cookies, Chinese style, 1 cookie (8 g)	1
Twix	
Cookie bars, 1 cookie bar (34 g)	8
Cookie bars, minis, 3 pieces (30 g)	7

Udi's

Cookies, chocolate chip, gluten free, 2 cookies (45 g)	10
Cookies, soft-baked, salted caramel cashew, 1 cookie (26 g)	5

Vienna Fingers

Cookies, sandwich, creme filled, 2 cookies (30.2 g)	6

Voortman

Cookies, coconut, 1 cookie (18 g)	4
Cookies, iced almonette, 2 cookies (28.38 g)	5
Cookies, sugar free, oatmeal, 1 cookie (18.92 g)	2
Oatmeal raisin cookies, 1 each (18.92 g)	3
Wafer cookies, sugar free, chocolate, 3 cookies (27 g)	4
Wafer cookies, sugar free, vanilla, 3 cookies (27 g)	4
Wafers, strawberry, 3 cookies (30 g)	6
Wafers, vanilla, 3 cookies (30 g)	6

Walker's

Shortbread, assorted, pure butter, 2 pieces (21.82 g)	5
Shortbread, pure butter, 1 piece (19 g)	4
Shortbread, rounds, pure butter, 1 piece (17 g)	4

Wegman's

Cookies, spritz, 3 cookies (34 g)	7

Wegman's Italian Classics

Cookies, almond paste, amaretti, 3 cookies (34 g)	6
Cookies, jelly, 2 cookies (34.67 g)	7

Custards

Gilles

Frozen custard, vanilla, ½ cup	9

Kozy Shack

Flan, creme caramel, 1 snack cup (113 g)	7

Dessert Toppings

Breyers

Hot fudge ice cream sauce, 2 Tbsp	4
Ice cream sauce, caramel flavored, 2 Tbsp	4

Cool Whip

Frosting, whipped, chocolate, 2 Tbsp	4
Frosting, whipped, cream cheese, 2 Tbsp	4
Frosting, whipped, vanilla, 2 Tbsp	4
Whipped topping, extra creamy, with real cream, 2 Tbsp	2
Whipped topping, fat free, 2 Tbsp	1
Whipped topping, lite, 2 Tbsp	1
Whipped topping, original, 2 Tbsp	1
Whipped topping, regular, 2 Tbsp	1
Whipped topping, strawberry, 2 Tbsp	1
Whipped topping, sugar free, 2 Tbsp	1

Cool Whip Lite

Whipped topping, 2 Tbsp	1

Essential Everyday

Whipped topping, fat free, 2 Tbsp	1
Whipped topping, lite, 2 Tbsp	1

Fit & Active

Fat free whipped topping, 2 Tbsp	1

Hershey's

Topping, hot fudge, 2 Tbsp	7

Hood

Light whipped cream, sugar free, 2 Tbsp	0

Kroger

Whipped topping, fat free, 2 Tbsp	1
Whipped topping, lite, 2 Tbsp	1

Lucerne

Whipped topping, 2 Tbsp	1
Whipped topping, extra creamy, 2 Tbsp	1
Whipped topping, fat free, 2 Tbsp	0

Desserts, Cakes, Candy & Cookies

	SmartPoints™ value
Martha's	
Chocolate sauce, killer, 2 Tbsp	5
Mrs. Richardson's	
Hot fudge topping, 2 Tbsp	8
Reddi Wip	
Dairy whipped topping, chocolate topper, 2 Tbsp	1
Dairy whipped topping, extra creamy, 2 Tbsp	1
Dairy whipped topping, fat free, 2 Tbsp	0
Dairy whipped topping, original, 2 Tbsp	1
Safeway Kitchens	
Whipped topping, fat free, 2 Tbsp	1
ShopRite	
Whipped topping, fat free, 2 Tbsp	1
Smucker's	
Topping, caramel flavored, 2 Tbsp	6
Topping, hot fudge, 2 Tbsp	6
Topping, sugar free, caramel, 2 Tbsp	3
Smucker's Magic Shell	
Flavored topping, chocolate fudge, 2 Tbsp	10
Topping, chocolate, 2 Tbsp	10
Smucker's Simple Delight	
Salted caramel ice cream topping, 2 Tbsp	7
Smucker's Sugar Free	
Topping, hot fudge, 2 Tbsp	3
Smucker's Toppings	
Hot fudge, 2 Tbsp	6
Torani	
Sauce, white chocolate, 2 Tbsp	6
Tru Whip	
Whipped topping, 2 Tbsp	2
Whipped topping, the natural, light, 2 Tbsp	1

	SmartPoints™ value

Eclairs
Private Selection
Mini eclairs, 5 eclairs (70 g)	8

Frozen Yogurt
Ben & Jerry's Fro Yo
Frozen yogurt, cherry Garcia, ½ cup	9
Frozen yogurt, chocolate fudge brownie, ½ cup	8
Frozen yogurt, lowfat, half baked, ½ cup	9
Frozen yogurt, phish food, ½ cup	11

Ben & Jerry's Greek
Frozen yogurt, blueberry vanilla graham, ½ cup	9

Breyers Blasts!
Frozen dairy dessert, chocolate, ½ cup	6

Edy's Slow Churned Yogurt Blends
Cappuccino chip frozen dairy dessert, ½ cup	6
Caramel praline crunch frozen dairy dessert, ½ cup	6
Chocolate fudge brownie frozen dairy dessert, ½ cup	6
Chocolate vanilla swirl frozen dairy dessert, ½ cup	5
Vanilla fat free frozen yogurt, ½ cup	4

Fit & Active
Cherry Greek yogurt smoothie bar, 1 bar (74 ml)	4

Friendly's
Fat free chocolate frozen yogurt, ½ cup	5
Fat free vanilla frozen yogurt, ½ cup	5

Friendly's Frozen Yogurt
Vienna mocha swirl, ½ cup	7

Green's

Lowfat frozen yogurt, vanilla, ½ cup	6

Haagen Dazs

Frozen yogurt, low fat, coffee, ½ cup	7
Frozen yogurt, low fat, vanilla, ½ cup	8

Healthy Choice

Frozen yogurt, Greek, raspberry, 1 container (71 g)	4

Healthy Choice Greek Frozen Yogurt

Dark fudge swirl, 1 container (112 ml)	4

Hood Smooth & Creamy

Frozen yogurt, low fat, chocolate fudge brownie, ½ cup	6

Kemps

Chocolate caramel brownie premium frozen yogurt, ½ cup	7
Cookies and cream frozen yogurt, ½ cup	6
Frozen yogurt, caramel praline crunch, fat free, ½ cup	6
Frozen yogurt, chocolate chip cookie dough, ½ cup	7
Frozen yogurt, chocolate peanut butter cup, ½ cup	6
Frozen yogurt, Denali original moose tracks, ½ cup	8
Frozen yogurt, fat free, chocolate, ½ cup	4
Frozen yogurt, fat free, wild blueberries 'n sweet cream, ½ cup	4
Frozen yogurt, vanilla, ½ cup	2
Low fat, black Jack cherry frozen yogurt, ½ cup	5
Mint chocolate chip smooth and creamy lowfat frozen yogurt, ½ cup	5
Sea salt caramel truffle frozen yogurt, ½ cup	7

Strawberry low fat frozen yogurt, ½ cup	5
Vanilla bean smooth and creamy lowfat frozen yogurt, ½ cup	6
Vanilla fat free frozen yogurt, ½ cup	4
Yogurt parfait, vanilla, with granola, 1 container (127 g)	12

Kroger Deluxe

Frozen yogurt, chocolate, ½ cup	5
Frozen yogurt, vanilla, ½ cup	5

Kroger Party Pail

Frozen yogurt, lowfat, vanilla, ½ cup	4

Oikos

Cafe latte flavored Greek frozen yogurt, ½ cup	7
Chocolate flavored Greek frozen yogurt, ½ cup	7
Key lime flavored Greek frozen yogurt, ½ cup	7

Publix Premium

Frozen yogurt, lowfat, black Jack cherry, ½ cup	6
Frozen yogurt, lowfat, butter pecan, ½ cup	6
Frozen yogurt, lowfat, chocolate, ½ cup	5
Frozen yogurt, lowfat, cookies & cream, ½ cup	6
Frozen yogurt, lowfat, peanut butter cup, ½ cup	5
Frozen yogurt, lowfat, toffee candy crunch, ½ cup	6
Frozen yogurt, lowfat, vanilla, ½ cup	5

Stonyfield Farm Organic

Frozen yogurt, nonfat, after dark chocolate, ½ cup	5

Stonyfield Farm Organic Oikos

Frozen yogurt, Greek, nonfat, vanilla, ½ cup	5

Desserts, Cakes, Candy & Cookies

Desserts, Cakes, Candy & Cookies

	SmartPoints™ value
TCBY Fruit n' Yogurt	
Low fat orange and vanilla sherbert and frozen yogurt bars, 1 bar (74 g)	6
Turkey Hill	
Frozen yogurt, chocolate marshmallow, ½ cup	5
Frozen yogurt, mint cookies 'n cream, ½ cup	5
Frozen yogurt, neapolitan, ½ cup	4
Frozen yogurt, vanilla bean, ½ cup	4
Yasso	
Frozen Greek yogurt bar, blueberry, 1 bar (75 g)	3
Frozen Greek yogurt bar, chocolate fudge, 1 bar (70 g)	4
Frozen Greek yogurt bar, dark chocolate raspberry, 1 bar (60 g)	5
Frozen Greek yogurt bar, mint chocolate chip, 1 bar (70 g)	4
Frozen Greek yogurt bar, peanut butter cup, 1 bar (60 g)	6
Frozen Greek yogurt bar, raspberry, 1 bar (75 g)	3
Frozen Greek yogurt bar, sea salt caramel, 1 bar (70 g)	4
Frozen Greek yogurt bar, strawberry, 1 bar (70 g)	3
Yoplait	
Raspberry flavored Greek low fat frozen yogurt bar, 1 bar (61 g)	4

Fruit Cobblers

	SmartPoints™ value
Mrs. Smith's	
Cobbler, blackberry, ⅛ cobbler (113 g)	10
Cobbler, peach, ⅛ pie (113 g)	10

Gelatin

	SmartPoints™ value
Jell-O	
Black cherry low calorie sugar free gelatin snack, 1 snack (89 g)	0
Gelatin and pudding, sugar free, variety pack (gelatin flavors), 1 snack (89 g)	0
Gelatin dessert, lemon, ¼ package (22 g)	5
Gelatin dessert, lime, ¼ package (22 g)	5
Gelatin dessert, low calorie, cherry, ¼ package (2.5 g)	0
Gelatin dessert, low calorie, sugar free, lemon, unprepared, ¼ package (2 g)	0
Gelatin dessert, low calorie, sugar free, orange, ⅛ package (2.5 g)	0
Gelatin dessert, low calorie, sugar free, raspberry, ¼ package (2.1 g)	0
Gelatin dessert, orange, ¼ package (22 g)	5
Gelatin dessert, peach, ¼ package (22 g)	5
Gelatin dessert, raspberry, ¼ package (22 g)	5
Gelatin dessert, strawberry, ¼ package (22 g)	5
Gelatin dessert, strawberry kiwi, sugar free, ⅛ package (2.5 g)	0
Gelatin snacks, low calorie, cherry pomegranate, 1 snack (89 g)	0
Gelatin snacks, low calorie, orange, 1 snack (89 g)	0
Gelatin snacks, low calorie, strawberry, 1 snack (89 g)	0
Gelatin snacks, low calorie, strawberry-kiwi, 1 snack (89 g)	0
Gelatin snacks, low calorie, sugar free, black cherry, 1 snack (89 g)	0

Gelatin snacks, low calorie, sugar free, cherry, 1 snack (89 g)	0
Gelatin snacks, low calorie, sugar free, cherry & black cherry, 1 snack (92 g)	0
Gelatin snacks, low calorie, sugar free, lemon-lime & orange, 1 snack (92 g)	0
Gelatin snacks, low calorie, sugar free, raspberry, 1 snack (89 g)	0
Gelatin snacks, low calorie, sugar free, raspberry & orange, 1 snack (92 g)	0
Gelatin snacks, low calorie, sugar free, strawberry, 1 snack (92 g)	0
Gelatin snacks, low calorie, sugar free, strawberry, 8 pack, 1 container (89 g)	0
Gelatin snacks, original, orange, 1 snack (96 g)	4
Gelatin snacks, original, raspberry, 1 snack (96 g)	4
Gelatin snacks, original, strawberry, 1 snack (96 g)	4
Lemon lime low calorie sugar free gelatin snack, 1 snack (89 g)	0
Low calorie gelatin dessert, sugar free, black cherry, ¼ package (2.1 g)	0
Low calorie gelatin dessert, sugar free, orange, ¼ package (2.1 g)	0
Low calorie gelatin dessert, sugar free, strawberry banana, ¼ package (2.1 g)	0
Original strawberry gelatin snack, 1 snack (96 g)	4
Snacks, low calorie gelatin, sugar free, variety pack, 1 snack (92 g)	0
Sugar free lemon-lime gelatin snacks, 1 snack (89 g)	0

Sugar free low calorie gelatin dessert, cranberry, ⅛ package (2.1 g)	0
Kroger	
Gel bites, strawberry, ½ cup	0
Snack Pack	
Cherry juicy gels, 1 container (92 g)	0
Juicy gels, strawberry & orange, sugar free, 1 gel snack (92 g)	0
Juicy gels, sugar free, cherry, 1 gel snack (99 g)	0

Ice Cream

Almond Dream Lil' Dreamers

Dessert sandwiches, vanilla, 1 sandwich (40 g)	4
Arctic Zero	
Gluten free lactose free cappuccino creamy frozen dessert, ½ cup	1
Gluten free lactose free chocolate frozen dessert, ½ cup	1
Gluten free lactose free chocolate peanut butter frozen dessert, ½ cup	1
Gluten free lactose free creamy cookies and cream frozen dessert, ½ cup	1
Gluten free lactose free hint of mint creamy frozen dessert, ½ cup	1
Gluten free lactose free vanilla maple frozen dessert, ½ cup	1
Arctic Zero Chunky	
Cookie dough chip fit frozen dessert, ½ cup	3
Ben & Jerry's	
Ice cream, cherry Garcia, ½ cup	12
Ice cream, chocolate chip cookie dough, ½ cup	13
Ice cream, chocolate fudge brownie, ½ cup	13
Ice cream, chocolate therapy, ½ cup	12

Desserts, Cakes, Candy & Cookies

Desserts, Cakes, Candy & Cookies

	SmartPoints™ value
Ice cream, chubby hubby, ½ cup	15
Ice cream, chunky monkey, ½ cup	14
Ice cream, coffee heath bar crunch, ½ cup	14
Ice cream, cookie dough, 1 container (96 g)	12
Ice cream, everything but the…, ½ cup	15
Ice cream, half baked, ½ cup	13
Ice cream, limited batch key lime pie, ½ cup	12
Ice cream, mint chocolate cookie, ½ cup	12
Ice cream, New York super fudge chunk, ½ cup	15
Ice cream, peanut butter cup, ½ cup	17
Ice cream, phish food, ½ cup	14
Ice cream, pistachio pistachio, ½ cup	12
Ice cream, red velvet cake, ½ cup	12
Ice cream, Stephen Colbert's Americone dream, ½ cup	13

Ben & Jerry's Core

Ice cream, hazed and confused, ½ cup	14
Ice cream, karamel sutra, ½ cup	13
Ice cream, peanut butter fudge, ½ cup	14
Ice cream, salted caramel, ½ cup	13
Ice cream, that's my Jam, ½ cup	13

Blue Bunny

Ice cream, fat free, no sugar added, brownie sundae, ½ cup	3
Ice cream, fat free, no sugar added, vanilla, ½ cup	3

	SmartPoints™ value
Blue Bunny Blue Ribbon Classics	
Fudge bars, freezer pack, 1 bar (61 g)	4
Star bar, freezer pack, 1 bar (42 g)	6
Blue Bunny Cadbury	
Ice cream bar, caramello, snack size, 1 bar (48 g)	8
Blue Bunny Mini Swirls	
Birthday party ice cream cone, 1 cone (46 g)	8
Caramel ice cream cones, 1 (44 g)	7
Mini cones, chocolate, 1 cone (43 g)	7
Vanilla cone, 1 cone (43 g)	6
Blue Bunny Premium	
Ice cream, mint chocolate chip, ½ cup	8
Ice cream, peanut butter panic, ½ cup	9
Ice cream, vanilla, ½ cup	7
Bomb Pop	
Frozen confection, the original, 1 bar (47 g)	2
Breyers	
All natural ice cream, calcium rich, natural vanilla with real vanilla bean specks, ½ cup	6
Homemade vanilla ice cream, ½ cup	7
Ice cream, black raspberry chocolate, ½ cup	8
Ice cream, butter pecan, ½ cup	7
Ice cream, cherry vanilla, ½ cup	7
Ice cream, chocolate, ½ cup	7
Ice cream, chocolate chip, ½ cup	8
Ice cream, chocolate chip cookie dough, ½ cup	8
Ice cream, coffee, ½ cup	7
Ice cream, cookies & cream, ½ cup	8

	SmartPoints™ value
Ice cream, extra creamy vanilla, ½ cup	7
Ice cream, French vanilla, ½ cup	7
Ice cream, homemade vanilla, ½ cup	7
Ice cream, lactose free, vanilla, ½ cup	7
Ice cream, light, chocolate, lactose free, ½ cup	5
Ice cream, mint chocolate chip, ½ cup	8
Ice cream, natural vanilla, ½ cup	6
Ice cream, rocky road, ½ cup	8
Ice cream, strawberry, ½ cup	6
Ice cream, vanilla, ½ cup	6
Ice cream, vanilla, chocolate, ½ cup	7
Ice cream, vanilla, chocolate, strawberry, ½ cup	7

Breyers Blasts!

Frozen dairy dessert, Girl Scouts samoas, ½ cup	7
Frozen dairy dessert, heath milk chocolate English toffee, ½ cup	7
Frozen dairy dessert, oreo cookies & cream chocolate, ½ cup	6
Frozen dairy dessert, thin mints, ½ cup	7
Frozen dairy dessert, waffle cone with Hershey's semi-sweet chocolate chips, ½ cup	7
Ice cream, cookies & cream, oreo, ½ cup	7
Ice cream, milk chocolate Reese's peanut butter cups, ½ cup	8
Ice cream, snickers caramel swirl chunk, ½ cup	8
M&M's chocolate light ice cream, ½ cup	7
The original brand creamsicle frozen dairy dessert, ½ cup	5

	SmartPoints™ value
Breyers Carb Smart	
Frozen dairy dessert, chocolate, ½ cup	4
Frozen dairy dessert, vanilla, ½ cup	4
Fudge bar, 1 bar (56 g)	4
Ice cream bar, almond bar, 1 bar (56 g)	8
Ice cream bars, 1 bar (55 g)	9
Breyers Gelato Indulgences	
Raspberry cheesecake, ½ cup	8
Triple chocolate, ½ cup	8
Vanilla caramel ice cream, ½ cup	9
Breyers No Sugar Added	
Salted caramel swirl frozen dairy dessert, ½ cup	4
Ice cream, extra creamy, no sugar added, butter pecan, ½ cup	4
Ice cream, fat free, creamy vanilla, ½ cup	4
Ice cream, fat free, French chocolate, ½ cup	4
Ice cream, light, creamy vanilla, ½ cup	6
Ice cream, light, no sugar added, vanilla, ½ cup	4
Ice cream, reduced fat, no sugar added, vanilla, chocolate, strawberry, ½ cup	4
Carvel	
Ice cream cake, celebration, 1 serving (118 ml)	9
Country Fresh	
Fudge bars, 1 bar (74 ml)	4
Creamsicle	
Cream bars, original, low fat, orange, raspberry, 1 bar (74 ml)	5
Dean's	
Ice cream, moose tracks, ½ cup	9

Desserts, Cakes, Candy & Cookies

Ice Cream (cont'd)

SmartPoints™ value

Diana's

Banana babies, dark chocolate, 1 piece (60 g)	5

Dole

Banana dippers with almonds covered in dark chocolate, 4 slices (48 g)	5
Vanilla or chocolate ice cream with dark chocolate, 5 pieces (88 g)	16

Dove Miniatures

Ice cream bars, flavor collection, 5 pieces (118.33 g)	16

Drumstick

Ice cream cone, vanilla caramel, 1 drumstick (136 ml)	17
Ice cream cone, vanilla fudge, 1 drumstick (136 ml)	17
Sundae cone, the original, vanilla, 1 drumstick (93 g)	13
Sundae cones, vanilla, 1 drumstick (93 g)	13
Sundae ice cream cones, fudge sundae, 1 cone (127 ml)	15

Drumstick Lil' Drums

Frozen dairy dessert cones, assorted, snack size, 1 cone (45 g)	6

Eating Right

Fudge bars, 1 bar (76 g)	5
Ice cream bars, dark chocolate raspberry, 1 bar (36 ml)	4
Ice cream bars, English toffee crunch, 1 bar (35 ml)	4
Ice cream sandwiches, low fat, vanilla and chocolate, 1 sandwich (68 g)	5

Edy's Grand

Chocolate ice cream, ½ cup	7
Mint chocolate chip ice cream, ½ cup	8
Vanilla bean ice cream, ½ cup	7
Vanilla rich and creamy ice cream, ½ cup	7

Edy's Limited Edition

Peppermint wonderland grand ice cream, ½ cup	7

Edy's Slow Churned

Butter pecan light ice cream, ½ cup	5
Caramel delight light ice cream, ½ cup	5
Chocolate chip light ice cream, ½ cup	6
Chocolate light ice cream, ½ cup	5
Coffee light ice cream, ½ cup	5
Cookie dough light ice cream, ½ cup	6
Cookies 'n cream light ice cream, ½ cup	5
Double fudge brownie light ice cream, ½ cup	6
French silk light ice cream, ½ cup	7
French vanilla light ice cream, ½ cup	5
Fudge tracks light ice cream, ½ cup	6
Mint chocolate chip light ice cream, ½ cup	6
Mint cookie crunch light ice cream, ½ cup	5
Mud pie light ice cream, ½ cup	5
Neapolitan light ice cream, ½ cup	5
Nestlé drumstick light ice cream, ½ cup	6
Peanut butter cup light ice cream, ½ cup	6
S'mores light ice cream, ½ cup	6
Strawberry light ice cream, ½ cup	5
The original rocky road light ice cream, ½ cup	5
Vanilla bean light ice cream, ½ cup	5

Edy's Slow Churned No Sugar Added

Butter pecan light ice cream, ½ cup	4
Fudge tracks light ice cream, ½ cup	4
Mint chocolate chip light ice cream, ½ cup	5
Neapolitan light ice cream, ½ cup	3
Triple chocolate light ice cream, ½ cup	4
Vanilla bean light ice cream, ½ cup	4
Vanilla light ice cream, ½ cup	4

Edy's Slow Churned Yogurt Blends

Cultured key lime pie frozen dairy dessert, ½ cup	6
Vanilla frozen dairy dessert, ½ cup	5

Enlightened

Ice cream bars, low fat, coffee, 1 bar (74 g)	2
Ice cream bars, low fat, fudge, 1 bar (74 g)	2

Enlightened The Good-For-You Ice Cream

Peanut butter low fat ice cream bars, 1 bar (73 g)	2

Fat Boy

Ice cream sandwich, premium vanilla, 3 oz	9

Fit & Active

Chocolate fudge ice cream bar, 1 bar (76 g)	5
Cookies and cream ice cream sandwich, 1 sandwich (71 g)	6

Fit & Active Sundae Shoppe

Mint ice cream sandwich, 1 sandwich (78 g)	6

Friendly's

100 calories fudgealicious bar, 1 bar (67 g)	5
Premium ice cream, mint chocolate chip, ½ cup	7
Premium ice cream, vanilla, ½ cup	7

Friendly's Smooth Churned

Ice cream, light, vanilla, ½ cup	5
Light ice cream, chocolate chip cookie dough, ½ cup	6
Light ice cream, mint chocolate chip, ½ cup	6
Light ice cream, purely pistachio, ½ cup	5

Fudgsicle

Fudge bars, low fat, the original, 1 bar (65 g)	5
Fudge bars, original, 1 pop (43 g)	3
Fudge pops, low fat, the original, 1 bar (43 g)	3
Original fudge bar, 1 bar (74 ml)	5
Original fudge bar, fat free, 1 piece (52 ml)	3

Good Humor

Ice cream bar, strawberry shortcake, 1 bar (83 g)	10
Ice cream bars, birthday cake, 1 bar (47 g)	6
Ice cream bars, chocolate eclair, 1 each (89 ml)	7
Ice cream bars, strawberry shortcake, 1 bar (60 g)	7

Graeter's

Ice cream, black raspberry chocolate chip, ½ cup	14

Great Value

Ice cream cones, mini, chocolate dipped, 1 cone (44 g)	6
Ice cream cups, chocolate & vanilla, 1 unit (49 g)	5
Ice cream cups, vanilla, 1 unit (49 g)	5

Desserts, Cakes, Candy & Cookies

Desserts, Cakes, Candy & Cookies

	SmartPoints™ value
Ice cream sandwich, no sugar added, vanilla, 1 sandwich (64 g)	4
Ice cream sandwiches, 100 calorie minis, vanilla flavored, 1 sandwich (40 g)	4
Ice cream sandwiches, chocolate & vanilla flavored, 1 sandwich (60 g)	7
Ice cream sandwiches, vanilla flavored, 1 sandwich (60 g)	7
Ice cream, chocolate chip cookie dough, ½ cup	8
Haagen Dazs	
Gelato, sea salt caramel, 1 container (97 g)	12
Ice cream bars, vanilla milk chocolate almond, 1 bar (87 g)	14
Ice cream bars, vanilla milk chocolate almond, snack size, 1 bar (52 g)	9
Ice cream, all natural, chocolate peanut butter, ½ cup	15
Ice cream, butter pecan, ½ cup	13
Ice cream, caramel cone, ½ cup	16
Ice cream, chocolate, ½ cup	12
Ice cream, chocolate chocolate chip, ½ cup	14
Ice cream, chocolate peanut butter, 1 container (95 g)	14
Ice cream, coffee, ½ cup	12
Ice cream, dulce de leche caramel, ½ cup	14
Ice cream, vanilla, ½ cup	12
Ice cream, vanilla, Swiss almond, ½ cup	14
Hannaford	
Ice cream, cookies and cream, ½ cup	8
Healthy Choice	
Fudge bars, 1 bar (64 g)	3
Fudge bars, premium, 1 bar (74 ml)	3

	SmartPoints™ value
Premium ice cream bars, vanilla ice cream dipped in fudge, 1 bar (74 ml)	3
Premium mocha swirl bars, 1 bar (74 ml)	5
Hood	
Ice cream sandwiches, mini, vanilla flavored, 1 sandwich (31 g)	4
Hood Hoodsie Cups	
Vanilla and chocolate ice cream, 1 cup	5
Joy	
Classic waffle cones, 1 cone (16.58 g)	3
Sugar cones, old-fashioned, 1 cone (142 g)	2
Kirkland Signature	
Super premium vanilla ice cream, ½ cup	14
Klondike	
Ice cream bar, caramel pretzel, 1 bar (85 g)	14
Ice cream bar, dark chocolate, 1 bar (86 g)	13
Ice cream bar, double chocolate, 1 bar (86 g)	13
Ice cream bar, heath, 1 bar (74 g)	12
Ice cream bar, krunch, 1 bar (83 g)	13
Ice cream bar, mint chocolate chip, 1 bar (78 g)	13
Ice cream bar, oreo, cookies & cream, 1 bar (75 g)	13
Ice cream bar, Reese's, 1 bar (76 g)	13
Ice cream bars, neopolitan, 1 bar (86 g)	13
Ice cream bars, no sugar added, vanilla, 1 bar (78 g)	8
Ice cream bars, the original, 1 bar (86 g)	13

	SmartPoints™ value
Ice cream cookie sandwiches, mrs. fields, 1 sandwich (67 g)	10
Ice cream sandwich cookies, oreo, 1 sandwich (69 g)	8
Ice cream sandwiches, classic vanilla, 1 sandwich (73 g)	8
Ice cream, rocky road, 1 bar (77 g)	12
Klondike 100 Calorie	
Ice cream sandwiches, vanilla, 1 sandwich (46 g)	4
Klondike Kandy Bars	
Fudge krunch ice cream bar, 1 bar (54 g)	9
Klondike Slim-a-Bear	
Chocolate low fat ice cream bars, 100 calorie bars, chocolate fudge, 1 bar (104 ml)	5
Kroger	
Deluxe ice cream, neopolitan, ½ cup	7
Kroger Arctic Blasters	
Fudge bars, 1 bar (68 g)	5
Fudge bars, fat free, 1 bar (67 g)	4
Kroger Deluxe	
Ice cream, vividly vanilla, ½ cup	7
Kroger Deluxe Churned	
Ice cream, light, artisan vanilla bean, ½ cup	5
Ice cream, light, death by chocolate, ½ cup	6
Ice cream, light, French silk, ½ cup	7
Ice cream, light, fun munch cookies n' cream, ½ cup	6
Ice cream, light, mint chocolate chip, ½ cup	6
Ice cream, light, vividly vanilla, ½ cup	5
Ice cream, reduced fat, no sugar added, cherry cordial, ½ cup	5

	SmartPoints™ value
Ice cream, reduced fat, no sugar added, peanut butter fudge swirl, ½ cup	5
Ice cream, reduced fat, no sugar added, vividly vanilla, ½ cup	4
Kroger Ice Cream Sammies	
Ice cream sandwiches, mini, vanilla, 1 bar (41 g)	5
Ice cream sandwiches, vanilla, 1 sandwich (63 g)	7
Lactaid	
Ice cream, lactose free, chocolate, ½ cup	7
Ice cream, lactose free, vanilla, ½ cup	7
Lucerne	
Ice cream, low fat, cookies 'n cream, ½ cup	6
Ice cream, low fat, vanilla flavored, ½ cup	5
Magnum	
Ice cream bars, double caramel, 1 bar (95 g)	18
Ice cream bars, double caramel, mini, 2 bars (114 g)	19
Ice cream bars, mini, almond, 2 bars (91 g)	16
Ice cream bars, mini, classic, 2 bars (87 g)	15
Mini classic white ice cream bars, 2 bars (87 ml)	15
Magnum Infinity	
Ice cream bars, chocolate, 1 bar (84 g)	13
Mayfield	
Dessert bars, brown cow juniors, 1 bar (37 g)	5
Fudge bars, 1 bar (65 g)	4
Ice cream sandwiches, mini, 1 sandwich (34 g)	4
Ice cream, moose tracks, ½ cup	9

Desserts, Cakes, Candy & Cookies

Desserts, Cakes, Candy & Cookies

	SmartPoints™ value
Mochi	
Ice cream, chocolate, 1 ½ oz	5
Ice cream, green tea, 2 pieces (85 g)	10
Ice cream, mango, 2 pieces (85 g)	10
Ice cream, strawberry, 1 ½ oz	5
Nestlé Drumstick	
Drumstick, vanilla, 1 drumstick (136 g)	16
Vanilla fudge crunch dipped sundae cones, 1 cone (94 g)	14
Oreo	
Premium ice cream cake (serves 12), 1 serving (76 g)	10
Private Selection	
Ice cream, cookies and cream, ½ cup	10
Publix Premium	
Ice cream, light, no sugar added, creamy churned style, vanilla, ½ cup	4
Ice cream, lowfat, Denali original moose tracks, ½ cup	7
Reese's	
Ice cream cup, peanut butter, 1 bar (70 g)	13
Safeway Select	
Ice cream cake, vanilla ice cream & chocolate cake, 1 serving (78 g)	11
Skinny Cow	
Cookies 'n dough ice cream bars, 1 bar (48 g)	8
Double caramel swirl ice cream bars, 1 bar (67 g)	8
Fudge bars, low fat, 1 bar (74 g)	4
Ice cream bars, caramel truffle, 1 bar (63 g)	5
Ice cream bars, chocolate truffle, 1 bar (64 g)	5
Ice cream bars, French vanilla truffle, 1 bar (63 g)	5

	SmartPoints™ value
Ice cream bars, low fat, chocolate truffle, value pack, 1 bar (64 g)	5
Ice cream cones, chocolate mint ganache, 1 cone (72 g)	7
Ice cream cones, chocolate mousse ganache, 1 cone (72 g)	7
Ice cream cone, low fat, chocolate with fudge, 1 cone (75 g)	7
Ice cream cone, low fat, mint with fudge, 1 cone (75 g)	7
Ice cream cone, low fat, vanilla with caramel, 1 cone (75 g)	7
Ice cream sandwich, low fat, vanilla, 1 sandwich (71 g)	6
Ice cream sandwich, low fat, vanilla & chocolate combo, 1 sandwich (71 g)	6
Ice cream sandwiches, low fat, chocolate peanut butter, 1 sandwich (71 g)	6
Ice cream sandwiches, low fat, cookies 'n cream, 1 sandwich (72 g)	6
Ice cream sandwiches, low fat, mint, 1 sandwich (71 g)	6
Ice cream sandwiches, low fat, no sugar added, vanilla, 1 sandwich (71 g)	4
Ice cream sandwiches, low fat, vanilla, 1 sandwich (71 g)	6
Ice cream sandwiches, low fat, vanilla and cookies 'n cream, 1 sandwich (71 g)	6
Ice cream, low fat, caramel cone, 1 container (99 g)	8
Ice cream, low fat, cookies 'n cream, 1 container (94 g)	7
Low fat ice cream bars, cookies and cream, 1 bar (118.3 ml)	5
Low fat vanilla and chocolate ice cream sandwich (variety pack), 1 sandwich (71 g)	6
Low fat vanilla ice cream sandwich, 1 sandwich (71 g)	6

	SmartPoints™ value
Salted caramel pretzel ice cream bars, 1 bar (50 g)	8
Skinny carb ice cream bars, fudge, 1 bar (118.3 ml)	5
Truffle, cookies 'n cream, 1 bar (66 g)	5
Vanilla almond crunch ice cream bars, 1 bar (66 g)	8
Skinny Cow Limited Editions	
Snickerdoodle ice cream sandwiches, 1 sandwich (71 g)	6
Snickers	
Ice cream bar, 1 bar (50 g)	9
Ice cream, vanilla with snickers, ½ cup	9
So Delicious Minis	
Frozen dessert, non-dairy, sandwiches, vanilla, 1 sandwich (37 g)	4
Non-dairy frozen dessert, coconut sandwich, 1 sandwich (37 ml)	4
Vanilla flavored coconut milk non dairy frozen dessert bar, 1 bar (50 g)	7
Gelato, Tahitian vanilla bean, ½ cup	10
Talenti Gelato Pop	
Double dark chocolate gelato pop, 1 bar (75 g)	9
Sea salt caramel ice cream sticks, 1 bar (78 g)	9
Tillamook	
Premium ice cream, vanilla bean, ½ cup	7
Trader Joe's	
12 mini mint ice cream mouthfuls, 2 sandwiches (40 g)	5
4 low fat ice cream sandwiches, 1 sandwich (72 g)	6
Hold the cone! mini ice cream cones, chocolate, 1 cone (21 g)	3
Hold the cone! mini ice cream cones, vanilla, 1 cone (29 g)	3

	SmartPoints™ value
Ice cream bon bons, 1 bon bon (18 g)	3
Salted caramel gelato, ½ cup	9
Sublime ice cream sandwiches, 1 sandwich (148 ml)	21
Turkey Hill	
Ice cream, fat free, Dutch chocolate, ½ cup	2
Ice cream, fat free, vanilla bean, ½ cup	3
Ice cream, light, Denali original, moose tracks, ½ cup	4
Ice cream, premium, original recipe, butter pecan, ½ cup	7
Ice cream, premium, original recipe, choco mint chip, ½ cup	8
Ice cream, premium, original recipe, chocolate chip cookie dough, ½ cup	8
Ice cream, premium, original recipe, chocolate peanut butter cup, ½ cup	8
Ice cream, premium, original recipe, cookies 'n cream, ½ cup	7
Ice cream, premium, original recipe, double dunker, ½ cup	8
Ice cream, premium, original recipe, Dutch chocolate, ½ cup	7
Ice cream, premium, original recipe, French vanilla, ½ cup	7
Ice cream, premium, original recipe, vanilla & chocolate, ½ cup	7
Ice cream, premium, original vanilla, ½ cup	7
Ice cream, vanilla bean, ½ cup	7
Turkey Hill Light Recipe	
Ice cream, chocolate chip cookie dough, ½ cup	6
Ice cream, chocolate, Denali nutty moose tracks, ½ cup	6
Ice cream, Denali original moose tracks, ½ cup	6

Desserts, Cakes, Candy & Cookies

Desserts, Cakes, Candy & Cookies

	SmartPoints™ value
Ice cream, extreme cookies 'n cream, ½ cup	6
Ice cream, vanilla bean, ½ cup	5
Turkey Hill Philadelphia Style	
Ice cream, all natural recipe, mint chocolate chip, ½ cup	8
Twix	
Ice cream bar, 1 bar (75 g)	14
Wegman's	
Ice cream sandwiches, light, vanilla, 1 sandwich (61 g)	7
Ice cream sandwiches, vanilla, 1 sandwich (61 g)	7
Wonka Push-Up	
Orange frozen dairy dessert pop, 1 pop (52 g)	4
Yoplait	
Strawberry flavored with granola Greek frozen yogurt bar, 1 bar (52 g)	6

Ice Cream Cones

	SmartPoints™ value
Keebler	
Cones, sugar, 1 cone (13 g)	2
Cones, waffles, 1 cone (12 g)	2
Kroger	
Cones, sugar, 1 cone (13 g)	2
Cones, waffle, 1 cone (22 g)	3

Ices, Sherbets, Sorbets & Frozen Fruit Bars

	SmartPoints™ value
Almond Dream	
Frozen dessert bites, non-dairy, vanilla, 15 pieces (67 g)	12
Blue Bell	
All natural fruit bars, 1 bar (69 g)	4
Bullets, sugar free, 1 bar (56 g)	0
Fruit bars, ice, strawberry, 1 bar (67 g)	4
Fruit bars, mixed berries, 1 bar (68 g)	5

	SmartPoints™ value
Mixed berries sherbet, ½ cup	6
Rainbow sherbet, ½ cup	7
Budget Saver	
Monster pops, slushed, cherry-pineapple, 3 ½ fl oz pop	4
Twin pops, assorted, 2 ⅓ oz	3
Twin pops, banana, 2 ⅓ fl oz twin pop	3
Creamsicle	
Ice cream pop, orange & raspberry sherbet, 1 pop (43 g)	3
Diana's	
Banana babies, dark chocolate, 1 piece (60 g)	5
Banana babies, milk chocolate, 1 piece (60 g)	6
Dreyer's Outshine	
Cranberry ice bars, 1 bar (84 g)	4
Edy's Outshine	
Blueberry medley fruit and veggie bars, 1 bar (76 g)	4
Coconut waters with banana fruit bar, 1 bar (83 g)	3
Coconut waters with pineapple fruit bar, 1 bar (84 g)	4
Creamy coconut fruit bar, 1 bar (87 g)	6
Grape fruit bar, 1 bar (84 g)	4
Lemon fruit bar, 1 bar (85 g)	4
Lime fruit bar, 1 bar (46 g)	2
Mango fruit bar, 1 bar (85 g)	5
Peach fruit bar, 1 bar (86 g)	5
Pineapple fruit bar, 1 bar (85 g)	5
Pomegranate fruit bar, 1 bar (77 g)	4
Raspberry fruit bar, 1 bar (84 g)	5
Strawberry fruit bar, 1 bar (85 g)	4
Strawberry rhubarb fruit and veggie ice bar, 1 bar (46 g)	2

Tangerine carrot fruit and veggie bars, 1 bar (76 g)	4
Tangerine fruit bar, 1 bar (85 g)	5
Edy's Outshine Seasonal Picks	
Peach fruit bar, 1 bar (86 g)	5
Fruttare	
Black cherry ice bars, 1 bar (57 g)	3
Frozen dessert bars, banana and milk, 1 bar (72 g)	6
Frozen dessert bars, coconut and milk, 1 bar (72 g)	7
Frozen dessert bars, strawberry and milk, 1 bar (73 g)	7
Ice bars, mango, 1 bar (53 g)	3
Ice bars, strawberry, 1 bar (56 g)	4
Great Value	
Sherbet, fat free, orange, ½ cup	6
Sherbet, fat free, rainbow, ½ cup	6
Haagen Dazs	
Sorbet, all natural, zesty lemon, ½ cup	7
Sorbet, mango, ½ cup	9
Sorbet, raspberry, ½ cup	7
ICEE	
Freeze, blue raspberry, 1 cup	5
Freeze, cherry, 4 fl oz cup	5
Freeze, wild cherry, 1 cup	5
Kroger Deluxe	
Sherbet, fat free, rainbow, ½ cup	6
Lindy's	
Italian ice, lemon, 1 cup	6
Italian ice, orange, 1 cup	5
Italian ice, strawberry & watermelon, 1 cup	5
Luigi's	
Mango tropical real Italian ice, 1 tube (118 ml)	5
Real Italian ice, blue raspberry, watermelon, 1 cup	9
Real Italian ice, cherry, 1 cup	7

Real Italian ice, lemon, 1 cup	5
Real Italian ice, lemon, cherry, 1 cup	2
Real Italian ice, lemon, strawberry, 1 cup	5
Market Pantry	
Fat free fudge bars, 1 bar (75 g)	5
Mayfield	
Banana pops, 1 pop (56 g)	2
Philly Swirl	
Italian ice, swirl stix, assorted flavors, frozen bar, 1 bar (43 g)	3
Popsicle	
A-C-E juice pops, assorted flavors, 1 piece (47 ml)	2
All natural real fruit juice bars, 1 bar (52 ml)	3
Big stick, cherry pineapple swirl, 1 piece (80 g)	4
Firecracker ice pop, 1 pop (44 g)	2
Flavored ice pops, assorted, 1 piece (53 g)	2
Ice bars, orange, grape & cherry, 1 bar (52 ml)	3
Ice pop, red classics, 1 pop (51 g)	2
Ice pops, assorted, 1 pop (53 g)	2
Ice pops, banana mania!, 1 pop (53 g)	2
Ice pops, jolly rancher, assorted flavors, 1 pop (53 g)	2
Ice pops, rainbow, 1 piece (53 g)	2
Ice pops, sugar free, assorted, 1 pop (50 g)	0
Ice pops, sugar free, orange, cherry, grape, 1 pop (50 g)	0
Ice pops, sugar free, tropicals, 1 piece (51 g)	0
Popsicle Sugar Free	
Ice pops, tropicals, 1 piece (48.75 ml)	0

Desserts, Cakes, Candy & Cookies

SmartPoints™ value

Private Selection

Fruit bar, premium, strawberry, 1 bar (86 g)	5

So Delicious

Non-dairy frozen dessert, coconut milk, chocolate, ½ cup	5

So Delicious Minis

Frozen dessert, non-dairy, almond milk, mocha almond fudge, 1 bar (52 g)	6
Non-dairy frozen dessert, coconut almond, 1 bar (52 g)	8
Non-dairy frozen dessert,low fat, vanilla sandwich, 1 sandwich (68 ml)	4

Sobe Lifewater

Pacific coconut frozen bar, 1 bar (48 g)	2

Talenti

Sorbetto, roman raspberry, ½ cup	7

Trader Joe's

12 classic lemon bars, 1 bar (25 g)	4
Gone bananas!, 4 pieces (43 g)	7

Pies

Edwards

Pie, Hershey's creme, 1 serving (120 g)	22
Pie, turtle, ⅛ pie (108 g)	19

Edwards Singles

Pie, chocolate creme, made with Hershey's, 1 piece (76 g)	14
Pie, key lime, 1 piece (92 g)	17
Pie, turtle, 1 piece (77 g)	14

Hostess Snack Classics

Fruit pie, apple, 1 pie (128 g)	22
Fruit pie, cherry, 1 pie (128 g)	22

SmartPoints™ value

Jell-O Temptations

Pie snacks, double chocolate pie flavor, 1 container (95 g)	5
Pie snacks, key lime pie, 1 container (95 g)	4
Pie snacks, lemon meringue pie, 1 container (95 g)	4

Marie Callender's

Chocolate satin pie (serves 6), 1 serving (132 g)	26
Pie, banana cream, 1 serving (107 g)	13
Pie, coconut cream, 1 serving (107 g)	14
Pie, Dutch apple, 1 serving (128 g)	14
Pie, key lime, 1 serving (102 g)	16
Pie, lemon meringue, 1 serving (110 g)	12
Razzleberry pie (serves 9), 1 serving (126 g)	14
Very berry blackberry pie, 1 serving (119 g)	13

Mrs. Smith's

Apple pie (serves 6), 1 serving (128 g)	14

Mrs. Smith's Classic

Dutch apple crumb pie (serves 6), 1 serving (128 g)	14

Mrs. Smith's Singles

Pie, mixed berry, 1 slice (99 g)	9

Pepperidge Farm

Turnovers, puff pastry, apple, 1 turnover (89 g)	11

Trader Joe's

Apple pie with loverly lattice crust (⅙ of pie), 1 serving (133 g)	10
Cherry pie (serves 6), 1 serving (94 g)	12

Pudding & Pudding Mixes

Aunty's

Steamed puddings, sticky toffee, 1 container (100 g)	13

Fiber One 90 Calorie

Instant chocolate pudding mix, ½ package (17 g)	1

Hunt's

Pudding, sugar free, chocolate, 1 pudding cup (99 g)	3

Hunt's Snack Pack

Fat free pudding, vanilla, 1 cup	4
Pudding cups, chocolate vanilla, 3 ½ oz	6
Pudding, reduced calorie, vanilla, 1 pudding cup (99 g)	2

Jell-O

Cool and classic strawberries and creme pudding snacks, 1 pudding cup (110 g)	6
Fat free chocolate pudding snacks, 1 snack (110 g)	5
Fat free chocolate vanilla swirls pudding snacks, 1 snack (110 g)	5
Instant pudding & pie filling, oreo cookies 'n creme, ¼ package (31 g)	6
Instant reduced calorie pudding & pie filling, sugar free/fat free, banana cream, ¼ package (6.3 g)	1
Ooey gooey chocolatey fudge brownie pudding snack, 1 pudding cup (110 g)	6
Pudding & pie filling, instant, banana cream, ¼ package (25 g)	5
Pudding & pie filling, instant, chocolate flavor, ¼ cup	5
Pudding & pie filling, instant, chocolate fudge, ¼ package (26.8 g)	5

Pudding & pie filling, instant, fat free, sugar free, disney pixar toy story, unprepared, 1 serving (8 g)	1
Pudding & pie filling, instant, pistachio, ¼ package (25 g)	5
Pudding & pie filling, instant, pumpkin spice, seasonal release, /4 package (25 g)	5
Pudding & pie filling, instant, reduced calorie, vanilla, ¼ package (8 g)	1
Pudding snacks, chocolate vanilla swirls, 1 snack (110 g)	6
Pudding snacks, oreo dirt cup, 1 snack (96 g)	6
Pudding snacks, original, butterscotch, 1 container (110 g)	6
Pudding snacks, original, chocolate flavor, 1 snack (110 g)	6
Pudding snacks, original, chocolate vanilla swirls, 1 snack (110 g)	6
Pudding snacks, original, oreo cookies, 1 container (110 g)	6
Pudding snacks, original, rice pudding, vanilla, 1 container (103 g)	5
Pudding snacks, original, vanilla, 1 snack (110 g)	6
Pudding snacks, reduced calorie, Boston cream pie, 1 snack (106 g)	2
Pudding snacks, reduced calorie, dark chocolate flavor, 1 snack (106 g)	2
Pudding snacks, reduced calorie, rice pudding, creme brulee, 1 snack (106 g)	2
Pudding snacks, reduced calorie, rice pudding, original, 1 snack (106 g)	2
Pudding snacks, reduced calorie, rice, creme brulee, 1 container (103 g)	2

Desserts, Cakes, Candy & Cookies

	SmartPoints™ value
Pudding snacks, reduced calorie, rice, original, 1 container (103 g)	2
Pudding snacks, reduced calorie, sugar free, chocolate flavor, 8 pack, 1 snack (103 g)	2
Pudding snacks, reduced calorie, sugar free, chocolate vanilla swirl, 8 pack, 1 snack (103 g)	2
Pudding snacks, reduced calorie, sugar free, double chocolate flavor, 1 snack (106 g)	2
Pudding snacks, reduced calorie, sugar free, rice pudding, cinnamon, 1 snack (106 g)	2
Pudding snacks, rice pudding, original, cinnamon, 1 container (103 g)	5
Pudding snacks, s'more, 1 snack (93 g)	6
Pudding snacks, tapioca, 1 container (110 g)	5
Pudding, tapioca, original, 1 snack (110 g)	6
Pumpkin spice cheesecake snack, 1 snack (92 g)	6
Reduced calorie sugar free chocolate vanilla swirls pudding, 1 pudding cup (103 g)	2
Sugar free dark chocolate pudding snacks, 1 snack (103 g)	2
Sugar free double chocolate pudding snack, 1 snack (103 g)	2

Jell-O 100 Calorie Packs

Pudding snacks, chocolate flavor, 1 snack (113 g)	5
Pudding snacks, chocolate, chocolate vanilla swirls, 1 snack (113 g)	5
Pudding snacks, fat free, chocolate vanilla swirls, 1 snack (113 g)	5
Pudding snacks, tapioca, 1 snack (113 g)	5

	SmartPoints™ value

Jell-O 60 Calorie, Sugar Free

Boston cream pie pudding snacks, 1 snack (103 g)	2

Jell-O Chocolate Lovers

Pudding snacks, reduced calorie, dark chocolate desire, 1 snack (106 g)	2
Pudding snacks, reduced calorie, milk chocolate dream, 1 snack (106 g)	2

Jell-O Cook & Serve

Pudding & pie filling, chocolate, ¼ package (25 g)	4
Reduced calorie pudding & pie filling, sugar free/fat free, chocolate, unprepared, 1 serving (9 g)	1
Reduced calorie pudding & pie filling, sugar free/fat free, vanilla, ¼ package (5.5 g)	1
Tapioca fat free pudding and pie filling mix, ¼ package (21 g)	5

Jell-O Live Active

Milk chocolate bliss sugar free pudding snacks, 1 snack (103 g)	2

Jell-O Reduced Calorie

Pudding snacks, chocolate flavor, 1 snack (103 g)	2
Pudding snacks, dulce de leche, 1 snack (103 g)	2
Pudding snacks, vanilla, 1 snack (103 g)	2

Jell-O Temptations

Dessert mix, chocolate truffle indulgence, ⅛ package (21 g)	5

Kozy Shack

All natural pudding, original rice, 1 snack cup (113 g)	6
Kozy shack lactose free dairy pudding rice snack cups, 1 snack cup (113 g)	5
Original rice pudding, 1 pudding cup (118 g)	6

Pudding, old fashioned tapioca, ½ cup	6
Pudding, original rice, ½ cup	6
Pudding, real chocolate, ½ cup	7
Pudding, tapioca, 1 cup	6
Kozy Shack Simply Well	
Pudding, dark chocolate, 1 cup	4
Rice pudding no sugar added (gluten free), 4 oz	3
Tapioca pudding no suagr added (gluten free), 4 oz	3
Señor Rico	
Mexican style rice pudding, ½ cup	7
Snack Pack	
Butterscotch pudding, 1 container (92 g)	5
Chocolate fudge pudding, 1 pudding cup (92 g)	5
Chocolate pudding, 1 snack cup (92 g)	5
Fat free tapioca pudding, 1 container (92 g)	4
Pudding cups, chocolate vanilla, 1 pudding cup (92 g)	6
Pudding cups, chocolate, fat free, 1 pudding cup (92 g)	4
Pudding cups, chocolate, sugar free, 1 pudding cup (92 g)	2
Pudding cups, lemon, 1 pudding cup (92 g)	6
Pudding cups, tapioca, 1 pudding cup (92 g)	5
Pudding cups, vanilla, 1 pudding cup (92 g)	5

Pudding cups, vanilla, sugar free, 1 pudding cup (92 g)	2
Pudding, banana cream pie, 1 pudding cup (99 g)	5
Pudding, chocolate caramel, 1 cup	6
Pudding, chocolate cupcake, 1 pudding cup (92 g)	5
Pudding, chocolate fudge & milk chocolate swirl, family pack, 1 pudding cup (99 g)	6
Pudding, ice cream sandwich, 1 pudding cup (92 g)	6
Pudding, milk chocolate variety, 1 cup	6
Pudding, sugar free, caramel, 1 pudding cup (92 g)	2
Pudding, vanilla, chocolate, family pack, 1 cup	5
Sugar free chocolate pudding cup, 1 pudding cup (92 g)	2
Snack Pack Bakery Shop	
Pudding, banana cream pie, 1 pudding cup (92 g)	5
Snack Pack Pudding	
Pudding, vanilla and chocolate, family pack, 1 cup	6
The Chia Co.	
Vanilla bean chia pod, 1 container (170 g)	8
Wegman's	
Pudding, sugar free, chocolate, 1 snack (106 g)	2
Pudding, sugar free, chocolate vanilla swirl, 1 snack (106 g)	2
Pudding, sugar free, dark chocolate with calcium, 1 snack (106 g)	2
Zensoy	
Pudding, chocolate, 1 container (108 g)	5

Desserts, Cakes, Candy & Cookies

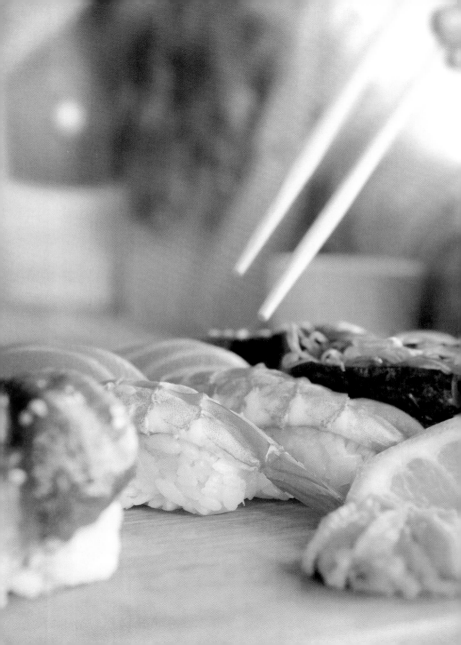

fish
& Seafood

Barramundi

Giant

Barramundi fillets, 4 oz	0

Calamari

Kroger

Calamari rings, 15 pieces (90 g)	6

Clams

Matlaw's

Clams casino, 2 clams (37 g)	2
Stuffed clams, 1 (62 g)	3

Sea Pak Shrimp & Seafood Co.

Clam strips, oven crispy, 3 oz	7

Snows

Clams, chopped, in clam juice, ¼ cup	0

Cod

Copper River Seafoods Fisherman Favorites

Zesty grill wild Alaska cod portions, 1 portion (170 g)	5

Goya

Salted codfish, bacalao, pre-priced, 2 oz	0

Icelandic

All natural wild caught cod loins, 1 fillet (140 g)	1
Beer battered cod fillets, 2 fillets (112 g)	7

Kroger

Wild-caught cod fillets, 4 oz	1

Sea Cuisine

Cod, loins, Atlantic, premium, 3 oz	1
Cod, potato crusted, 1 fillet (140 g)	6
Cod, potato crusted, 1 fillet (140 g)	6

Sea Cuisine Chef Inspired Recipe

Cod, breaded, 1 fillet (85 g)	6

Trader Joe's

Oven ready breaded cod fillets, 2 pieces (149 g)	7

Trident Seafoods

Cod, pubhouse battered, 2 pieces (85 g)	3

Crab

Aquamar

Imitation crab meat, ½ cup	3

Kroger Crab Select

Flake style imitation crab meat, ¼ cup	2
Leg style imitation crab meat, 3 pieces (90 g)	2

Louis Kemp Seafood Co. Crab Deli Delights

Chesapeake bay flake style crabmeat, ½ cup	2
Crab delights, flake style, ½ cup	3
Crab delights, leg style, 3 legs (91 g)	2
Imitation crabmeat, flake style, 4 oz	2
Imitation king crabmeat, flake style, ½ cup	2
Leg style imitation crab, 3 (85 g)	2

Mrs. Friday's

Immitation crab meat, chunk style, ⅔ cup	2

Omaha Steaks

King crab legs, 3 ½ oz	1

Original Rangoon

Crab rangoons, 2 pieces (57 g)	5

Pagoda Express

Crab rangoon, 5 pieces (85 g)	10

Private Selection

King crab, legs & claws, 6 oz	1

Seafest

Imitation crab meat, salad style, ½ cup	3

Trans Ocean

	SmartPoints™ value
Crab classic, chunk style, ½ cup	2
Crab classic, flake style, ½ cup	2
Crab classic, leg style, 3 pieces (90 g)	3
Crab supreme, flake style, ½ cup	2

Fish Cakes

Daily Chef Gourmet Foods

Handmade crab cakes, 1 (85 g)	5

Dockside Classics

Lobster cakes, gourmet, 3 oz	7

Phillips Seafood Restaurants

Crab cakes, Maryland style, 1 cake (85 g)	4
Salmon cakes, 1 cake (85 g)	5

Fish Sticks & Fillets

Dr. Praeger's

Fish sticks, lightly breaded, 3 sticks (81 g)	4

Fisher Boy

Fish sticks, 6 sticks (85 g)	6

Gorton's

Crunchy breaded fish fillets, southern fried country style, 2 fillets (104 g)	7
Fish fillets, battered, lemon pepper, 2 fillets (104 g)	9
Fish fillets, battered, skillet crisp tilapia, 1 fillet (99 g)	6
Fish fillets, battered, skillet crisp tilipia, 1 fillet (99 g)	5
Fish fillets, beer battered, 2 fillets (103 g)	8
Fish fillets, breaded, crunchy, 2 fillets (108 g)	8
Fish fillets, breaded, crunchy golden, 2 fillets (108 g)	8
Fish fillets, breaded, potato crunch, 2 fillets (103 g)	8

	SmartPoints™ value
Fish fillets, crispy battered, 2 fillets (108 g)	7
Fish fillets, crunchy breaded, 2 fillets (108 g)	8
Fish fillets, crunchy breaded, garlic and herb, 2 fillets (104 g)	7
Fish portions, value pack, 1 portion (70 g)	5
Fish sandwich fillets, 1 fillet (65 g)	5
Fish sticks, 6 sticks (107 g)	8
Fish sticks, 100% Alaska pollock, super crunchy, 6 sticks (91 g)	7
Fish sticks, crunchy, 6 sticks (94 g)	7
Fish sticks, value pack, 6 sticks (91 g)	7
Grilled fillets, Cajun blackened, 1 fillet (107 g)	1
Grilled fillets, garlic butter, 1 fillet (107 g)	1
Grilled fillets, Italian herb, 1 fillet (107 g)	1
Grilled fillets, lemon butter, 1 fillet (107 g)	1
Grilled fillets, lemon pepper, 1 fillet (107 g)	1
Tenders, beer battered, 3 pieces (95 g)	8

Gorton's Smart & Crunchy

Breaded fish fillets, 2 fillets (108 g)	6
Breaded fish sticks, 5 sticks (86 g)	6
Fish sticks, 100% wild-caught Alaska pollock, 5 sticks (86 g)	6

Gorton's Tenders

Fish fillets, original batter, 3 pieces (100 g)	7

Healthy Choice

Herb crusted fish, 1 meal (312 g)	8

Healthy Choice Complete Meals

Lemon pepper fish, 1 meal (303 g)	10

Fish & Seafood

Fish Sticks & Fillets (cont'd)

SmartPoints™ value

SmartPoints™ value

Lean Cuisine Culinary Collection

Lemon pepper fish, 1 package (255 g)	9
Parmesan crusted fish, 1 package (255 g)	9
Tortilla crusted fish, 1 package (226 g)	9

Mrs. Paul's

Beer battered fillets, 2 fillets (108 g)	7
Crunchy fish sticks, xtra large, 4 sticks (84 g)	5
Fish sandwich fillets, 1 fillet (85 g)	6
Fish sticks, crunchy, 6 sticks (95 g)	7

Mrs. Paul's 90 Calorie

Crunchy fish fillets, 1 fillet (50 g)	2

Stouffer's Homestyle Classics

Fish filet, 1 package (255 g)	12

Trader Joe's

Battered fish nuggets, 4 pieces (113 g)	5
Lightly breaded fish sticks reduced fat, 6 pieces (114 g)	6

Trident Seafoods

The ultimate fish stick, 3 pieces (85 g)	4

Van de Kamps

Crispy fish fillets, 2 fillets (110 g)	7
Fish fillets, beer battered, 2 fillets (108 g)	7
Fish sandwich fillets, 1 fillet (85 g)	6
Fish sticks, x-large crunchy, 4 sticks (84 g)	6

Flounder

Mrs. Paul's

Flounder fillets, lightly breaded, 1 fillet (75 g)	5

Treasures from the Sea by Odyssey Wild Alaska

Skinless boneless flounder, 4 oz	1

Haddock

Gorton's

Grilled haddock, signature grilled, 1 fillet (89 g)	1
Haddock fillets, crispy battered, 2 fillets (108 g)	10

Hake

Kirkland Signature

Wild caught hake loins, 5 oz	1

Lobster

Louis Kemp Seafood Co. Lobster Delights

Imitation lobster meat, chunk style, fat free, ½ cup	2
Imitation lobster meat, flake style, ½ cup	2

Omaha Steaks

Lobster tails (warm water), 6 oz	3

Trans Ocean Lobster Classic

Chunk style imitation lobster, ½ cup	2

Mahi Mahi

Kirkland Signature

Pacific wild mahi mahi, 4 oz	1

Trader Joe's

Mahi mahi burgers, 1 patty (91 g)	2

Mussels

Atlantic

Maine mussels, whole, shelled, ¼ cup	2

Bantry Bay

Mussels in a garlic butter sauce, 8 oz	4

Private Selection

Mussels, gourmet, natural, 10 mussels (226 g)	3

Fish & Seafood

Roland

Mussels, ⅓ cup	1
Mussels, in tomato sauce, ⅓ cup	1

Waterfront Bistro

Mussels, garlic butter sauce, 8 oz	4
Mussels, tomato & garlic sauce, 8 oz	3

Oysters

Chicken Of The Sea

Smoked oysters in oil, smoked, 1 can (106 g)	5

Salmon

Acme

Salmon, smoked nova, 2 slices (57 g)	1

Aqua Star

Wild pacific salmon, pre-portioned fillet, 4 oz	2

Bear & Wolf

Pink salmon, ¼ cup	1

Bumble Bee

Pink salmon, skinless & boneless, premium wild, ¼ cup	0

C. Wirthy & Co.

Blackened salmon, 1 fillet (142 g)	7
Blackened salmon, 1 fillet (170 g)	8
Salmon, atlantic, 1 fillet (170 g)	6

Chicken Of The Sea

Pink salmon, skinless & boneless, 1 pouch (74 g)	1
Salmon, pink, ¼ cup	1
Salmon, pink, in water, chunk style, ¼ cup	1
Salmon, smoked, 1 pouch (85 g)	2

Cuisine Solutions

Crab stuffed salmon fillets, lemon herb sauce, 1 entrée (210 g)	10

Gorton's

Grilled salmon, classic grilled, 1 fillet (89 g)	2
Grilled salmon, lemon butter, 1 fillet (89 g)	2

Gorton's Simply Bake

Salmon, roasted garlic & butter, 1 fillet (126 g)	2

Kirkland Signature

Atlantic salmon, 1 portion (196 g)	9
Wild Alaskan sockeye salmon, 1 piece (170 g)	6

Kroger

Wild caught pink salmon, 4 oz	2

Lean Cuisine Spa Collection

Salmon with basil, 1 package (272 g)	7

Morey's

Marinated wild Alaskan salmon, 1 fillet (170 g)	5

Morey's Fish Creations

Salmon, wild pacific, seasoned grill, 1 fillet (142 g)	5

Salmolux

Smoked salmon, nova lox, 3 oz	3

Sea Cuisine

Salmon, applewood smoked, fire roasted, 1 fillet (112 g)	4

Simply Balanced

Chipotle barbecue glazed salmon fillets, 1 fillet (126 g)	3
Sea salt & cracked pepper glazed salmon fillets, 1 fillet (126 g)	2

Trader Joe's

Premium salmon burgers, 1 patty (91 g)	2

Trident Seafoods

Burgers, Alaskan salmon, 1 piece (79 g)	3
Pacific salmon burgers, 1 piece (113 g)	3

Fish & Seafood

SmartPoints™ value

Waterfront Bistro

Salmon, blackened rubbed, 1 fillet (112 g)	3

Whole Foods

Wild caught Alaskan salmon burgers, 1 burger (91 g)	3

Sardines

Beach Cliff

Sardines in mustard sauce, 1 can (106 g)	3
Sardines in water, 1 can (92 g)	3

Bumble Bee

Sardines in water, 1 can drained (106 g)	3

Chicken Of The Sea

Sardines, in water, 1 can (106 g)	4

King Oscar

Sardines, in extra virgin olive oil, 1 can (106 g)	4

Season

Sardines in pure olive oil, imported, ¼ cup	4

Scallops

Omaha Steaks

Bacon wrapped scallops, 2 pieces (77 g)	4

Trader Joe's

Jumbo sea scallops, 4 pieces (113 g)	1

Shrimp

Atkins

Shrimp scampi, 1 tray (255 g)	10

Birds Eye Voila!

Garlic shrimp, 2 cups	7

Daily Chef

Jumbo cooked shrimp, 3 oz	1

Giant/Stop & Shop

Large raw shrimp (ready to eat), 10 shrimp (113 g)	1

Gorton's

Scampi grilled shrimp, 8 shrimp (112 g)	2
Shrimp scampi, garlic butter, 4 oz	3
Shrimp, grilled, classic grilled, 8 shrimp (113 g)	2

Gorton's Select Shrimp

Popcorn shrimp, 22 shrimp (99 g)	8

Gorton's Shrimp Temptations

Shrimp, jumbo butterfly, 5 shrimp (99 g)	8

Hooters

Buffalo shrimp, breaded, 4 oz	8

Kroger

Shrimp, cocktail, cooked, peeled, tail-on, 18 shrimp (90 g)	1
Shrimp, cocktail, peeled & deveined, with sauce, 9 shrimp (85 g)	2
Shrimp, cocktail, peeled, tail-on, 10 shrimp (90 g)	1

Lean Cuisine Culinary Collection

Shrimp Alfredo, 1 package (255 g)	6
Shrimp and angel hair pasta, 1 package (283 g)	7

Michelina's Lean Gourmet

Shrimp scampi, 1 package (227 g)	8

Omaha Steaks

Blackened shrimp, 4 oz	3
Coconut shrimp, 3 pieces (84 g)	6
Jumbo shrimp (fully cooked), 4 pieces (84 g)	0

Sea Pak Shrimp & Seafood Co.

Coconut shrimp, oven crispy, family size, 4 shrimp, sauce (102 g)	10
Popcorn shrimp, 14 shrimp (70 g)	6
Popcorn shrimp, 15 shrimp (84 g)	7
Popcorn shrimp, oven crispy, family size, 15 shrimp (85 g)	7
Shrimp scampi, 6 pieces (113 g)	9
Shrimp scampi, 8 pieces (113 g)	11

Fish & Seafood

Shrimp, butterfly, 7 shrimp (80 g)	6
Shrimp, butterfly, jumbo, 3 shrimp (84 g)	6
Tiger Thai	
Tempura shrimp, jumbo, 1 shrimp (28 g)	2
Trader Joe's	
Coconut shrimp, 5 shrimp (113 g)	8
World Classics	
Shrimp cocktail ring, with cocktail sauce, 3 oz	2

Swai

Baltimore Crab Company	
Swai fillets, 4 oz	2
Clear Value	
Fillets, swai, 4 oz	1
Kroger	
Farm-raised swai fillets, 1 fillet (113 g)	4
Paramount Reserve	
Swai fillets, 1 fillet (170 g)	1
Safeway	
Swai fillets, boneless & skinless, value pack, 3 oz	4
Simply Balanced	
Swai fillets, 4 oz	1
Trader Joe's	
Swai striped pangasius, 4 oz	1
Valu Time	
Swai fillets, 4 oz	1

Tilapia

Dr. Praeger's	
Tilapia fillets, lightly breaded, 1 piece (128 g)	6
Fishin'	
Tilapia fillets, 4 oz	1
Gorton's	
Tilapia with signature seasoning, 1 fillet (128 g)	2

Tilapia, grilled, roasted garlic & butter, 1 fillet (89 g)	1
Tilapia, grilled, signature grilled, 1 fillet (89 g)	1
Kroger	
Farm-raised tilapia fillets, 1 fillet (113 g)	1
Morey's	
Marinated tilapia fillets, 1 fillet (140 g)	4
Morey's Fish Creations	
Tilapia, seasoned grill, 1 fillet (142 g)	4
Odyssey Treasures from the Sea	
Tilapia, boneless fillets, 4 oz	1
Sea Cuisine	
Parmesan crusted tilapia, 1 fillet (140 g)	7
Tilapia, basil pesto, 1 fillet (101 g)	2
Tilapia, cracked peppercorn, fire roasted, 1 fillet (112 g)	2
Tilapia, tortilla crusted, 1 fillet (105 g)	4
Tortilla crusted tilapia, 1 fillet (140 g)	6
Simply Balanced	
Tilapia fillets, 4 oz	1
Trader Joe's	
Panko breaded tilapia fillets, 1 fillet (110 g)	10
Treasures from the Sea	
Parmesan encrusted tilapia, 4 oz	6
Trident	
Panko breaded tilapia, 4 oz	6

Trout

Omaha Steaks	
Lemon parm steelhead trout, 6 oz	4

Tuna

Ace of Diamonds

Fancy albacore solid white tuna in water, ¼ cup	1

Bumble Bee

Chunk light tuna in water, 2 oz drained	0
Chunk white albacore tuna in water, 2 oz drained	1
Solid white albacore tuna in water, ¼ cup	1
Tuna, chunk light, in water, 2 oz	0
Tuna, light, premium, in water, ¼ cup	1
Tuna, premium albacore, in water, ¼ cup	1
Tuna, premium, solid white albacore in oil, ¼ cup	1

Bumble Bee Sensations

Tuna medley, seasoned, lemon & pepper, 4 oz	3
Tuna medley, seasoned, spicy Thai chili, 4 oz	5

Chicken Of The Sea

Albacore tuna, solid white, ¼ cup	1
Chunk light tuna, in water, 1 can (84 g)	1
Premium albacore tuna in water, 1 pouch (85 g)	1
Premium light tuna in water, 1 pouch (85 g)	1
Solid white tuna, albacore in water, 1 can (84 g)	1
Tuna, albacore in water, solid white, ¼ cup	1
Tuna, albacore, chunk light, in water, ¼ cup	0
Tuna, albacore, in water, to go cups, 1 cup	1

Tuna, albacore, solid white, in water, ¼ cup	1
Tuna, chunk light, in oil, ¼ cup	1
Tuna, chunk light, in water, 2 oz	0
Tuna, chunk light, to go cups, 1 cup	1
Tuna, in water, chunk light, ¼ cup	0

Essential Everyday

Tuna, chunk light, in water, ¼ cup	0

Genova

Tuna, tonno, solid light, premium yellowfin, in olive oil, ¼ cup	3

Hawaiian Select

Tuna steak, ahi, 1 piece (113 g)	1

Kirkland

Signature solid white albacore tuna packed in water, ¼ cup	1

Kirkland Signature

Solid white albacore tuna, ¼ cup	1

Kroger

Chunk light tuna, ¼ cup	1
Chunk white albacore tuna, ¼ cup	1
Tuna, chunk light, in water, 2 oz	1
Tuna, solid white, in water, fancy albacore, ¼ cup drained	1

Market Pantry

Chunk light tuna in water, ¼ cup drained	0

Omaha Steaks

Ahi tuna steaks, 6 oz	2

Orca Bay

Ahi tuna, wild caught, 4 oz	1

ShopRite

Tuna, albacore, solid white, in water, ¼ cup	1

StarKist

Albacore white tuna in water single serve, 1 pouch (74 g)	1
Chunk white albacore in water, ¼ cup drained	0
Low sodium chunk white tuna in water, 1 pouch (74 g)	0
Tuna, albacore white, in water, 2 oz	1
Tuna, albacore, solid white, in water, ¼ cup	0
Tuna, chunk light, in water, ¼ cup	0
Tuna, solid white albacore, in vegetable oil, 2 oz	2
Tuna, white albacore, 2 oz	0
Tuna, white albacore, white, 2 oz	1

StarKist Chunk Light

Tuna in vegetable oil, ¼ cup	2

StarKist Flavor Fresh Pouch

Chunk light tuna in water, ¼ cup	1

StarKist Gourmet Selects

Mediterranean style tuna, 1 pouch (74 g)	4
Mexican style tuna, 1 pouch (74 g)	2
Thai style tuna, 1 pouch (74 g)	4

StarKist Lunch To-Go

Tuna, albacore, in water, 1 kit (116 g)	8
Tuna kit, chunk light, in water, 1 kit (116 g)	7

StarKist Selects

Tuna, solid light, in extra virgin olive oil, ¼ cup	3
Very low sodium chunk white albacore tuna in water, ¼ cup	1

Starkist Tuna Creations

Ranch flavor chunk light tuna, 1 pouch (74 g)	1
Sweet and spicy chunk light tuna, ¼ cup	1
Tuna, chunk light, herb & garlic, single serve, 1 pouch (74 g)	2
Tuna, chunk light, hickory smoked, single serve, 1 pouch (74 g)	2
Tuna, chunk light, sweet & spicy, single serve, 1 pouch (74 g)	2
Tuna, chunk light, zesty lemon pepper, single serve, 1 pouch (74 g)	1
Tuna, premium chunk light, lightly marinated, sweet and spicy, 2 oz	1

Trader Joe's

Half salt albacore solid white tuna in water, 2 oz drained	1
SkipJack tuna in water with sea salt, ¼ cup drained	0

Wegman's

Tuna, solid white albacore, in water, ¼ cup	1

Wild Planet

Tuna, light, wild skipJack, 2 oz	1
Tuna, wild albacore, 2 oz	2

Fish & Seafood

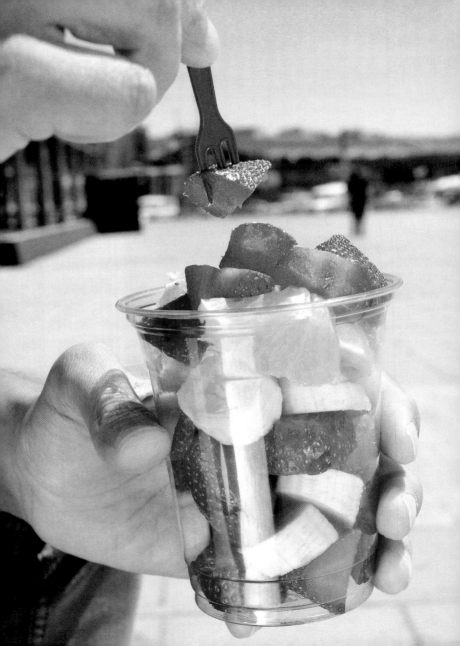

fruits

Apple

Crunch Pak Dipperz

Sweet apples with low fat caramel dip, 1 container (78 g)	4

Dippin Stix

Apples & caramel, sliced, 1 package (78 g)	5
Apples & caramel, sliced, with peanuts, 1 package (78 g)	7
Apples & peanut butter, sliced, 1 package (78 g)	6
Apples & yogurt fruit dip, sliced, 1 package (78 g)	5

Applesauce

Dole Fruit Squish 'Ems!

Apple pineapple squeezable fruit pouch, 1 pouch (90 g)	0

Eden Organic

Apple sauce, 1 cup	0

Essential Everyday

Apple sauce, unsweetened, 1 container (113 g)	0

Gefen

Apple sauce, unsweetened, ½ cup	0

GoGo Squeez

Apple pear applesauce on the go, 1 pouch (90 g)	0

Great Value

Cinnamon apple sauce, ½ cup	6
Unsweetened apple sauce, 1 container (113 g)	0

Kroger

Apple sauce, classic, 1 container (113 g)	4
Apple sauce, no sugar added, ½ cup	0
Applesauce, natural, ½ cup	0
Cinnamon applesauce, ½ cup	5
No added sugar natural applesauce, ½ cup	0

Lunch Buddies

Natural applesauce, 1 container (113 g)	0

Materne GoGo Squeez

Applesauce on the go, apple apple, 1 pouch (90 g)	3
Applesauce on the go, apple banana, 1 pouch (90 g)	3
Applesauce on the go, apple cinnamon, 1 pouch (90 g)	3
Applesauce on the go, apple peach, 1 pouch (90 g)	3
Applesauce on the go, apple strawberry, 1 pouch (90 g)	3

Meijer

Applesauce, cinnamon, ½ cup	5
Applesauce, strawberry, 4 oz	5

Mott's

Apple sauce, ½ cup	6
Apple sauce, cinnamon, ½ cup	7
Apple sauce, mango peach, 1 cup	5
Apple sauce, original, ½ cup	6
Apple sauce, peach medley, 1 cup	3
Apple sauce, pear, 1 cup	5
Apple sauce, strawberry, 1 cup	5
Applesauce original, ½ cup	6
Applesauce, mixed berry, 1 cup	5
Applesauce, original, 1 container (113 g)	6
Cinnamon applesauce, ½ cup	7
Natural applesauce, ½ cup	0
Natural applesauce (individual containers), 1 container (111 g)	0

Mott's Healthy Harvest

Apple sauce, country berry, 1 cup	3
Blueberry delight naturally flavored applesauce, 1 cup	0
Granny smith flavored applesauce no sugar added, 1 cup	0
Summer strawberry applesauce, 1 container (111 g)	3

Mott's Organics

Apple sauce, unsweetened, 1 cup	0

Mott's Plus Calcium

Apple sauce, harvest apple, 1 container (111 g)	0

Mott's Snack & Go!

Applesauce, no sugar added, natural, portable pouch, 1 pouch (90 g)	0
Applesauce, portable pouch, natural, 1 pouch (90 g)	0
Applesauce, portable pouch, strawberry, 1 pouch (90 g)	2
Cinnamon applesauce, 1 pouch (90 g)	5

Musselman's

Apple sauce, ½ cup	5
Apple sauce, cinnamon, 1 each (113 g)	5
Apple sauce, cinnamon, big cup, 1 container (170 g)	7
Apple sauce, lite, 1 unit (113 g)	0
Apple sauce, lite, cinnamon, 4 oz	0
Apple sauce, natural, unsweetened, big cup, 1 container (170 g)	0
Apple sauce, unsweetened, natural, 1 container (113 g)	0

Safeway Kitchens

Apple sauce, unsweetened, ½ cup	0

Santa Cruz Organic

Apple sauce, 1 container (113 g)	0

Seneca

Apple sauce, natural, no sugar added, ½ cup	0

Simply Nature

Unsweetened applesauce, ½ cup	3

Trader Joe's

Organic unsweetened apple sauce, ½ cup	0

Tree Top

Apple sauce, apple, no sugar added, 1 pouch (90 g)	0
Apple sauce, no sugar added, ½ cup	0

Dates

Bard Valley Natural Delights

Dates, medjool, 2 (46 g)	8
Dates, pitted medjool, 2 dates (46 g)	8

Hadley

Dates, pitted, deglet noor, 5 dates (40 g)	7

Sun Date

Dates, pitted, 5 dates (40 g)	7

Tree Of Life Organic

Dates, medjool, 1 oz	5

Fruit Cocktail, Salad & Mixed Fruit

Big Valley

Frozen mixed fruit, ⅔ cup	0

Del Monte

Cherry mixed fruit cups, 1 cup	4
Fruit cocktail, 100 calorie, ½ cup	3
Fruit cocktail, lite, ½ cup	4
Mixed fruit, cherry, in cherry flavored light syrup, 1 cup	4
Mixed fruit, in light syrup, 1 cup	4
Mixed fruit, no sugar added, 1 cup	0
No sugar added citrus salad, ½ cup	0
Plastic fruit cups, variety pack, 1 cup	4

Del Monte 100 Calorie

Mixed fruit, cherry, ½ cup	3

Del Monte Fruit Naturals

Cherry mixed fruit in extra light syrup, ½ cup	4
Citrus salad in 100% juice, ½ cup	4

Fruits

	SmartPoints™ value
Del Monte Fruit Naturals, Fruit Cup	
Mixed fruit in fruit juices from concentrates, pop-top, 1 can (112 g)	3
Del Monte Fruit To-Go	
Fruit cup, tropical fruit in lightly sweetened fruit juices from concentrate, 1 container (113 g)	4
Del Monte No Sugar Added	
Fruit cocktail, ½ cup	0
Very cherry mixed fruit, ½ cup	0
Dole	
Cherry mixed fruit in 100% fruit juice, 1 container (113 g)	5
Fruit bowls, 16 cup variety pack, 1 container (112 g)	5
Mixed fruit, 1 container (113 g)	4
Mixed fruit, cherry, 1 container (113 g)	4
Mixed fruit, in 100% fruit juice, 1 container (198 g)	7
Mixed fruit, in black cherry gel, 1 container (123 g)	6
Mixed fruit, in cherry gel, sugar free gel, 1 container (123 g)	2
Pineapple, in strawberry gel, sugar free gel, 1 container (123 g)	3
Tropical fruit, ½ cup	5
Tropical fruit, in 100% fruit juice, 1 container (113 g)	5
Dole Chef-Ready Cuts	
Diced pineapple and mango, 1 cup	0
Dole Harvest Best	
Tropical fruit, in 100% fruit juices, ½ cup	4
Dole Ready-Cut Fruit	
Strawberries & bananas, 1 cup	0
Strawberries, peaches & bananas, 1 cup	0
Strawberries, sliced, 1 cup	0

	SmartPoints™ value
Dole Wildly Nutritious	
Frozen mixed fruit, ¾ cup	0
Tropical fruit, immunity blend, ¾ cup	0
Dole Wildly Nutritious Signature Blends	
Mandarin sunshine blend frozen fruit, 1 cup	0
Essential Everyday	
Fruit cocktail, no sugar added, ½ cup	0
Great Value	
Fruit cocktail, ½ cup	0
Great Value Fruit Selections	
Mixed fruit, 1 bowl (108 g)	0
Happy Squeeze	
Fruit and veggie twist, apple mango kale, 1 pouch (99 g)	4
Hy-Vee	
Fruit cups, mixed fruit, 1 cup	4
Libby's Skinny Fruits	
Tropical fruit salad, ½ cup	1
Market Pantry	
Antioxidant blend of frozen fruit, 1 cup	4
Our Family Fresh Frozen	
Mixed fruit, 1 cup	0
Private Selection	
Fruit blend, for smoothies, frozen, ¾ cup	0
Mixed fruit, frozen, ¾ cup	0
Publix	
Mixed fruit, frozen, ¾ cup	0
Ready Pac	
Fresh fruit mix, 9 pieces (140 g)	0
Safeway	
Fruit medley, ¾ cup	0
Signature Cafe	
Fresh mixed fruit, 1 ½ cups	0
Simple Truth Organic	
Frozen mixed fruit medley, 1 cup	0

Wawona Frozen Foods

Festival blend frozen fruit, 1 cup	0
Spectrum blend mixed fruit, 1 cup	0

Wegman's Food You Feel Good About

Just picked quickly frozen mixed fruit, 1 cup	0

Whole Foods 365 Organic

Tropical blend frozen strawberries, bananas and mango, 1 cup	0

Wymans

Blueberries, strawberries, and mango chunks, fresh frozen, 1 cup	0

Fruit Parfait

Dole

Parfait, apples & creme, 1 container (123 g)	7
Parfait, peaches & creme, 1 container (123 g)	6

Fruit, Dried

Bare Fruit

Apple chips, crunchy, fuji red, 1 bag (15 g)	3

Brothers-All-Natural

Crisps, Asian pear, 1 bag (10 g)	2
Crisps, fuji apple, 1 bag (10 g)	2
Crisps, strawberry banana, 1 package (12 g)	2

Crispy Green Crispy Fruit

Crispy apples, 1 package (10 g)	2

Fresh Gourmet

Cranberries, 1 Tbsp	1

Kirkland Signature

Dried tart cherries, ⅓ cup	7
Whole dried blueberries, ⅓ cup	7

Kirkland Signature Sunsweet

Dried plums, 5 dried plums (40 g)	5

Kroger

Raisins, seedless, 3 boxes (42 g)	7

Mariani

Premium raisins, vanilla flavored yogurt, ¼ cup	8

Navita's Naturals Goji Power

Goji berries, 1 oz	4

Ocean Spray

Dried cranberries, original, sweetened, ⅓ cup	7

Ocean Spray Craisins

Cranberries, sweetened dried, original, ⅓ cup	7
Dried cranberries, blueberry, ⅓ cup	7
Dried cranberries, cherry, ⅓ cup	7
Dried cranberries, cherry juice infused, ⅓ cup	7
Dried cranberries, original, ⅓ cup	7
Dried cranberries, pomegranate, ⅓ cup	7
Dried cranberries, pomegranate juice infused, ⅓ cup	7
Dried cranberries, sweetened, original, 1 box (28 g)	5
Dried cranberries, sweetened, reduced sugar, ¼ cup	5
Original sweetened dried cranberries, ¼ cup	7
Reduced sugar dried cranberries, ¼ cup	5
Sweetened dried cranberries, ⅓ cup	7

Seneca

Original crispy apple chips, 12 chips (28 g)	6

Stretch Island

Fruit leather, wild apple, 1 each (14 g)	2

Sun-Maid

California organic raisins, ¼ cup	7
Dark chocolate yogurt raisins, 1 box (28 g)	6
Figs, mission, California, 4 figs (40 g)	6

Fruits

	SmartPoints™ value
Natural California raisins, mini - snacks, 1 box (14 g)	3
Raisins, golden, California, ¼ cup	7
Raisins, natural California, 1 box (28 g)	5
Sun-Maid Mini-Snacks	
Natural California raisins, 1 box (14 g)	3
Raisins, natural California, 1 box (40 g)	3
Sunsweet	
Pitted prunes, 5 prunes (40 g)	5
Prunes, d'noir, pitted, 4 prunes (40 g)	4
Prunes, pitted, bite size, petite, 7 prunes (40 g)	5
Prunes, pitted, cherry essence, 5 prunes (40 g)	5
Prunes, pitted, family size, 5 prunes (40 g)	5
Prunes, pitted, orange essence, 5 prunes (40 g)	5
Prunes, premium, 4 prunes (42 g)	4
Sunsweet Gold Label	
Prunes, pitted dried plums, ones, 4 prunes (40 g)	4
Sunsweet Gold Label Smart 60 Calorie Packs	
Dried plums, pitted prunes, 1 bag (26 g)	3
Sunsweet Ones	
California prunes, 4 prunes (40 g)	5
Sunsweet Plum Amazins	
Diced dried plums, ¼ cup	5
That's It	
Fruit bar, apple + blueberry, 1 bar (35 g)	5
Trader Joe's	
Dried apricots, 6 pieces (40 g)	5
Pitted prunes, 5 pieces (40 g)	4
Roasted coconut chips, ½ package (28 g)	9

	SmartPoints™ value
Vacaville Fruit Company	
California natural dry apples, 7 slices (17 g)	2

Grapefruit

	SmartPoints™ value
Del Monte	
Red grapefruit, in water, ½ cup	0
Red grapefruit, ½ cup	0
Red grapefruit, no sugar added, 1 container (184 g)	0
Del Monte SunFresh	
Grapefruit, red, ½ cup	3
No sugar added red grapefruit, ½ cup	0
Dole	
Red grapefruit sunrise, 1 container (113 g)	4
Red grapefruit sunrise cups, 1 container (112 g)	4
Kirkland Signature	
Red grapefruit pieces, ½ cup	3
Sundia True Fruit	
Grapefruit, ruby, 1 container (198 g)	5

Mango

	SmartPoints™ value
Del Monte	
Diced mangos in light syrup, 1 cup	4
Mango pineapple in light syrup, 1 container (113 g)	4
Del Monte Fruit Naturals	
Mango, chunks, in extra light syrup, 1 container (198 g)	6
Dole	
Mango chunks, 1 cup	0
Great Value	
Frozen mango chunks, 1 cup	0
Trader Joe's	
Just mango slices, 4 pieces (38 g)	6

Fruits

Peach

Big Valley

Frozen freestone peaches, ⅔ cup	0

Del Monte

No sugar added California sliced peaches, ½ cup	0
Peach cup, 1 (28 g)	5
Peaches, diced, in light syrup, 1 cup	4
Peaches, sliced, ½ cup	4
Peaches, sliced, lite, ½ cup	4

Del Monte 100 Calorie

Sliced peaches, ½ cup	3

Del Monte Fruit Naturals

Peach chunks, yellow cling, in 100% juice, ½ cup	3
Peach, yellow cling, chunks, no sugar added, 1 container (184 g)	0

Del Monte Lite

Peaches, diced, 1 can (113 g)	3

Del Monte No Sugar Added

Peach chunks, ½ cup	0
Peaches, California, diced, no sugar added, 1 container (106 g)	0

Del Monte Orchard Select

Cling peaches, in water, sliced, ½ cup	0
Peaches, no sugar added, ½ cup	0

Dole

Diced peaches in light syrup, 1 container (113 g)	5
Peaches, diced, yellow cling, 1 container (113 g)	5
Peaches, diced, yellow cling, no sugar added, 1 container (113 g)	0
Peaches, in strawberry gel, 1 container (123 g)	5
Peaches, yellow cling, sliced, in 100% fruit juice, 1 container (198 g)	7
Sliced peaches, all natural fruit, ¾ cup	0

Sliced peaches, yellow cling, in 100% juice, ½ cup	4
Yellow cling diced peaches in 100% fruit juice, 1 container (113 g)	5

Dole Harvest Best

Peaches, yellow cling, sliced, in 100% fruit juices, ½ cup	5

Great Value

Peaches, sliced, 1 cup	0
Sliced peaches sweetened with splenda, ½ cup	0

Kirkland

Peaches, sliced, cling, yellow, in extra light syrup, ½ cup	4

Kirkland Signature

Diced peaches in juice, ½ cup	3

Kroger Lite

Peaches, yellow cling, sliced, ½ cup	3

Kroger No Sugar Added

Yellow cling diced peaches snack bowls, 1 bowl (108 g)	0

Market Pantry

No sugar added diced peaches fruit cups, 1 snack cup (40 g)	0

Our Family Fresh Frozen

Sliced peaches, 1 cup	0

Private Selection

Peaches, sliced, ¾ cup	0

Pear

Del Monte

Pears, diced, 1 cup	4
Pears, diced, in water, no sugar added, 1 cup	0

Del Monte Lite

Pear, halves, lite, ½ cup	4
Pears, sliced, ½ cup	4

Del Monte No Sugar Added

Pears, northwest, sliced, no sugar added, ½ cup	0

Fruits

	SmartPoints™ value
Dole	
Pears, diced, 1 container (113 g)	5
Kroger No Sugar Added	
Diced pears snack bowls, 1 bowl (108 g)	0

Pineapple

Del Monte	
Pineapple in coconut flavored light syrup fruit cup, 1 cup	4
Del Monte Fruit Naturals	
Pineapple cup, 1 (113 g)	3
Dole	
Pineapple chunks, ½ cup	4
Pineapple tidbits, 1 container (113 g)	2
Pineapple tidbits, in 100% pineapple juice, 1 container (113 g)	3
Pineapple, crushed, ½ cup	4
Pineapple, in lime gel, 1 container (123 g)	5
Pineapple, slices, 2 slices (114 g)	3
Dole Dippers	
Pineapple covered in dark chocolate, 1 pouch (30 g)	4
Dole Harvest Best	
Pineapple chunks, in 100% pineapple juice, ½ cup	4
Kirkland Signature	
Frozen golden sweet pineapple chunks, ¾ cup	0
Libby's Skinny Fruits	
Pineapple, chunk, ½ cup	0
Pineapple, crushed, ½ cup	0
Pineapple, sliced, 2 slices (114 g)	0
Trader Joe's	
Pineapple tidbits, 1 cup	0

Plantain

	SmartPoints™ value
Goya	
Ripe plantains, 2 oz	5

Tangelo

Wegman's Food You Feel Good About	
Tangelos, minneola, California, 1 medium	0

Tangerine/Mandarin

Cuties	
California mandarins, 1	0
Del Monte	
Mandarin orange, segments in light syrup, 1 cup	4
Del Monte Fruit Naturals	
Mandarin oranges, in 100% juice, ½ cup	4
Del Monte No Sugar Added	
Mandarin oranges, in water, no sugar added, 1 container (113 g)	0
Dole	
Mandarin oranges, 1 container (113 g)	5
Mandarin oranges, in 100% fruit juice, 1 container (198 g)	7
Mandarin oranges, no sugar added, 1 container (113 g)	0
Mandarins in orange gel, 1 container (123 g)	5
Dole Harvest Best	
Mandarin oranges, in 100% fruit juices, ½ cup	5
Kroger No Sugar Added	
Mandarin oranges snack bowl, 1 container (108 g)	0
Libby's Skinny Fruits	
Mandarin oranges, ½ cup	0

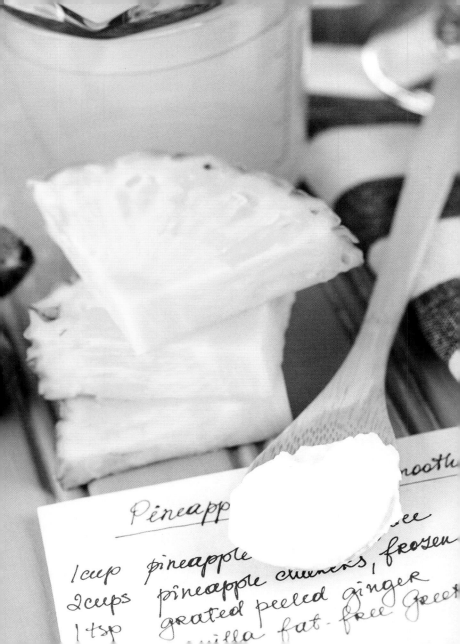

Pineapp___ ___ooth__

___ ___ee

1 cup   pineapple ___
2 cups   pineapple chunks, frozen
         grated peeled ginger
1 tsp   ___nilla fat-free gree___

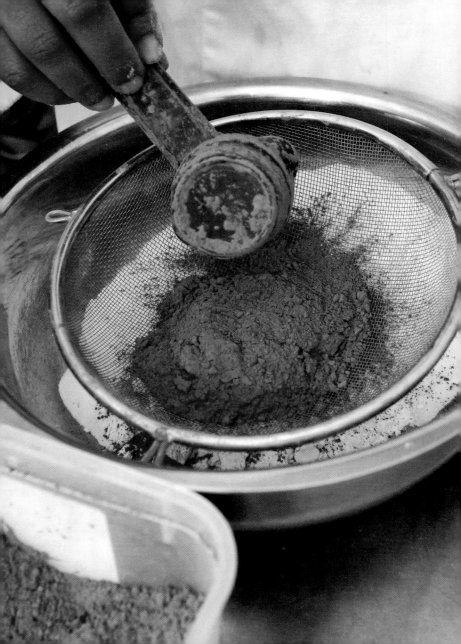

ingredients

Bread Crumbs

4C

Bread crumbs, seasoned,
100% whole wheat, ⅓ cup — 3

Kikkoman

Bread crumbs, panko, Japanese
style, ½ cup — 3

Kroger

Bread crumbs, Italian, ¼ cup — 3

Panko

Bread crumbs, Japanese style,
½ cup — 3

Private Selection

Bread crumbs, panko, ½ cup — 3

Progresso

Bread crumbs, crispy panko,
Italian style, ¼ cup — 3

Bread crumbs, crispy panko,
plain, ¼ cup — 3

Bread crumbs, garlic and herb,
¼ cup — 3

Bread crumbs, Italian, ¼ cup — 3

Bread crumbs, plain, ¼ cup — 3

Chocolate & Candy, Baking

Baker's

Baking chocolate bar, semi-sweet,
56% cacao, 2 pieces (14 g) — 4

Dipping chocolate, real milk
chocolate, 6 wafers (15 g) — 4

Dagoba

Cacao powder, organic
chocolate, 1 Tbsp — 0

Enjoy Life

Chocolate chips, semi-sweet,
½ oz — 4

Semi-sweet chocolate,
mega chunks, 1 Tbsp — 4

Ghirardelli Chocolate

60% cacao bittersweet chocolate
premium baking chips,
16 chips (15 g) — 4

Baking chips, premium, bittersweet
chocolate, 16 chips (15 g) — 4

Baking chips, premium, milk
chocolate, 16 chips (15 g) — 4

Baking chips, premium, mini,
semi-sweet chocolate,
115 chips (15 g) — 4

Baking chips, premium, semi-sweet
chocolate, 32 chips (15 g) — 4

Dark chocolate melting wafers,
18 wafers (41 g) — 13

Guittard

Chocolate chips, 63% cacao,
extra dark, 30 pieces (15 g) — 4

Chocolate chips, real milk,
12 pieces (15 g) — 4

Chocolate chips, real semisweet,
30 pieces (15 g) — 4

Hershey's

Baking bits, heath English toffee,
1 Tbsp — 4

Chips, butterscotch, 1 Tbsp — 4

Chocolate chips, semi-sweet,
1 Tbsp — 4

Cocoa, naturally unsweetened,
1 Tbsp — 0

Hershey's Bake Shoppe

Milk chocolate chips, 1 Tbsp — 4

Hershey's Kisses

Milk chocolate, mini,
11 pieces (15 g) — 4

Hershey's Special Dark

Chocolate chips, mildly sweet,
1 Tbsp — 4

Cocoa, 100% cacao, special dark,
1 Tbsp — 1

Kirkland Signature

Chocolate chips, 30 pieces (15 g) — 4

Kroger

Chocolate chips, semi-sweet,
mini, 1 Tbsp — 3

Ingredients

	SmartPoints™ value
M&M's	
Mini baking bits, milk chocolate, 1 Tbsp	4
M&M's Minis	
Chocolate candy baking bits, 1 Tbsp	4
Navita's Naturals	
Cacao powder, 2 ½ Tbsp	2
Nestlé Chocolatier	
Chocolate morsels, premium baking, dark chocolate, 53% cacao, 1 Tbsp	4
Nestlé Toll House	
Morsels, dark chocolate& mint, ½ oz	4
Saco Dolci Frutta	
Hard chocolate shell, 10 wafers (28 g)	9
Theo	
Cocoa nibs, roasted, ¼ cup	7
Toll House	
Cocoa, 1 Tbsp	0
Morsels, butterscotch, 1 Tbsp	4
Morsels, dark chocolate, 53% cacao, 1 Tbsp	4
Morsels, milk chocolate, 1 Tbsp	4
Morsels, premier white, 14 Tbsp	4
Original semi-sweet morsels, 1 Tbsp	4
Toll House Mini	
Semi-sweet chocolate morsels, 1 Tbsp	4
Trader Joe's	
Semi-sweet chocolate chips, 1 Tbsp	4

Coating Mixes
Kraft Shake 'n Bake

	SmartPoints™ value
Bbq glaze coating mix, ⅛ packet (11 g)	2
Coating mix for chicken or pork, seasoned, Italian, ⅛ packet (10 g)	1
Coating mix for chicken or pork, seasoned, parmesan crusted, ⅛ packet (10 g)	1
Coating mix, crunchy pretzel, ⅛ packet (8 g)	1
Coating mix, original, 1 serving (12 g)	1
Coating mix, seasoned panko, ⅛ packet (7 g)	1
Coating mix, seasoned, extra crispy, ⅛ packet (9 g)	1
Crispy buffalo seasoned coating mix, ⅛ packet (8 g)	1
Hot and spicy seasoned coating mix, ⅛ packet (8 g)	1
Original chicken seasoned coating mix, ⅛ packet (8 g)	1
Original chicken seasoned coating mix, ⅛ packet (8 g)	1
Parmesan crusted seasoned coating mix, ⅛ packet (8 g)	1
Pork seasoned coating mix, ⅛ packet (9 g)	1
Ranch and herb seasoned coating mix, ⅛ packet (8 g)	1
Oven Fry	
Extra crispy chicken seasoned coating mix, ⅛ packet (15 g)	2
Extra crispy pork seasoned coating mix, ⅛ package (15 g)	2

Coconut
Bob's Red Mill

Coconut, flaked, unsweetened, ¼ cup	6
Coconut, unsweetened, medium shredded, 3 Tbsp	6
Dang	
Toasted coconut chips (serves 2), 1 serving (20 g)	6
Toasted coconut chips (serves 4.5), 1 serving (20 g)	6
Kroger	
Coconut, flake, sweetened, 2 Tbsp	3

Cornmeal

Food Merchants

Traditional Italian polenta (1 serving one 2.5" slice), 1 serving (100 g)　2

Cornstarch

Acme

Corn starch, 1 Tbsp　1

Argo

Corn starch, 1 Tbsp　1

Flaxseed Meal

Bob's Red Mill Organic

Flaxseed meal, golden, 100% whole ground, 2 Tbsp　2

Golden flaxseed meal, whole ground, 2 Tbsp　2

Spectrum Essentials Organic

Flaxseed, whole premium, 1 ½ Tbsp　2

Frosting & Icing

Betty Crocker

Cupcake icing, decorating, chocolate, 2 Tbsp　7

Betty Crocker Whipped

Frosting, butter cream, 2 Tbsp　5

Frosting, chocolate, 2 Tbsp　5

Frosting, cream cheese, 2 Tbsp　5

Frosting, fluffy white, 2 Tbsp　5

Frosting, vanilla, 2 Tbsp　5

Duncan Hines Creamy Home-Style

Frosting, premium, classic chocolate, 2 Tbsp　7

Premium frosting, buttercream, 2 Tbsp　7

Pillsbury Creamy Supreme

Frosting, chocolate fudge, 2 Tbsp　7

Frosting, sugar free, chocolate fudge, 2 Tbsp　3

Pillsbury Funfetti

Frosting, vanilla, 2 Tbsp　8

Graham Cracker Crumbs

Keebler

Graham cracker crumbs, 3 Tbsp　2

Honey

Aunt Sue's

Honey, raw-wild, 1 Tbsp　4

Fischer's

Natural pure raw honey, 1 Tbsp　4

Golden Blossom Honey

Genuine natural pure honey, 1 Tbsp　4

Great Value

Clover honey, 1 Tbsp　4

Kirkland Signature

Clover honey, 1 Tbsp　4

Kroger

Clover honey, 1 Tbsp　4

Naturally Healthy Mountain Ridge

100% pure raw honey, 1 Tbsp　4

Nature Nate's

Honey, 100% pure raw & unfiltered, 1 Tbsp　2

Really Raw

Honey, 1 Tbsp　4

Simply Balanced

Honey, organic, 1 Tbsp　4

Honey, organic, raw, wildflower, 1 Tbsp　4

SueBee

Suebee premium clover honey, 1 Tbsp　4

Trader Joe's

Clover honey, 1 Tbsp　4

Organic raw honey, 1 Tbsp　4

Trader Joe's Organic

Wild collected raw honey, 1 Tbsp　4

Wedderspoon

Honey, manuka honey, 1 Tbsp　4

Wholesome Sweeteners

Honey, raw, organic, 1 Tbsp　4

Pie Crust

Keebler

Pie crusts, mini graham cracker,
1 crust (19 g) — 5

Pillsbury

Pie crusts, ⅛ crust (25 g) — 4

Pizza Crust

Betty Crocker

Pizza crust mix, ¼ crust (46 g) — 5

Boboli

Pizza crust, 100% whole wheat,
1 serving (47 g) — 4

Pizza crust, mini 8",
½ shell (71 g) — 6

Pizza crust, original,
1 serving (66 g) — 5

Pizza crust, thin, 1 serving (47 g) — 4

Jiffy

Mix, pizza crust, 1 serving (37 g) — 4

Mama Mary's

Pizza crusts, 100% whole wheat,
with honey, 12",
¼ pizza crust (57 g) — 5

Pizza crusts, gourmet thin
& crispy, 1 serving (38 g) — 4

Pizza crusts, thin & crispy, 7",
½ pizza crust (43 g) — 4

Pizza crusts, traditional,
½ pizza crust (57 g) — 5

Pillsbury

Pizza crust, classic,
1 serving (65 g) — 5

Pizza crust, thin, 1 serving (62 g) — 6

Pizza dough, gluten free thin crust,
1 serving (61 g) — 6

Udi's

Pizza crust, ¼ package (56 g) — 5

Pizza Kit

Chef Boyardee

Pizza kit, cheese, ¼ package
(115 g) — 8

Pizza kit, cheese, family size,
⅛ of package (113 g) — 8

Puff Pastry

Pepperidge Farm

Puff pastry sheets, 1 serving (41 g) — 7

Sugar & Sugar Substitutes

Agave In The Raw

Agave nectar, organic, 1 Tbsp — 4

BetterBody Foods

Organic coconut palm sugar, 1 tsp — 1

C&H

Agave nectar, blue, organic,
light, 1 Tbsp — 4

Organic sugar, certified,
pure cane, 1 tsp — 1

Pure cane sugar cubes,
1 cube (4 g) — 1

Pure cane sugar, granulated, 1 tsp — 1

Pure cane sugar, individual
packets, 1 packet (4 g) — 1

C&H Light

Sugar & stevia blend, ½ tsp — 0

Sugar & stevia blend, packets,
1 packet (1.7 g) — 0

Domino

Agave nectar, organic, light, 1 Tbsp — 4

Brown sugar, light, 1 tsp — 1

Cane sugar, washed raw,
demerara, 1 tsp — 1

Certified organic sugar, 1 tsp — 1

Dark brown sugar, 1 tsp — 1

Light brown sugar, 1 tsp — 1

Premium pure cane sugar, extra
fine granulated, 1 packet (4 g) — 1

Ingredients

	SmartPoints™ value
Premium pure cane sugar, granulated, 1 tsp	1
Pure cane sugar, premium, granulated, 1 tsp	1
Sugar 'n cinnamon, 1 tsp	1
Sugar, dark brown, 1 tsp	1
Sugar, pourable, light brown, 1 tsp	1
Sugar, premium, granulated, pure cane, 1 tsp	1
Sugar, pure cane, granulated, 1 tsp	1
Domino Brownulated	
Sugar, light brown, 1 tsp	1
Domino Dots	
Sugar cubes, premium pure cane sugar, 1 each (2 g)	1
Domino Pure D'Lite	
Sugar blend, 1 tsp	1
Equal	
Artificial sweetener, 1 tsp	0
Original zero calorie sweetener, 1 packet (1 g)	0
Sugar lite, 1 tsp	0
Sweetener, 0 calorie, 1 packet (1 g)	0
Sweetener, sucralose, 1 packet (1 g)	0
Florida Crystals	
Cane sugar, natural, 1 tsp	1
Demerara sugar, 1 tsp	1
Organic cane sugar, 1 tsp	1
Great Value	
Pure cane sugar, 1 tsp	1
Zero calorie sweetener, 1 packet (2 g)	0
Great Value Altern	
No calorie sweetener, 1 tsp	0
Hain	
Sugar, organic, 1 tsp	1

	SmartPoints™ value
Imperial Sugar	
Sugar, pure cane, extra fine granulated, 1 tsp	1
Sugar, turbinado, gold'n natural, 1 tsp	1
Kroger	
Sugar, light brown, 1 tsp	1
Sweetener, stevia blend, 1 packet (2 g)	0
Kroger Apriva	
Sweetener, no calorie, 1 packet (1 g)	0
Madhava	
Coconut sugar, organic, 1 tsp	1
Sugar, coconut, organic, 1 tsp	1
Mccormick	
Cinnamon sugar, 1 tsp	1
Monk Fruit In The Raw	
All natural sugar substitute, 1 packet (0.8 g)	0
Nectresse	
No calorie sweetener, 1 packet (2.4 g)	0
No calorie sweetener, natural, ¼ tsp	0
O Organics	
Sugar, light brown, organic, 1 tsp	1
Sugar, turbinado, organic, 1 tsp	1
Private Selection	
Sugar, natural cane turbinado, 1 packet (4.5 g)	1
Sugar, natural cane turbinado, bulk, 1 tsp	1
Sugar, organic, 1 tsp	1
Pure Via	
Stevia, 1 packet (1 g)	0
Sugar and stevia blend, raw cane, turbinado, 1 packet (1.7 g)	0
Sweetener, zero calorie, 1 packet (2 g)	0

Ingredients

Pure Via Stevia

Sugar and stevia blend, raw cane, turbinado, ½ tsp	0

Pyure

Sweetener, stevia, organic, 1 packet (1 g)	0

Safeway

Stevia, 1 packet (47 g)	0

ShopRite

Sugar substitute, sucralose, packets, 1 tsp	0

Simply Nature Organic

Light agave nectar, 1 Tbsp	4

Skinny Girl

Sweetener, stevia extract blend, organic, 1 packet (1 g)	0

Splenda

Brown sugar blend, ½ tsp	1
No calorie sweetener, granulated, 1 tsp	0
Sweetener packets, 1 packet (1 g)	0
Sweetener, no-calorie, 1 packet (1 g)	0
Sweetener, sugar blend, ½ tsp	1

Splenda Flavors For Coffee

No calorie sweetener, French vanilla, 1 packet (1 g)	0

Stearns & Lehman

Turbinado sugar, 1 tsp	1

Stevia In the Raw

Sweetener, zero calorie, granulated, 1 tsp	0
Zero calorie sweetener, 1 packet (1 g)	0

Sugar In The Raw

Sugar in the raw, liquid, turbinado cane, 1 tsp	1

Sweet Additions

Natural calorie-free sweetener, 1 packet (1 g)	0

Sweet Leaf

Sweetener, 1 packet (1 g)	0
Sweetener, stevia plus, ⅛ tsp	0

Sweet 'N Low

Granulated sugar substitute, 1 packet (1 g)	0
Sweetener, 1 packet (1 g)	0
Sweetener, zero calorie, 1 packet (1 g)	0

Trader Joe's

Fair trade turbinado raw cane sugar, 1 tsp	1
Organic blue agave sweetner, 1 Tbsp	4
Organic coconut sugar, 1 tsp	1
Organic liquid stevia, 4 drops (0.13 ml)	0
Stevia extract, ⅓ tsp	0
Stevia packets, 1 packet (1 g)	0

Trader Joe's Organic

Raw blue agave sweetener, 1 Tbsp	4

Truvia

Baking blend, ½ tsp	0
Natural sweetener with brown sugar blend, ½ tsp	0
Sweetener. calorie-free, 1 packet (4 g)	0

Wholesome Sweeteners

Blue agave, organic, light, 1 Tbsp	4
Coconut palm sugar, organic, 1 tsp	1
Organic sugar, 1 tsp	1
Organic turbinado, raw cane sugar, 1 tsp	1
Stevia, organic, 1 packet (1 g)	0

Woodstock Farms

Sugar, pure cane, organic, 1 tsp	1

Xagave

Organic agave, 1 Tbsp	3

Ingredients

Syrup

Aunt Jemima

	SmartPoints™ value
Original lite syrup, ¼ cup	6
Syrup, butter lite, ¼ cup	6
Syrup, butter rich, ¼ cup	10

Aunt Jemima Country Rich Lite

Country rich lite syrup, ¼ cup	6

Aunt Maple's

Lite syrup, ¼ cup	7

Cary's

Syrup, sugar free, artificial maple flavor, ¼ cup	1

Country Kitchen

Butter flavored syrup, ¼ cup	10
Original syrup, ¼ cup	10

DaVi

Vanilla syrup, classic, 2 Tbsp	4
Vanilla syrup, sugar free, 2 Tbsp	0

DaVi Gourmet

Original hazelnut syrup, sugar free, 2 Tbsp	0

Essential Everyday

Syrup, light, ¼ cup	6

Finest Call

Triple sec syrup, premium, 1 fl oz	2

Full Circle Organic

Maple syrup, 4 Tbsp	12

Giant/Stop & Shop

Syrup lite, ¼ cup	6

Great Value

Syrup, sugar free, chocolate flavored, 2 Tbsp	0

Hershey's

Chocolate syrup, lite, 2 Tbsp	3
Sundae syrup, double chocolate, 2 Tbsp	6
Syrup, plus calcium, chocolate flavor, 2 Tbsp	5
Syrup, caramel, 2 Tbsp	6
Syrup, chocolate flavor, 2 Tbsp	5

	SmartPoints™ value
Syrup, strawberry, 2 Tbsp	6
Syrup, sugar free, chocolate, 2 Tbsp	0

Hershey's Special Dark

Syrup, 2 Tbsp	5

Hungry Jack

Lite syrup, ¼ cup	6
Sugar free breakfast syrup, ¼ cup	1
Syrup, original, ¼ cup	10

IHOP At Home

Syrup, original, ¼ cup	10
Syrup, sugar free, ¼ cup	0

Izzys Organic

Blue agave, 1 Tbsp	3

Joseph's

Syrup, sugar free, maple flavor, ¼ cup	1

Kirkland Signature

Grade A dark amber maple syrup, ¼ cup	12
Grade A dark amber organic maple syrup, ¼ cup	12

Kroger

Syrup, chocolate flavored, 2 Tbsp	5
Syrup, lite, ¼ cup	5
Syrup, sugar free, ¼ cup	1

Log Cabin

Lite syrup no high fructose corn syrup, ¼ cup	0
Original syrup, ¼ cup	9
Original syrup no high fructose corn syrup, ¼ cup	9
Syrup, all natural, ¼ cup	11
Syrup, sugar free, ¼ cup	1

Madhava

Agave nectar, light, 1 Tbsp	4
Coffee syrup, organic, salted caramel, 1 Tbsp	4

Ingredients

Maple Grove Farms

	SmartPoints™ value
Syrup, sugar free, butter flavor, ¼ cup	1
Syrup, sugar free, maple flavor, ¼ cup	1

Maple Mountain

Sugar free syrup, 2 Tbsp	0

Market Pantry

Sugar-free syrup in original flavour, ¼ cup	1

Mrs. Butterworth's

Original syrup, ¼ cup	11
Syrup, sugar free, ¼ cup	1
Reduced calorie syrup, ¼ cup	6

Nesquik

Syrup, chocolate, 2 Tbsp	6

Private Selection

Syrup, maple, 100% pure, ¼ cup	6

ShopRite

Syrup, reduced calorie, lite, ¼ cup	6
Syrup, sugar free, ¼ cup	1
Syrup, sugar free, pancake & waffle, ¼ cup	1

Smucker's

Syrup, blueberry, ¼ cup	11
Syrup, breakfast, sugar free, ¼ cup	1

Smucker's Sugar Free

Sundae syrup, caramel, 2 Tbsp	3
Sundae syrup, chocolate, 2 Tbsp	3

Smucker's Sundae Syrup

Sundae syrup, caramel flavored, 2 Tbsp	5
Syrup, chocolate flavored, 2 Tbsp	6

Spring Tree

Syrup, sugar free, ¼ cup	1

Starbucks

Starbucks syrup, vanilla, 2 Tbsp	4

Stirring's

	SmartPoints™ value
Simple syrup, 1 oz	3

Torani

Syrup, classic, caramel, 2 Tbsp	5
Syrup, classic, hazelnut, 2 Tbsp	5
Syrup, sugar free, caramel, 1 oz	0
Syrup, sugar free, chocolate, 1 fl oz	0
Syrup, sugar free, classic hazelnut, 2 Tbsp	0
Syrup, sugar free, salted caramel, 2 Tbsp	0
Syrup, sugar free, vanilla, 2 Tbsp	0
Syrup, vanilla, 2 Tbsp	4

Trader Joe's

Simple syrup, 2 Tbsp	4

Trader Joe's Organic

Maple agave syrup blend, ¼ cup	10
Maple syrup, ¼ cup	13

Vermont

Low calorie syrup, sugar free, ¼ cup	0
Syrup, low calorie, sugar free, butter flavor, ¼ cup	1
Syrup, sugar free, ¼ cup	0

Vermont Maid

Syrup, sugar free, ¼ cup	1

Walden Farms

Syrup, chocolate, 2 Tbsp	0
Syrup, pancake, ¼ cup	0

Wholesome Sweeteners

Blue agave, organic, raw, 1 Tbsp	4

Wine, Cooking

Holland House

Cooking wine, sake, 2 Tbsp	1
Cooking wine, white, 2 Tbsp	1

Ingredients

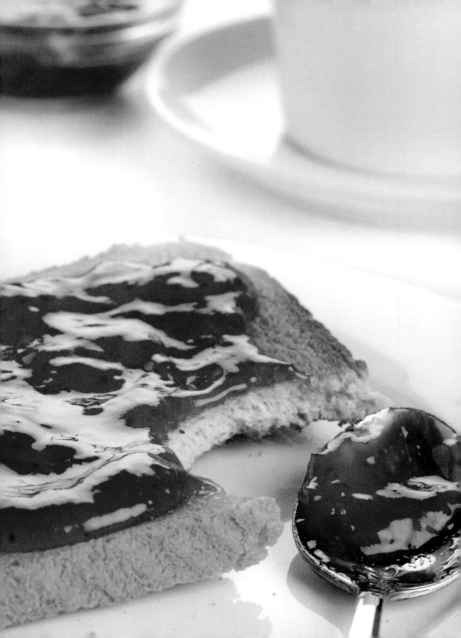

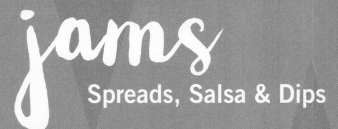

jams

Spreads, Salsa & Dips

Almond Butter

Barney Butter

Almond butter, crunchy, 2 Tbsp	6
Almond butter, smooth, 2 Tbsp	6

Jif

Almond butter, creamy, 2 Tbsp	6
Almond butter, crunchy, 2 Tbsp	6

Justin's

Almond butter, chocolate, 2 Tbsp	7
Almond butter, classic, 1 pack (14 g)	3
Almond butter, honey, 2 Tbsp	6
Almond butter, honey peanut butter blend, 2 Tbsp	6
Classic almond butter, 2 Tbsp	6
Classic almond butter, 2 Tbsp	6

Kroger

Creamy almond butter, 2 Tbsp	6

MaraNatha

All natural no stir creamy almond butter, 2 Tbsp	6
Almond butter, creamy, 2 Tbsp	5
Almond butter, creamy, coconut, 2 Tbsp	7
Almond butter, crunchy, no stir, 2 Tbsp	6

Naturally More

Almond butter, 2 Tbsp	5

Nature's Promise Organics

Almond butter, smooth, unsalted, 2 Tbsp	6

Trader Joe's

Almond butter, raw, creamy, unsalted, 2 Tbsp	5
Almond butter, raw, crunchy, unsalted, 2 Tbsp	5
Creamy almond butter with sea salt, 2 Tbsp	5

Wegman's Food You Feel Good About

Almond butter, organic, smooth, unsalted, 2 Tbsp	6

Woodstock Farms Natural

Almond butter, smooth/unsalted, 2 Tbsp	6

Bruschetta

Sabra

Bruschetta, 2 Tbsp	1

Trader Joe's

Bruschetta, 2 Tbsp	1

Cashew Butter

Jif

Cashew butter, creamy, 2 Tbsp	7

Trader Joe's

Creamy salted cashew butter, 2 Tbsp	6

Cheese Spread

Green Mountain Farms

Cream cheese & Greek yogurt, whipped, blueberry, 2 Tbsp	2

Kraft

Sharp cheese spread, old English, 2 Tbsp	4

Kroger

Greek cream cheese and Greek yogurt, 2 Tbsp	2

Merkts

Cheese spread, port wine, 2 Tbsp	4
Cheese spread, sharp cheddar, 2 Tbsp	4

Price's

Cheese spread, lite, pimiento, ¼ cup	4

Trader Joe's

Feta cheese spread, 1 oz	2

Chocolate Spread

Hershey's

Chocolate spread, 2 Tbsp	8

Hershey's Snacksters

Spread, chocolate, served with graham dippers, 1 package (51 g)	11

Hershey's Spreads

Chocolate with almond, 2 Tbsp	9
Chocolate, with hazelnut, 2 Tbsp	9

Cookie Spread

Lotus

Creamy biscoff spread, 1 Tbsp	4

Trader Joe's

Cookies & creme cookie butter, 1 oz	7
Speculoos cookie and cocoa swirl spread, 1 Tbsp	4
Speculoos cookie butter, 1 Tbsp	4
Speculoos crunchy cookie butter, 1 Tbsp	4

Dips

Artisan Fresh

Spinach artichoke dip, 2 Tbsp	4

Bubbas Back 9 Dips

Chicken dip, buffalo blue cheese, 2 oz	3

Casa Mamita

Salsa con queso, original, medium, 2 Tbsp	2

Cedar's

Cucumber garlic tzatziki, 2 Tbsp	1
Spinach dip, 2 Tbsp	3

Central

Chip 'n dip, French onion, 2 Tbsp	1

Cheez Whiz

Dip, cheese, original, 2 Tbsp	3

Cool Whip Dips

Dip, whipped, chocolate, 2 Tbsp	2

Dean's

Dip, French onion, 2 Tbsp	3
Dip, guacamole flavored, 2 Tbsp	3
Dip, ranch, 2 Tbsp	3
Ranch dip, lite, 2 Tbsp	2

El Terrifico Tamale Co.

White cheese dip, 2 Tbsp	4

French's

Dipping sauce, honey mustard, 2 Tbsp	3

Friendly Farms

Ranch dip, 2 Tbsp	3

Frito Lay

French onion dip, 2 Tbsp	2

Fritos

Bean dip, 1 serving (35 g)	1
Hot bean dip with jalapeño peppers, 2 Tbsp	1
Jalapeño cheddar flavored cheese dip, 2 Tbsp	1
Mild cheddar flavored cheese dip, 2 Tbsp	1
Original flavor bean dip, 2 Tbsp	1

From Grammas Kitchen

Taco dip, 2 Tbsp	3

GoodFoods Tableside

Chunky guacamole with garlic onions and tomatoes, 2 Tbsp	1

Gordo's

Cheese dip, mild, with jalapeño, 2 Tbsp	3

Hannah

Dip, tzatziki, yogurt, Greek style, 1 Tbsp	1

Heluva Good!

Dip, Greek style yogurt, French onion, 2 Tbsp	2
Dip, Greek style yogurt, herb ranch, 2 Tbsp	2
Dip, sour cream, buffalo wing, 2 Tbsp	3

Jams, Spreads, Salsa & Dips

	SmartPoints™ value
Dip, sour cream, buttermilk ranch, 2 Tbsp	3
Dip, sour cream, French onion, 2 Tbsp	2
Dip, sour cream, jalapeño cheddar, 2 Tbsp	3
Jimmy's	
Dip, dill vegetable, 2 Tbsp	5
Joseph's	
Cucumber & garlic yogurt dip, tzatziki, 1 Tbsp	1
Kraft	
Dip, creamy ranch, 2 Tbsp	3
Dip, French onion, 2 Tbsp	3
Kroger	
Dip, French onion, 2 Tbsp	3
Dip, French onion, fat free, 2 Tbsp	1
Dip, sour cream, French onion, 2 Tbsp	3
Dip, sour cream, ranch, 2 Tbsp	3
Spinach dip, 2 Tbsp	2
La Terra Fina	
Chunky artichoke and jalapeño dip, 2 Tbsp	3
Spinach, artichoke and parmesan dip, 2 Tbsp	3
Lay's	
French onion dip, 2 Tbsp	2
Smooth ranch dip, 2 Tbsp	2
Litehouse	
Veggie dip, homestyle ranch, 2 Tbsp	4
Luisa's	
Mild five layered fiesta dip, 2 Tbsp	1
Marketside	
Low fat buttermilk ranch dip, 2 Tbsp	2
Marzetti	
Apple dip, old fashioned, caramel, 2 oz	11
Dill veggie dip, 2 Tbsp	4

	SmartPoints™ value
Dip, fat free, caramel, 2 Tbsp	5
Dip, old fashioned, caramel, 2 Tbsp	6
Dip, ranch, 2 Tbsp	2
Fruit dip, cream cheese, natural strawberry flavored, 2 Tbsp	4
Fruit dip, light yogurt, French vanilla, 2 Tbsp	2
Fruit-dip, cream cheese, 2 Tbsp	4
Light dill veggie dip, 2 Tbsp	2
Light French onion veggie dip, 2 Tbsp	2
Light ranch veggie dip, 2 Tbsp	2
Light southwest ranch veggie dip, 2 Tbsp	2
Ranch veggie dip, 2 Tbsp	4
Southwest ranch veggie dip, 2 Tbsp	4
Spinach veggie dip, 2 Tbsp	4
Veggie dip, light dill, 2 Tbsp	2
Veggie dip, light, ranch, 2 Tbsp	2
Veggie-dip, fat free, ranch, 2 Tbsp	1
Veggie-dip, ranch, 2 Tbsp	5
Marzetti 100 Calorie Packs	
Veggie-dip, light ranch, 1 ½ oz	4
Marzetti Otria	
Caramelized onion Greek yogurt veggie dip, 2 Tbsp	2
Roasted red pepper Greek yogurt veggie dip, 2 Tbsp	2
Veggie dip, Greek yogurt, spinach artichoke, 2 Tbsp	2
Mission	
Salsa con queso, medium, 2 Tbsp	2
Oasis	
Baba ghannouj, 2 Tbsp	1
Oikos	
Cucumber and dill yogurt dip, 2 Tbsp	1
French onion Greek yogurt dip, 2 Tbsp	1

Jams, Spreads, Salsa & Dips

On The Border

Monterey Jack creamy queso, 2 Tbsp — 2

Opadipity By Litehouse

Chipotle ranch Greek yogurt dip, 2 Tbsp — 2

Cucumber dill Greek yogurt dip, 2 Tbsp — 1

Otria Otria

Veggie dip, Greek yogurt, cucumber dill feta, 2 Tbsp — 2

Veggie dip, Greek yogurt, garden herb ranch, 2 Tbsp — 2

Pancho's

Dip, white cheese, 1 oz — 3

Peloponnese

Spread, baba ganoush, eggplant & tahini, 2 Tbsp — 1

Phillips

Dip, crab, Maryland style, 2 Tbsp — 3

Prairie Farms

Dip, French onion, 2 Tbsp — 1

Ruffles

Dip, creamy buffalo ranch, 2 Tbsp — 1

Sabra

Babaganoush, 2 Tbsp — 3

Crisp bell pepper Greek yogurt dip, 2 Tbsp — 1

Cucumber dill tzatziki Greek yogurt dip, 2 Tbsp — 2

Guacamole, classic, 2 Tbsp — 2

Mediterranean herb Greek yogurt dip, 2 Tbsp — 1

Veggie dip, cucumber & dill, 2 Tbsp — 1

Veggie dip, onion, 2 Tbsp — 2

Skotidakis

Jalapeño yogurt dip, 2 Tbsp — 2

Smilin Bobs

Original smoked fish dip, ½ oz — 2

Stonemill Kitchens

Dip, artichoke & jalapeño, 2 Tbsp — 3

T. Marzetti

Caramel apple-dip, light, 2 Tbsp — 5

T.G.I. Friday's

Cheese dip, spinach & artichoke, 2 Tbsp — 1

Queso dip, Mexican style, 2 Tbsp — 2

Taco Bell

Dip, sour cream, creamy jalapeño, 2 Tbsp — 3

Spicy ranch dressing and dip, 2 Tbsp — 5

The Fresh Hummus Co.

Olive hummus, 2 Tbsp — 2

Tostitos

Dip, creamy spinach, 2 Tbsp — 2

Dip, nacho cheese, medium, 1 cup — 6

Dip, nacho cheese, spicy, 2 Tbsp — 1

Dip, smooth & cheesy flavored, mild, 2 Tbsp — 2

Dip, zesty bean & cheese, medium, 2 Tbsp — 1

Queso blanco dip, 2 Tbsp — 2

Salsa con queso, medium, 2 Tbsp — 2

Tostitos Cantina

Roasted garlic thick and chunky salsa, 2 Tbsp — 0

Tostitos Dip-etizers

Mexican style four cheese queso dip, 2 Tbsp — 2

Trader Joe's

Cilantro & chive yogurt dip, 1 oz — 2

Creamy spinach and artichoke dip, 2 Tbsp — 2

Jalapeño Greek yogurt dip, 2 Tbsp — 2

Reduced guilt spinach and kale Greek yogurt dip, 1 oz — 2

Tzatziki, 1 oz — 1

Trader Joe's Reduced Guilt

Chunky guacamole, 2 Tbsp — 1

Jams, Spreads, Salsa & Dips

Jams, Spreads, Salsa & Dips

	SmartPoints™ value
Velveeta Bowls	
Dip, cheese & chili, with beef, 2 Tbsp	1
Dip, cheese & salsa, 2 tsp	1
Walden Farms	
Chocolate dip, 2 Tbsp	0
Dip, ranch, veggie, 2 Tbsp	0
Wegman's	
Dip, tzatziki, 2 Tbsp	2
Wholly	
Guacamole, classic, 2 Tbsp	2
Guacamole, Classic, 2 Tbsp	2
Wholly 100 Calorie Cups	
Guacamole, classic, minis, 1 cup	3
Guacamole, spicy, minis, 1 cup	3
Wholly 100 Calorie Snack Packs	
Classic flavor guacamole, 1 pouch (57 g)	3
Wholly Guacamole	
Guacamole, all natural classic, 2 Tbsp	2
Wholly Guacamole 100 Calories	
Avocado ranch guacamole snack packs, 1 pouch (57 g)	3
Spicy guacamole snack packs, 1 pouch (57 g)	3
Wholly Guacamole Minis	
Avocado ranch guacamole, 1 container (57 g)	3
Yucatan	
Authentic guacamole, 2 Tbsp	2

Fruit Butter/Spread

	SmartPoints™ value
Dalmatia	
Fig spread, 1 Tbsp	4
Dickinson's	
Curd, lemon, 1 Tbsp	3
Kirkland Signature Organic	
Strawberry spread, 1 Tbsp	2

	SmartPoints™ value
Kroger Just Fruit	
Spreadable fruit, seedless blackberry, 1 Tbsp	3
Spreadable fruit, strawberry, 1 Tbsp	2
Musselman's	
Apple butter, 1 Tbsp	2
Polaner	
Fruit spread, strawberry, seedless, 1 Tbsp	2
Polaner All Fruit	
Fruit spread, boysenberry, 1 Tbsp	2
Fruit spread, orange marmalade, 1 Tbsp	2
Spreadable fruit, raspberry, 1 Tbsp	2
Spreadable fruit, with fiber, apricot, 1 Tbsp	2
Spreadable fruit, with fiber, cherry, 1 Tbsp	2
Spreadable fruit, with fiber, grape, 1 Tbsp	2
Spreadable fruit, with fiber, seedless raspberry, 1 Tbsp	2
Strawberry spreadable fruit, 1 Tbsp	2
Polaner All Fruit with Fiber	
Fruit spread, apricot, 1 Tbsp	2
Fruit spread, blackberry seedless, 1 Tbsp	2
Fruit spread, grape, 1 Tbsp	2
Spreadable fruit, blueberry, 1 Tbsp	2
Spreadable fruit, peach, 1 Tbsp	2
Spreadable fruit, seedless, strawberry, 1 Tbsp	2
Spreadable fruit, strawberry, 1 Tbsp	2
Simple Truth Organic	
Spread, strawberry fruit, 1 Tbsp	2

Smucker's Natural

Concord grape fruit spread, 1 Tbsp	3
Fruit spread, concord grape, 1 Tbsp	3
Fruit spread, red raspberry, 1 Tbsp	2
Red raspberry fruit spread, 1 Tbsp	2
Strawberry fruit spread, 1 Tbsp	2
Strawberry fruit spread, 1 Tbsp	2

Smucker's Simply 100% Fruit

Apricot spreadable fruit, 1 Tbsp	2
Concord grape spreadable fruit, 1 tsp	2
Red raspberry spreadable fruit, 1 Tbsp	2
Seedless blackberry spreadable fruit, 1 Tbsp	2
Spreadable fruit, seedless, blackberry, ⅔ oz	2
Spreadable fruit, seedless, strawberry, ⅔ oz	2
Strawberry spreadable fruit, 1 Tbsp	2

Smucker's Simply Fruit

Spreadable fruit, apricot, 1 Tbsp	2
Spreadable fruit, black cherry, 1 Tbsp	2
Spreadable fruit, black raspberry, 1 Tbsp	2
Spreadable fruit, blueberry, 1 Tbsp	2
Spreadable fruit, red raspberry, 1 Tbsp	2
Spreadable fruit, strawberry, 1 Tbsp	2

Smucker's Squeeze

Fruit spread, reduced sugar, strawberry, 1 Tbsp	1
Fruit spread, strawberry, 1 Tbsp	3

Tap N' Apple

Apple butter spread, 1 Tbsp	1

Trader Joe's

Fig butter, 1 Tbsp	3

Welch's Natural

Spread, concord grape, 1 Tbsp	2
Spread, strawberry, 1 Tbsp	2
Raspberry spread, 1 Tbsp	2
Strawberry spread, 1 Tbsp	2

Garlic Spread

Stonewall Kitchen

Aioli, roasted garlic, 1 Tbsp	3

Hazelnut Butter/Spread

Jif

Hazelnut spread, chocolate flavored, 2 Tbsp	10
Hazelnut spread, salted caramel, 2 Tbsp	10

Justin's

Hazelnut butter, chocolate, 1 pack (14 g)	3
Hazelnut butter, chocolate, 2 Tbsp	7

Kroger

Hazelnut spread, with cocoa, 2 Tbsp	8

Nutella

Hazelnut spread with skim milk and cocoa, 2 Tbsp	10

Nutella & Go!

Hazelnut spread and breadsticks, 1 unit (52 g)	12

Nutella Mini Cups

Hazelnut spread, 1 (15 g)	4

Honey Butter

Downey's

Honey butter, cinnamon, 1 Tbsp	3
Honey butter, original, 1 Tbsp	3

Jams, Spreads, Salsa & Dips

Jams, Spreads, Salsa & Dips

Hummus

Archer Farms

Spinach and artichoke hummus, 2 Tbsp	2

Athenos

Hummus, artichoke & garlic, 2 Tbsp	2
Hummus, black olive, 2 Tbsp	2
Hummus, original, 2 Tbsp	2
Hummus, roasted eggplant, 2 Tbsp	1
Hummus, roasted garlic, 2 Tbsp	2
Hummus, roasted red pepper, 2 Tbsp	2
Hummus, spicy three pepper, 2 Tbsp	1

Basha

Original premium hommus, 1 oz	2

Boar's Head

Roasted red pepper hummus, 2 Tbsp	2
Traditional hummus, 2 Tbsp	3

Cedar's

Hommus, artichoke kalamata, 2 Tbsp	2
Hommus, artichoke spinach, 2 Tbsp	2
Hommus, classic original, 2 Tbsp	3
Hommus, garlic lovers, 2 Tbsp	1
Hommus, garlic lovers, family size, 2 Tbsp	1
Hommus, red pepper, roasted, party size, 2 Tbsp	2
Hommus, roasted garlic, 2 Tbsp	2
Hommus, roasted red pepper, 2 Tbsp	2
Hommus, tahini, original, 2 Tbsp	2
Hommus, zesty lemon, 2 Tbsp	2
Original hommus tahini, party size, 2 Tbsp	1
Original organic hommus, 2 Tbsp	2

Eat Well Enjoy Life

Hummus, black bean, sweet & spicy, with spicy roasted corn relish topping, medium, 2 Tbsp	1
Hummus, edamame, 2 Tbsp	3
Hummus, edamame (baby soybean), with roasted red peppers and toasted sesame, 2 Tbsp	3
Hummus, red lentil chipotle spicy, with poblano pepper & corn topping, medium, 2 Tbsp	2
Hummus, spicy yellow lentil, with sunflower seeds and apricot, medium, 2 Tbsp	2
Hummus, tuscan white bean, with roasted garlic tapenade, 2 Tbsp	3
Hummus, tuscan white bean, with roasted pine nuts & herbs, 2 Tbsp	3
Hummus, with Greek yogurt, roasted red pepper, 2 Tbsp	1

Eating Right

Hummus, artichoke spinach, 2 Tbsp	1
Hummus, garlic, 2 Tbsp	1
Hummus, roasted red pepper, 2 Tbsp	1
Hummus, traditional, 2 Tbsp	1

Fountain of Health

Roasted garlic hummus dip, 2 Tbsp	2
Roasted red pepper hummus, 2 Tbsp	1

Hannah Organic Singles

Hommus, 2 Tbsp	2

Hope Foods

Spicy avocado hope hummus, 2 Tbsp	2
Thai coconut curry hummus, 2 Tbsp	2

Joseph's

Hommus tahini, garlic lovers, party size!, 2 Tbsp	1
Hommus tahini, original, party size!, 2 Tbsp	1
Hommus tahini, roasted red pepper, 2 Tbsp	2
Hommus tahini, roasted red pepper, party size!, 2 Tbsp	1
Hommus, spinach & artichoke, 2 Tbsp	2

Marzetti Otria

Veggie dip, hummus, roasted garlic, 2 Tbsp	2
Veggie dip, hummus, roasted red pepper, 2 Tbsp	2

Oasis

Hommus, jalapeño, hot, 2 Tbsp	1
Hommus, original, 2 Tbsp	1
Hommus, roasted garlic, 2 Tbsp	1
Hommus, roasted red pepper, 2 Tbsp	1
Hommus, with roasted red pepper, 2 Tbsp	1

Oasis Classic Cuisine

Hommus, mediterranean medley, 2 Tbsp	0

Pita Pal

Hummus, roasted red pepper, 2 Tbsp	2

Sabra

Basil pesto hummus, 2 Tbsp	3
Classic hummus, 2 Tbsp	2
Classic hummus with pretzels, 1 container (128 g)	12
Hummus, classic, 2 Tbsp	2
Hummus, classic, singles, ¼ cup	5
Hummus, jalapeño, 2 Tbsp	2
Hummus, luscious lemon, 2 Tbsp	2
Hummus, olive tapenade, 2 Tbsp	3

Hummus, roasted garlic, 2 Tbsp	2
Hummus, roasted garlic, 2 Tbsp	2
Hummus, roasted pine nut, 2 Tbsp	3
Hummus, roasted red pepper, 2 Tbsp	2
Hummus, spinach and artichoke, 2 Tbsp	2
Hummus, sun dried tomatoes, 2 Tbsp	2
Hummus, supremely spicy, 2 Tbsp	2
Hummus, tuscan herb garden, 2 Tbsp	2
Roasted garlic hummus with pretzels, 1 container (128 g)	11

Sabra Go Mediterranean

Hummus chipotle, 2 Tbsp	2

Summer Fresh

Hummus, avocado, 2 Tbsp	1

The Fresh Hummus Co.

Garlic hummus, 2 Tbsp	2
Roasted red pepper hummus, 2 Tbsp	2
Spinach artichoke hummus, 2 Tbsp	2

Trader Joe's

Beet hummus, 2 Tbsp	2
Hummus quartet, 2 Tbsp	1
Kalamata olive hummus, 1 oz	2
Mediterranean hummus, 1 oz	2
Mediterranean hummus snack pack with pita chips, 1 container (113 g)	10
Original hummus dip, 1 oz	1
Roasted garlic hummus, 1 oz	2
Smooth & creamy cilantro & jalapeño hummus, 1 oz	2
Smooth & creamy spicy hummus, 1 oz	2
Tomato basil hummus, 1 oz	1

Jams, Spreads, Salsa & Dips

SmartPoints™ value

Tribe

Everything hummus, 2 Tbsp	2
Hummus, classic, 1 serving (57 g)	4
Hummus, cracked chili peppers, 2 Tbsp	1
Hummus, forty spices, 2 Tbsp	1
Hummus, organic, classic, 2 Tbsp	1
Hummus, organic, sweet roasted red peppers, 2 Tbsp	1
Hummus, roasted garlic, 2 Tbsp	1
Hummus, roasted vegetables, 2 Tbsp	2
Hummus, spicy red pepper, 2 Tbsp	2
Hummus, zesty lemon, 2 Tbsp	1
Hummus, zesty spice & garlic, 2 Tbsp	2
Mediterranean olive hummus, 2 Tbsp	2
Mediterranean style hummus, 2 Tbsp	2
Sweet roasted red pepper hummus, 2 Tbsp	1

Tribe Origins

Hummus, classic, 2 Tbsp	2

Wegman's Food You Feel Good About

Hummus, 1 container (57 g)	4
Hummus, roasted garlic, 1 container (57 g)	4
Hummus, roasted red pepper, 1 container (57 g)	3
Hummus, roasted red pepper, snack packs, 1 container (57 g)	3
Hummus, snack packs, 1 snack pack (57 g)	4
Roasted garlic hummus, 2 Tbsp	2
Spicy chipotle hummus, 2 Tbsp	2
Vegetable hummus, 2 Tbsp	2

Whole Foods

Hummus, original, ⅛ package (28 g)	1

Wild Garden Snack Pack to Go

Traditional hummus dip and sea salt pita chips, 1 pack (85 g)	7

Jam

SmartPoints™ value

Bama

Jam, grape, 1 Tbsp	3

Bonnie's Jams

Fig preserves jam, 1 Tbsp	1

Knott's Berry Farm

Pure seedless jam, boysenberry, 1 Tbsp	3

Kroger

Jam, concord grape, 1 Tbsp	3

Polaner Sugar Free with Fiber

Jam, concord grape, 1 Tbsp	0

Smucker's

Black raspberry blackberry seedless jam, 1 Tbsp	3
Jam, black raspberry, 1 Tbsp	3
Jam, blackberry, 1 Tbsp	3
Jam, blackberry, seedless, ¾ oz	3
Jam, red plum, 1 Tbsp	3
Jam, red raspberry, 1 Tbsp	3
Jam, seedless blackberry, sugar free, 1 Tbsp	0
Jam, strawberry, seedless, 1 Tbsp	3
Jam, sugar free, seedless, blackberry, 1 Tbsp	0
Seedless boysenberry jam, 1 Tbsp	3
Strawberry jam, 1 Tbsp	3

Smucker's Sugar Free

Concord grape jam, 1 Tbsp	0
Seedless blackberry jam, 1 Tbsp	0
Seedless strawberry jam, 1 Tbsp	0

Stonewall Kitchen

Jam, wild Maine blueberry, 1 Tbsp	2

Welch's

Jam, concord grape, 1 Tbsp	3

Whole Foods

Jam, wild blueberry (serves 16), 1 serving (21 g)	3

Ziyad

Jam, fig, 1 tsp	3

Jelly

Bama

Jelly, grape, 1 Tbsp	3

Berryhill

Grape jelly, 1 Tbsp	3

Bonne Maman

Jelly, blackberry, 1 Tbsp	3

Bonnie's Jams

Red pepper jelly, 1 Tbsp	2

Clover Valley

Concord grape jelly, 1 Tbsp	2

Crofters Organic

Conserve, raspberry, 1 Tbsp	2

Great Value

Squeezable grape jelly, 1 Tbsp	2

Hannaford

Jelly, strawberry, 1 Tbsp	3

Kroger

Jelly, concord grape, 1 Tbsp	2

Our Family Jellies

Jelly, grape, 1 Tbsp	3

Palmalito

Jelly, jalapeño pepper, 1 Tbsp	3

Polaner

Jelly, grape, 1 Tbsp	2

Reese

Jelly, pepper, hot, 1 Tbsp	3

ShopRite

Jelly, strawberry, 1 Tbsp	3

Smucker's

Blackberry jelly, 1 Tbsp	3
Jelly, apple, 1 Tbsp	3
Jelly, black raspberry, 1 Tbsp	3
Jelly, blackberry, 1 Tbsp	3
Jelly, cherry, 1 Tbsp	3
Jelly, concord grape, 1 Tbsp	3
Jelly, low sugar, concord grape, 1 Tbsp	1
Jelly, mixed fruit, 1 Tbsp	3

Jelly, red raspberry, 1 Tbsp	3
Jelly, strawberry, 1 Tbsp	3

Smucker's Low Sugar

Jelly, reduced sugar, concord grape, 1 Tbsp	1

Smucker's Squeeze

Jelly, grape, 1 Tbsp	3

Trader Joe's

Organic concord grape jelly, 1 Tbsp	3

Trappist Preserves

Jelly, hot pepper, 1 Tbsp	3

Welch's

Jelly, concord grape, 1 Tbsp	3
Jelly, reduced sugar, concord grape, 1 Tbsp	1

Margarine

Blue Bonnet

46% vegetable oil spread, 1 Tbsp	2
65% vegetable oil spread, 1 Tbsp	3
Vegetable oil spread with calcium and vitamin D, 1 Tbsp	2
Vegetable oil spread, 53%, 1 Tbsp	3

Blue Bonnet Light

Vegetable oil spread, 31%, 1 Tbsp	1

Brummel & Brown

Spread, 1 Tbsp	2
Spread made with yogurt, 1 Tbsp	2

Country Crock

35% vegetable oil & 25% yogurt spread, 1 Tbsp	1
39% vegetable oil spread, 1 Tbsp	2

Countryside Creamery

Homestyle spread, country recipe, 1 Tbsp	2

Earth Balance

Buttery spread, organic, whipped, 1 Tbsp	3
Vegan buttery sticks, 1 Tbsp	4

Jams, Spreads, Salsa & Dips

	SmartPoints™ value
Fleischmann's	
Light margarine, 1 Tbsp	1
Margarine spread, 1 Tbsp	3
Margarine, original, 1 Tbsp	4
Vegetable oil spread, 60% whipped, 1 Tbsp	2
Vegetable oil spread, 60%, whipped, original, 1 Tbsp	2
Gold n Soft	
Spread, 40% vegetable oil, 1 Tbsp	2
Great Value	
Spreadable butter with canola oil, 1 Tbsp	4
I Can't Believe It's Not Butter!	
45% vegetable oil spread made with olive oil, 1 Tbsp	2
Garlic spread, 1 Tbsp	2
Light 30% vegetable oil spread, 1 Tbsp	1
Light vegetable spread, 1 Tbsp	1
Original 45% vegetable oil spread, 1 Tbsp	2
Original spread, 1 Tbsp	2
I Can't Believe It's Not Butter! Deliciously Simple	
Vegetable oil spread, 1 serving (14 g)	4
Imperial	
Vegetable oil spread, 65%, cholesterol free, 1 Tbsp	3
Kroger	
Butter it's not!, 1 Tbsp	3
Land O' Lakes	
Margarine, 1 Tbsp	4
Spread, fresh buttery taste, 1 Tbsp	3
Land O' Lakes Fresh Buttery Taste	
Spread with olive oil, 1 Tbsp	3
Melt	
Buttery spread, organic, 1 Tbsp	3

	SmartPoints™ value
Move Over Butter	
Vegetable oil spread, whipped with sweet cream buttermilk, 1 Tbsp	2
Parkay	
60% vegetable oil spread, original, 1 Tbsp	3
Vegetable oil spread, 60%, 1 Tbsp	3
Vegetable oil spread, whipped, 1 Tbsp	3
Whipped vegetable oil spread, 1 Tbsp	3
Promise	
Margarine, nonfat, 1 Tbsp	0
Spread, 60% vegetable oil, buttery, 1 Tbsp	3
Spread, Vegetable oil, buttery light, 1 Tbsp	2
Promise Activ	
Spread, 35% vegetable oil, light, 1 Tbsp	2
Shedd's	
39% vegetable oil spread, calcium plus vitamin D, 1 Tbsp	2
39% vegetable oil spread, light, 1 Tbsp	2
48% vegetable oil spread, 1 Tbsp	2
51% vegetable oil spread, 1 Tbsp	2
51% vegetable oil spread, churn style, 1 Tbsp	2
53% vegetable oil spread, original, 1 Tbsp	3
Vegetable oil spread, 52%, soft, country crock, 1 Tbsp	2
Vegetable oil spread, shedd's spread, 1 Tbsp	2
Shedd's Spread Country Crock	
Original vegetable oil spread, 1 Tbsp	2
Smart Balance	
Buttery spread, omega plus, non-hydrogenated, 1 Tbsp	3
Light buttery spread, 1 Tbsp	2

Smart Beat
Super light margarine, 1 Tbsp	1

Smart Beat Smart Squeeze
Nonfat margarine spread, 1 Tbsp	0

Marmalade

Albertson's
Marmalade, orange, 1 Tbsp	3

Polaner
Marmalade, orange, with fiber, sugar free, 1 Tbsp	0

Smucker's
Marmalade, sweet orange, 1 Tbsp	3
Sweet orange marmalade, 1 Tbsp	3

Smucker's Low Sugar
Marmalade, reduced sugar, sweet orange, 1 Tbsp	1

Smucker's Simply 100% Fruit
Orange marmalade spreadable fruit, 1 Tbsp	2

Smucker's Sugar Free
Marmalade, orange, 1 Tbsp	0

Trader Joe's
Seville orange marmalade, 1 Tbsp	3

Peanut Butter

Adams
Organic peanut butter, creamy, 2 Tbsp	6
Peanut butter, creamy, 2 Tbsp	6
Peanut butter, unsalted, creamy, 2 Tbsp	6
Peanut butter, unsalted, crunchy, 2 Tbsp	6

BetterBody Foods PB Fit
Peanut butter powder, 2 Tbsp	2

Better'n Peanut Butter
Banana, 2 Tbsp	3
Chocolate, 2 Tbsp	3
Low sodium, 2 Tbsp	3
Original, 2 Tbsp	3

Betty Lou's Just Great Stuff
Organic powdered chocolate peanut butter, 2 Tbsp	1

Crazy Richard's
Peanut butter, chunky, 2 Tbsp	6
Peanut butter, creamy, 2 Tbsp	6

Cream Nut
Peanut butter, natural, smooth, 2 Tbsp	6

Earth Balance
Crunchy natural peanut butter, 2 Tbsp	6
Peanut butter, natural, and flaxseed, creamy, 2 Tbsp	6

Essential Everyday
Peanut butter spread, creamy, reduced fat, 2 Tbsp	6
Peanut butter, creamy, 2 Tbsp	7

Full Circle Organic
Peanut butter, creamy, no sugar added, 2 Tbsp	7

Great Value Natural
Crunchy no stir peanut butter spread, 2 Tbsp	6

Hilton
Replacement, peanut butter, 2 Tbsp	7

Jif
Creamy peanut butter, 2 Tbsp	6
Extra crunchy peanut butter, 2 Tbsp	6
Omega-3 creamy peanut butter, 2 Tbsp	6
Peanut butter spread, creamy, reduced fat, 2 Tbsp	6
Peanut butter spread, natural, creamy, 2 Tbsp	6
Peanut butter, creamy, 2 Tbsp	6
Peanut butter, creamy, family size, 2 Tbsp	5
Peanut butter, creamy, omega-3, 2 Tbsp	6

Jams, Spreads, Salsa & Dips

Jams, Spreads, Salsa & Dips

	SmartPoints™ value
Peanut butter, creamy, with honey, 2 Tbsp	7
Peanut butter, reduced fat, crunchy, 2 Tbsp	6
Reduced fat creamy peanut butter, 2 Tbsp	6
To go, creamy natural peanut butter spread, 1 container (43 g)	8
Whipped peanut butter and pumpkin pie spice, 2 Tbsp	5
Jif Natural	
Peanut butter spread & honey, creamy, 2 Tbsp	6
Peanut butter spread, creamy, 2 Tbsp	6
Peanut butter spread, crunchy, 2 Tbsp	6
Peanut butter, crunchy, 2 Tbsp	6
Jif Simply	
Peanut butter, creamy, 2 Tbsp	6
Jif To Go	
Creamy peanut butter, 1 snack cup (43 g)	8
Creamy peanut butter spread, 1 container (43 g)	8
Peanut butter, crunchy, 1 cup	8
Reduced fat creamy peanut butter spread, 1 container (48 g)	8
Jif To Go Chocolate Silk	
Peanut butter and chocolate flavored spread, 1 container (43 g)	10
Jif To Go Dippers	
Creamy peanut butter with pretzels, 1 pack (48 g)	8
Jif Whips	
Peanut butter, whipped, & chocolate flavored spread, 2 Tbsp	6
Peanut butter, whipped, creamy, 2 Tbsp	5
Whipped peanut butter and chocolate mint spread, 2 Tbsp	6
Whipped peanut butter and maple brown sugar spread, 2 Tbsp	5

	SmartPoints™ value
Just Great Stuff	
Peanut butter, organic, powdered, 2 Tbsp	1
Krema	
Peanut butter, natural, crunchy, 2 Tbsp	6
Peanut butter, natural, smooth & creamy, 2 Tbsp	6
Kroger	
Crunchy peanut butter, 2 Tbsp	6
Crunchy roasted peanuts and honey, 2 Tbsp	6
Natural creamy peanut butter, 2 Tbsp	6
Natural crunchy peanut butter, 2 Tbsp	6
Peanut butter, creamy, 2 Tbsp	6
Peanut butter, crunchy, 2 Tbsp	6
Peanut butter, natural creamy, 2 Tbsp	6
Peanut butter, natural crunchy, 2 Tbsp	6
Peanut butter, with honey, creamy, 2 Tbsp	7
Laura Scudder's	
Old fashioned peanut butter, smooth, 2 Tbsp	6
Peanut butter, old fashioned, nutty, 2 Tbsp	6
Peanut butter, smooth, 2 Tbsp	6
MaraNatha Organic	
Peanut butter, no stir, creamy, 2 Tbsp	6
Market Pantry	
Creamy no stir peanut butter spread, 2 Tbsp	6
Meijer Naturals	
Peanut butter, creamy, 2 Tbsp	6

Nature's Promise Organics

Organic crunchy peanut butter, 2 Tbsp	6
Peanut butter, organic smooth, salted, 2 Tbsp	6
Peanut butter, smooth/unsalted, organic, 2 Tbsp	7

O Organics

Peanut butter, no stir creamy, 2 Tbsp	7
Peanut butter, no stir crunchy, 2 Tbsp	7

Olde Style

100% natural peanut butter, unsalted, 2 Tbsp	6
Fresh ground peanut butter, unsalted, 2 Tbsp	6
Peanut butter, honey roasted, 2 Tbsp	7

Open Nature

Peanut butter, creamy, old fashioned, 2 Tbsp	6

Our Family Natural

Peanut butter, creamy, 2 Tbsp	6

PB2

Powdered peanut butter, 2 Tbsp	1
Powdered peanut butter with premium chocolate, 2 Tbsp	1

Peanut Butter & Co.

Crunch time peanut butter, 2 Tbsp	6

Peanut Delight

Peanut butter, creamy, 2 Tbsp	6

Peter Pan

Peanut butter, 100% natural, crunchy, 2 Tbsp	7
Peanut butter, creamy, 2 Tbsp	7
Peanut butter, creamy, 2 Tbsp	7
Peanut butter, creamy, reduced fat, 2 Tbsp	6
Peanut butter, crunchy, 2 Tbsp	6

Peanut butter, whipped creamy, ⅓ less sugar, 2 Tbsp	5
Peanut butter, whipped, creamy, 2 Tbsp	5

Peter Pan 100% Natural

Peanut butter, honey roast, creamy, 2 Tbsp	8

Planters

Peanut butter, creamy, 2 Tbsp	6

Publix

Peanut butter, creamy, all natural, 2 Tbsp	6

Reese's

Peanut butter chips, 1 Tbsp	4
Peanut butter chocolate spread, 2 Tbsp	8
Peanut butter, creamy, 2 Tbsp	6

Safeway Kitchens

Peanut spread, reduced fat, creamy, 2 Tbsp	6

Santa Cruz Organic

Peanut butter, creamy, 2 Tbsp	6

Santa Cruz Organic

Peanut butter, dark roasted, creamy, 2 Tbsp	6

ShopRite

Peanut butter, natural, super chunky, 2 Tbsp	6

Simply Jif

Fresh roasted peanut butter, low sodium, creamy, 2 Tbsp	6
Peanut butter, creamy, 1 serving (31 g)	6

Skippy

Natural peanut butter spread, creamy, 2 Tbsp	6
Peanut butter spread, reduced fat, creamy, 2 Tbsp	6
Peanut butter spread, super chunk, reduced fat, 2 Tbsp	6
Peanut butter, creamy, 2 Tbsp	6

Jams, Spreads, Salsa & Dips

Jams, Spreads, Salsa & Dips

	SmartPoints™ value
Peanut butter, creamy, roasted honey nut, 2 Tbsp	7
Peanut butter, extra crunchy, super chunk, 2 Tbsp	6
Skippy Natural	
Creamy peanut butter spread (⅓ less sodium and sugar), 2 Tbsp	7
Extra crunchy peanut butter with honey, 2 Tbsp	7
Peanut butter spread with dark chocolate, 2 Tbsp	7
Peanut butter spread, creamy, ⅓ less sodium & sugar, 2 Tbsp	7
Peanut butter spread, creamy, with honey, 2 Tbsp	7
Peanut butter spread, extra crunchy, super chunk, 2 Tbsp	6
Peanut butter spread, super chunk, 2 Tbsp	6
Peanut butter spread, super chunk, extra chunky, 2 Tbsp	6
Peanut butter spread, with honey, creamy, 2 Tbsp	7
Skippy Natural Super Chunk	
Extra crunchy peanut butter, 2 Tbsp	6
Skippy Singles	
Creamy peanut butter, 1 container (42 g)	9
Natural creamy peanut butter spread, 1 container (42 g)	9
Smart Balance	
Peanut butter, natural, chunky, rich roast, 2 Tbsp	6
Peanut butter, real, chunky, 2 Tbsp	6
Smart Balance Natural	
Creamy peanut butter, 2 Tbsp	6
Smart Balance Omega	
Natural peanut butter, and omega-3 from flax oil, extra creamy, 2 Tbsp	6

	SmartPoints™ value
Smucker's	
Goober, strawberry, 3 Tbsp	9
Reduced fat peanut butter, creamy, 1 oz	6
Smucker's Goober	
Peanut butter and grape jelly stripes, 3 Tbsp	10
Smucker's Natural	
Chunky peanut butter, 2 Tbsp	6
Creamy peanut butter, 2 Tbsp	6
Peanut butter, chunky, 2 Tbsp	6
Smucker's Organic	
Peanut butter, chunky, 2 Tbsp	6
Peanut butter, creamy, 2 Tbsp	6
Stop & Shop All Natural	
Peanut butter, creamy, 2 Tbsp	6
Teddie	
Peanut butter, all natural, smooth, 2 Tbsp	6
Peanut butter, old fashioned, super chunky, 32 Tbsp	6
Peanut butter, old fashioned, unsalted, smooth, 2 Tbsp	6
Peanut butter, smooth, all natural organic, 2 Tbsp	6
Peanut butter, unsalted, super chunky, 2 Tbsp	6
Peanut butter, with flaxseed, chunky, 2 Tbsp	5
Peanut butter, with flaxseed, smooth, 2 Tbsp	5
Trader Joe's	
Crunchy salted peanut butter with flax & chia seeds, 1 oz	5
Peanut butter, creamy salted, 2 Tbsp	6
Peanut butter, creamy unsalted, 2 Tbsp	6
Peanut butter, crunchy salted, 2 Tbsp	6
Peanut butter, crunchy unsalted, 2 Tbsp	6

Trader Joe's Organic

Creamy salted peanut butter, 2 Tbsp	6
Creamy unsalted peanut butter, 2 Tbsp	6
Crunchy salted peanut butter, 2 Tbsp	6
Crunchy unsalted peanut butter, 2 Tbsp	6

Wegman's

Peanut butter, creamy, 2 Tbsp	7
Peanut spread, reduced fat, creamy, 2 Tbsp	6

Wegman's Food You Feel Good About

Peanut butter, natural, creamy, 2 Tbsp	6
Peanut butter, natural, organic, creamy, 2 Tbsp	7
Peanut butter, organic, crunchy, 2 Tbsp	7

Welch's

Pb&j creamy peanut butter with concord grape bite size snacks, 1 pouch (23 g)	5
Pb&j creamy peanut butter with strawberry bite size snacks, pouch (23 g)	5

Whole Foods 365 Everyday Value

All natural crunchy peanut butter, 2 Tbsp	6

Whole Foods 365 Organic

Creamy peanut butter, 2 Tbsp	6

Wonder Natural Foods

Better'n peanut butter, original, 2 Tbsp	3

Pimiento Spread

Kraft

Pimento spread, 2 Tbsp	4

Trader Joe's

Pimento cheese spread, 1 oz	5

Preserves

Berryhill
Preserves, strawberry, 1 Tbsp	3

Bonne Maman
Preserves, apricot, 1 Tbsp	3
Preserves, cherry, 1 Tbsp	3
Preserves, fig, 1 Tbsp	3
Preserves, four fruits, 1 Tbsp	3
Preserves, peach, 1 Tbsp	3
Preserves, raspberry, 1 Tbsp	3
Preserves, strawberry, 1 Tbsp	3
Preserves, wild blueberry, 1 Tbsp	3

Braswell's
Fig preserves, 1 Tbsp	2

Dickinson's
Preserves, pure pacific mountain strawberry, 1 Tbsp	3
Preserves, pure seedless, marion blackberry, 1 Tbsp	3

E.D. Smith
Michigan cherry preserve, 1 Tbsp	1

Fit & Active Sugar Free
Red raspberry preserves, 1 Tbsp	0

Galil
Preserve, strawberry, 1 Tbsp	3

Giant
Peach preserves, 1 Tbsp	3

Hafi
Preserves, lingonberry, 1 Tbsp	2

Kroger
Preserves, apricot, 1 Tbsp	2
Preserves, peach, 1 Tbsp	2
Preserves, red raspberry, 1 Tbsp	2
Preserves, reduced sugar, strawberry, 1 Tbsp	1
Preserves, strawberry, 1 Tbsp	3

Jams, Spreads, Salsa & Dips

	SmartPoints™ value
Polaner	
Preserves, apricot, with fiber, sugar free, 1 Tbsp	0
Preserves, with fiber, seedless blackberry, sugar free, 1 Tbsp	0
Preserves, with fiber, strawberry, sugar free, 1 Tbsp	0
Smucker's	
Light boysenberry preserves, sugar free, 1 Tbsp	0
Preserves, blueberry, 1 Tbsp	3
Preserves, light, sugar free, strawberry, 1 Tbsp	0
Preserves, strawberry, 1 Tbsp	3
Preserves, strawberry, sugar free, 1 Tbsp	0
Preserves, strawberry-blackberry, 1 Tbsp	3
Red raspberry preserves, organic, 1 Tbsp	3
Red raspberry reduced sugar preserves, 1 Tbsp	1
Strawberry preserves, low sugar, 1 Tbsp	1
Smucker's Low Sugar	
Preserves, reduced sugar, apricot, 1 Tbsp	1
Preserves, strawberry, reduced sugar, 1 Tbsp	1
Smucker's Orchard's Finest	
Preserves, Michigan red tart cherry, 1 Tbsp	3
Preserves, northwest triple berry, 1 Tbsp	3
Preserves, northwoods blueberry, 1 Tbsp	3
Preserves, pacific mountain strawberry, 1 Tbsp	3
Smucker's Special Recipe	
Strawberry preserves, 1 Tbsp	3

	SmartPoints™ value
Smucker's Sugar Free	
Preserves, apricot, 1 Tbsp	0
Preserves, cherry, 1 Tbsp	0
Preserves, peach, 1 Tbsp	0
Red raspberry preserves, 1 Tbsp	0
Strawberry preserves, 1 Tbsp	0
Trader Joe's	
Organic reduced sugar strawberry preserves, 1 Tbsp	2
Raspberry preserves made with fresh raspberries, 1 Tbsp	3
Strawberry preserves made with real strawberries, 1 Tbsp	3

Pumpkin Butter
Trader Joe's	
Pumpkin butter, 1 Tbsp	2

Salsa
Casa Mamita	
Salsa, thick & chunky, medium, 2 Tbsp	0
Salsa, thick & chunky, mild, 2 Tbsp	0
Chachies	
Mango peach salsa, 2 Tbsp	1
East Coast Fresh Cuts	
Salsa, fresh, 2 Tbsp	0
Garden Fresh Gourmet	
Salsa, artichoke garlic, mild, 2 Tbsp	1
Salsa, Jack's special, medium, 2 Tbsp	1
Salsa, Jack's special, medium hot, 1 oz	1
Salsa, Jack's special, mild, 2 Tbsp	0
Salsa, sweet onion, mild, 1 oz	1
Salsa, thick & chunky, medium, 2 Tbsp	0
Giant/Stop & Shop	
Mild salsa, 2 Tbsp	0

Green Mountain Gringo

Salsa, medium, 2 Tbsp	0

Herdez

Salsa, casera, 2 Tbsp	0
Salsa, mild, 2 Tbsp	0
Salsa, verde, 2 Tbsp	0

Italian Rose

Fresh salsa, 1 Tbsp	0
Fresh salsa with cilantro, 2 Tbsp	0

Kirkland Signature Organic

Salsa, 2 Tbsp	0

La Mexicana

Hot salsa, 2 Tbsp	0
Salsa, medium, 2 Tbsp	0
Salsa, mild, 2 Tbsp	0

La Victoria

Salsa verde, thick 'n chunky, medium, 2 Tbsp	0

Newman's Own

Salsa, all natural chunky, mild, 2 Tbsp	0
Salsa, farmer's garden, medium, 2 Tbsp	1
Salsa, mango, medium chunky, 2 Tbsp	1
Salsa, medium chunky, 2 Tbsp	0
Salsa, medium chunky, black bean & corn, 2 Tbsp	1

Newman's Own All Natural

Salsa, peach, 2 Tbsp	1
Salsa, pineapple, medium, chunky, 2 Tbsp	1

On The Border

Medium salsa, 2 Tbsp	0
Salsa, mild, 2 Tbsp	0

On The Border Mexican Grill & Cantina

Salsa, medium, 2 Tbsp	0

Ortega

Salsa, thick & chunky, medium, 2 Tbsp	0
Salsa, thick & chunky, mild, 2 Tbsp	0

Pace

Chunky medium salsa, 2 Tbsp	1
Chunky mild salsa, 2 Tbsp	1
Chunky salsa, hot, 2 Tbsp	0
Chunky salsa, medium, 2 Tbsp	0
Chunky salsa, mild, 2 Tbsp	0
Salsa, chipotle, medium, 2 Tbsp	1
Salsa, restaurant style, medium, 2 Tbsp	0
Salsa, restaurant style, peach mango, medium, 2 Tbsp	1

Sabra

Salsa, chunky pico de gallo, medium, 2 Tbsp	0
Salsa, homestyle, medium, with tostitos tortilla chips, 1 serving (116 g)	4
Salsa, mango peach, medium, 2 Tbsp	1

Specially Selected

All natural black bean & corn salsa, 2 Tbsp	1

Tostitos

Salsa, chunky, hot, 2 Tbsp	0
Salsa, chunky, mild, 2 Tbsp	0
Salsa, con queso, medium, 2 Tbsp	2
Salsa, medium, 2 Tbsp	1
Salsa, restaurant style, medium, 2 Tbsp	1

Tostitos Cantina

Chipotle restaurant style salsa, 2 Tbsp	0

Trader Jose's

Salsa verde, 2 Tbsp	0

Wholly

Salsa, guacamole & spicy pico, 2 Tbsp	1

Jams, Spreads, Salsa & Dips

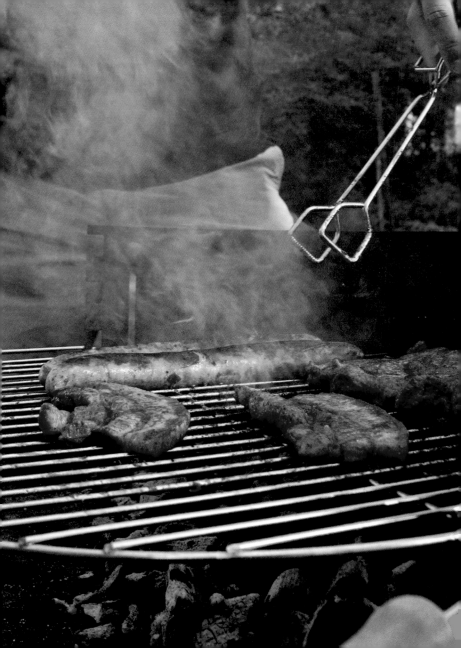

meat
& Poultry

Bacon & Canadian Bacon

Applegate

Bacon, turkey, uncured,
2 slices (28 g) — 1

Applegate Naturals

Bacon, Sunday, uncured,
2 slices (14 g) — 2

Bacon, uncured, good morning,
2 slices (14 g) — 1

Appleton Farms

Bacon, fully cooked, 3 slices (15 g) — 2

Boar's Head

Bacon, imported, naturally smoked,
fully cooked, 3 slices (14 g) — 2

Bacon, naturally smoked,
2 slices (45 g) — 2

Bob Evans

Canadian bacon, smoked,
4 slices (57 g) — 1

Butterball Everyday

Turkey bacon, original,
1 slice (14 g) — 1

Turkey bacon, thin & crispy,
2 slices (18 g) — 1

Coleman

Bacon, uncured, hickory smoked,
2 slices (15 g) — 2

Eating Right

Canadian bacon, sliced,
4 slices (57 g) — 1

Eating Right For Calorie Counting

Bacon, turkey, 1 slice (28 g) — 1

Farmland

Bacon, classic cut, naturally
hickory smoked,
2 pan fried slices (15 g) — 3

Fit & Active

Turkey bacon, 1 slice (14 g) — 1

Giant

Bacon, fully cooked, hickory
smoked, 3 slices (15 g) — 2

Center cut bacon, 2 slices (15 g) — 1

Godshall's

Turkey bacon, 1 slice (28 g) — 1

Turkey bacon slices, 2 slices (12 g) — 1

Turkey bacon, smoked sliced,
1 slice (28 g) — 1

Turkey bacon, smoked sliced,
maple, 1 slice (28 g) — 1

Great Value

Bacon, hickory smoked,
fully cooked, 2 slices (15 g) — 3

Bacon, lower sodium,
2 slices (15 g) — 3

Bacon, naturally hardwood
smoked, 2 slices (15 g) — 2

Bacon, real pieces (serves 10),
1 serving (7 g) — 1

Turkey bacon, 1 slice (14 g) — 1

Gwaltney

Bacon, beef, 1 slice (9 g) — 1

Bacon, premium sliced, hardwood
smoked, 2 fried slices (14 g) — 2

Habbersett

Bacon, Canadian, 3 slices (51 g) — 1

Hatfield

Bacon, hardwood smoked, classic,
3 slices (76 g) — 2

Ham, Canadian brand,
1 slice (28 g) — 1

Hempler's

Bacon, center cut, applewood
smoked, 2 slices (20 g) — 2

Hormel

Bacon pieces, fully cooked, ½ oz — 2

Bacon, applewood smoked, 1 Tbsp — 1

Bacon, crumbled, 1 Tbsp — 1

Bacon, fully cooked, 2 slices (14 g) — 2

Bacon, microwave ready,
lower sodium, 2 slices (15 g) — 3

Bacon, microwave ready,
original, 2 slices (15 g) — 3

Canadian bacon, pizza style,
22 slices (56 g) — 2

Meat & Poultry

	SmartPoints™ value
Canadian bacon, thick sliced, 2 slices (56 g)	1
Real bacon bits, 1 Tbsp	1
Hormel Black Label	
Bacon, 2 slices (21 g)	3
Bacon, original, 2 fried slices (15 g)	3
Bacon, thick sliced, applewood smoked, 2 slices (23 g)	4
Hormel Natural Choice	
Bacon, uncured, original, sliced, 2 slices (15 g)	3
Canadian bacon, sliced, 2 slices (56 g)	1
Jennie-O	
Turkey bacon, 1 slice (15 g)	1
Turkey bacon, lean, thick cut, 1 slice (28 g)	1
Turkey bacon, smoked and cured, 1 slice (17 g)	1
Jimmy Dean	
Bacon slices, premium precooked, harvest maple, 3 slices (16 g)	4
John Morrell Ready Crisp	
Bacon, fully cooked, premium, 3 slices (13 g)	2
Jones Dairy Farm	
Canadian bacon, naturally hickory smoked, 3 slices (51 g)	1
Kirkland Signature	
Bacon, crumbled, 1 Tbsp	1
Bacon, sliced, 2 slices (15 g)	2
Bacon, thick sliced, fully cooked, 2 slices (18 g)	3
Kroger	
Bacon, fully cooked, lower sodium, 3 slices (15 g)	3
Bacon, hardwood smoked, thick cut, 1 slice (12 g)	2
Bacon, lower sodium, hardwood smoked, 2 slices (15 g)	3
Bacon, turkey, 1 slice (14 g)	1

	SmartPoints™ value
Canadian bacon, sliced, 4 slices (57 g)	1
Real bacon bits, hickory smoke flavor, 1 Tbsp	1
Real turkey bacon pieces, hickory smoke flavor added, 1 Tbsp	1
Kroger Meals Made Simple	
Bacon, fully cooked, 3 slices (15 g)	2
Land O'Frost	
Canadian bacon, natural hickory smoked, 2 oz	1
Land O'Frost Breakfast Cuts	
Canadian bacon, thick sliced, natural hickory smoked, 3 slices (60 g)	1
Canadian bacon, thick sliced, sweet country maple, 3 slices (60 g)	1
Meijer	
Bacon bits, real, original, 1 Tbsp	1
Canadian bacon, 3 slices (61 g)	1
Turkey bacon, 1 slice (17 g)	1
Niman Ranch	
Canadian bacon, uncured, 2 slices (66 g)	2
Omaha Steaks	
Bacon slice, precooked (80 ct.), 4 pieces (30 g)	3
Oscar Mayer	
Bacon, applewood smoked, thick cut, 1 cooked slice (12 g)	2
Bacon, center cut, original, 2 slices (13 g)	2
Bacon, fully cooked, family size, 3 slices (18 g)	2
Bacon, fully cooked, original, 3 slices (18 g)	2
Bacon, fully cooked, thick cut, 2 slices (14 g)	2
Bacon, hickory smoked, butcher thick cut, 1 cooked slice (12 g)	2
Bacon, maple, 2 slices (18 g)	3
Bacon, naturally hardwood smoked, 2 slices (19 g)	3

Meat & Poultry

	SmartPoints™ value
Bacon, thick cut, 1 slice (38 g)	2
Real bacon, bits, 1 Tbsp	1
Real bacon, recipe pieces, 1 Tbsp	1
Turkey bacon, lower sodium, with sea salt, 1 slice (15 g)	1
Oscar Mayer Selects	
Bacon, turkey, 1 slice (15 g)	1
Bacon, uncured, smoked, 2 slices (15 g)	3
Plumrose	
Bacon, center cut, 3 slices (49 g)	2
Private Selection	
Bacon, center cut, 2 slices (15 g)	1
Publix	
Bacon, hickory smoked fully cooked, 3 slices (12 g)	2
Red Label	
Canadian bacon, 2 oz	1
Rose	
Canadian bacon, sliced, smoked, 3 slices (62 g)	1
Rose Private Stock	
Canadian bacon, sliced, 4 slices (57 g)	1
Shady Brook Farms	
Turkey bacon, smoked, 1 slice (14 g)	1
ShopRite	
Bacon, turkey, 1 slice (14 g)	1
Smithfield	
Bacon, hometown original, pouch pack, 2 slices (17 g)	3
Bacon, naturally hickory smoked, lower sodium, 2 slices (17 g)	3
Bacon, naturally hickory smoked, thick sliced, 1 slice (12 g)	2
Specially Selected	
Bacon, center cut, 3 slices (15 g)	2
Sugardale	
Bacon, regular sliced, 2 slices (16 g)	3

	SmartPoints™ value
Trader Joe's	
Bacon, uncured, apple smoked, 1 slice (15 g)	3
Turkey bacon, uncured, 1 slice (28 g)	0
Tyson	
Bacon, naturally hardwood smoked, 2 slices (15 g)	3
Bacon, thick cut, naturally hardwood smoked, 2 fried slices (24 g)	5
W Brand All Natural	
Bacon, classic sliced, dry rubbed uncured, 2 slices (12 g)	2
Wegman's	
Bacon, center cut, 3 slices (16 g)	2
Bacon, center cut, regular slice, 3 slices (16 g)	2
Bacon, center cut, thick slice, 3 slices (18 g)	2
Wright	
Bacon, applewood, 2 slices (15 g)	3
Bacon, naturally hickory smoked, 1 slice (14 g)	2

Beef

	SmartPoints™ value
Ball Park	
Beef patty, flame grilled, 1 patty (85 g)	8
Boar's Head	
Prime rib of beef, seasoned, 3 oz	9
Bubba	
Burger, ¼ pound, 1 burger (114 g)	7
Burger, original, 1 burger (151 g)	14
Burgers, certified angus chuck, 1 burger (150 g)	15
Burgers, with sweet onions, 1 burger (150 g)	11
Butchers Cut	
Ground beef, angus, grass fed, 4 oz	4
Cargill Meat Solutions	
Ground beef, 96/4, 4 oz	2

Castle Wood Reserve

Beef, angus, 2 oz	3

Century Farm

Beef, ground, extra lean, 96%, 4 oz	2

Great American Hamburgers

Hamburgers, 3 oz, 1 patty (63 g)	6
Hamburgers, 6 oz, 1 patty (114 g)	10
Homestyle burgers, sirloin steak, ⅓ lb, 1 patty (135 g)	9

Great Value

100% pure beef burgers, 1 burger (113 g)	9

Hormel

Beef roast, au jus, 5 oz	5

Inter-American Products, Inc.

Ground beef, 93/7, 4 oz	3

Jack Daniel's

Beef brisket, with Jack Daniel's glaze, ⅓ package (151 g)	7

John Soules Foods Fully Cooked

Angus beef steak seasoned and thinly sliced, 3 oz	2

Kirkland Signature

Ground beef patty, 1 patty (112 g)	10
Ground sirloin and loin of beef patty, 1 patty (151 g)	10

Kroger

Beef patties, ground, 4 oz	3
Burgers, sliders, 1 patty (56 g)	4
Ground sirloin, 4 oz	5
Patties, ground chuck, 1 patty (112 g)	9
Sirloin patties, ground, 4 oz	5

Landis

Beef tip steak, sirloin, 4 oz	4

Laura's Lean Beef

Beef, ground, 4 oz	4
Patties, ground beef, 1 patty (112 g)	4

Marcela Valladolid

Beef flank steak, for arrachera, 4 oz	5
Beef skirt steak, for carne asada, 4 oz	6

Market Pantry

Beef patties, 93% lean, ground, 4 oz	4
Beef, 93% lean, ground, 4 oz	4

Meal Mart

Corned beef, cooked, 2 oz	3

Old Neighborhood

Beef, steak, shaved, 2 oz	3

Omaha Steaks

4 oz beef tenderloin steak (filet mignon), 1 (112 g)	9
4 oz beef top sirloin steaks, 1 (112 g)	7
4 oz gourmet style ground beef burgers, 1 (112 g)	7
4 oz ground beef burgers, 1 (112 g)	9
5 oz beef tenderloin steak (filet mignon), 1 (140 g)	11
5 oz beef top sirloin steaks, 1 (140 g)	9
5 oz ground beef burgers, 1 (140 g)	12
5 oz triple trim filet mignon, 1 (140 g)	5
6 oz beef ribeye steaks, 1 (168 g)	15
6 oz beef tenderloin steaks (filet mignon), 1 (168 g)	13
6 oz beef top sirloin steaks, 1 (168 g)	10
7 oz beef ribeye steaks, 1 (196 g)	18
8 oz beef ribeye steaks, 1 (224 g)	20
8 oz beef top sirloin steaks, 1 (224 g)	14
10 oz beef ribeye steaks, 1 (280 g)	26
Beef ribeye slices (fully cooked), 8 oz	19

Meat & Poultry

	SmartPoints™ value
Beef rib roast, bone in, 3 oz	8
Beef rib roast, boneless, 3 oz	8
Beef short ribs, braised, 6 ½ oz	7
Beef sirloin tips, 3 oz	5
Beef sirloin tri tip roast, 3 oz	5
Beef stroganoff with noodles, 1 cup	10
Beef tenderloin steaks, 5 oz	10
Beef tenderloin tips, 3 oz	6
Beef top sirloin roast, 3 oz	5
Hamburger steak, 8 oz	14
Individual homestyle meatloaves, 6 oz	11
London broil top sirloin steak, 10 oz	7
Sirloin supreme top sirloin steak, 4 oz	2
Oscar Mayer Selects	
Roast beef, slow roasted, 6 slices (51 g)	1
Philly-Gourmet	
Beef homestyle patties, 100% pure, quarter pound, 1 patty (73 g)	7
Quick 'n Eat	
Beef, fully cooked choice angus patties, 1 patty (113 g)	8
Sinai Kosher	
Corned beef, cooked, sliced, 2 oz	2
Steak Umm	
Sliced steak, 1 cooked portion (32 g)	4
Trader Joe's	
Carne asada autentica, 4 oz	4
Tyson	
Country fried steak, 1 patty (75 g)	8
Wegman's Food You Feel Good About	
Ribeye steak, beef, organic, 3 oz	5
White Castle	
Microwaveable, hamburgers, 2 sandwiches (90 g)	8

	SmartPoints™ value
## Bison	
Great Range	
Bison, ground, 4 oz	5
Tender Bison	
Bison burgers, 80/20, 1 (151 g)	13
## Chicken	
Aidells	
Meatballs, chicken, caramelized onion, 3 meatballs (64 g)	4
Meatballs, chicken, spicy mango and jalapeño, 3 meatballs (64 g)	4
Meatballs, chicken, teriyaki & pineapple, 3 meatballs (64 g)	4
al fresco	
Chicken burgers, sweet Italian style, 1 patty (98 g)	3
Applegate Farms	
Chicken strips, organic, 3 strips (90.4 g)	4
Bell & Evans	
Burgers, chicken, 4 oz	3
Chicken breast tenders, breaded, 4 oz	5
Chicken breasts, breaded, boneless, skinless, 1 fillet (149 g)	6
Boar's Head	
Roasted chicken breast, boneless, skinless, maple glazed, 2 oz	1
Boca	
Chicken nuggets, meatless, original, 4 nuggets (87 g)	4
Brookdale	
Premium white chunk chicken breast in water, 2 oz	1
Bumble Bee	
Premium white chicken chunk in water, 2 oz	1
Daily Chef	
Chicken breast in water, ⅓ cup	1
Chicken fillets, with rib meat, mesquite grilled, 3 oz	1

Empire Kosher

Chicken leg quarters, 4 oz	5

Gold N Plump

Original boneless skinless chicken breast fillet, 1 piece (170 g)	2

Great Value

Chicken breasts, 4 oz	1
Chunk chicken breast, 2 oz	1
Crispy chicken tenderloin strips, 3 oz	4
Grilled chicken breast fillet with rib meat, 1 fillet (99 g)	2

Hannaford

Chicken breast, premium chunk, in water, canned, 2 oz	1

Harvestland

Chicken breast, boneless, skinless, 1 breast (177 g)	2
Chicken burger, uncooked, 1 burger (112 g)	3

Hormel

Premium chicken breast in water, 2 oz drained	0

Jack Daniel's

Pulled chicken, with Jack daniel's barbeque sauce, ⅓ package (151 g)	9

Jennie-O

Ground turkey, 85% lean/15% fat, 4 oz	6

John Soules Foods

Chicken breast fajitas, 3 oz	2
Grilled chicken breast strips, 3 oz	1
Rotisserie seasoned chicken breast strips, with rib meat, 3 oz	2

Joy of Cooking

Chicken leg quarters, 5 oz	8

Just Bare

Hand trimmed boneless skinless chicken tenders, 4 oz	1

Kirkland Signature

Chicken tenderloins, 4 oz	1
Premium chunk chicken breast packed in water, 2 oz	1

Kirkwood

Chicken tenderloins, 1 serving (94 g)	1

Kirkwood Original

Grilled chicken breast strips, 3 oz	2

Kroger

Chicken, chunk, in water, ¼ cup	1

Lloyd's

Honey hickory barbeque sauce with shredded chicken, ¼ cup	4

Lloyd's Barbeque Company

Original bbq sauce with seasoned shredded chicken, ¼ cup	3

Market Day

Chicnsteakes, 1 piece (113 g)	1

Michael Angelo's

Chicken piccata, twin pack, ¾ cup	10

Nature's Promise Naturals

Chicken, boneless skinless breast with rib meat., 1 fillet (113 g)	1

Omaha Steaks

Bbq rubbed chicken breast, 3 oz	3
Buffalo chicken wing, 2 pieces (85 g)	5
Chicken breast, boneless skinless, 4 oz	2
Chicken fried steak, 4 ½ oz	9

Oscar Mayer Carving Board

Rotisserie seasoned chicken breast, 2 oz	1

Perdue

Chicken leg quarters, 3 oz	6
Chicken roast, boneless, 4 oz	2
Chicken strips, homestyle, 2 strips (81.9 g)	6
Chicken, fresh ground patties, 1 patty (112 g)	4

Meat & Poultry

	SmartPoints™ value
Perdue Oven Ready	
Chicken breast, roaster, bone-in, whole seasoned, 4 oz	3
Chicken, roaster, whole seasoned, 4 oz	6
Perdue Perfect Portions	
Chicken breast, boneless, skinless, Italian style, 99% fat free, 1 fillet (136 g)	2
Chicken breasts, boneless skinless, 1 fillet (136 g)	1
Perdue Short Cuts	
Chicken breast, grilled, ½ cup	1
Chicken breast, carved, grilled, ½ cup	1
Chicken breast, carved, grilled fajita style, ½ cup	1
Chicken breast, carved, original roasted, ½ cup	1
Chicken breast, carved, Southwestern style, ½ cup	2
Chicken breast, grilled Italian style, ½ cup	2
Chicken breast, original roasted, ½ cup	1
Chicken, breast original roasted, ½ cup	1
Perdue Simply Smart	
Breaded chicken chunks, 3 oz	3
Chicken chunks, lightly breaded, 3 oz	5
Chicken strips, lightly breaded, 1 serving (84 g)	3
Lightly breaded chicken filets, 1 fillet (115 g)	5
Original grilled chicken strips, 1 serving (84 g)	2
Perdue Whole Grain	
Chicken breast strips with rib meat, 3 oz	4
Pilgrim's	
Chicken breast, tenderloins, pieces (150 g)	6

	SmartPoints™ value
Pilgrim's Wing Dings	
Chicken wings, fully cooked, 3 oz	7
Simply Smart	
Lightly breaded chicken strips, 3 oz	4
Swanson	
White premium chunk chicken breast in buffalo style sauce, 2 oz	1
T.G.I. Friday's	
Chicken wings, buffalo, 3 pieces (96 g)	5
Tender Bird	
Chicken breasts filets, 4 oz	2
Trader Joe's	
Breaded chicken tenderloins, 1 oz	1
Chicken breast tenderloins, 4 oz	1
Just chicken, 3 oz	1
Just... grilled chicken strips, 3 oz	1
Tyson	
All natural chicken breast tenderloin, 4 oz	1
Boneless chicken wings, honey bbq, 3 pieces (98 g)	6
Boneless skinless chicken breast portions, 1 (168 g)	3
Boneless skinless chicken breast with rib meat, 4 oz	2
Breaded white meat chicken patties, 1 piece (76 g)	5
Chicken breast fillets, 1 piece (129 g)	6
Chicken breast tenders, honey battered, 5 pieces (84 g)	7
Chicken thigh strips, boneless skinless, 4 oz	4
Chicken wings, 4 pieces (120 g)	7
Crispy chicken breast strips, 3 oz	5
Fully cooked buffalo style tenders, 3 oz	4
Fully cooked lightly breaded chicken breast strips, 3 oz	4
Fully cooked spicy chicken breast patties, 1 piece (74 g)	5

Meat & Poultry

Premium white chicken in water, 2 oz	1
Smokey steakhouse seasoned boneless skinless chicken breasts, 4 oz	3
Tyson All Natural	
Chicken breasts, ice glazed, boneless skinless, 4 oz	1
Tyson Family Favorites	
Popcorn chicken bites, diced chicken breast fritters with rib meat, 6 pieces (87.1 g)	7
Tyson Grilled & Ready	
Chicken breast chunks, 3 oz	2
Chicken breast strips, 3 oz	1
Chicken fillets, teriyaki flavored, 3 oz	3
Diced chicken breast, oven roasted, 3 oz	2
Fajita chicken breast strips, 3 oz	1
Honey bbq seasoned chicken breast strips, 3 oz	2
Oven roasted diced chicken breast, 3 oz	1
Tyson Ready To Cook	
Chicken breast tenderloins, 4 ½ oz	1
Valley Fresh	
Chicken, breast, in water, 2 oz	0
Valley Fresh Organic	
Chicken breast, 2 oz	1

Cornish Hen

Tyson

Cornish game hens, split, 4 oz	4

Frankfurters/Hot Dogs

Applegate

Hot dog, the great organic uncured beef, 1 hot dog (57 g)	3
Hot dog, the great organic uncured, turkey, 1 hot dog (48 g)	1
Hot dogs, uncured turkey, 1 hot dog (42 g)	1

Applegate Naturals	
Gluten-free uncured beef corn dogs, 1 corn dog (71 g)	6
Ball Park	
Beef franks, 1 frank (53 g)	7
Franks, 1 frank (37 g)	6
Franks, beef, lean, bun size, 1 frank (50 g)	2
Franks, smoked white turkey, fat free, bun size, 1 frank (50 g)	1
Original angus beef frank, 1 frank (50 g)	6
Turkey frank, 1 frank (53 g)	4
Ball Park Angus	
Beef frank bun size, 1 frank (57 g)	6
Bar S	
Chicken, pork and beef franks, 1 frank (42 g)	4
Classic bun length frank, 1 link (56 g)	6
Jumbo frank, 1 link (56 g)	6
Boar's Head	
Lite skinless beef frankfurters (gluten free), 1 (45 g)	3
Fit & Active	
Hardwood smoked turkey franks, 1 frank (34 g)	2
Foster Farms	
Corn dogs, honey crunchy flavor, 1 corn dog (75 g)	6
Corn dogs, mini, honey crunchy flavor, 4 mini dogs (76 g)	8
Turkey franks, 1 frank (56 g)	5
Giant	
Pigs in a blanket, mini, 4 pieces (85 g)	10
Hebrew National	
Franks, beef, 97% fat free, 1 frank (45 g)	1
Franks, beef, bun length, 1 frank (57 g)	7
Franks, beef, in a blanket, 5 pieces (82 g)	10

Meat & Poultry

	SmartPoints™ value
Franks, beef, jumbo, 1 frank (85 g)	10
Franks, beef, quarter pound, 1 frank (113 g)	13
Franks, beef, reduced fat, 1 frank (45 g)	4
Kirkland Signature	
Beef dinner franks, 1 link (123 g)	13
Beef hot dogs, 1 link (57 g)	6
Louis Rich	
Premium turkey hot dogs, 1 link (45 g)	3
Nathan's Famous	
100% angus beef franks, 1 link (57 g)	6
Beef frank, 1 link (57 g)	6
Bigger than the bun skinless beef franks, 1 link (50 g)	6
Skinless beef franks, 1 link (50 g)	6
Oscar Mayer	
95% fat free wieners, 1 link (50 g)	1
Cheese dogs, 1 link (45 g)	5
Franks, beef, 1 link (45 g)	5
Franks, beef, classic, 1 link (45 g)	5
Franks, beef, light, 1 link (45 g)	3
Franks, beef, premium, 1 link (42 g)	5
Franks, beef, premium jumbo, 1 link (53 g)	6
Franks, beef, premium, bun-length, 1 link (53 g)	6
Franks, turkey, 1 (45 g)	3
Franks, turkey, bun-length, classic, 1 link (57 g)	4
Franks, turkey, classic, 1 link (45 g)	3
Hot dogs, turkey, 1 link (45 g)	3
Lean beef franks, 1 link (50 g)	2
Light wieners, 1 serving (50 g)	3
Smokies, 1 link (50 g)	5
Wieners, 1 link (45 g)	4
Wieners, bun-length, classic, 1 link (57 g)	6

	SmartPoints™ value
Oscar Mayer Selects	
Franks, angus beef, smoked uncured, 1 link (53 g)	7
Franks, angus beef, smoked uncured, bun length, 1 link (53 g)	7
Turkey franks, hardwood smoked, 1 link (57 g)	4
Wieners, premium, 1 link (57 g)	5
Sabrett	
Skinless beef frankfurters, 1 frank (50 g)	5
State Fair	
Corn dogs, beef, 1 corn dog (76 g)	8
Corn dogs, classic, 1 corn dog (75 g)	7
Trader Joe's	
Turkey corn dog, 1 (71 g)	5
Uncured all beef hotdog, 1 link (56 g)	6
Vienna Beef	
Beef franks, 1 frank (45 g)	4

Luncheon & Deli Meats

	SmartPoints™ value
Aidells	
Garlic and basil smoked chicken breast deli meat, 2 slices (56 g)	0
Applegate	
Chicken breast, roasted, 2 oz	1
Chicken breast, sliced, organic smoked, 2 oz	1
Ham, honey, uncured, 2 oz	2
Ham, slow cooked, uncured, 2 oz	1
Turkey breast, herb, 2 oz	0
Turkey breast, honey & maple, 2 oz	1
Uncured pepperoni, 1 oz	3
Applegate Farms	
Salami, genoa, 1 oz	4
Applegate Farms Organics	
Chicken breast, organic roasted, 2 oz	1

Applegate Naturals

Ham, black forest, uncured, 2 oz	1
Pepperoni, turkey, uncured, 1 oz	1
Turkey breast, oven roasted, 2 oz	0
Turkey breast, smoked, 2 oz	0

Applegate Organics

Genoa salami, organic, 1 oz	3
Turkey breast, roasted, 2 oz	1

Bar S

Bologna, 1 slice (32 g)	4
Classic cooked ham deli meat, 1 slice (37 g)	1
Thick sliced bologna, 1 slice (56 g)	6

Best Kosher

Sliced cooked corn beef, lean, 2 oz	2

Boar's Head

All natural roasted turkey breast (gluten free), 2 oz	1
All natural smoked turkey breast (gluten free), 2 oz	0
Bold blackened oven roasted turkey breast (gluten free), 2 oz	1
Bold Cajun style smoked oven roasted turkey breast (gluten free), 2 oz	1
Bold jerk turkey breast (gluten free), 2 oz	1
Bold salsalito roasted turkey breast (gluten free), 2 oz	1
Boneless smoked ham with natural juices, sweet slice, 3 oz	2
Cracked pepper mill smoked turkey breast (gluten free), 2 oz	1
Genoa salami, 8 slices (56 g)	6
Golden catering style oven roasted turkey breast - 43% lower sodium (gluten free), 2 oz	1
Ham, cooked, 2 oz	1
Ham, oven roasted, pesto-parmesan, 2 oz	1
Hard salami, 5 slices (28 g)	4

Hickory smoked black forest turkey breast - 40% lower sodium (gluten free), 2 oz	1
Honey smoked turkey breast, 2 oz	1
Lemon pepper roasted chicken breast, 2 oz	1
Lightly browned turkey breast, 2 oz	1
London broil, 2 oz	1
Maple glazed honey coat cured turkey breast (gluten free), 2 oz	1
Mesquite wood smoked roasted turkey breast (gluten free), 2 oz	1
No salt added oven roasted turkey breast (gluten free), 2 oz	1
Oven roasted seasoned beef, Italian style, 2 oz	1
Ovengold roasted breast of turkey (gluten free), 2 oz	1
Pastrami seasoned turkey breast (gluten free), 2 oz	1
Pepperoni, 1 oz	5
Pork shoulder butt roast, 3 oz	5
Premium 46% lower sodium oven roasted turkey breast - skinless (gluten free), 2 oz	1
Roasted turkey breast, tuscan brand, all natural, 2 oz	0
Smoked ham, 2 oz	1
Turkey breast, black forest, hickory smoked, 2 oz	1
Turkey breast, oven roasted, 3 oz	1
Turkey pepperoni, 1 oz	1
Virginia ham, 2 oz	1

Buddig

Beef, extra thin, original, 10 slices (56 g)	2
Beef, original, 1 package (56 g)	2
Chicken lunch meat, ⅛ package (56 g)	2
Chicken, original, 1 package (56 g)	2
Corned beef, original, 1 package (56 g)	2
Ham, 1 package (56 g)	2

Meat & Poultry

	SmartPoints™ value
Ham, honey, original, 1 package (56 g)	3
Original deli thin ham, 10 slices (56 g)	2
Turkey, extra thin, original, 9 slices (56 g)	2
Turkey, honey roasted, 1 package (56 g)	3
Turkey, original, 1 package (56 g)	2
Buddig Deli Cuts	
Ham, honey, baked, 6 slices (56 g)	2
Ham, honey, water added, baked, 6 slices (56 g)	2
Smoked ham, 6 slices (56 g)	2
Buddig The Original Deli Thin	
Pastrami, 1 package (56 g)	2
Butterball	
Deep fried Thanksgiving style turkey breast deli meat, 1 slice (28 g)	0
Honey roasted smoked turkey breast deli meat, 1 slice (28 g)	1
Turkey breast, deep fried, Thanksgiving style, 7 slices (56 g)	1
Turkey breast, honey roasted, 4 slices (54 g)	1
Turkey breast, oven roasted, 1 slice (28 g)	0
Turkey breast, oven roasted, deli thin slice, 4 slices (57 g)	1
Turkey breast, oven roasted, thin sliced, 4 slices (54 g)	1
Turkey breast, smoked, thin sliced, 97% fat free, 4 slices (56 g)	2
Butterball Deli Inspirations	
Maple honey turkey breast, 2 oz	1
Carando Classic Italian	
Hot capicola, thin sliced, 2 oz	2
Casa Italia	
Genoa salami, 6 slices (30 g)	3

	SmartPoints™ value
Castle Wood	
Herb roasted turkey breast, 2 oz	1
Oven roasted turkey deli meat, 2 oz	1
Thinly shaved black forest ham, 2 oz	1
Turkey pastrami, 2 oz	1
Castle Wood Heart Healthy	
Hickory smoked turkey breast, 2 oz	1
Oven roasted chicken breast, 2 oz	1
Castle Wood Reserve	
Buffalo style chicken breast, 2 oz	1
Castle Wood Thinly Shaved	
Applewood smoked ham, 2 oz	1
Citerio	
Mortadella, 3 slices (50 g)	4
Salame, genoa, 6 slices (28 g)	4
Columbus	
Rotisserie seasoned chicken breast, 2 oz	1
Salame, Italian dry, 1 oz	3
Columbus Salumeria San Francisco	
Peppered turkey breast, 2 oz	1
DAK	
Ham, premium, 1 slice (28 g)	0
Deli Select	
Chicken breast, oven roasted, thin sliced, 6 slices (57 g)	1
Corned beef, 6 slices (57 g)	0
Ham, baked, thin sliced, 6 slices (57 g)	1
Ham, honey, thin sliced, 6 slices (57 g)	1
Ham, smoked, thin sliced, 6 slices (57 g)	1
Hard salami, ultra thin, 5 slices (28 g)	4
Roast beef, thin sliced, 7 slices (58 g)	1
Turkey breast, honey roasted, thin sliced, 6 slices (57 g)	1

Meat & Poultry

	SmartPoints™ value
Turkey breast, oven roasted, thin sliced, 6 slices (57 g)	1
Turkey breast, smoked, thin sliced, 6 slices (57 g)	1
Deli Select Deli Select	
Chicken breast, rotisserie seasoned, ultra thin, 2 oz	1
Dietz & Watson	
Ham, maple & honey, 2 oz	1
Ham, peppered, 2 oz	2
Ham, smoked, black forest, 2 oz	2
Ham, tavern, 2 oz	1
Ham, virginia brand, 2 oz	1
Roast beef, London broil, 2 oz	1
Roast beef, London broil, top round, 2 oz	1
Salami, hard, 1 oz	4
Turkey breast, Cajun style, 2 oz	1
Turkey breast, homestyle black pepper, 2 oz	1
Turkey breast, maple & honey, 2 oz	1
Turkey breast, mesquite smoked, 2 oz	0
Turkey breast, oven classic, 2 oz	1
Turkey breast, smoked, black forest, 3 slices (54 g)	0
Dietz & Watson Classic	
Pork, shoulder butt, 3 oz	4
Dietz & Watson Gourmet Lite	
Chicken breast, 2 oz	1
Ham, cooked, 2 oz	1
Turkey breast, 2 oz	1
Turkey breast, no salt added, 2 oz	1
Eating Right	
Deli style oven roasted turkey, 6 slices (56 g)	1
Smoked turkey, 6 slices (56 g)	1
Eating Right For Calorie Counting	
Pepper turkey breast deli style luncheon meat, 2 oz	1

	SmartPoints™ value
Empire	
Turkey breast, smoked, slices, 4 slices (57 g)	0
Turkey pastrami, deli slices, 3 slices (57 g)	1
Turkey pastrami, slices, 4 slices (57 g)	1
Turkey slices, oven prepared, 4 slices (57 g)	0
Essential Everyday	
Turkey pepperoni, 15 slices (30 g)	2
Farmer John	
Ham, cooked, original, 1 slice (38 g)	1
Farmland	
Ham, deli style, 1 slice (28 g)	1
Field	
Bologna, sandwich, 1 slice (38 g)	4
Fiorucci	
Hard salami panino, 2 oz	9
Prosciutto panino, 4 pieces (85 g)	9
Fit & Active	
Smoked honey ham, 2 oz	2
Frick's	
Sliced ham, 2 oz	1
Gallo	
Italian dry salame deli thin sliced, 5 slices (28 g)	3
Light Italian dry salame deli thin sliced, 6 slices (28 g)	2
Great Value	
Deli sliced black forest smoked ham, 5 slices (53 g)	1
Deli sliced rotisserie seasoned chicken breast, 4 slices (51 g)	1
Thinly sliced roast beef, 6 slices (56 g)	2
Hannaford	
Turkey breast, oven roasted, thin deli sliced, 2 oz	1

Meat & Poultry

Meat & Poultry

	SmartPoints™ value
Hatfield	
Bologna, ring, 2 oz	3
Hebrew National	
Salami, beef, 2 slices (56 g)	5
Salami, beef, lean, thin sliced, 4 slices (56 g)	3
Hickory Farms	
Summer sausage, turkey, 2 oz	3
Hillshire Farm	
Chicken breast, chipotle, 3 slices (49 g)	1
Salami, hard, 4 Slices (28 g)	4
Turkey breast, black pepper, 3 slices (49 g)	1
Turkey breast, honey roasted, thin sliced, 2 oz	1
Turkey breast, oven roasted, 2 slices (53 g)	1
Turkey breast, oven roasted, thick sliced, 1 slice (28 g)	1
Hillshire Farm Deli Select	
Chicken breast, rotisserie seasoned, ultra thin, 2 oz	1
Ham, baked, Virginia brand, hearty slices, 1 slice (28 g)	1
Ham, black forest, ultra thin, 2 oz	1
Ham, brown sugar, ultra thin, 2 oz	2
Ham, honey, ultra thin, 2 oz	2
Ham, honey, ultra thin, lower sodium, 2 oz	2
Ham, smoked, lower sodium, 2 oz	2
Pastrami, ultra thin, 2 oz	1
Pastrami, ultra thin, 2 oz	1
Roast beef, ultra thin, 2 oz	1
Roast beef, ultra thin, 2 oz	1
Turkey breast, cracked black pepper, ultra thin, 2 oz	1
Turkey breast, honey roasted, lower sodium, 2 oz	2
Turkey breast, honey roasted, ultra thin, 2 oz	1

	SmartPoints™ value
Turkey breast, mesquite smoked, ultra thin, 2 oz	1
Turkey breast, oven roasted, lower sodium, 2 oz	1
Turkey breast, oven roasted, ultra thin, 2 oz	1
Hillshire Farm Farm Classics	
Deli meat, ham, black forest, 4 slices (50 g)	1
Deli meat, honey ham, 95% fat free, 4 slices (50 g)	2
Deli meat, turkey breast, honey roasted, 97% fat free, 4 slices (50 g)	2
Deli meat, turkey breast, oven roasted, 97% fat free, 4 slices (50 g)	1
Ham, hickory smoked, 4 slices (50 g)	1
Hillshire Farm Naturals	
Deli meat, ham, black forest, 3 slices (49 g)	1
Deli meat, ham, honey roasted, 3 slices (49 g)	2
Deli meat, turkey breast, hardwood smoked, 3 slices (52 g)	1
Deli meat, turkey breast, slow roasted, 3 slices (52 g)	0
Hillshire Farm Premium Deli	
Chicken breast, thin sliced, mesquite smoked, 3 slices (51 g)	1
Ham, honey, oven roasted, thin sliced, 3 slices (51 g)	2
Hormel Natural Choice	
Cherrywood smoked deli ham, 4 slices (56 g)	1
Chicken breast, deli, rotisserie style, 3 slices (56 g)	0
Ham, deli, honey, 4 slices (56 g)	2
Ham, deli, smoked, 4 slices (56 g)	1
Hard uncured salami, 6 slices (28 g)	4
Honey deli ham, 4 slices (56 g)	2

Oven roasted deli turkey, 3 slices (56 g)	1
Roast beef, deli, 4 slices (56 g)	1
Turkey breast, basil rosemary and olive oil, 3 slices (56 g)	1
Turkey, deli, cracked black pepper, 3 slices (56 g)	1
Turkey, deli, honey, 3 slices (57 g)	1
Turkey, deli, mesquite, 3 slices (56 g)	1
Turkey, deli, oven roasted, 3 slices (56 g)	1
Turkey, deli, smoked, 3 slices (56 g)	1

Jack Link's

Original crinkle cut turkey pepperoni, 8 slices (28 g)	2

John Morrell

Ham, cubed, 2 oz	2

John Morrell Off The Bone

Turkey breast, oven roasted, 2 oz	2

Johnsonville

Ring bologna, original, 2 oz	6
Summer sausage, beef, 2 oz	6

Jones Dairy Farm

Sliced braunschweiger, liverwurst with bacon added, 2 slices (45 g)	5

Kahns

Genuine baked ham, 2 oz	1

Kirkland Signature

Extra lean ham sliced 98% fat free, 1 slice (28 g)	0
Rotisserie seasoned chicken breast, 2 oz	1
Turkey breast slices, 2 slices (56 g)	1

Kroger

Ham, cubed, ½ cup	1
Ham, diced, ½ cup	1
Ham, honey, deli thin sliced, 2 oz	2
Ham, smoked, deli thin sliced, 2 oz	2
Hard salami, sliced, 4 slices (28 g)	4

Pepperoni, deli thin sliced, 8 slices (28 g)	5
Roast beef, deli thin sliced, 2 oz	1
Sliced pepperoni, 15 slices (30 g)	5
Turkey breast & white turkey, oven roasted, 1 slice (28 g)	1
Turkey breast & white turkey, oven roasted, honey, 1 slice (28 g)	1
Turkey breast, honey, deli thin sliced, 2 oz	1
Turkey breast, mesquite, deli thin sliced, 2 oz	1
Turkey breast, oven roasted, deli thin sliced, 2 oz	1
Turkey breast, smoked, deli thin sliced, 2 oz	1

Kroger Deli Style

Chicken breast, oven roasted, value pack, 6 slices (56 g)	2
Ham, smoked, value pack, 6 slices (56 g)	2
Honey ham, smoked, value pack, 6 slices (56 g)	2
Turkey breast, honey smoked, value pack, 6 slices (56 g)	3
Turkey breast, oven roasted, value pack, 6 slices (57 g)	2
Turkey breast, smoked, value pack, 6 slices (57 g)	2

Kroger Private Selection

Oven roasted breast of turkey, 1 oz	0

Land O'Frost

Sub sandwich kit, honey ham & honey smoked white turkey, 6 slices (57 g)	2

Land O'Frost Bistro Favorites

Beef, cracked black pepper, 7 slices (57 g)	1
Ham, smoked, honey glazed, 6 slices (57 g)	2
Roast beef, 7 slices (57 g)	1
Turkey breast, cured, rotisserie seasoned, 5 slices (57 g)	2

Meat & Poultry

	SmartPoints™ value
Land O'Frost Deli Shaved	
Chicken, 9 slices (57 g)	2
Ham, black forest, 10 slices (57 g)	3
Honey ham with natural juices, 10 slices (57 g)	2
Land O'Frost Simply Delicious	
Black forest ham, 5 slices (51 g)	1
Chicken breast, rotisserie seasoned, 5 slices (51 g)	1
Honey cured ham, 5 slices (51 g)	1
Honey roasted turkey breast, 5 slices (51 g)	1
Slow roasted turkey breast, 5 slices (51 g)	1
Lunch Mate	
Hard salami, 3 slices (28 g)	4
Lunch Mate Deli Style	
Oven roasted turkey breast, 2 oz	1
Lunch Mate Premium Deli Slices	
Oven roasted cured chicken breast, 2 oz	2
Smoked honey ham, 2 oz	2
Mama Cozzi's Pizza Kitchen	
Original pepperoni pizza, 14 slices (30 g)	5
Margherita	
Pepperoni, sliced, 16 slices (30 g)	5
Turkey pepperoni, 14 slices (28 g)	1
Market Pantry	
Ham, black forest, ultra thin deli slices, 2 oz	1
Honey ham, deli slices, 3 slices (56 g)	1
Honey ham, healthy, ultra thin deli slices, 2 oz	2
Turkey breast, oven-roasted, deli slices, 3 slices (56 g)	1
Turkey breast, oven-roasted, ultra-thin deli slices, 2 oz	1
Turkey breast, smoked honey ultra-thin deli slices, 2 oz	2
Ultra thin black forest ham deli slices, 2 oz	1

	SmartPoints™ value
Nature's Promise Naturals	
Breast of turkey, oven roasted, 2 slices (56 g)	1
Oscar Mayer	
98% fat free bologna, 1 slice (28 g)	0
Black forest chopped ham, 1 slice (28 g)	2
Bologna, 1 slice (28 g)	3
Bologna, beef, 1 slice (28 g)	3
Bologna, beef, light, 1 slice (28 g)	2
Bologna, hearty thick cut, 1 slice (41 g)	5
Bologna, jalapeño, 1 slice (28 g)	3
Bologna, light, 1 slice (28 g)	2
Bologna, thick cut, 1 slice (43 g)	5
Chicken breast, rotisserie seasoned, 1 package (57 g)	1
Chicken breast, thin sliced, oven roasted, 5 slices (57 g)	1
Chicken, white, homestyle, oven roasted, 1 slice (28 g)	1
Chopped ham, 1 slice (28 g)	1
Chopped ham, smoke flavor, 1 slice (28 g)	1
Combos, oven roasted turkey breast, smoked ham, 2 oz	1
Cotto salami, 1 slice (28 g)	2
Ham, baked cooked, 3 slices (63 g)	1
Ham, baked, cooked, 3 slices (63 g)	1
Ham, boiled, 3 slices (63 g)	1
Ham, honey, 3 slices (57 g)	1
Ham, lower sodium, 3 slices (63 g)	2
Ham, smoked, 3 slices (64 g)	1
Ham, thin sliced, honey, 5 slices (57 g)	1
Ham, thin sliced, smoked, 5 slices (57 g)	1
Hard salami, cracked black pepper, 3 slices (28 g)	4
Honey ham, 3 slices (57 g)	1

Jalapeño and cheese white turkey lunch meat, 1 slice (28 g)	1
Loaf, ham & cheese, 1 slice (28 g)	2
Oven roasted shaved white turkey 95% fat free, 2 oz	1
Oven roasted, extra lean turkey breast and white turkey, 3 slices (62 g)	2
Premium shaved oven roasted turkey breast & white turkey, 2 oz	1
Roast beef, cured, slow roasted, 1 slice (28 g)	1
Salami, cotto, louis rich turkey, 1 slice (28 g)	1
Salami, hard, 3 slices (27 g)	3
Smoked ham, 3 slices (64 g)	1
Smoked shaved ham 97% fat free, 2 oz	1
Turkey & cheese, oven roasted white, 1 slice (28 g)	1
Turkey bologna, louis rich, lower fat, 1 slice (28 g)	1
Turkey breast & white turkey, honey smoked, family size, 1 slice (28 g)	1
Turkey breast & white turkey, mesquite smoked, extra lean, family size, 1 slice (28 g)	1
Turkey breast & white turkey, smoked, 3 slices (63 g)	1
Turkey breast & white turkey, smoked, 1 slice (28 g)	1
Turkey breast, applewood smoked, 2 oz	1
Turkey breast, honey smoked, 3 slices (64 g)	1
Turkey breast, smoked, thin sliced, 5 slices (57 g)	1
Turkey breast, thin sliced, honey smoked, 5 slices (57 g)	1
Turkey breast, thin sliced, mesquite, 5 slices (57 g)	1
Turkey breast, thin sliced, oven roasted, 5 slices (57 g)	1

Turkey, lean white, honey smoked, 1 slice (28 g)	1
Turkey, white, oven roasted, 1 slice (28 g)	1
White turkey, Italian herb seasoned, 1 slice (28 g)	1
Oscar Mayer Carving Board	
Roast beef, cured, slow roasted, 2 oz	1
Oscar Mayer Deli Fresh	
Black forest ham water added, 2 oz	1
Bold Cajun style turkey breast, 2 oz	1
Bold chipotle seasoned chicken breast, 2 oz	1
Bold honey maple ham, 2 oz	1
Bold Italian style herb turkey breast, 2 oz	1
Chicken breast, barbecue seasoned, 6 slices (51 g)	1
Chicken breast, buffalo style, 3 oz	1
Chicken breast, Cajun seasoned, shaved, 6 slices (51 g)	1
Chicken breast, chipotle seasoned, bold, 2 oz	1
Chicken breast, grilled, strips, 3 oz	1
Chicken breast, oven roasted, 3 slices (65 g)	1
Chicken breast, oven roasted, cuts, ⅔ cup	1
Chicken breast, shaved, rotisserie style, 6 slices (51 g)	1
Chicken breast, southwestern seasoned, strips, 3 oz	1
Classic combo oven roasted turkey breast & smoked ham, 2 oz	1
Cracked black pepper turkey breast, 2 oz	1
Ham, black forest, 2 oz	1
Ham, shaved, brown sugar, 6 slices (51 g)	1
Ham, smoked, shaved, family size, 6 slices (56 g)	1

Meat & Poultry

SmartPoints™ value

Ham, virginia brand, shaved, 6 slices (51 g)	1
Honey ham water added, 2 oz	1
Honey ham water added deli meat, 2 oz	1
Honey smoked turkey breast, 2 oz	1
Honey smoked turkey breast, 2 oz	1
Mesquite turkey breast (family size), 2 oz	1
Oven roasted turkey breast, 2 oz	1
Rotisserie seasoned chicken breast, 2 oz	1
Slow roasted cured roasted beef, 2 oz	1
Smoked ham, 2 oz	1
Smoked ham water added, 2 oz	1
Smoked turkey breast, 2 oz	1
Turkey breast, cracked black pepper, shaved, 6 slices (51 g)	1
Turkey breast, honey smoked, 1 slice (28 g)	1
Turkey breast, shaved, oven roasted, 6 slices (51 g)	1
Turkey breast, smoked, 6 slices (51 g)	1

Oscar Mayer Deli Fresh Combos

Honey smoked turkey breast and honey ham, 2 oz	1

Oscar Mayer Natural

Turkey breast, oven roasted, 3 slices (63 g)	1

Oscar Mayer Premium Deli Meat

Ham, smoked, shaved, 4 slices (56 g)	1

Oscar Mayer Selects

Slow roasted turkey breast, 2 oz	1
Turkey breast, slow roasted, 2 oz	1

Plumrose

Ham, baked, premium, deli sliced, 1 slice (28 g)	0
Ham, deli sliced, 1 slice (28 g)	0
Ham, lower sodium, 1 slice (28 g)	0

SmartPoints™ value

Prima Della

Chicken, breast, sliced oven roasted, 2 oz	1

Primo Taglio

Chicken, breast, oven roasted, 3 slices (50 g)	1
Ham, applewood honey, 4 slices (56 g)	2
Turkey breast, oven roasted, 2 slices (56 g)	1

Private Selection

Capicola, hot, sliced, 8 slices (56 g)	3
Roast beef, homestyle, slow roasted, 3 slices (59 g)	1

Private Selection Sliced Deli Meats

Honey cured ham water added, 1 serving (59 g)	2

Publix

Turkey breast, smoked, 1 slice (28 g)	0

Russer

Ham, cooked, water added, reduced sodium, 1 slice (28 g)	0

Safeway

Ham, cooked, 1 slice (28 g)	1
Ham, deli style, thin sliced, honey, 2 oz	1
Turkey breast, oven roasted, 1 slice (28 g)	1

Safeway Deli Style

Roast beef, thin sliced, 2 oz	1

Safeway Farms

Ham, deli style, thin sliced, smoked, 2 oz	1
Roast beef, slow roasted, thin sliced, 6 slices (56 g)	2
Thin sliced oven roasted turkey breast, 2 oz	1
Turkey breast, deli style, thin sliced, smoked, 2 oz	1

Meat & Poultry

Sara Lee Premium Meats

Hardwood smoked turkey breast deli meat, 2 slices (47 g)	1
Honey ham deli meat, 2 slices (47 g)	2
Honey roasted turkey breast deli meat, 2 slices (47 g)	1
Lower sodium honey ham deli meat, 2 slices (47 g)	1
Lower sodium honey roasted turkey breast deli meat, 2 slices (47 g)	1
Lower sodium oven roasted turkey breast deli meat, 2 slices (57 g)	1
Lower sodium virginia brand ham deli meat, 2 slices (45 g)	1
Oven roasted chicken breast deli meat, 2 slices (57 g)	1
Oven roasted turkey breast deli meat, 2 slices (57 g)	1

ShopRite

Cooked ham, with natural juices, deli style, 2 oz	1
Turkey breast, smoked, deli style, 2 oz	1

Simple Truth

Oven roasted turkey, 2 oz	1
Smoked turkey, 2 oz	1
Uncured black forest ham, 2 oz	1

Simply Nature

Oven roasted turkey breast, 2 oz	1

Smithfield

Ham, black forest, 2 oz	1
Ham, cooked, 1 slice (28 g)	1
Ham, cooked, deli thin, 2 oz	1
Ham, virginia brand, 2 oz	1

Spam

Spam, classic, 2 oz	6
Spam, oven roasted turkey, 2 oz	2

The Deli Counter

Smoked ham, 2 oz	2
Turkey breast, oven roasted shaved, family size, 2 oz	1

Tofurky

Deli slices, hickory smoked, 5 slices (52 g)	2
Deli slices, oven roasted, 5 slices (52 g)	2
Deli slices, peppered, 5 slices (52 g)	2

Trader Joe's

All natural uncured sliced corned beef, ¼ package (57 g)	2
Oven roasted turkey breast, 4 slices (56 g)	1
Smoked turkey breast, 4 slices (56 g)	1

Wegman's

Ham, thin shaved, club pack, 2 oz	1
Sliced turkey pepperoni, 16 slices (28 g)	2
Turkey breast, oven roasted, thin shaved, club pack, 2 oz	1
Turkey breast, oven roasted, thin sliced, 5 slices (57 g)	1

Wegman's Food You Feel Good About

Turkey breast, honey roasted, 2 oz	1

Winn Dixie

Ham, brown sugar baked, 2 oz	2

World Classics

Turkey breast, honey maple flavored, 2 oz	2

Wunderbar German

Bologna, 2 oz	6

Pork & Ham

Armour

Pepperoni slices, 16 slices (30 g)	5

Boar's Head

Ham, 2 oz	1

Bob Evans

Ham steaks, 1 steak (112 g)	2

Brookwood Farms

Barbeque pork, 5 oz	7

Pork & Ham (cont'd)

SmartPoints™ value

Carando
Hickory smoked sprial ham (without glaze), 3 oz	4

Corky's
Bar-b-q pork ribs, 5 ribs (140 g)	11

Cumberland Gap
Diced ham, 2 oz	1

Curly's
Baby back pork ribs, 3 oz	7
Hickory smoked pulled pork, 2 oz	4
Pulled pork, barbecue sauce, ¼ cup	3

DAK
Premium sliced ham, 1 slice (28 g)	0

Del Duca Gourmet Selection
Prosciutto, 1 oz	1

Del Real
Pork in green sauce, chile verde, 5 oz	3

Dietz & Watson
Spare ribs, pork, Canadian center cut, with tangy barbecue sauce, 5 oz	10

Farmer John
Ham, smoked, classic, 2 oz	1

Farmland
Cherrywood smoked uncured Canadian bacon, 4 slices (60 g)	1
Ham, fully cooked, cubed, 2 oz	2
Hickory smoked ham steaks, 1 slice (65 g)	1
Salt pork belly, sliced, 2 oz	12
Spiral sliced ham, hickory smoked, 3 oz	4

Farmland Nutrition Wise
Center cut pork loin roast, boneless, 4 oz	2
Sirloin tip pork roast, boneless, 4 oz	2

Fletcher's
Ham, black forest, 3 oz	2

Goya
Ham croquettes, 3 croquettes (109 g)	9

Great Value
97% fat free cooked ham, 1 slice (28 g)	0

Habbersett
Scrapple, 2 oz	4

Healthy Ones
Ham, black forest, deli thin sliced, 6 slices (54 g)	1

Hillshire Farm
Ham, smokey bourbon, 3 slices (49 g)	1
Polska kielbasa, 2 oz	7
Pulled pork, barbeque, 2 oz	2

Hormel
Bacon, real crumbled, peppered, 1 Tbsp	1
Ham, extra lean, 2 oz	1
Pork loin filet, center cut, extra lean, lemon garlic, 4 oz	3
Pork loin filet, center cut, extra lean, mesquite barbecue flavor, 4 oz	2
Pork tenderloin, extra lean, peppercorn, 4 oz	2
Pork tenderloin, extra lean, teriyaki, 4 oz	3
Slow simmered pork roast, au jus, 5 oz	4
Smoked ham, lean, water added, 2 oz	2
Smoked pork chops, original, 3 oz	2

Hormel Always Tender
Apple bourbon flavor pork tenderloin, 4 oz	3
Boneless pork chops, 4 oz	4
Boneless pork roast, 4 oz	4

Meat & Poultry

	SmartPoints™ value
Onion garlic flavored boneless pork roast, 4 oz	4
Pork center cut loin filet, extra lean, original, 4 oz	3
Hormel Thin Cut Bone-In	
Smoked pork chops, 3 oz	4
Jack Daniel's	
Pulled pork, with Jack daniel's barbeque sauce, ⅓ package (151 g)	10
Jimmy Dean	
Breakfast bowls, ham, 1 bowl (227 g)	14
John Morrell	
Diced ham, 2 oz	2
Ham steaks, 3 oz	2
Ham, mini cubed, 2 oz	2
Jones Dairy Farm	
Ham slices, naturally hickory smoked, 2 slices (45 g)	1
Ham steak, naturally hickory smoked, extra lean, 3 oz	2
Liverwurst, braunschweiger, light, 2 oz	2
Kirkland Signature	
Smoked pulled pork, 2 oz	4
Krakus	
Sliced imported polish ham with natural juices, 1 slice (28 g)	0
Land O'Frost Bistro Favorites	
Ham, black forest, 6 slices (57 g)	1
Land O'Frost Premium	
Black forest ham, old world style, 4 slices (50 g)	1
Lloyd's	
Ribs, babyback pork with original bbq sauce, 2 ribs (212 g)	12
Ribs, pork, babyback, with original bbq sauce, 5 oz	12
Shredded pork, seasoned, in original bbq sauce, 1 bowl (112 g)	6

	SmartPoints™ value
Lloyd's Barbeque Company	
Original bbq sauce with seasoned shredded pork, ¼ cup	3
Marcela Valladolid	
Pork, al pastor, 4 oz	7
New York Style Sausage	
Ground pork, 4 oz	2
Omaha Steaks	
Bbq pulled pork, 2 oz	3
Boneless pork chop, 5 oz	6
Carnitas pork roast, 4 oz	4
Oscar Mayer	
Ham, honey, shaved, the one pounder, 2 oz	1
Oscar Mayer Carving Board	
Slow cooked ham with natural juices, 2 oz	1
Oscar Mayer Selects	
Ham, applewood smoked, 6 slices (51 g)	1
Plumrose	
Ham steaks, smoked, 1 steak (170 g)	3
Pork baby back ribs, with smoky barbeque sauce, 5 oz	11
PrimoTaglio	
Ham off the bone, with natural juices, hickory smoked, 4 slices (57 g)	2
Rapa	
Scrapple, our original, 2 oz	4
Signature Cafe	
Bbq pork loin, 5 oz	8
Smithfield	
Ham steak, boneless, hickory smoked, 3 oz	2
Ham steak, boneless, honey cured, 3 oz	3
Ham steak, boneless, maple flavored, 3 oz	3
Pork loin filet, garlic & herb, 4 oz	3
Pork tenderloin, teriyaki, 4 oz	2

	SmartPoints™ value
Smithfield Anytime Favorites	
Ham, diced, 97% fat free, 2 oz	2
Spam	
Spam, singles, lite, 1 package (85 g)	5
Spartan	
Ham loaf, ready to cook, 4 oz	8
Stubb's	
Pork, pulled, ½ cup	8
Sweet Baby Ray's	
Shredded pork, with sauce, 5 oz	10
Taylor	
Pork roll, 1 slice (56 g)	5
Trader Joe's	
Bbq shredded pork with barbeque sauce, ¼ cup	2
Sliced prosciutto, ¼ pack (28 g)	3
Tyson	
Ham cubes, extra lean, 2 oz	1
Tyson Heat 'N Eat	
Baked ham, sweet glaze with honey, 3 oz	4

Sausage

	SmartPoints™ value
Aidells	
Artichoke and garlic smoked chicken sausage, 1 link (85 g)	4
Chicken & apple smoked chicken sausage, 1 link (85 g)	5
Mango smoked chicken sausage, 1 link (85 g)	5
Organic chicken & apple smoked sausage, 1 link (85 g)	4
Sausage, smoked, chicken & apple, minis, 5 links (56 g)	4
Sausage, smoked, habanero & green chile, 1 each (85 g)	4
Sausage, smoked, Italian style with mozzarella cheese, 1 link (85 g)	5
Sausage, smoked, pork, Cajun style, 1 link (85 g)	5

	SmartPoints™ value
Sausage, smoked, portobello mushroom, 1 link (85 g)	4
Sausage, smoked, roasted garlic & gruyere cheese, 1 link (85 g)	6
Sausage, smoked, spicy mango with jalapeño, 1 link (85 g)	6
Sausage, smoked, sun-dried tomato, 1 link (85 g)	4
Spinach and feta smoked chicken sausage, 1 link (85 g)	4
al fresco	
Chicken sausage, breakfast patties, country style, 1 patty (50 g)	2
Chicken sausage, buffalo style, 1 link (85 g)	3
Chicken sausage, chipotle chorizo, 1 link (85 g)	4
Chicken sausage, country style, 1 link (32 g)	1
Chicken sausage, garden primavera, 1 link (85 g)	3
Chicken sausage, jalapeños and roasted red peppers, 1 link (85 g)	3
Chicken sausage, roasted garlic, 1 link (85 g)	3
Chicken sausage, roasted pepper and asiago, 1 link (85 g)	3
Chicken sausage, smoked andouille, 1 link (85 g)	3
Chicken sausage, spinach and feta, 1 link (85 g)	3
Chicken sausage, sundried tomato, 1 link (85 g)	4
Chicken sausage, sweet apple, 1 link (80 g)	3
Chicken sausage, sweet Italian style, 1 link (85 g)	3
Applegate Farms Naturals	
Chicken and maple breakfast sausage patty, 1 patty (33 g)	2
Applegate Farms Organic	
Chicken & apple sausage, mild, 1 link (85 g)	4

Meat & Poultry

Applegate Naturals

Breakfast patty, chicken and apple, 1 patty (33 g)	2
Breakfast sausage patty, savory turkey, 1 patty (33 g)	2
Breakfast sausage, chicken & apple, 3 links (59 g)	3
Breakfast sausage, classic pork, 3 links (59 g)	6
Breakfast sausage, savory turkey, 3 links (59 g)	3

Armour

Vienna sausage, original, 3 sausages (50 g)	4

Banquet Brown 'N Serve

Fully cooked sausage links, lite original, 3 each (57 g)	4
Sausage links, beef, 3 links (54 g)	7
Sausage links, fully cooked, hot & spicy, 3 links (54 g)	6
Sausage links, fully cooked, lite original, 3 links (54 g)	3
Sausage links, fully cooked, maple, 3 links (54 g)	6
Sausage links, fully cooked, original, 3 links (54 g)	6
Sausage links, original, family pack, 3 links (54 g)	6
Sausage links, turkey, 3 links (60 g)	3
Sausage patties, fully cooked, maple, 2 patties (45 g)	5
Sausage patties, fully cooked, original, 2 patties (45 g)	5
Sausage patties, fully cooked, original, family pack, 2 pieces (45 g)	5
Sausage patties, turkey, 2 patties (45 g)	3

Bilinski's

Sausage, chicken, spinach & garlic, 1 link (68 g)	1

Bob Evans

Fully cooked turkey sausage links, 2 links (45 g)	1
Fully cooked turkey sausage patties, 2 patties (68 g)	2
Links, maple, 3 links (51 g)	5
Links, original, 3 links (51 g)	5
Links, sweet Italian, 1 cooked link (40 g)	4
Pork sausage links, maple, 3 links (51 g)	6
Pork sausage links, original, 3 links (51 g)	5
Pork sausage patties, original, 2 patties (59 g)	5
Sausage links, turkey, 2 links (45 g)	1
Sausage, zesty hot, 2 oz	6
Turkey sausage patties, 2 patties (56 g)	2

Breakfast Best Heat-n-Serve

Turkey sausage links, 3 links (54 g)	3

Bridgford

Pepperoni, turkey, sliced, 12 slices (30 g)	2

Butterball

Turkey polska kielbasa, extra tender, 2 oz	3
Turkey smoked sausage, extra tender, 2 oz	3

Butterball Everyday

Hardwood smoked turkey sausage, 2 oz	3
Turkey breakfast sausage patties, 2 patties (71 g)	3
Turkey sausage polska kielbasa, 2 oz	3

Cacique

Chorizo, beef, 2 ½ oz	12
Chorizo, pork, 2 ½ oz	10
Chorizo, soy, 2 oz	2

Meat & Poultry

SmartPoints™ value

Daily Chef

Mozzarella and roasted garlic chicken sausage (serves 15), 1 serving (91 g)	4
Spinach and asiago chicken sausage (serves 15), 1 serving (91 g)	4

Eckrich

Li'l smokies cocktail smoked sausages, 5 links (76 g)	6
Polska kielbasa, natural hardwood smoked, 2 oz	7
Sausage, smoked, 2 oz	7
Skinless smoked sausage, 2 oz	7
Skinless smoked turkey sausage, 2 oz	4
Smoked sausage, turkey, skinless, 2 oz	4
Turkey smoked sausage, 2 oz	4

Eckrich Smok-Y

Breakfast sausage, original, 2 links (47 g)	6

Eckrich Smok-Y Breakfast Links

Sausage, lite, 2 links (47 g)	3

Eckrich Traditional Rope

Smoked sausage, 2 oz	7

EverGood

Sausage, hot link, Louisiana brand, 2 oz	6

Farmer John

Pork links, classic, 2 links (37 g)	5
Pork links, original, 2 links (56 g)	5

Field Roast Original

Grain meat sausages, vegetarian, Mexican chipotle, hot & spicy, 1 sausage (92 g)	7
Grain meat sausages, vegetarian, smoked apple sage, 1 sausage (92 g)	5

Field Roast Original Field Roast

Grain meat sausages, vegetarian, Italian, 1 sausage (92 g)	5

SmartPoints™ value

Fit & Active

Fresh sweet Italian turkey sausage, 1 link (112 g)	4
Lean turkey polish kielbasa, 2 oz	2

Fletcher's

Sausage, pork, ground, 2 oz pan fried	5

Galileo

Salami, hard, deli thin sliced, 5 slices (28 g)	4
Salami, Italian dry, deli thin sliced, 5 slices (28 g)	4
Salami, Italian dry, light, deli thin sliced, 5 slices (28 g)	2

Gallo

Salame, light, Italian dry, 5 slices (28 g)	2

Great Value

Pork sausage patties, spicy, 1 patty (50 g)	7

Guy Fieri

Fajita seasoned chicken sausage, 1 link (85 g)	3
Sausage, chicken, smoked tequila lime, 1 link (85 g)	3

Gwaltney

Sausage patties, turkey, original flavor, 2 patties (56 g)	3

Hatfield

Sausage, pork roll, 1 slice (41 g)	3

Hickory Farms

Summer sausage, 2 oz	7

Hillshire Farm

Hot links, beef, 1 link (64 g)	7
Polska kielbasa (beef hot smoked, beer brat, cheddarwurst, hot and spicy Italian), 1 link (64 g)	7
Polska kielbasa, lite, 2 oz	3
Polska kielbasa, turkey, 2 oz	2
Sausage, beef, smoked, 2 oz	6
Sausage, hardwood smoked, chicken, 2 oz	3

	SmartPoints™ value
Sausage, smoked, 2 oz	7
Sausage, smoked, cheddar wurst, 1 link (64 g)	8
Sausage, smoked, lite, 2 oz	3
Sausage, smoked, turkey, 2 oz	2
Sausage, summer, 2 oz	6
Sausage, turkey pepper Jack, 1 link (64 g)	3
Wurst, cheddar, 1 link (66 g)	8
Hillshire Farm American Craft	
Sausage, smoked, jalapeño and cheddar cheese, 1 link (82 g)	9
Hillshire Farm Lit'l Smokies	
Sausage, smoked, 5 links (50 g)	6
Sausage, smoked, cheddar, 5 links (50 g)	6
Sausage, smoked, turkey, 5 links (50 g)	2
Honeysuckle White	
Fresh breakfast sausage, 2 ½ oz	2
Italian sausage, 1 link (112 g)	4
Hormel	
Original extra lean pork tenderloin, 4 oz	2
Pepperoni stix, 1 stick (28 g)	5
Pepperoni, minis, 1 oz	5
Pepperoni, original, 14 slices (28 g)	5
Pepperoni, turkey, 17 slices (30 g)	2
Pepperoni, turkey, minis, 1 oz	2
Hormel Little Sizzlers	
Pork sausage, maple, 3 links (46 g)	8
Pork sausage, original, 3 links (46 g)	7
Isernio's	
Sausage, premium, breakfast chicken, 2 ½ oz	1
Sausage, premium, Italian chicken, 2 ½ oz	1

	SmartPoints™ value
Jennie-O	
Breakfast sausage, turkey, mild, lean, 2 oz	2
Hardwood smoked turkey kielbasa, 2 oz	2
Hot turkey breakfast sausage, 2 oz	2
Italian turkey sausage, hot, lean, 1 link (109 g)	4
Italian turkey sausage, sweet, lean, 1 link (109 g)	4
Smoked turkey sausage, lean, 2 oz	2
Turkey bratwurst, original, lean, 1 link (109 g)	5
Jennie-O Lean	
Turkey breakfast sausage links, 2 links (48 g)	1
Turkey breakfast sausage links, 3 links (68 g)	3
Jimmy Dean	
Breakfast bowls, sausage & gravy, 1 bowl (226 g)	12
Chorizo chicken sausage links, 3 links (64 g)	3
Fully cooked turkey sausage crumbles, ½ cup	1
Fully cooked turkey sausage links, 3 links (68 g)	3
Fully cooked turkey sausage patties, 2 patties (68 g)	3
Maple turkey sausage links, 3 links (68 g)	3
Original fresh pork sausage patties, 2 patties (53 g)	6
Original pork sausage patties, 2 patties (68 g)	9
Pork sausage links, maple, 3 links (68 g)	10
Pork sausage links, original, 3 links (68 g)	9
Pork sausage, premium, hot, 2 oz cooked	6

Meat & Poultry

	SmartPoints™ value
Pork sausage, premium, maple, 2 oz cooked	6
Pork sausage, premium, original, reduced fat, 2 oz cooked	4
Pork sausage, premium, regular, 2 oz	6
Pork sausage, premium, sage, 2 oz cooked	6
Sausage crumbles, hearty, original, ⅔ cup	7
Sausage patties, maple turkey, 2 patties (68 g)	3
Sausage patties, pork, maple, 2 patties (68 g)	9
Sausage, pork, regular, 2 oz cooked	6
Jimmy Dean Delights	
Applewood smoke chicken sausage links, 3 links (64 g)	3
Applewood smoke chicken sausage patties, 2 patties (64 g)	3
Maple and brown sugar chicken sausage patties, 2 patties (64 g)	3
Jimmy Dean Fully Cooked Sausage	
Turkey sausage links, 3 links (68 g)	3
Jimmy Dean Heat 'N Serve	
Sausage links, turkey, 3 links (55 g)	4
Sausage patties, original, 2 patties (52 g)	7
Sausage patties, turkey, 2 patties (52 g)	3
Johnsonville	
Andouille, 2 oz	6
Beddar with cheddar smoked sausage, 1 link (66 g)	7
Beer brats, 1 link (76 g)	9
Brats, beef, 1 link (57 g)	7
Brats, beer, 1 link (66 g)	8
Brats, beer 'n bratwurst, 1 link (85 g)	9
Brats, cheddar, 1 link (85 g)	9
Brats, original, 1 link (85 g)	9
Brats, stadium, 1 link (66 g)	8

	SmartPoints™ value
Breakfast sausage, hickory smoke, 3 pan-fried links (68 g)	7
Breakfast sausage, patties, original recipe, 1 patty (32 g)	3
Breakfast sausage, pork & chicken, maple, 4 links (83 g)	5
Breakfast sausage, pork & chicken, original recipe, 4 links (83 g)	5
Chicken sausage, Cajun style, 1 link (85 g)	5
Chicken sausage, Italian style with cheese, single sealed links, 2 oz	3
Fully cooked turkey breakfast sausage, 2 links (45 g)	2
Hot links, 1 link (76 g)	8
Hot links, beef, 1 link (57 g)	7
Italian sausage, mild, 1 link (81 g)	9
Italian sausage, mild Italian, sliced, 2 oz	7
Kielbasa, polish, 1 link (66 g)	8
Luck of the Irish o'garlic sausage, 1 grilled link (82 g)	9
Original recipe fully cooked breakfast sausage, 2 links (45 g)	5
Polish kielbasa, 2 oz	6
Sausage, chicken, 3 cheese Italian style, 1 link (85 g)	6
Sausage, chicken, apple, 1 link (85 g)	5
Sausage, chicken, chipotle Monterey Jack cheese, 1 link (85 g)	5
Sausage, Italian, hot, 2 oz cooked	6
Sausage, Italian, mild, 1 link (85 g)	9
Sausage, Italian, mild, ground, 2 oz	6
Sausage, Italian, sweet, 1 grilled link (85 g)	9
Sausage, smoked, jalapeño & cheese, 1 link (66 g)	8
Smoked brats, 1 link (66 g)	7
Smoked sausage, new orleans brand, andouille recipe, 1 link (66 g)	7

Meat & Poultry

	SmartPoints™ value
Summer sausage, beef, 2 oz	6
Turkey sausage, smoked, 1 link (64 g)	3
Turkey with cheddar, 1 link (64 g)	3
Vermont maple syrup breakfast sausage, 2 links (45 g)	5
Johnsonville Brats	
Cheddar cheese and bacon flavor sausage, 1 link (82 g)	9
Original bratwurst, 1 link (85 g)	9
Jones Dairy Farm	
Fully cooked & browned sausage, mild, 1 patty (38 g)	5
Sausage links, turkey, golden brown, 4 links (56 g)	2
Jones Dairy Farm All Natural	
Golden brown turkey sausage patties, 1 patty (35 g)	2
Little turkey sausage, 2 links (53 g)	2
Jones Dairy Farm All Natural Golden Brown	
Fully cooked sausage links, 3 links (59 g)	9
Jones Dairy Farm Golden Brown	
Sausage, 10 links, maple, 2 links (45 g)	7
Sausage, 10 links, mild, 2 links (227 g)	7
Kiolbassa	
Sausage, beef smoked, 2 oz	7
Kroger	
Breakfast sausage, 2 oz	6
Fully cooked turkey sausage patties, 2 patties (56 g)	3
Pepperoni, turkey, sliced, 15 slices (30 g)	2
Reduced fat turkey sausage patties, 1 patty (51 g)	2
Sausage, mild ground, Italian, 2 oz	6
Traditional turkey sausage links, 3 links (74 g)	5

	SmartPoints™ value
Meijer	
Roasted garlic and asiago chicken sausage, 1 link (85 g)	2
Spinach and mozzarella chicken sausage, 1 link (85 g)	2
Morningstar Farms	
Original veggie sausage patty, 1 patty (38 g)	2
Morningstar Farms Breakfast	
Sausage links, veggie, 2 links (45 g)	2
New York Style Sausage	
Pork sausage, breakfast links, 2 links (57 g)	4
Odom's Tennessee Pride	
Mild sausage patties, 2 patties (48 g)	6
Turkey sausage patties, 2 patties (62 g)	3
Old Folks	
Sausage patties, country, medium, 2 patties (56 g)	8
Old Smokehouse	
Summer sausage, 2 oz	8
Old Wisconsin	
Sausage sticks, turkey, 1 stick (20 g)	1
Snack bites, turkey sausage, 6 pieces (30 g)	2
Snack sticks, turkey sausage, 1 stick (16 g)	1
Open Nature	
Chicken sausage, chicken & apple, 1 link (85 g)	5
Sausage, chicken, mild Italian, 1 link (85 g)	3
Sausage, chicken, roasted red pepper & garlic, 1 link (85 g)	3
Sausage, chicken, smoked andouille, 1 link (85 g)	4
Sausage, chicken, spinach & feta, 1 link (85 g)	3

Meat & Poultry

SmartPoints™ value

SmartPoints™ value

Oscar Mayer

Kielbasa, polska, turkey, 2 oz	2
Liver sausage, braunschweiger, authentic, 2 oz	7
Sausage, smoked, turkey, 2 oz	3
Sausages, little smokies, 6 links (57 g)	6

Owen's

Pork sausage patties, original, 2 patties (56 g)	5
Sausage patties, turkey, 2 patties (56 g)	2

Premio

Sausage chicken, Italian, with cheese & garlic, 1 link (60 g)	3
Sausage, chicken, Italian, hot & spicy, 1 link (60 g)	3
Sausage, chicken, Italian, sweet, 1 link (60 g)	3
Sausage, Italian, sweet, 1 link (70 g)	6

Roger Wood

Smoked sausage, 2 ½ oz	5

Saag's Naturals

Sausage, chicken brats, 1 link (85 g)	5

Sausages by Amylu

Sausage, chicken, apple & gouda cheese, smoked, 1 link (63 g)	3

Silva

Linguica, 2 oz	6

Simply Balanced

Sausage, chicken, spinach & garlic, 1 link (68 g)	2

Simply Nature

Country style chicken breakfast sausage with sage and thyme, 1 link (32 g)	1

Smithfield

Sausage patties, restaurant style, 1 patty (50 g)	7

Swaggerty's Farm

Premium sausage patties, 1 patty (34 g)	5

Tennessee Pride

Country sausage, mild, 2 oz	7
Sausage patties, biscuit size, original flavor, 1 patty (42 g)	6
Sausage patties, original, 2 patties (51 g)	6

Tennessee Pride Homestyle

Sausage balls, 4 (72 g)	10

Tillamook

Pepperoni stick, 1 piece (41 g)	7

Tofurky

Kielbasa, 3 ½ oz	5
Sausage, Italian, with sun-dried tomatoes and basil, 3 ½ oz	6

Trader Joe's

Roasted garlic chicken sausage, 1 link (68 g)	3
Smoked apple chardonnay chicken sausage, 1 link (85 g)	3
Spicy chicken sausage, 1 link (85 g)	5
Spicy Italian chicken sausage, 1 link (85 g)	3
Spicy jalapeño chicken sausage, 1 link (68 g)	3
Sun-dried tomato basil chicken sausage, 1 link (68 g)	3
Sweet apple with pure vermont maple syrup chicken sausage, 1 link (68 g)	4
Sweet Italian style red & green pepper chicken sausage, 1 link (68 g)	3

Williams

Sausage patties, country, mild, 1 patty (40 g)	6

Turkey

Applegate Farms

Turkey burgers, organic, 1 burger (112 g)	4

Ball Park

Flame grilled turkey patty, 1 patty (85 g)	2

Bubba

Burgers, turkey, 1 burger (112 g)	3

Butterball

Ground turkey breast, 4 oz	1
Turkey breast roast, boneless, 4 oz	2
Turkey burger patties with natural flavoring, 1 patty (114 g)	2

Butterball Everyday

Sweet onion seasoned turkey burgers, 1 patty (151 g)	5
Turkey burgers, 1 patty (151 g)	5
Turkey, ground, 93/7, lean, 4 oz	3

Essential Everyday Premium Deli

Shaved oven roasted turkey breast, 2 oz	1

Fit & Active

Oven roasted turkey breast, 2 oz	1

Foster Farms Savory Servings

Turkey tenderloins, island teriyaki, 4 oz	2
Turkey tenderloins, lemon peppercorn, 4 oz	2

Great Value

Breakfast patties, turkey, 1 patty (50 g)	2

Harvestland

Turkey burgers, ground, fresh, 1 burger (112 g)	4

Hillshire Farm

Turkey breast, Tuscan style herb, 3 slices (49 g)	1

Homestyle

Meatballs, turkey, Italian style, 3 meatballs (85 g)	5

Hormel Natural Choice

Sun dried tomato deli turkey, 3 slices (56 g)	1

Jennie-O

90%/10% fat lean turkey burger patties, 1 patty (112 g)	4
93% lean/7% fat all white meat turkey burgers, 1 burger (149 g)	4
All natural turkey breast tenderloin, 4 oz	1
Applewood smoke flavor turkey breast tenderloin, 4 oz	2
Ground turkey breast, with natural flavorings, extra lean, 4 oz	1
Ground turkey, 85/15, 4 oz	6
Ground turkey, 90/10, 4 oz	4
Ground turkey, Italian seasoned, 4 oz	3
Ground turkey, lean, 4 oz	4
Ground turkey, taco seasoning, 4 oz	4
Jalapeño and Monterey Jack turkey burgers, 1 burger (149 g)	6
Seasoned turkey burger patties with onion and garlic seasoning, lean, 1 patty (114 g)	4
Turkey breast tenderloin, savory roast, 4 oz	1
Turkey breast tenderloins, roast turkey, 4 oz	1
Turkey burgers, 1 burger (112 g)	6
Turkey burgers, all natural, 93/7, with seasonings, 1 burger (149 g)	4
Turkey burgers, lean, original, 1 burger (112 g)	4
Turkey burgers, lean, savory seasoned, 1 burger (112 g)	4
Turkey patties, white, seasoned, 95/5, 1 patty (112 g)	2

Jennie-O All Natural

Turkey burger, 1 burger (149 g)	2

Jennie-O So Easy

Turkey meatloaf, lean, 5 oz	4

Meat & Poultry

Meat & Poultry

	SmartPoints™ value
Jennie-O Turkey Store	
Ground turkey, 4 oz	4
Turkey breast slices, extra lean, 4 oz	1
Turkey burgers, with seasonings, 95/5, 1 burger (149 g)	2
Kirkland Signature	
Turkey burgers, 1 burger (151 g)	3
Kroger	
85% lean fresh ground turkey, 4 oz	7
Fresh ground turkey patties, 1 patty (112 g)	7
Fresh lean ground turkey, 4 oz	3
Thinly sliced chicken breast cutlets, 1 piece (142 g)	2
Kroger Meals Made Simple	
Reduced fat turkey meatballs, 6 meatballs (85 g)	5
Land O'Frost Premium	
Turkey breast & white turkey, mesquite, 4 slices (50 g)	2
Member's Mark	
Seasoned rotisserie chicken, 4 oz	5
Nature's Promise Naturals	
Turkey, ground, 4 oz	3
On-Cor Traditionals	
Gravy and sliced turkey, dark & white, family size, 3 slices (123 g)	2
Oscar Mayer	
Smoked turkey breast, 4 slices (57 g)	1
Turkey breast & white turkey, mesquite smoked, 3 slices (61 g)	1
Turkey breast & white turkey, oven roasted, family size, 1 slice (28 g)	0
Perdue	
Ground turkey, lean, 4 oz	4
Turkey, ground, lean patties, 1 patty (112 g)	4

	SmartPoints™ value
Perdue Short Cuts	
Oven roasted carved turkey breast, ½ cup	1
Philly-Gourmet	
Turkey, homestyle patties, 1 patty (112 g)	3
Plainville Farms	
Turkey, ground, 94% lean 6% fat, 4 oz	3
Shady Brook Farms	
Ground turkey, 4 oz	3
Ground turkey, seasoned, Italian style, 4 oz	3
Lean ground turkey, 4 oz raw	3
Turkey breast tenderloin, lean, homestyle, 4 oz	2
Turkey breast tenderloins, rotisserie, 4 oz	2
ShopRite Deli Style	
Turkey breast, oven roasted, thin sliced, 2 oz	1
Signature Cafe	
Turkey meatloaf, 1 slice (85 g)	3
Sommer's Organic	
Turkey burgers, 100% organic turkey, 1 burger (114 g)	1
Specially Selected	
Bacon wrapped turkey filet, 1 (142 g)	6
Stouffer's Homestyle Classics	
Roast turkey, 1 package (272 g)	8
Trader Joe's	
Turkey burger, 1 patty (113 g)	4

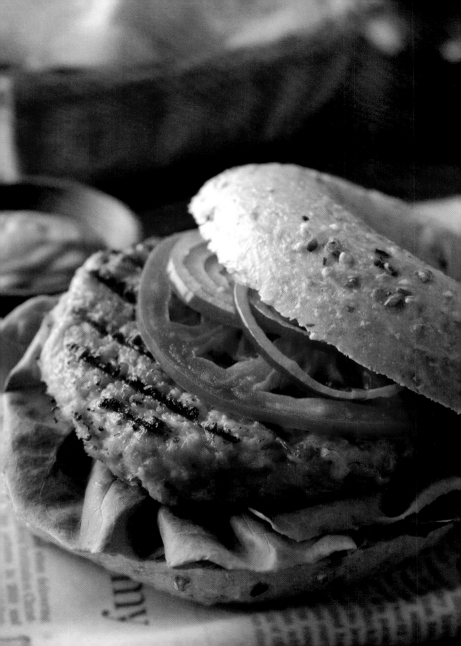

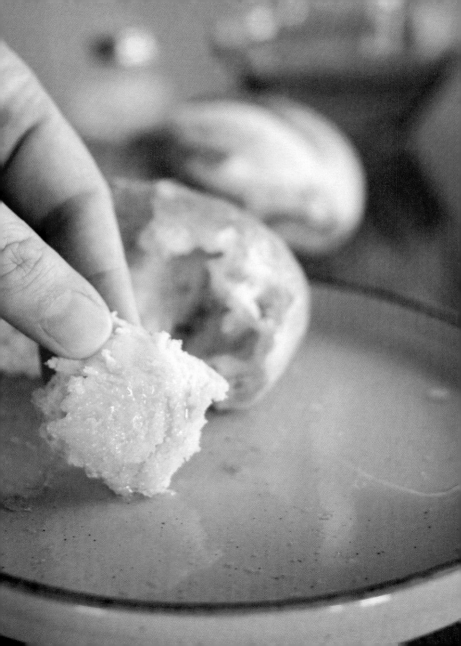

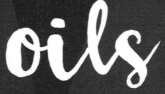

oils

& Dressings

Oils & Dressings

Oils

Bellino

Extra virgin olive oil, 1 Tbsp	4

Bertolli

Olive oil, extra virgin, 1 Tbsp	4
Olive oil, tasting, extra light, 1 Tbsp	4

BetterBody Foods

Coconut, extra virgin oil, organic, 1 Tbsp	7

California Olive Ranch

Olive oil, extra virgin, fresh California, 1 Tbsp	4

Carlini

100% extra virgin olive oil, 1 Tbsp	4

Carrington Farms

Coconut oil, 1 Tbsp	7
Coconut oil, 100% organic, extra virgin, 1 Tbsp	7

Colavita

Extra virgin olive oil, 1 Tbsp	4

Crisco

Olive oil, extra virgin, 1 Tbsp	4
Olive oil, light, tasting, 1 Tbsp	4
Vegetable oil, pure, 1 Tbsp	4

Filippo Berio

Extra virgin olive oil, 1 Tbsp	4
Olive oil, extra light tasting, 1 Tbsp	4

GrapeOla

Grape seed oil, all natural, 1 Tbsp	4

Great Value

Olive oil, 100% extra virgin, 1 Tbsp	4
Olive oil, extra light tasting, 1 Tbsp	4
Olive oil, pure, 1 Tbsp	4

Hollywood

Oil, safflower, enriched expeller pressed, 1 Tbsp	4

International Collection

Flax-seed oil, virgin, with cinnamon flavor, 1 Tbsp	4

Kelapo

Coconut oil, extra virgin, organic, 1 Tbsp	7

Kirkland Signature

Organic extra virgin olive oil, 1 Tbsp	4

Kroger

Canola oil, pure, 1 Tbsp	4
Olive oil, extra virgin, 1 Tbsp	4
Olive oil, lighter flavor, 1 Tbsp	4

LouAna

100% pure coconut oil, 1 Tbsp	7

Nature's Way EfaGold

Organic extra virgin coconut oil, 1 Tbsp	7

Nutiva

Coconut oil, organic extra virgin, 1 Tbsp	7

Pompeian

Olive oil, extra virgin, 1 Tbsp	4

Pompeian OlivExtra

Oil, canola and extra virgin olive, value size, 1 Tbsp	4

Smart Balance Omega

Oil, natural blend of canola, soy & olive, 1 Tbsp	4

Spectrum Naturals

Coconut oil, organic, unrefined, 1 Tbsp	7

Spectrum Organic

Coconut oil, refined, 1 Tbsp	7

Trader Joe's

Extra virgin olive oil, 1 Tbsp	4
Organic extra virgin coconut oil, 1 Tbsp	7

Wesson

Canola oil, 1 Tbsp	4

Salad Dressing

Alessi
Premium balsamic reduction, 1 Tbsp	3

America's Choice
Dressing, lite, Caesar, 2 Tbsp	3
Dressing, lite, Italian, 2 Tbsp	2

Annie's
Dressing, Asian sesame, 2 Tbsp	4
Dressing, cowgirl ranch, 2 Tbsp	4
Dressing, goddess, lite, 2 Tbsp	2
Dressing, goddess, natural, 2 Tbsp	4
Dressing, poppy seed, lite, 2 Tbsp	3
Dressing, tuscany Italian, natural, 2 Tbsp	3
Vinaigrette, balsamic, 2 Tbsp	4
Vinaigrette, fat free, raspberry balsamic, 2 Tbsp	2
Vinaigrette, honey mustard, 2 Tbsp	2
Vinaigrette, lite, herb balsamic, 2 Tbsp	2

Annie's Lite
Vinaigrette, gingerly, 2 Tbsp	1
Vinaigrette, raspberry, 2 Tbsp	2

Annie's Naturals
Dressing, organic, goddess, 2 Tbsp	4
Dressing, roasted red pepper, 2 Tbsp	3
Vinaigrette, shitake sesame, 2 Tbsp	4

Archer Farms
Light Italian dressing, 2 Tbsp	3

Biltmore
Salad dressing, honey mustard, 2 Tbsp	6

Bob's Famous
Salad dressing & dip, bleu cheese, 2 Tbsp	5
Salad dressing & dip, roquefort, 2 Tbsp	5

Bolthouse Farms
Bold blue cheese Greek yogurt dressing, 2 Tbsp	1
Caesar parmigiano yogurt dressing, 2 Tbsp	2
Chunky blue cheese yogurt dressing, 2 Tbsp	1
Cilantro avocado yogurt dressing, 2 Tbsp	2
Classic ranch yogurt dressing, 2 Tbsp	2
Cucumber dill Greek yogurt dressing, 2 Tbsp	1
Dressing, yogurt, salsa ranch, 2 Tbsp	2
Honey mustard yogurt dressing, 2 Tbsp	2
Italian vinaigrette dressing (serves 14), 1 serving (30 g)	1
Mango chipotle yogurt dressing, 2 Tbsp	2
Miso ginger vinaigrette dressing (serves 14), 1 serving (30 g)	2
Peppercorn ranch Greek yogurt dressing, 2 Tbsp	1
Vinaigrette, extra virgin olive oil, chunky blue cheese, 2 Tbsp	2
Vinaigrette, extra virgin olive oil, classic balsamic, 2 Tbsp	2
Vinaigrette, extra virgin olive oil, raspberry merlot, 2 Tbsp	2
Yogurt dressing, creamy, thousand island, 2 Tbsp	3

Bragg
Salad dressing, ginger & sesame, 2 Tbsp	1

Bragg Healthy Organic
Vinaigrette, 2 Tbsp	5

Braswell's
Dressing, raspberry vinaigrette, 2 Tbsp	3
Dressing, vidalia onion summer tomato, 2 Tbsp	3

Oils & Dressings

Oils & Dressings

	SmartPoints™ value
Briannas	
Dressing, home style, blush wine vinaigrette, 2 Tbsp	5
Dressing, home style, champagne caper vinaigrette, 2 Tbsp	5
Dressing, home style, chipotle cheddar, 2 Tbsp	4
Dressing, home style, classic buttermilk ranch, 2 Tbsp	5
Dressing, home style, creamy balsamic, 2 Tbsp	6
Dressing, home style, Dijon honey mustard, 2 Tbsp	6
Dressing, home style, real French, vinaigrette, 2 Tbsp	4
Dressing, home style, rich poppy seed, 2 Tbsp	6
Home style dressing, asiago Caesar, 2 Tbsp	5
Special request dressing, lively lemon tarragon, 2 Tbsp	2
Cains	
Dressing, fat free, raspberry vinaigrette, 2 Tbsp	2
Reduced calorie dressing, blush wine vinaigrette, light, 1 oz	3
Vinaigrette, raspberry, 1 oz	1
Cardini's	
Dressing, balsamic vinaigrette, 2 Tbsp	4
Dressing, Caesar, 2 Tbsp	5
Dressing, Caesar vinaigrette, light, 2 Tbsp	2
Dressing, Caesar, fat free, 2 Tbsp	2
Dressing, Caesar, light, 2 Tbsp	3
Dressing, Greek vinaigrette, light, 2 Tbsp	2
Dressing, the original Caesar, large size, 2 Tbsp	5
Cardini's Light	
Dressing, light balsamic vinaigrette, 2 Tbsp	2

	SmartPoints™ value
Christie's	
Dressing, Greek, 2 Tbsp	5
Dressing, lite, Greek, 2 Tbsp	3
The original Greek dressing, 2 Tbsp	5
Cole Farms	
Dressing, cole slaw, 2 Tbsp	5
Cookwell	
Salad dressing, Asian ginger vinaigrette, 2 Tbsp	2
Salad dressing, olive and lemon vinaigrette, 2 Tbsp	3
Dorothy Lynch	
Fat free home style dressing, 2 Tbsp	4
Home style dressing, 2 Tbsp	5
Edelweiss	
Dressing, creamy cesar, 2 Tbsp	4
Emeril's	
Dressing, bleu cheese, 2 Tbsp	3
Essential Everyday	
Dressing, reduced fat, creamy ranch, light, 2 Tbsp	3
Dressing, reduced fat, Italian, light, 2 Tbsp	1
Thousand island light reduced fat dressing, 2 Tbsp	3
Fanny's Lite	
Italian dressing, 2 Tbsp	3
Farmer Boy	
Dressing, Greek, lite, 2 Tbsp	2
Dressing, house recipe Greek, 2 Tbsp	1
Feast from the East	
Sesame dressing, 2 Tbsp	4
Fit & Active	
Buffalo ranch light dressing, 2 Tbsp	3
Fat free zesty Italian dressing, 2 Tbsp	1
Light poppyseed dressing, 2 Tbsp	3

	SmartPoints™ value
Reduced fat light balsamic vinaigrette, 2 Tbsp	2
Reduced fat light ranch dressing, 2 Tbsp	3
Follow Your Heart	
Dressing, ranch, low fat, 2 Tbsp	1
Giant/Stop & Shop	
Light honey mustard dressing, 2 Tbsp	4
Girard's	
Dressing, Caesar, light, 2 Tbsp	3
Dressing, champagne, 2 Tbsp	5
Dressing, champagne, light, 2 Tbsp	2
Dressing, Greek feta vinaigrette, 2 Tbsp	4
Dressing, olde venice, Italian, 2 Tbsp	5
Dressing, spinach salad, 2 Tbsp	3
Dressing, white balsamic vinaigrette, 2 Tbsp	4
Vinaigrette, creamy balsamic, 2 Tbsp	4
Golding Farms	
Salad dressing, vidalia onion vinegarette, creamy, 2 Tbsp	5
Good Seasons	
Asian sesame with ginger dressing, 2 Tbsp	4
Balsamic dressing and recipe mix, ⅛ envelope (2 g)	0
Italian all natural salad dressing and recipe mix, ⅛ packet dry (2.5 g)	0
Great Value	
Fat free Italian dressing, 2 Tbsp	1
Gregg's	
Savory ranch dressing, 2 Tbsp	5
Hannaford	
Dressing, light ranch, 2 Tbsp	3
Heinz	
Dressing, salad cream, original, 1 Tbsp	2
Ranch dressing, light, 1 packet (42 g)	4

	SmartPoints™ value
Hellmann's	
Dressing, ranch, creamy, 1 packet (43 g)	4
Dressing, ranch, light, 2 Tbsp	3
Vinaigrette, light, raspberry, 2 Tbsp	4
Hendrickson's	
Salad dressing, classic Italian, 2 Tbsp	1
Salad dressing, marinade & seasoning, original, sweet vinegar & olive oil, 2 Tbsp	4
Henris	
Dressing, honey mustard, homestyle, fat free, 2 Tbsp	3
Hidden Valley	
Dressing, BBQ ranch, 2 Tbsp	4
Dressing, coleslaw, 2 Tbsp	6
Dressing, ranch, light, BLT ranch with bacon & tomato, 2 Tbsp	3
Dressing, ranch, light, buttermilk, 2 Tbsp	3
Dressing, ranch, spicy, 2 Tbsp	5
Dressing, ranch, with garlic, 2 Tbsp	5
Hidden Valley Farmhouse Originals	
Dressing & dip, creamy parmesan, 2 Tbsp	5
Dressing and dip, Southwest chipotle, 2 Tbsp	4
Dressing, Italian with herbs, 2 Tbsp	3
Dressing, pomegranate vinaigrette, 2 Tbsp	2
Vinaigrette dressing, mango chipotle, 2 Tbsp	3
Hidden Valley The Original Ranch	
Dressing, avocado, 2 Tbsp	3
Dressing, buttermilk, old fashioned, 2 Tbsp	5
Dressing, fat free, 1 packet (42.5 g)	1
Dressing, fiesta salsa, 2 Tbsp	4
Dressing, fiesta salsa, light, 2 Tbsp	2
Dressing, Italian ranch, 2 Tbsp	5
Dressing, light, 2 Tbsp	3

Oils & Dressings

SmartPoints™ value

Dressing, ranch, 2 Tbsp	5
Dressing, to go, 1 container (44 ml)	7
Mix, salad dressing and seasoning, ½ tsp	0
Hidden Valley To Go	
Dressing, light, thick & creamy, single cups, 1 container (44 ml)	4
Hy-Vee	
Dressing, light French, 2 Tbsp	3
Dressing, reduced fat, light, ranch, 2 Tbsp	2
JES	
Peanut dressing, Thai style, 2 Tbsp	3
John The Greek	
Salad dressing, original, 1 Tbsp	3
Ken's Steak House	
Balsamic with honey dressing, 2 Tbsp	4
Dressing & marinade, Italian, 2 Tbsp	5
Dressing, balsamic & basil vinaigrette, 2 Tbsp	4
Dressing, balsamic vinaigrette, lite, 1 ½ oz	3
Dressing, blue cheese vinaigrette, 2 Tbsp	4
Dressing, buttermilk ranch, 2 Tbsp	6
Dressing, chunky blue cheese, 2 Tbsp	5
Dressing, chunky blue cheese, lite, 2 Tbsp	3
Dressing, country French, 2 Tbsp	6
Dressing, creamy parmesan with cracked peppercorn, lite, 2 Tbsp	3
Dressing, fat free, raspberry pecan, 2 Tbsp	3
Dressing, Italian with aged romano, 2 Tbsp	4
Dressing, lite, balsamic vinaigrette, 2 Tbsp	2
Dressing, lite, raspberry walnut vinaigrette, 2 Tbsp	4

SmartPoints™ value

Dressing, lite, creamy Caesar, 2 Tbsp	3
Dressing, lite, northern Italian with basil & romano, 2 Tbsp	2
Dressing, lite, olive oil vinaigrette, 2 Tbsp	2
Dressing, lite, poppy seed, 2 Tbsp	4
Dressing, lite, raspberry pomegranate, 2 Tbsp	3
Dressing, lite, sweet vidalia onion, 2 Tbsp	4
Dressing, lite, thousand island, 2 Tbsp	3
Dressing, ranch, fat free, 1 packet (42.52 g)	2
Dressing, ranch, lite, 2 Tbsp	3
Dressing, red wine vinegar & olive oil, 2 Tbsp	2
Dressing, sweet vidalia onion, 2 Tbsp	5
Dressing, thousand island, 2 Tbsp	5
Dressing, topping & spread, squeezable, honey mustard, 2 Tbsp	5
Dressing, zesty Italian, 2 Tbsp	3
Fat free raspberry pecan dressing, 2 Tbsp	3
Greek dressing, 2 Tbsp	4
Honey mustard dressing, 2 Tbsp	5
Lite Asian sesame with ginger & soy dressing, 2 Tbsp	3
Lite honey mustard dressing, 2 Tbsp	4
Lite honey mustard dressing, topping & spread, 2 Tbsp	4
Lite strawberry vinaigrette dressing, 2 Tbsp	3
Ken's Steak House Chef's Reserve	
Dressing, blue cheese with gorgonzola, 2 Tbsp	5
Dressing, Italian with garlic & asiago cheese, 2 Tbsp	4
Dressing, tableside Caesar, 2 Tbsp	5

Oils & Dressings

Ken's Steak House Dressing Fat Free

Italian dressing pounch, 1 packet (42.5 g)	1

Ken's Steak House Healthy Options

Dressing, Caesar vinaigrette, 2 Tbsp	3
Dressing, honey Dijon, 2 Tbsp	3
Dressing, honey French, 2 Tbsp	3
Dressing, olive oil & vinegar, 2 Tbsp	2
Dressing, ranch, 2 Tbsp	3
Dressing, raspberry walnut, 2 Tbsp	3
Dressing, vinaigrette, sweet vidalia onion, 2 Tbsp	3

Ken's Steak House Light Options

Dressing, balsamic vinaigrette, 2 Tbsp	2
Dressing, Italian, 2 Tbsp	2
Parmesan & peppercorn dressing, 2 Tbsp	3

Ken's Steak House Lite

Apple cider vinaigrette dressing, 2 Tbsp	3
Dressing, sun-dried tomato, 2 Tbsp	2

Kraft

Anything dressing, balsamic vinaigrette, 2 Tbsp	3
Anything dressing, buttermilk ranch, 2 Tbsp	1
Anything dressing, coleslaw, 2 Tbsp	4
Anything dressing, fat free, French style, 2 Tbsp	2
Anything dressing, fat free, ranch, 2 Tbsp	2
Anything dressing, fat free, thousand island, 2 Tbsp	2
Balsamic vinaigrette with tomato and basil, 2 Tbsp	3
Dressing, creamy Italian, 2 Tbsp	3
Dressing, ranch with bacon, 2 Tbsp	4
Dressing & marinade, lime cilantro vinaigrette, 2 Tbsp	2

Dressing, Asian toasted sesame, 2 Tbsp	4
Dressing, Caesar vinaigrette with parmesan, 2 Tbsp	2
Dressing, catalina (1.5 oz pouch), 1 pouch (42 g)	6
Dressing, catalina, lite, 2 Tbsp	3
Dressing, chunky blue cheese, 2 Tbsp	4
Dressing, classic Caesar, 2 Tbsp	4
Dressing, classic ranch, 2 Tbsp	4
Dressing, classic, catalina, 2 Tbsp	4
Dressing, creamy balsamic, 2 Tbsp	3
Dressing, creamy French, 2 Tbsp	5
Dressing, creamy Italian, 2 Tbsp	4
Dressing, creamy poppyseed, 2 Tbsp	5
Dressing, cucumber ranch, 2 Tbsp	4
Dressing, golden Italian (1.5 oz pouch), 1 pouch (42 g)	4
Dressing, Greek vinaigrette, 2 Tbsp	4
Dressing, green goddess, 2 Tbsp	5
Dressing, honey mustard, 2 Tbsp	5
Dressing, Italian roasted red pepper with parmesan, 2 Tbsp	2
Dressing, lite, Asian toasted sesame, 2 Tbsp	2
Dressing, lite, balsamic vinaigrette, 2 Tbsp	1
Dressing, lite, creamy Caesar, 2 Tbsp	1
Dressing, lite, French style, 2 Tbsp	3
Dressing, lite, house Italian, 2 Tbsp	2
Dressing, lite, parmesan asiago balsamic vinaigrette, 2 Tbsp	2
Dressing, lite, ranch, 2 Tbsp	2
Dressing, lite, thousand island, 2 Tbsp	3
Dressing, lite, three cheese ranch, 2 Tbsp	2
Dressing, lite, zesty Italian, 2 Tbsp	1
Dressing, mango chipotle, 2 Tbsp	3

Oils & Dressings

Oils & Dressings

	SmartPoints™ value
Dressing, peppercorn ranch, 2 Tbsp	4
Dressing, ranch (1.5 oz pouch), 1 pouch (42 g)	7
Dressing, raspberry vinaigrette, lite, 2 Tbsp	2
Dressing, raspberry vinaigrette, with poppyseeds, 2 Tbsp	2
Dressing, raspberry with poppy seeds, 2 Tbsp	2
Dressing, roka blue cheese, 2 Tbsp	4
Dressing, strawberry balsamic vinaigrette, 2 Tbsp	2
Dressing, sun dried tomato vinaigrette, 2 Tbsp	2
Dressing, sweet balsamic, 2 Tbsp	4
Dressing, sweet honey catalina, 2 Tbsp	4
Dressing, tangy catalina bacon, 2 Tbsp	4
Dressing, thousand island, 2 Tbsp	5
Dressing, three cheese ranch, 2 Tbsp	4
Dressing, tuscan house, Italian, 2 Tbsp	2
Dressing, zesty catalina, 2 Tbsp	5
Dressing, zesty Italian, 2 Tbsp	2
Dressing, zesty lime vinaigrette, 2 Tbsp	2

Kraft Free

Dressing, fat free, Italian, 2 Tbsp	1
Fat free dressing, French style (1.5 oz pouch), 1 pouch (42 g)	3
Fat free dressing, Italian (1.5 oz pouch), 1 pouch (42 g)	1
Fat free dressing, ranch (1.5 oz pouch), 1 pouch (42 g)	2
Fat free dressing, raspberry vinaigrette (1.5 oz pouch), 1 pouch (43 g)	2
Fat free dressing, thousand island (1.5 oz pouch), 1 pouch (42 g)	2

Kroger

	SmartPoints™ value
Dressing, balsamic vinaigrette, 2 Tbsp	3
Dressing, balsamic vinaigrette, lite, 2 Tbsp	2
Dressing, California French, 2 Tbsp	4
Dressing, chunky bleu cheese, 2 Tbsp	5
Dressing, creamy Caesar, lite, 2 Tbsp	3
Dressing, creamy Italian, 2 Tbsp	4
Dressing, creamy ranch, 2 Tbsp	5
Dressing, Greek, 2 Tbsp	4
Dressing, lite creamy ranch, 2 Tbsp	3
Dressing, lite, southwest ranch, 2 Tbsp	3
Dressing, olive oil & vinegar, 2 Tbsp	4
Dressing, poppyseed, 2 Tbsp	6
Dressing, ranch, 2 Tbsp	5
Dressing, ranch, creamy, fat free, 2 Tbsp	1
Dressing, roasted red pepper vinaigrette, 2 Tbsp	2
Dressing, thousand island, 2 Tbsp	3
Dressing, zesty Italian, 2 Tbsp	3
Dressing, zesty Italian, fat free, 2 Tbsp	1
Dressing, zesty Italian, lite, 2 Tbsp	2
Honey mustard dressing and marinade, 2 Tbsp	4
Lite raspberry vinaigrette dressing and marinade, 2 Tbsp	3

Kroger Value

Dressing, salad, ranch, 2 Tbsp	4

LaRosa's Family Recipe

Salad dressing, creamy garlic, 2 Tbsp	6

Litehouse

Buttermilk ranch, 2 Tbsp	4
Chunky bleu cheese, 2 Tbsp	5
Dressing & sauce, creamy cilantro, 2 Tbsp	4

Dressing, blue cheese Greek style yogurt, 2 Tbsp	2
Dressing, sauce & marinade, Thai peanut flavored, mild, 2 Tbsp	2
Dressing, sauce & marinade, toasted sesame ginger, 2 Tbsp	2
Dressing, vinaigrette, lite, honey Dijon, 2 Tbsp	3
Dressing, vinaigrette, raspberry walnut, 2 Tbsp	4
Dressing, vinaigrette, red wine & olive oil, 2 Tbsp	3
Dressing, yogurt, bleu cheese, 2 Tbsp	3
Dressing, yogurt, ranch, 2 Tbsp	2
Homestyle ranch, 2 Tbsp	4
Vinaigrette dressing, pear gorgonzola, 2 Tbsp	2
Vinaigrette dressing, pomegranate blueberry, 2 Tbsp	1

Litehouse Lite

Dressing & dip, creamy ranch, 2 Tbsp	2

Litehouse Naturals

Balsamic vinaigrette, 2 Tbsp	3
Vinaigrette, blue cheese, 2 Tbsp	4

Makoto

Ginger dressing, 2 Tbsp	3
Honey ginger dressing, 2 Tbsp	3

Maple Grove Farms

All natural dressing, strawberry balsamic, 2 Tbsp	1
Balsamic vinaigrette dressing with pure maple syrup, 2 Tbsp	2
Dressing, all natural, sesame ginger, 2 Tbsp	2
Dressing, balsamic, 2 Tbsp	1
Dressing, balsamic vinaigrette, fat free, 2 Tbsp	0
Dressing, Caesar, fat free, 2 Tbsp	0
Dressing, citrus vinaigrette, 2 Tbsp	3
Dressing, cranberry balsamic vinaigrette, fat free, 2 Tbsp	2

Dressing, fat free, raspberry vinaigrette, 2 Tbsp	2
Dressing, fat free, vidalia onion, 2 Tbsp	1
Dressing, lime basil vinaigrette, fat free, 2 Tbsp	1
Dressing, fat free, Greek, 2 Tbsp	1
Dressing, honey Dijon, 2 Tbsp	2
Dressing, honey mustard, lite, 2 Tbsp	4
Dressing, poppyseed, 2 Tbsp	2
Fat free honey Dijon dressing, 2 Tbsp	2
Fat free poppyseed dressing, 2 Tbsp	2
Fat free wasabi Dijon dressing, 2 Tbsp	2
Vinaigrette, balsamic, sugar free, 2 Tbsp	0
Vinaigrette, raspberry, 2 Tbsp	2
Vinaigrette, raspberry, sugar free, 2 Tbsp	0

Marie's

Dressing, balsamic vinaigrette, 2 Tbsp	2
Dressing, blue cheese vinaigrette, 2 Tbsp	5
Dressing, buttermilk ranch, 2 Tbsp	5
Dressing, Caesar, 2 Tbsp	6
Dressing, chunky blue cheese, 2 Tbsp	6
Dressing, coleslaw, 2 Tbsp	6
Dressing, creamy chipotle ranch, 2 Tbsp	6
Dressing, creamy Italian garlic, 2 Tbsp	6
Dressing, creamy ranch, lite, 2 Tbsp	3
Dressing, Italian vinaigrette, 2 Tbsp	3
Dressing, lemon herb vinaigrette, 2 Tbsp	5
Dressing, poppy seed, 2 Tbsp	6

Oils & Dressings

Salad Dressing, Marie's (cont'd)

	SmartPoints™ value
Dressing, premium, super blue cheese, 2 Tbsp	6
Dressing, raspberry vinaigrette, 2 Tbsp	2
Dressing, red wine, vinaigrette, 2 Tbsp	3
Dressing, thousand island, 2 Tbsp	6
Dressing, yogurt, ranch, 2 Tbsp	2
Yogurt dressing, blue cheese, 2 Tbsp	3
Yogurt dressing, feta cheese, 2 Tbsp	3
Yogurt dressing, parmesan Caesar, 2 Tbsp	2
Marzetti	
Buttermilk ranch dressing, 1 ½ oz	7
Dressing, asiago peppercorn, 2 Tbsp	6
Dressing, blue cheese, 1 ½ oz	8
Dressing, chunky blue cheese, 2 Tbsp	5
Dressing, classic ranch, 2 Tbsp	6
Dressing, Dijon honey mustard, 1 ½ oz	7
Dressing, fat free, ranch, 1 ½ oz	2
Dressing, honey Dijon, 2 Tbsp	5
Dressing, honey French, 1 ½ oz	9
Dressing, light chunky blue cheese, 2 Tbsp	3
Dressing, light honey French, 2 Tbsp	4
Dressing, light, balsamic vinaigrette, 2 Tbsp	2
Dressing, light, classic ranch, 2 Tbsp	3
Dressing, light, original slaw, 2 Tbsp	4
Dressing, light, supreme Caesar, 2 Tbsp	3
Dressing, light, vinaigrette, Caesar, 2 Tbsp	3
Dressing, light, vinaigrette, raspberry cabernet, 2 Tbsp	3

	SmartPoints™ value
Dressing, original slaw, 2 Tbsp	6
Dressing, poppyseed, 2 Tbsp	6
Dressing, slaw, lite, 2 Tbsp	4
Dressing, spinach salad, 2 Tbsp	4
Dressing, supreme Caesar, 2 Tbsp	5
Dressing, sweet Italian, 2 Tbsp	6
Dressing, the ultimate blue cheese, 2 Tbsp	6
Poppyseed light dressing, 2 Tbsp	4
Ranch dressing, 1 oz	4
Vinaigrette, balsamic, 1 ½ oz	5
Vinaigrette, roasted garlic Italian, 2 Tbsp	3
Marzetti Light	
Italian dressing, 1 ½ oz	1
Ranch dressing, 1 ½ oz	3
Marzetti Salad Accents	
Fruit and nut salad toppings, 1 Tbsp	2
Marzetti Simply Dressed	
Cherry balsamic vinaigrette, 2 Tbsp	4
Dressing, blue cheese, 2 Tbsp	5
Dressing, Caesar, 2 Tbsp	4
Dressing, coleslaw, 2 Tbsp	4
Dressing, Greek feta, 2 Tbsp	4
Dressing, ranch, 2 Tbsp	4
Lemon vinaigrette dressing, 2 Tbsp	3
Light balsamic vinaigrette dressing, 2 Tbsp	2
Light roasted tomato vinaigrette dressing, 2 Tbsp	1
Light veggie ranch dressing, 2 Tbsp	2
Vinaigrette, balsamic, 2 Tbsp	3
Vinaigrette, champagne, 2 Tbsp	3
Vinaigrette, ginger sesame, 2 Tbsp	3
Vinaigrette, pomegranate, 2 Tbsp	3
Vinaigrette, strawberry poppyseed, 2 Tbsp	5
Marzetti Simply Dressed & Light	
Blue cheese dressing, 2 Tbsp	3
Red wine Italian vinaigrette, 2 Tbsp	1

Oils & Dressings

McCormick

Salad toppins, roasted garlic Caesar, 1 Tbsp	1

Meijer

Dressing, light, ranch, 2 Tbsp	3
Light balsamic vinaigrette, 2 Tbsp	2
Raspberry vinaigrette dressing, 2 Tbsp	2

Miracle Whip

Dressing, 1 Tbsp	1
Dressing, nonfat, fat free, 1 Tbsp	1
Dressing, nonfat, free, 1 Tbsp	1
Dressing, original, 1 Tbsp	1
Dressing, with olive oil, 1 Tbsp	1
Light dressing, 1 Tbsp	1
Salad dressing, 1 Tbsp	2

Muirhead

Balsamic vinaigrette, 1 Tbsp	3

Naturally Fresh

Dressing, classic ranch, 2 Tbsp	5
Dressing, ginger, 2 Tbsp	2
Dressing, light, bleu cheese, 2 Tbsp	4
Dressing, lite, ranch, 2 Tbsp	3
Jalapeño ranch dressing, 2 Tbsp	4
Poppy seed dressing, 2 Tbsp	6

Naturally Fresh Lite

Dressing, ranch, 2 Tbsp	3

Newman's Own

Balsamic vinaigrette, 2 Tbsp	3
Dressing, Caesar, 2 Tbsp	5
Dressing, creamy balsamic, 2 Tbsp	4
Dressing, creamy Caesar, 2 Tbsp	6
Dressing, family recipe Italian, 2 Tbsp	4
Dressing, honey French, 2 Tbsp	5
Dressing, light Caesar, 2 Tbsp	3
Dressing, olive oil & vinegar, 2 Tbsp	5
Dressing, poppy seed, 2 Tbsp	5
Dressing, ranch, 2 Tbsp	5

Dressing, red wine vinegar & olive oil, lite, 2 Tbsp	2
Family recipe Italian dressing, 2 Tbsp	4
Light Italian dressing, 2 Tbsp	2
Ranch dressing, 2 Tbsp	5
Vinaigrette, Greek, 2 Tbsp	4

Newman's Own Lighten Up!

Dressing, light honey mustard, 2 Tbsp	3
Dressing, light raspberry & walnut, 2 Tbsp	3
Dressing, low fat sesame ginger, 2 Tbsp	2
Italian dressing, light sun dried tomato, 2 Tbsp	2
Light balsamic vinaigrette, 2 Tbsp	2
Light Italian dressing, 2 Tbsp	2
Vinaigrette, light lime, 2 Tbsp	2
Vinaigrette, light roasted garlic balsamic, 2 Tbsp	2

Newman's Own Organic

Dressing, low fat Asian, 2 Tbsp	2
Light balsamic vinaigrette, 2 Tbsp	2

Olde Cape Cod

Dressing, balsamic vinaigrette, 2 Tbsp	2
Dressing, fat free, balsamic vinaigrette, 2 Tbsp	1
Dressing, lite, sweet & sour poppyseed, 2 Tbsp	4

Olde Cape Cod Local Favourites

Dressing, sweet & sour poppy seed, lite, 2 Tbsp	4

Olive Garden

Italian dressing, 2 Tbsp	3
Light Italian dressing, 2 Tbsp	1
Signature Italian dressing, 2 Tbsp	3

Olive Garden Signature Dressing

Italian dressing, 2 Tbsp	3

Oils & Dressings

	SmartPoints™ value
OPA	
Feta dill Greek style yogurt dressing, 2 Tbsp	1
Ranch Greek style yogurt dressing, 2 Tbsp	2
OPA by Litehouse	
Kalamata feta flavor Greek yogurt dressing, 2 Tbsp	2
Roasted pepper Greek yogurt dressing, 2 Tbsp	1
OPA by Litehouse Greek Style Yogurt	
Caesar dressing, 2 Tbsp	2
Open Nature	
Dressing, Asian sesame ginger, 2 Tbsp	2
Ott's	
Fat free dressing, poppy seed, 2 Tbsp	3
Our Family	
Salad dressing, light, 1 Tbsp	1
Panera Bread	
Dressing, Asian sesame vinaigrette, 2 Tbsp	2
Dressing, balsamic vinaigrette, low sodium, 2 Tbsp	4
Dressing, fuji apple vinaigrette, 2 Tbsp	4
Dressing, poppyseed, fat free, low calorie, low sodium, 2 Tbsp	1
Dressing, raspberry vinaigrette, fat free, 2 Tbsp	1
Private Selection	
Dressing, creamy Cesar, 2 Tbsp	5
Publix	
Dressing, salad, fat free thousand island, 2 Tbsp	2
Salad dressing, lite ranch, 2 Tbsp	3
Safeway	
Dressing, light, ranch, 2 Tbsp	3
Dressing, light, thousand island, 2 Tbsp	3

	SmartPoints™ value
Safeway Select	
Dressing, Greek feta vinaigrette, 2 Tbsp	2
ShopRite	
Dressing, Caesar, light, 2 Tbsp	3
Dressing, Italian, fat free, 2 Tbsp	1
Dressing, light French style, 2 Tbsp	2
Dressing, light ranch, 2 Tbsp	3
Ranch dressing, fat free, 2 Tbsp	2
Smart Balance Omega Plus	
Dressing, light mayonnaise, 1 Tbsp	2
Specially Selected	
All natural house vinaigrette, 2 Tbsp	4
Sushi Chef	
Salad dressing, sesame soy, Japanese style, 2 Tbsp	3
T. Marzetti	
Dressing, white balsamic vinaigrette, 2 Tbsp	4
Taco Bell	
Dressing & dip, southwest ranch, 2 Tbsp	5
The Ojai Cook	
Lemonaise, light, 1 Tbsp	1
Trader Giotto's	
Balsamic vinaigrette, 2 Tbsp	3
Trader Joe's	
Asian style spicy peanut vinaigrette, 2 Tbsp	3
Champagne pear vinaigrette, 2 Tbsp	2
Champagne pear vinaigrette with gorgonzola, 2 Tbsp	2
Cilantro salad dressing, 2 Tbsp	2
Cranberry walnut & gorgonzola salad dressing, 2 Tbsp	3
Fat free balsamic vinaigrette, 2 Tbsp	1
Goddess dressing, 2 Tbsp	4
Greek style feta dressing, 2 Tbsp	4
Light champagne vinaigrette, 2 Tbsp	2

	SmartPoints™ value
Low fat parmesan ranch dressing, 2 Tbsp	1
Raspberry dressing, 2 Tbsp	2
Sweet poppy seed dressing, 2 Tbsp	4
Trader Ming's	
Fat free sesame soy ginger vinaigrette, 2 Tbsp	2
Tuscan Garden	
Balsamic vinaigrette dressing, 2 Tbsp	2
Buttermilk ranch dressing, 2 Tbsp	5
Vidalia	
Dressing, creamy vidalia, 2 Tbsp	3
Virginia Brand	
Salad dressing, vidalia onion, vinaigrette, 2 Tbsp	4
Vidalia onion vinegarette salad dressing, 2 Tbsp	4
Walden Farms	
Dressing & dip, chipotle ranch, 2 Tbsp	0
Dressing, bacon ranch, 2 Tbsp	0
Dressing, balsamic vinaigrette, 2 Tbsp	0
Dressing, bleu cheese, calorie free, 2 Tbsp	0
Dressing, Caesar, 2 Tbsp	0
Dressing, honey Dijon, 1 packet (30 ml)	0
Dressing, honey Dijon vinaigrette, 2 Tbsp	0
Dressing, raspberry vinaigrette, 2 Tbsp	0
Dressing, sesame ginger, 2 Tbsp	0
Dressing, zesty Italian, 2 Tbsp	0
Dressing/vinaigrette, chipotle ranch, 2 Tbsp	0
Vinaigrette, raspberry, 2 Tbsp	0
Walden Farms Low Fat	
Dressing, ranch, 2 Tbsp	1
Dressing, thousand island, 2 Tbsp	1

	SmartPoints™ value
Wegman's	
Dressing, balsamic vinaigrette, 2 Tbsp	2
Dressing, fat free, parmesan Italian, 2 Tbsp	2
Light dressing, garlic Italian, 2 Tbsp	1
Light dressing, parmesan peppercorn ranch, 2 Tbsp	3
Light dressing, ranch, 2 Tbsp	3
Vinaigrette, white balsamic, 2 Tbsp	4
Wegman's Food You Feel Good About	
Dressing, yogurt, Greek feta, 2 Tbsp	2
Dressing, yogurt, ranch, 2 Tbsp	3
Vinaigrette, lemon, 2 Tbsp	3
Western	
Dressing, fat free sweet and smooth, 2 Tbsp	3
Dressing, lite, 2 Tbsp	3
Dressing, sweet & smooth, 2 Tbsp	7
Whole Foods Organic	
Roquefort blue cheese dressing, 2 Tbsp	3
Wish-Bone	
Dressing, balsamic vinaigrette, 2 Tbsp	2
Dressing, buffalo blue cheese, with frank's red hot, 2 Tbsp	5
Dressing, buffalo ranch, 2 Tbsp	5
Dressing, chipotle ranch, 2 Tbsp	5
Dressing, classic ranch, 2 Tbsp	4
Dressing, creamy Italian, 2 Tbsp	4
Dressing, deluxe French, 2 Tbsp	5
Dressing, fat free, chunky blue cheese, 2 Tbsp	1
Dressing, fat free, Italian, 2 Tbsp	1
Dressing, Greek vinaigrette, 2 Tbsp	2
Dressing, guacamole ranch, 2 Tbsp	5
Dressing, house Italian, 2 Tbsp	4
Dressing, Italian, 2 Tbsp	3
Dressing, Italian, 2 Tbsp	3

Oils & Dressings

SmartPoints™ value

Dressing, Italian balsamic vinaigrette, 2 Tbsp	3
Dressing, light balsamic & basil, vinaigrette, 2 Tbsp	2
Dressing, light buffalo ranch, 2 Tbsp	3
Dressing, light ranch, 2 Tbsp	3
Dressing, light raspberry walnut, vinaigrette, 2 Tbsp	3
Dressing, light, deluxe French, 2 Tbsp	2
Dressing, light, Italian, 2 Tbsp	1
Dressing, low fat, parmesan peppercorn ranch, 2 Tbsp	2
Dressing, mediterranean Italian, 2 Tbsp	2
Dressing, olive oil, vinaigrette, 2 Tbsp	2
Dressing, original, chunky blue cheese, 2 Tbsp	5
Dressing, original, ranch, 2 Tbsp	3
Dressing, ranch, 2 Tbsp	6
Dressing, raspberry hazelnut, vinaigrette, 2 Tbsp	3
Dressing, red wine, vinaigrette, 2 Tbsp	3
Dressing, robusto Italian, 2 Tbsp	3
Dressing, romano basil, vinaigrette, 2 Tbsp	2
Dressing, superfruit berry, vinaigrette, 2 Tbsp	3
Dressing, sweet & smooth western, 2 Tbsp	7
Dressing, sweet & spicy honey mustard, 2 Tbsp	4
Dressing, Thousand Island, 2 Tbsp	5
Wish-Bone Just 2 Good!	
Low fat dressing, ranch, 2 Tbsp	2
Low fat dressing, thousand island, 2 Tbsp	2

SmartPoints™ value

Wish-Bone Light!	
Asian with sesame and ginger vinaigrette dressing, 2 Tbsp	3
Dressing, Italian, 2 Tbsp	2
Dressing, sweet & spicy French, 2 Tbsp	2
Low fat dressing, creamy Caesar, 2 Tbsp	2
Low fat dressing, Italian, 2 Tbsp	2
Low fat dressing, western, 2 Tbsp	4
Yasou	
Dressing, Greek, the original, 2 Tbsp	6
Zia's	
Dressing, fat free, sweet Italian, 2 Tbsp	2

Vinegar

Bragg	
Apple cider vinegar, raw, unfiltered, organic, 1 Tbsp	0
Bragg Organic	
Apple cider vinegar, raw, unfiltered, 1 Tbsp	0
Colavita	
Balsamic vinegar, of modena, 1 Tbsp	1
Monari Federzoni	
Balsamic vinegar, modena, 1 Tbsp	1
Nakano	
Seasoned rice vinegar, roasted garlic, 1 Tbsp	1
Vinegar, rice, seasoned, 1 Tbsp	1
Newman's Own Organic	
Balsamic vinegar, organic, 1 Tbsp	1
Pompeian	
Vinegar, balsamic, 1 Tbsp	0
Vinegar, red wine, 1 Tbsp	0
Trader Giotto's	
Balsamic glaze, 1 Tbsp	2

Oils & Dressings

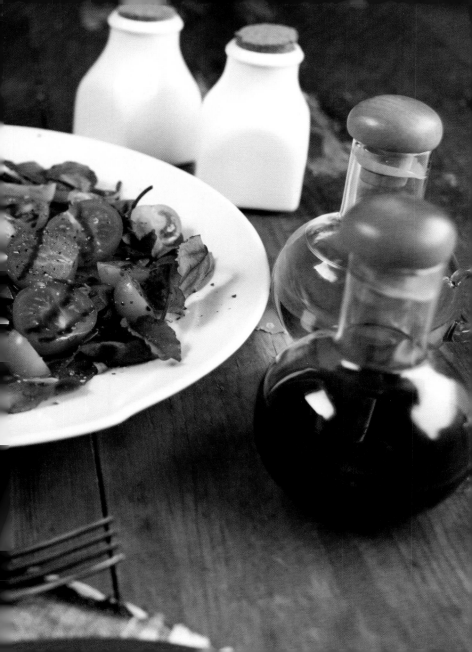

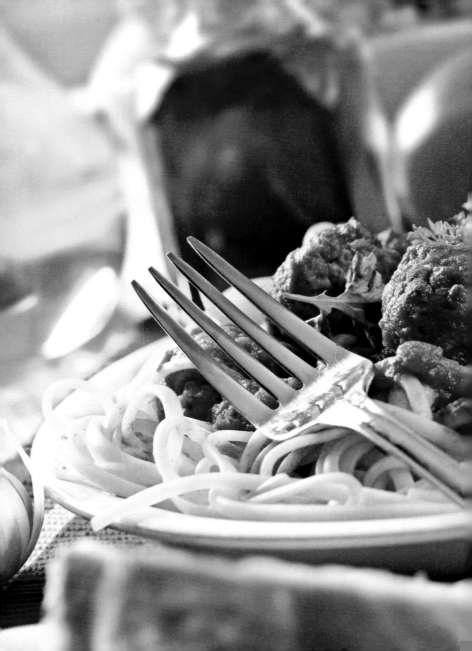

pasta
Rice & Grains

Pasta, Rice & Grains

Grains

Ancient Harvest	
Quinoa, inca red, ¼ cup dry	5
Quinoa, traditional, ¼ cup dry	5
Bob's Red Mill	
Wheat germ, natural raw, 2 Tbsp	1
DHC Fine Foods	
Organic quinoa, 1 bowl (120 g)	5
Finest	
Kiepe ble bulgar wheat, ¼ cup	4
Flax USA	
Golden flax, 2 Tbsp	2
Freekah Foods Original	
Roasted green wheat, ¼ cup	3
Hodgson Mill	
Quinoa and brown rice, Mediterranean, ¼ cup	4
Kretschmer	
Wheat germ, honey crunch, 2 Tbsp	1
Wheat germ, original toasted, 2 Tbsp	1
Nature's Earthly Choice	
Quinoa, 100% whole grain, organic, ¼ cup dry	4
Quinoa Ancient Harvest	
Quinoa, harmony, tri-color blend, ¼ cup dry	5
Roland	
Quinoa, garden vegetable, ¼ cup	4
Quinoa, roasted garlic, ¼ cup dry	4
Simple Truth	
Quinoa, ¼ cup dry	4
Spectrum	
Chia seed, ground, 2 Tbsp	2
Supremo	
Sopes, corn, Mexican style, 1 ⅔ oz	3

Trader Joe's	
Fully cooked organic quinoa, 1 oz	1
Harvest grains blend, ¼ cup	5
Organic polenta (serves 5), 1 serving (102 g)	2
Whole wheat cous cous, ⅓ cup	6
Tru Roots Organic	
100% wholegrain quinoa, ¼ cup dry	5
Village Harvest	
Quinoa, ¼ cup	4
Wild Oats Marketplace Organic	
Organic quinoa & brown rice blend (unprepared), ¼ cup	5

Noodles

Ah-So	
Chinese noodles, ½ cup	3
Al Dente Carba-Nada	
Noodles, egg fettuccine, 1 ½ cups	3
Annie Chun's	
Brown rice noodles, maifun, 2 oz	6
Asian Gourmet	
Chinese noodles, extra crispy, 1 oz	4
Chinese wide lo mein noodles, ½ cup	6
China Boy	
Chow mein noodles, ½ cup	4
Hokan	
Rice sticks, rice vermicelli noodles, py mai fun, 1 cup	6
House Foods	
Shirataki, traditional, 1 ⅔ oz	0
KA-ME	
Hokkien noodles, stir fry, ½ pouch (100 g)	5
Lo mein noodles, wide, Chinese, ¼ package (56 g)	6

Kroger

Egg noodles, whole wheat, wide, 1 cup dry	6

La Choy

Chow mein noodles, ½ cup	4
Noodles, chow mein, ½ cup	4
Rice noodles, ½ cup	4

Light N Fluffy

Egg noodles, extra wide, 2 oz	6
Egg noodles, wide, enriched, ¼ package (56 g)	6

Maruchan Yakisoba

Teriyaki beef flavor, ½ container (57 g)	9

Mee Tu

Chinese noodles, 1 oz	4

Miracle Noodle

Noodles, angel hair, 3 oz	0
Noodles, fettuccini, 3 oz	0

Mrs. Grass

Noodles, goulash, 1 ½ cups dry	6

Nissin Original

Chow mein noodles, teriyaki beef flavor, ½ container (57 g)	9
Chow mein noodles, with shrimp, ½ container (57 g)	9

No Yolks

Noodles, extra broad, 2 oz	6
Whole grain extra broad egg white pasta, 1 ½ cups	6

Pennsylvania Dutch

Egg noodles, homestyle, 1 ½ cups	6

Ronzoni Healthy Harvest

Wide noodle, 2 oz	5

Safeway

Chow mein noodles, ½ cup	4

Thai Kitchen

Stir-fry rice noodles, 2 oz	5
Thin rice noodles, vermicelli-style, 2 oz	5

Thai Kitchen Asian Creations

Stir-fry rice noodles, brown rice noodles, 2 oz	6

Wel Pac

Stir fry noodles, chow mein, 2 oz dry	5

Pasta

Ancient Harvest

Gluten-free garden pagodas quinoa pasta, 2 oz dry	6
Gluten-free quinoa pasta, linguine, 2 oz	6
Gluten-free quinoa pasta, penne, 2 oz	6
Gluten-free quinoa pasta, elbows, 2 oz dry	6
Gluten-free quinoa pasta, rotelle, 2 oz dry	6
Gluten-free quinoa pasta, shells, 2 oz dry	6

Barilla

100% whole wheat angel hair pasta, 2 oz	5
Campanelle, n. 99, 2 oz	6
Cellentani, n. 97, ⅛ box (56 g)	6
Ditalini, ⅛ box (56 g)	6
Elbows, no. 41, 2 oz	6
Elbows, veggie, 2 oz	6
Farfalle, no. 65, 2 oz	6
Fettuccine, n. 6, 2 oz	6
Linguine, n. 13, 2 oz	6
Mezze penne, no. 369, 2 oz	6
Mezzi rigatoni, ⅛ box (56 g)	6
Mini farfalle, 2 oz dry	6
Mostaccioli, no. 71, 2 oz	6
Orzo, n. 26, ⅛ box (56 g)	6
Pastina, 2 oz dry	6
Penne, tri-color, 2 oz	6
Rigatoni, no. 83, 2 oz	6
Rotini, n. 81, 2 oz	6

	SmartPoints™ value
Rotini, tri-color, n. 381, 2 oz	6
Shells, jumbo, no. 333, 5 pieces (50 g)	5
Shells, medium no. 393, 2 oz	6
Spaghetti, no. 5, 2 oz	6
Thick spaghetti, no 7, 2 oz	6
Thin spaghetti, no. 3, 2 oz	6
Thin veggie spaghetti, 1 serving (56 g)	6
Veggie spaghetti, 1 serving (56 g)	6
Ziti, ⅛ box (56 g)	6
Barilla Gluten Free	
Elbows, 2 oz	6
Penne, 2 oz	6
Rotini, 2 oz	6
Spaghetti, 2 oz	6
Barilla Plus	
Elbows, 2 oz	6
Penne, 2 oz	6
Spaghetti, 2 oz	6
Barilla Veggie	
Pasta, penne, 2 oz	6
Rotini, 2 oz	6
Barilla White Fiber	
Mini shells pasta, 2 oz dry	6
Barilla Whole Grain	
100% whole wheat linguine pasta, 2 oz dry	5
100% whole wheat penne, 1 serving (56 g)	5
100% whole wheat spaghetti, 1 serving (56 g)	5
100% whole wheat thin spaghetti, 1 serving (56 g)	5
Elbows, 100% whole wheat, 2 oz	6
Medium shells pasta, 2 oz	6
Rotini, 100% whole wheat pasta, 1 serving (56 g)	5

	SmartPoints™ value
Bonavita	
Penne rigate pasta, gluten free, 1 cup	6
Buitoni	
Fettuccine pasta, 1 ¼ cups	7
Linguine pasta, 1 ¼ cups	7
Mixed cheese tortellini, 1 cup	10
Ravioli, four cheese, 1 ¼ cups	10
Tortellini, herb chicken, 1 cup	10
Tortellini, three cheese, 1 cup	10
Tortellini, three cheese, 100% whole wheat, 1 cup	10
Buitoni Riserva	
Agnolotti, wild mushroom, 1 cup	9
Creamette	
Elbow macaroni, ½ cup dry	6
Spaghetti, ½ cup	6
Thin spaghetti, 2 oz	6
DaVi	
100% whole wheat angel hair pasta, 2 oz	5
100% whole wheat penne pasta, ¾ cup	5
Dreamfields	
Angel hair, 2 oz dry	5
Elbows, ½ cup dry	5
Linguine, 2 oz	5
Penne rigate, ½ cup dry	5
Rotini, ¾ cup	5
Spaghetti, 2 oz (56 g)	5
Eating Right	
Whole grain penne pasta, ⅔ cup	6
Essential Everyday	
Whole wheat penne rigate pasta, ¾ cup dry	5
Whole wheat rotini pasta, ¾ cup dry	5
Whole wheat thin spaghetti, 2 oz dry	5

Explore Asian Authentic Cuisine

Organic black bean spaghetti pasta, 2 oz	4

Ferrara

Pastina, no. 75, 1 cup	6

Fit & Active

Whole grain rotini pasta, ¾ cup	6

Fresh Creative Foods

Orzo feta salad, orzo, mediterranean, ⅔ cup	8

Garofalo

Spaghetti, 2 oz dry	6

Garofalo Organic

Variety pack pasta, ⅔ cup dry	6

Golden Grain

100% whole grain penne pasta, ⅔ cup dry	5
100% whole grain spaghetti pasta, 2 oz	5

Goya

Fidelini/fideo, ½ cup	6

Great Value

Whole wheat elbow macaroni, ½ cup	6
Whole wheat spaghetti, 2 oz	5

Kroger

Capellini, angel hair, ⅛ package dry (56 g)	6
Elbow macaroni, ½ cup dry	6
Fettuccini, 1 serving (56 g)	6
Penne rigate, ¾ cup dry	5
Rotini, salad, ¾ cup dry	5
Spaghetti, thin, 2 oz dry	5
Thin spaghetti, ⅛ package dry (56 g)	6
Whole wheat, whole grain, spaghetti, dry, 2 oz dry	5

La Moderna

Fideo, ½ cup	6

Mueller's

Angel hair, 100% whole grain, 2 oz dry	5
Bowties, ¾ cup dry	6
Elbow macaroni, ½ cup	6
Penne pasta, ¾ cup	6
Penne, 100% whole grain, 2 oz dry	5
Spaghetti, 2 oz	6
Spaghetti, 100% whole grain, 2 oz dry	6
Thin spaghetti, 2 oz	6

Mueller's Pot-Sized

Thin spaghetti, 2 oz dry	6

Nasoya

Pasta zero plus, shirataki fettuccine, ⅔ cup	1
Pasta zero plus, shirataki spaghetti, ⅔ cup	1

No Yolks

Egg white pasta, cholesterol free, broad, 2 oz	6
Egg white pasta, cholesterol free, dumplings, 2 oz	6
Egg white pasta, cholesterol free, extra broad, 2 oz	6

Pacific

Mac & cheese, 1 cup	9

Pasta Prima

Ravioli, spinach and cheese, 1 cup	6

Pasta Roni

Angel hair pasta with herbs, 2 oz	6

Ronzoni

Bow ties, 1 cup dry	6
Rotini, garden delight, ¾ cup	5
Spaghetti, no. 8, 2 oz	6
Thin spaghetti, no. 9, 2 oz	6

Ronzoni 150 Calories

Penne pasta, ¾ cup	4
Spaghetti, thin, 2 oz	4
Spaghetti, thin, 2 oz	4

Pasta, Rice & Grains

	SmartPoints™ value
Ronzoni Garden Delight	
Fettuccine, 2 oz	5
Spaghetti, ¾ cup	5
Trio Italiano pasta blend, ¾ cup dry	6
Ronzoni Gluten Free	
Penne rigate pasta, ⅔ cup	6
Rotini pasta, ¾ cup	6
Spaghetti, 2 oz dry	6
Ronzoni Healthy Harvest	
Linguine, whole wheat blend, 2 oz	5
Spaghetti, whole wheat blend, 2 oz	5
Thin spaghetti, whole wheat blend, 2 oz	5
Whole wheat blend pasta, penne rigate, 2 oz	5
Ronzoni Smart Taste	
Angel hair, 2 oz	5
Elbows, 2 oz	5
Noodle style pasta, extra wide, 1 ½ cups dry	5
Penne rigate, ⅔ cup	5
Rotini, 2 oz	5
Spaghetti, ⅙ package (56 g)	5
Thin spaghetti, 2 oz	5
Thin spaghetti, 2 oz	5
San Giorgio Healthy Harvest	
Rotini, 2 oz	5
Simply Asia Asian Creations	
Street noodles, singapore, classic curry, hot, 1 cup	8
Tinkyada	
Brown rice pasta, with rice bran, spirals, 2 oz	6
Tinkyada Pasta Joy	
Brown rice pasta, penne, 2 oz dry	6
Tinkyada Pasta Joy Ready	
Pasta, brown rice, spaghetti style, 2 oz	6

	SmartPoints™ value
Trader Giotto's	
Gnocchi alla sorrentina, 1 cup	6
Trader Joe's	
Organic brown rice & quinoa fusilli pasta, ½ cup	6
Organic brown rice penne pasta, 1 cup cooked	6
Organic brown rice spaghetti pasta, 1 cup cooked	6
Organic gluten free brown rice & quinoa spaghetti pasta, 2 oz	6
Organic whole wheat penne pasta, ¾ cup	6
Sweet potato gnocchi with butter and sage, 1 cup	9
Wegman's	
Pasta, elbows, ½ cup	6
Pasta, shells, ¾ cup	6
Pasta, small shells, ½ cup	6

Rice

	SmartPoints™ value
Annie Chun's Rice Express	
Sticky white rice, ½ tray (105 g)	4
Bombay	
Basmati rice, ¼ cup	5
Carolina	
Jasmine rice, ¼ cup	5
Long grain brown rice, ¼ cup	4
Casa Fiesta	
Mexican style rice, mild, ⅔ cup	4
Fit & Active	
Instant brown rice, ½ cup	4
Giant	
Rice, boil-in-bag, brown, ½ cup	4
Go Go Rice	
Steamed rice bowl, organic brown rice, ½ container (105 g)	4
Golden Star	
Jasmine rice, brown, ⅔ cup dry	2

Goya

Low sodium yellow rice, ¼ cup	4
Mexican rice, chicken flavor, ¼ cup	5
Rice & red beans, ¼ cup	4
Spanish rice, ¼ cup	5
Spanish style yellow rice, ¼ cup	5
Yellow rice, Spanish style, multi-pack, ¼ cup	4

Idahoan

Mashed potatoes, original, ⅓ cup dry	2

Kikkoman

Baste & glaze, teriyaki, 2 Tbsp	3

Kroger

Brown rice, ½ cup	4
Brown rice, boil-in-bag, ½ cup	4
Rice, white, original instant, ½ cup	4

Lundberg

Wild blend rice, ¼ cup dry	5

Lundberg Essences

Organic California basmati brown rice, ¼ cup dry	4

Mahatma

Brown rice, ¼ cup	4
Enriched rice, extra long grain, ¼ cup	4
Rice, basmati, naturally fragrant, ¼ cup	5
Rice, jasmine, long grain, ¼ cup	4

Mahatma Jasmine

Long grain rice, ¼ cup dry	5

McCormick

Rice, Mexican, ⅓ cup dry	7

Minute

Enriched premium long grain instant rice, ½ cup dry	5
Whole grain instant brown rice, ½ cup	5

Minute Ready To Serve!

Black beans and rice, 1 container (132 g)	5
Long grain white rice, 1 container (125 g)	6
Natural whole grain brown rice, 1 container (125 g)	7
White jasmine rice, 1 container (125 g)	7

Minute® Rice

Brown rice, ½ cup	4
Premium white rice, ½ cup	5
White rice, ½ cup	6
White, instant rice, premium long grain, prepared, 1 cup	5
White, long grain rice, instant, prepared, 1 cup	5
Whole grain brown rice, instant, prepared, ⅔ cup	5

Minute® Rice Ready to Serve

Brown & wild rice mix, 1 container (125 g)	7
Brown rice, 1 container (125 g)	5
Multi-grain medley, 1 serving (125 g)	6
White rice, 1 container (125 g)	5

Rice A Roni

Rice, beef flavor, family size, 2 ½ oz	7
Rice, cheddar broccoli flavor, 1 cup	7

Rice A Roni Quick Serve

Rice, beef flavor, ½ cup dry	5
Rice, chicken flavor, ½ cup dry	5

Rice Expressions

Organic brown rice, whole grain, 1 cup	5

Pasta, Rice & Grains

	SmartPoints™ value
Rice Select	
Brown rice, texmati, long grain American basmati, ¼ cup dry	5
Rice, jasmati, long grain American jasmine, ¼ cup dry	4
Rice Select Royal Blend	
Rice blend, ⅓ cup	4
Rice, light brown, texmati, with red quinoa, ¼ cup	5
Texmati, light brown rice, with flaxseed, ¼ cup	5
Riceland	
Brown rice, natural, extra long grain, ¼ cup	4
Royal	
Rice, basmati, ¼ cup	4
Seeds Of Change	
Tigris seven whole grain organic rice, 1 cup	8
Success Boil-in-Bag	
Basmati white rice, ¾ cup dry	5
Brown rice, whole grain, precooked, ½ cup	4
Precooked whole grain brown rice, ½ cup dry	4
Rice, white, jasmine, ¼ cup dry	4
White rice, enriched precooked, ½ cup	5
Trader Joe's	
Basmati rice from india, ¼ cup	5
Brown rice, 1 cup	7
Frozen cooked organic brown rice, 1 cup	4
Japanese style fried rice, 1 cup	8
Organic jasmine rice, 1 cup	5
Sprouted organic California rice (brown, red & black rice), ¼ cup	5
Uncle Ben's	
Enriched parboiled long grain converted rice, 1 cup	5
Fast & natural whole grain instant brown rice, 1 cup	5

	SmartPoints™ value
Long grain & wild rice original recipe, 1 cup	6
Natural whole grain brown rice, ¼ cup (dry)	5
Natural whole grain instant brown rice, ¼ cup dry	5
Original long grain converted rice, ¼ cup	5
Spanish style rice, 1 container (125 g)	5
Whole grain long grain white rice, ¼ cup dry rice	5
Uncle Ben's Boil-In-Bag	
Enriched long grain rice, ¼ cup dry	5
Natural whole grain brown rice, ¼ cup dry	5
Uncle Ben's Country Inn	
Rice pilaf, 1 cup	6
Uncle Ben's Original	
Enriched parboiled long grain, ¼ cup dry	5
Uncle Ben's Ready Rice	
Basmati rice, 1 cup	6
Jasmine, 1 cup	7
Natural whole grain brown, 1 cup	5
Original enriched long grain white rice, 1 cup	6
Red beans and rice, 1 cup	6
Basmati rice, 1 cup	6
Pouch whole grain brown, 1 cup	5
Rice pilaf, 1 cup	6
Uncle Ben's Ready Whole Grain Medley	
Pouch brown & wild brown rice, wild rice & red rice perfectly seasoned with herbs & spices, 1 cup	6
Zatarain's	
Rice mix, caribbean, new orleans style, ⅓ cup dry	8
Zatarain's New Orleans Style	
Yellow rice, ¼ cup dry	5

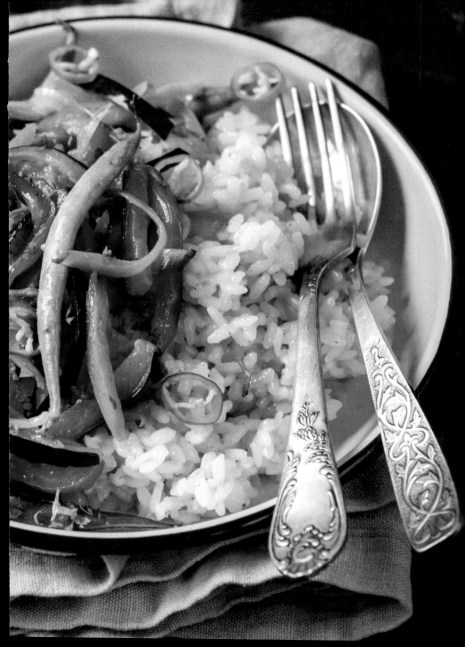

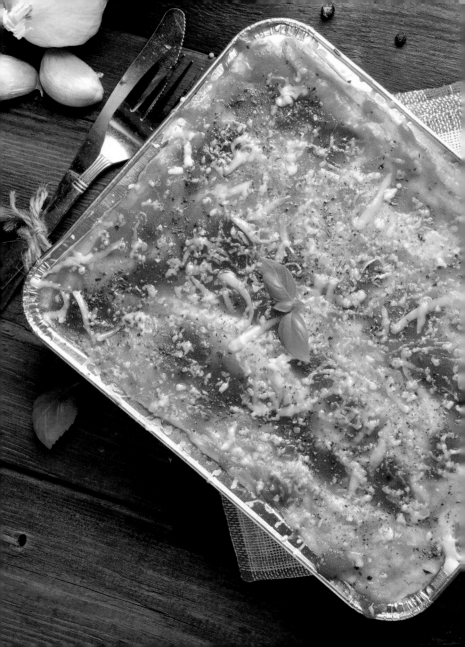

prepared

Foods, Salads & Sides

Prepared Foods, Salads & Sides

Appetizers

Banquet

Sliders, cheese-burger, 2 sandwiches (110 g)	11

Chung's

Egg rolls, mini, vegetable, 2 eggrolls (66 g)	4
Egg rolls, vegetable, 1 eggroll, sauce (88 g)	5
Egg rolls, white meat chicken, 1 egg roll, sauce	5
Spring rolls, vegetable, 2 rolls & sauce (122 g)	6

CJ Bibigo

Chicken and cilantro all natural mini wontons, 4 pieces (36 g)	1

Don Miguel

Chipotle chicken flautas, 2 (142 g)	9
Mini tacos with chicken and cheese, 4 mini tacos (79 g)	5

FarmRich

Breaded mozzarella sticks, 2 sticks (57 g)	6
Breaded mushrooms, 8 pieces (85 g)	6
Crispy dill pickles, 7 pieces (79 g)	6

Foster Farms

Hot'n spicy chicken wings, 3 wing sections (92 g)	6

Frankly Fresh

Stuffed grape leaves, 1 piece (42 g)	2

Galil

Stuffed grape leaves, homemade style, 5 each (133 g)	7

Giant

Spring rolls, vegetable, 1 spring roll (56 g)	3

Giorgio

Mozzarella sticks, Italian breaded, 2 pieces (37.8 g)	4
Portabella mushrooms stuffed with parmesan cheese artichoke and spinach (serves 2), ½ package (114 g)	4

Golden

Filled crepes, cheese blintzes, 1 blintz	3

Kroger

Garlic bread sticks, 1 breadstick (49 g)	5

Lean Cuisine Culinary Collection

Fajita style chicken spring rolls, 3 spring rolls (113 g)	5
Garlic chicken spring rolls, 3 spring rolls (113 g)	6
Thai style chicken spring rolls, 3 spring rolls (113 g)	6
Three cheese and spinach stuffed pretzels, 1 pouch (99 g)	7

Ling Ling

Vegetable mini spring rolls, 3 rolls (102 g)	5

Ling Ling Asian Kitchen

Chicken and vegetable dumplings with sauce, 5 pieces (162 g)	9

Mediterranean Organic

Grape leaves, stuffed, organic, 5 pieces (142 g)	4

Michelina's Lean Gourmet

Chicken snackers, buffalo-style, 11 snacks (85 g)	6

Minh

Egg rolls, mini, chicken, 4 egg rolls	7
Pork & vegetable egg rolls, 1 egg roll	6

New York

Garlic knots, hand-tied, 1 knot (35 g)	4

P.F. Chang's Home Menu

Chang's cream cheese wontons, ½ package (85 g)	11
Chicken mini egg rolls (with sauce), ½ package (125 g)	8
Vegetable mini egg rolls (with sauce), 4 pieces (125 g)	8

Pagoda Cafe Sensations

Egg rolls, vegetable, Asian style, 1 egg roll	5

Pagoda Express

Egg rolls, pork & shrimp, 1 eggroll (87 g)	5
Egg rolls, white meat chicken, 1 egg roll	4

Raphy's

Stuffed grape leaves, 1 piece (20 g)	1

Safeway Select

Arancini, three cheese, 2 pieces (42 g)	3

Sea Pak Shrimp & Seafood Co.

Spring rolls, shrimp, with dipping sauce, 3 rolls (85 g)	3

Sister Schubert's

Rolls, sausage wrap, 1 roll (32 g)	4

T.G.I. Friday's

Buffalo wings, 4 pieces (89 g)	5
Chicken wings with honey bbq sauce (3 oz wings with 2 tbsp sauce), 1 serving (115 g)	6
Green bean fries, crispy, with dipping sauce, 12 pieces (84 g)	6
Honey bbq sauce boneless chicken bites, 6 pieces (80 g)	3
Mozzarella sticks, with marinara sauce, 1 piece (32 g)	3
Potato skins, cheddar & bacon, 3 pieces (96 g)	7

T.G.I. Friday's Loaded!

Potato skins, cheddar & bacon, 1 piece (81 g)	7

T.G.I. Friday's Poppers

Stuffed jalapeños with cream cheese, 3 pieces (70 g)	8

T.G.I. Friday's Restaurant Crispy Style

Boneless buffalo style chicken bites (without sauce), 6 pieces (84 g)	4

Tai Pei

Egg rolls, chicken, 1 roll (85 g)	5

Totino's Pizza Rolls

Pepperoni pizza snack, 6 rolls (85 g)	7

Trader Joe's

Arancini bites, 2 (42 g)	4
Chicken gyoza potstickers, 7 (140 g)	6
French onion soup, 1 bag (283.49 g)	7
Spanakopita - filled with spinach, ricotta & feta cheese, 3 pieces (85 g)	5

Tyson

Honey bbq flavored chicken wings, 2 pieces (69 g)	5

Tyson Any'tizers

Chicken fries, homestyle, 7 pieces (90 g)	6

Van

Authentic egg rolls, 1 egg roll	3

Wegman's

Mini quiches, 3 assorted flavors, 4 quiches (80 g)	9

Egg Entrées

Atkins Breakfast Bowls

Bacon scramble, 1 bowl (184 g)	12

Atkins Day Break

Farmhouse-style sausage scramble, 1 bowl (198 g)	12

Aunt Jemima

Scrambled eggs and bacon, with hash brown potatoes, 1 package (149 g)	10

Prepared Foods, Salads & Sides

SmartPoints™ value

SmartPoints™ value

Bob Evans Breakfast Bake

Bacon, egg, cheese and hash browns, 1 patty (99 g)	5
Sausage, egg, cheese and hash browns, 1 patty (99 g)	5
Southwest with peppers, egg, cheese and hash browns, 1 patty (99 g)	4

Camilla's Kitchen

Ham and cheddar waffle sandwich, 1 sandwich (105 g)	10

CedarLane

Omelette, egg white, garden vegetable & mozzarella, 8 oz	7
Omelette, egg white, spinach and mushroom, 1 omelet (227 g)	8

CedarLean

Frittata, egg white, broccoli & cheddar, 6 oz	6
Frittata, egg white, spinach & roasted tomato, 6 oz	6

Cuisine Adventures

Mini quiche assortment - florentine flavor only, 4 mini quiches (80 g)	8

Eating Right

Cheesy scramble, 1 tray (187 g)	6
Ham & cheese scramble, 1 tray (197 g)	6

Eggo

Bacon egg and cheese breakfast sandwich, 1 sandwich (77 g)	7
Egg and cheese breakfast sandwich, 1 sandwich (92 g)	7
Sausage egg and cheese breakfast sandwich, 1 sandwich (98 g)	10

Elisa's

Omelette, cheddar cheese, 6 oz	11

Evol

Uncured spicy bacon and egg burrito, 1 burrito (142 g)	11

Good Food Made Simple

Burrito, egg white, southwestern veggie, mildly spicy, 1 burrito (142 g)	7

Good Food Made Simple Breakfast in a Bowl

Southwestern veggies entrée, 1 bowl (198 g)	6
Uncured bacon and turkey sausage entrée, 1 bowl (198 g)	9

Home Made Brand

Quiche, spinach, crustless, ¼ quiche (114 g)	11

IHOP At Home

Applewood bacon, egg and cheese flatbread breakfast sandwich, 1 sandwich (89 g)	8
Breakfast sandwich, French toast, egg, Canadian bacon and cheese, 1 sandwich (122 g)	6

Jimmy Dean

Breakfast bowls, bacon, 1 bowl (227 g)	16
Breakfast bowls, meat lovers, 1 bowl (198 g)	15
Breakfast bowls, sausage, 1 bowl (227 g)	16
Casserole, country breakfast, sausage, family size, 1 cup	12
Omelets, ham and cheese, 1 omelet (122 g)	8

Jimmy Dean Delights

Breakfast bowl, garden blend, 1 bowl (198 g)	7
Canadian bacon egg white and cheese on honey wheat English muffin sandwich, 1 sandwich (128 g)	6
Southwest style breakfast bowl, 1 bowl (198 g)	7
Turkey sausage breakfast bowl, 1 bowl (198 g)	6
Turkey sausage egg white and cheese whole grain muffin sandwich, 1 sandwich (145 g)	7

Prepared Foods, Salads & Sides

Lean Cuisine Morning Collection

Turkey sausage scramble, 1 package (198 g)	5
Veggie scramble, 1 package (198 g)	5

Market Day

Mini omelets with reduced fat cheese, 1 omelet (57 g)	2

Mrs. Smith's Pour-A-Quiche

Quiche filling, broccoli & cheddar, 1 serving (123 g)	7

Pillsbury Toaster Scrambles

Pastry, toaster, bacon, 1 pastry (51 g)	6
Toaster pastries, sausage, 1 pastry (51 g)	6

Timber Ridge Farms

Scrambled egg patties, 1 patty (43 g)	2

Trader Joe's

Spicy ranchero egg white salad, ½ container (85 g)	1

Ethnic Entrées

Ajinomoto

Yakitori chicken with Japanese-style fried rice, cooked, 1 cup	10

Ajinomoto Yakisoba

Japanese style stir fried noodles with vegetables and sauce, ½ pack (128 g)	8

Amy's

Asian noodle, stir fry, 1 meal (284 g)	10
Breakfast burrito, 1 burrito (170 g)	7
Burrito, black bean, 1 burrito (170 g)	8
Burrito, especial, 1 burrito (170 g)	8
Burrito, non-dairy, 1 burrito (170 g)	9

Burrito, southwestern, 1 burrito (156 g)	9
Cheddar cheese burrito, 1 burrito (170 g)	9
Cheese enchilada, 1 enchilada (127 g)	8
Enchilada verde, 1 meal (284 g)	13
Enchilada, black bean vegetable, 1 enchilada (135 g)	5
Enchilada, cheese, 1 enchilada (127 g)	8
Mexican casserole family size, 1 cup	9
Pad Thai, 1 entrée (269 g)	15
Tamale verde, black bean, 1 entrée (291 g)	10
Tamale verde, cheese, 1 entrée (291 g)	12
Tamale, roasted vegetables, 1 package (292 g)	8
Thai red curry, 1 meal (284 g)	16

Amy's Bowls

Mexican casserole, 1 entrée (269 g)	12
Teriyaki, 1 entrée (269 g)	10
Tortilla casserole & black beans, 1 bowl (269 g)	13

Amy's Gluten Free

Burrito, cheddar cheese, 1 burrito (156 g)	8
Burrito, non-dairy, 1 burrito (156 g)	7
Indian aloo mattar wrap, 1 wrap (156 g)	8

Amy's Indian

Samosa wrap, 1 each (142 g)	7
Vegetable korma, 1 each (269 g)	10

Amy's Light & Lean

Enchilada, black bean & cheese, 1 entrée (227 g)	8
Mattar paneer, 1 entrée (227 g)	8
Soft taco fiesta, 1 bowl (227 g)	7

Prepared Foods, Salads & Sides

Prepared Foods, Salads & Sides

	SmartPoints™ value
Amy's Whole Meals	
Enchilada dinner, cheese, 1 meal (255 g)	12
Enchilada, with Spanish rice & beans, 1 meal (284 g)	10
Atkins	
Beef fiesta taco bowl, 1 bowl (241 g)	12
Mexican-style chicken and vegetables, 1 tray (255 g)	11
Birds Eye	
Stir fry vegetables, aparagus sir-fry, 2 cups	3
Birds Eye Voila!	
Beef lo mein, 2 ¼ cups	8
Chicken stir fry, 2 cups frozen	6
Fajita chicken, 7 ½ oz	4
Sweet & sour chicken, 1 ⅓ cups frozen	8
Teriyaki chicken, 1 cup cooked	8
Bob Evans	
Burrito, homestyle, sausage, egg & cheese, 2 burritos (136 g)	12
Casablanca	
Tabouli, mediterranean salad, ⅓ cup	2
CedarLane	
Breakfast burrito, scrambled egg, vegetable & cheese, 1 burrito (170 g)	9
Burrito, beans, rice & cheese style, 1 burrito (170 g)	7
Chili's	
Chicken fajita rice bowl, 1 package (284 g)	11
Chung's	
Potstickers, vegetable, 3 potstickers (52 g)	4
CJ Bibigo	
Fully cooked chicken and cilantro mini wontons, 4 pieces (36 g)	1

	SmartPoints™ value
Contessa	
Crispy chicken, with general tsao sauce, 2 ½ cups	14
Crazy Cuizine	
Mandarin orange chicken, 5 oz	9
Deep Indian Gourmet Indian Gourmet	
Samosa, punjabi style, with chutney, jumbo, 1 piece (71 g)	7
Delimex	
Beef and cheddar rolled tacos, 3 tacos (85 g)	7
Beef taquitos, 3 taquitos (85 g)	7
Chicken and cheese large taquitos, 2 taquitos (68 g)	6
White meat chicken taquitos, 3 taquitos (85 g)	6
Eating Right	
Chicken enchilada, 1 tray (255 g)	9
Chicken tamale, with green chile verde sauce, 1 tray (237 g)	9
Chicken with peanut sauce, 1 tray (255 g)	8
Sante Fe style rice & beans, 1 tray (284 g)	9
El Monterey	
Burrito, beef & bean, 1 burrito (113 g)	9
Burrito, chicken, rice & beans, 1 burrito (113 g)	7
Burritos, bean & cheese, family pack, 1 burrito (113 g)	7
Burritos, beef & bean, family pack, 1 burrito (113 g)	10
Burritos, spicy taco picante, family pack, 1 burrito (113 g)	9
Chimichanga, chicken & Monterey Jack cheese, 1 chimichanga (142 g)	9
Chimichangas, beef & bean, family pack, 1 chimichanga (113 g)	10

Chimichangas, spicy jalapeño bean & cheese, family pack, 1 chimichanga (113 g)	7
Taquitos, chicken & cheese, 2 taquitos (85 g)	6

El Monterey All Natural

Chicken and Monterey Jack cheese chimichanga, 1 chimichanga (142 g)	8
Shredded steak and cheese burrito, 1 burrito (142 g)	9

El Monterey Breakfast Supreme

Burritos, egg & bacon, 1 burrito (128 g)	8
Burritos, jalapeño, egg & cheese, 1 burrito (128 g)	8
Burritos, Mexican-style skillet, 1 burrito (128 g)	8

Evol

Chicken bean and rice burrito, 1 burrito (170 g)	10
Chicken tikka masala, 1 bowl (255 g)	8
Chipotle chicken burrito, 1 (312 g)	16
Shredded beef burrito, 1 burrito (170 g)	11

Evol Bowls

Chicken enchilada, 1 bowl (255 g)	11

Evol Burrito

Burrito, cilantro lime chicken, 1 burrito (170 g)	9
Burrito, pork & green chile, 1 burrito (227 g)	10

Evol Lean & Fit

Chicken apple sausage egg and smoked gouda burrito, 1 burrito (142 g)	9
Chicken tandoori, 1 bowl (241 g)	7
Egg white and spinach burrito, 1 burrito (142 g)	8

Evol Street Tacos

Shredded chicken and caramelized onion tacos, 1 package (181 g)	6

Exceline

Chicken and cheese quesadillas, 1 quesadilla (113 g)	8

Full Circle

Thai red curry chicken, 9 oz	9

Gardein

Crispy fingers, chipotle lime, 2 pieces (90 g)	4

Good Food Made Simple

Breakfast burrito, eggs, cheese & potato, 1 burrito (142 g)	10
Breakfast burrito, eggs, cheese & turkey sausage, 1 burrito (142 g)	9
Burrito, egg white, chicken apple sausage, 1 burrito (142 g)	10
Eggs cheese and Canadian bacon breakfast burrito, 1 burrito (142 g)	9

Goya

Empanadas, beef, 2 empanadas (135 g)	11

Healthy Choice

Chicken enchilada bake, 1 meal (252 g)	10

Healthy Choice Cafe Steamers

Asian pineapple chicken, 1 entrée (280 g)	10
Asian sweet and spicy orange zest chicken, 1 entrée (269 g)	8
Beef teriyaki, Asian, 1 entrée (269 g)	9
Cajun style chicken and shrimp, 1 meal (280 g)	6
Kung pao chicken entrée, 1 meal (269 g)	8
Potstickers, Asian, 1 meal (280 g)	12
Simply chicken fried rice, 1 entrée (283 g)	9

Healthy Choice Complete Meals

Sweet & sour chicken, 1 meal (340 g)	16

Herdez

Bowl, carnitas & charro beans, 1 bowl (283 g)	8

Prepared Foods, Salads & Sides

SmartPoints™ value

Hormel

Tamales, beef in chili sauce, 2 tamales (142 g)	5

InnovAsian Cuisine

Chicken and broccoli family style entrée kit, 1 cup	9
Entrée kit, family style, general tso's chicken breast, ⅓ package (170 g)	14

John Soules Foods

Beef fajitas, 3 oz	2
Chicken fajitas, 3 oz	1

Jose Ole

Chimichanga, chicken & cheese, 1 chimichanga (142 g)	10
Chimichanga, steak & cheese, 1 chimichanga (142 g)	11
Mini tacos, beef & cheese, 4 mini tacos (85 g)	7
Taquitos, large, chicken & cheese, 2 taquitos (85 g)	7
Taquitos, shredded steak, 3 taquitos (85 g)	6

Joyce Chen

Potstickers, Chinese-style, pork & vegetable, ravioli peking, 6 dumplings (114 g)	5

KA-ME

Stir-fry noodles, udon, 3 ½ oz	4

Kashi

Enchilada, spicy black bean, 1 entrée (255 g)	8
Southwest style chicken, 1 entrée (283 g)	9

Knorr Sides Plus

Teriyaki noodles, with Asian style vegetables, 1 cup	9

Lean Cuisine

Sesame chicken, 1 entrée (255 g)	7

SmartPoints™ value

Lean Cuisine Cafe Classics Asian Style Cuisine

Chicken fried rice, 1 package (340 g)	9

Lean Cuisine Culinary Collection

Fiesta grilled chicken, 1 package (240 g)	7
Orange chicken, 1 package (255 g)	10
Sesame chicken, 1 package (255 g)	10
Sweet and sour chicken, 1 package (283 g)	9

Lean Cuisine Market Collection

Chicken pot stickers, 1 package (283 g)	10

Lean Cuisine Simple Favorites

Asian style pot stickers, 1 package (255 g)	9
Chicken chow mein, 1 package (255 g)	6
Chicken fried rice, 1 package (255 g)	7
Chicken teriyaki stir fry, 1 package (255 g)	7
Vegetable eggroll, 1 package (255 g)	10

Lean Cuisine Spa Collection

Ginger garlic stir fry with chicken, 1 package (280 g)	10
Szechuan style stir fry with shrimp, 1 package (255 g)	7
Thai style noodles with chicken, 1 package (276 g)	9

Ling Ling

Potstickers, chicken & vegetable dumplings, 5 pieces (148 g)	9
Potstickers, chicken & vegetable dumplings with sauce, 8 pieces (156.8 g)	8
Potstickers, pork & vegetable dumplings, 5 pieces (145 g)	8

Prepared Foods, Salads & Sides

Marie Callender's

Sweet & sour chicken, 1 meal (397 g)	19

Michelina's Authentico

Chicken fried rice, 1 package (227 g)	12

Michelina's Lean Gourmet

Rice & beans, Santa Fe style, 1 package (241 g)	9
Shrimp with pasta & vegetables, 1 package (227 g)	8

Minh

White meat chicken mini egg rolls, 3 egg rolls with sauce	5

Morningstar Farms

Asian veggie patties, 1 burger (67 g)	3

Mr. Kook's Indian Food Express

Chicken tikka masala, with rice, medium spice, 1 container (85 g)	9

Mrs. T's

Pierogies, mini, potato & 4 cheese blend, 7 pierogies (91 g)	5
Pierogies, mini, potato & cheddar, 7 pierogies (91 g)	4
Pierogies, potato & 4 cheese blend, 3 pierogies (114 g)	7
Pierogies, potato & cheddar, 3 pierogies (117.6 g)	5
Pierogies, potato & cheddar, family pack, 3 pierogies (114 g)	5
Pierogies, potato & cheddar, low fat, 3 pierogies (114 g)	5
Pierogies, potato & onion, 3 pierogies (114 g)	5
Pierogies, potato & onion, low fat, 3 pierogies (114 g)	4
Pierogies, potato, cheddar & jalapeño, 3 pierogies (114 g)	5
Pierogies, potato, spinach & feta, 3 pierogies (114 g)	5

Old El Paso

Enchiladas, chicken, ½ package (283 g)	10
Enchiladas, shredded beef, ½ package (283 g)	10
Fajitas, chicken, ½ package (283 g)	8

Organic Bistro Bowls

Thai style yellow curry with chicken, 10 oz	10

Owen's Border Breakfasts

Tacos, sausage, egg & cheese, 2 tacos (136 g)	12

P.F. Chang's Home Menu

Chicken fried rice, meal for two, ½ package (312 g)	11
Chicken, General Chang's, ½ package (312 g)	15
Chicken, Kung pao, meal for two, ½ package (312 g)	10
Chicken, orange, Meals for 2, ½ package (312 g)	16
Chicken, sesame, meal for two, ½ package (312 g)	13
Garlic chicken with dan dan noodles, ½ package (312 g)	11

P.F. Chang's Home Menu Meals for 2

Chicken, Mongolian style, ½ package (312 g)	12
Grilled chicken teriyaki with lo mein noodles, ½ package (312 g)	11

Pagoda Express

Potstickers, 3 pieces (77 g)	4

Perdue

Chicken, General Tso's, 3 oz	6

PJ's Organics

Burrito, organic, chicken, 1 burrito (170 g)	8

Reds

Chicken and cheese burrito, 1 burrito (142 g)	7

Prepared Foods, Salads & Sides

	SmartPoints™ value
Saffron Road	
Chicken pad Thai with rice noodles, 1 entrée (312 g)	15
Chicken tikka masala with basmati rice, 1 entrée (312 g)	8
Lamb saag with basmati rice, 1 entrée (312 g)	8
Sea Pak Shrimp & Seafood Co.	
Oven crunchy shrimp poppers, 20 pieces (84 g)	6
Sonrito's	
Breakfast burrito, egg, sausage & cheese, Mexican style, 1 burrito (113 g)	9
Stouffer's	
Chicken enchiladas, with cheese sauce & rice, party size, 1 enchilada (201 g)	10
Stouffer's Family Size	
Chicken enchiladas, 7 ½ oz	9
Sweet Earth	
Burrito, big sur breakfast, 7 oz	7
Burrito, the curry tiger, 7 oz	9
Burrito, the peruvian, 7 oz	9
Taco Bell	
Crunchy taco dinner kit, 2 tacos (41 g)	4
Soft tortilla taco dinner kit (serves 5), 1 serving (82 g)	6
Tai Pei	
Beef & broccoli, 1 cup	5
Chicken fried rice, 1 cup	7
Chinese style bbq pork, 1 cup	7
Combination fried rice, 1 cup	6
General Tso's chicken, 1 cup	2
Orange chicken, 1 cup	8
Pork potstickers with sauce, 5 pieces (162 g)	10
Rice, shrimp fried, 1 cup	7
Tandoor Chef	
Chicken curry, 1 tray (283 g)	8

	SmartPoints™ value
Thai Kitchen	
Pad Thai noodle kit, ⅓ package (85 g)	9
Thai Kitchen Asian Creations	
Chicken pad Yhai, 1 entrée (283 g)	13
Tina's	
Burrito, bean & cheese, 1 burrito (113 g)	8
Trader Joe's	
Cheese & green chili tamales, 1 (140 g)	9
Chicken cilantro mini wontons, 4 pieces (36 g)	1
Chicken tikka masala, 1 tray (241 g)	9
Chile relleno, 1 tray (284 g)	13
Mini chicken tacos, 4 (79 g)	5
Palak paneer, ½ package (142 g)	8
Paneer tikka masala, 1 tray (255 g)	12
Pork gyoza potstickers, 7 (140 g)	7
Spicy California rolls, 3 pieces (90 g)	5
Thai shrimp gyoza, 5 pieces (140 g)	7
Thai vegetable gyoza, 5 pieces (140 g)	9
Vegetable biryani with vegetable dumplings, ½ tray (142 g)	8
Vegetable samosas, 2 (84 g)	5
Trader Jose's	
Breakfast burritos - eggs, potatoes, turkey bacon & cheese, 1 (170 g)	9
Handcrafted chicken & cheese tamales, 1 (140 g)	7
Trader Ming's	
Cha siu bao Chinese style pork buns, 1 (58 g)	5
Tyson	
Chicken, teriyaki, 3 oz	3
Fajita chicken strips, 3 oz	2

Meat & Poultry Entrées

Aidells

Chicken meatballs with carmelized onions, 3 meatballs (64 g)	4
Meatballs, chicken & turkey, Italian style with sun-dried tomato, 3 meatballs (64 g)	5

al fresco

Chicken meatballs, Italian style, 4 meatballs (85 g)	4
Chicken meatballs, tomato and basil, 4 meatballs (85 g)	4

Amylu

Sweet caramelized onion chicken burgers, 1 burger (112 g)	3

Applegate Farms

Chicken nuggets, 7 nuggets (88 g)	4

Applegate Naturals

Chicken nuggets, 7 nuggets (88 g)	5
Gluten free chicken breast tenders, 2 tenders (84 g)	3
Gluten free chicken nuggets, 7 nuggets (88 g)	4

Armour

Italian style meatballs, 6 meatballs (85 g)	10
Meatballs, turkey, 6 meatballs (91 g)	5
Original meatballs, 6 meatballs (85 g)	9
Potted meat, 1 can (85 g)	5
Turkey meatballs, 6 meatballs (84 g)	5

Atkins

Beef merlot, 1 tray (255 g)	9
Chicken margherita, 1 entrée (255 g)	12
Chili con carne, 1 bowl (255 g)	10
Crustless chicken pot pie, 1 bowl (255 g)	11

Meatloaf, with portobello mushroom gravy, 1 tray (255 g)	10
Sesame chicken stir fry, 1 tray (255 g)	10
Swedish meatballs, 1 tray (255 g)	11

Ball Park

Fully cooked flame grilled beef patty, 1 patty (77 g)	7

Banquet

Boneless pork rib shaped patty meal, 1 meal (283 g)	11
Chicken breast nuggets, family pack, 6 nuggets (85 g)	7
Chicken breast patties, family pack, 1 patty (68 g)	5
Chicken breast strips, breaded chicken breast patties, 2 strips (85 g)	5
Chicken breast tenders, family pack, 5 tenders (85 g)	6
Chicken nuggets, 6 nuggets (85 g)	8
Chicken nuggets, family pack, 6 nuggets (85 g)	6
Chicken patties, family pack, 1 patty (68 g)	6
Chicken, popcorn, 10 pieces (85 g)	6
Deep dish, sausage & gravy, 1 piece (198 g)	16
Meat loaf meal, 1 meal (269 g)	9
Popcorn chicken, 11 pieces (85 g)	6
Pot pie, beef, 1 pie (198 g)	14
Pot pie, chicken, 1 pie (198 g)	13
Pot pie, turkey, 1 pie (198 g)	13
Salisbury steak meal, 1 meal (269 g)	10
Turkey meal, 1 meal (262 g)	7

Banquet Family Size

Salisbury steaks & brown gravy, 1 steak/gravy (128 g)	6

Barber Foods

Stuffed chicken breasts, cordon bleu, fully cooked, 1 piece (140 g)	7
Stuffed chicken breasts, homestyle stuffing, 1 piece (170 g)	7
Stuffed chicken breasts, raw, broccoli & cheese, 1 piece (140 g)	6

Barber Foods Premium Entrées

Stuffed chicken breast, broccoli and cheese, raw, 1 piece (168 g)	7
Stuffed chicken breasts, creme brie and apple, 1 piece (140 g)	9

Barber Foods Seasoned Selects

Stuffed chicken breasts, broccoli & cheese, raw, 1 piece (140 g)	4
Stuffed chicken breasts, raw, mushroom & Swiss, 1 piece (140 g)	4
Stuffed chicken breasts, with rib meat, spinach florentine, 1 piece (140 g)	5

Bertolli Al Dente

Chicken florentine Alfredo, 1 meal (286 g)	13

Bertolli Classic Meal for 2

Chicken margherita and penne, 2 cups	7

Bertolli Rustico Bakes

Chicken parmigiana and penne, 1 meal (306 g)	13

Betty Crocker Ultimate Hamburger Helper

Creamy stroganoff dinner kit, ⅓ cup dry	4

Birds Eye

Garlic chicken, complete meal, 2 cups	9

Birds Eye Steamfresh Chef's Favorites

Pasta & broccoli, with bacon, in a cheese sauce, 1 ½ cups frozen	8

Birds Eye Voila!

Alfredo chicken, 1 ½ cups	10
Cheesy chicken, family size, 1 ¾ cups	8
Cheesy ranch chicken, 1 ½ cups	7
Chicken florentine, creamy parmesan, 1 cup cooked	7
Garlic chicken, family size, 1 ⅔ cups	8
Sweet and sour chicken stir fry, 1 cup	9
Three cheese chicken, 1 ⅔ cups frozen	7

Blake's All Natural

Shepherd's pie, 1 pie (227 g)	9

BMC

Beef meat balls, 4 (85 g)	3

Bob Evans

Beef pot roast, with gravy, 5 oz	4
Beef stew, with vegetables, slow roasted, 1 cup	5
Original sausage and gravy biscuits, ½ package (189 g)	13

Bob Evans Homestyle Recipe

Beef and gravy with noodles, 1 tray (255 g)	7
Chicken and noodles, 1 cup	5

Boston Market

Chicken parmesan, 1 tray (454 g)	17
Home style meals, oven roasted chicken, juicy breast quarter, 1 each (170 g)	4
Home style meals, oven roasted chicken, juicy leg & thigh pieces, 1 package (170 g)	7
Turkey breast medallions, 1 tray (425 g)	8

Bryan Food Service

Corn beef hash, 1 cup	15

Butcher's Prime

Spare ribs, pork, in bbq sauce, 5 oz	12

Butterball Everyday Chef Selects

Turkey meatloaf, 5 oz	8

Casa di Bertacchi

Authentic Italian style beef meatballs, 5 meatballs (88 g)	9
Turkey meatballs, 5 meatballs (88 g)	4

Casual Gourmet

Chicken sausage with roasted red pepper and spinach, 1 link (90 g)	3

CedarLane

Chicken tikka masala, with basmati rice and sauce, 1 package (284 g)	15

Chef Solutions

Cranberry pecan chicken salad, ½ cup	12

Chicken Helper

Rice & seasoning mix, chicken fried rice, 2 Tbsp	3

Chili's

Cajun style chicken Alfredo, 1 package (284 g)	12
Island chicken and rice, 1 package (284 g)	12

Coleman Natural

Florentine chargrilled chicken burger, 1 burger (106 g)	4

Cooked Perfect

Meatballs, homestyle, bite size, 6 meatballs (85 g)	7
Meatballs, Italian style, 6 meatballs (14 g)	8
Meatballs, Italian style, dinner size, 3 meatballs (85 g)	7

Cooked Perfect Angus Beef

Meatballs, 3 meatballs (85 g)	8

Cooked Perfect Gluten Free

Italian style meatballs, 3 meatballs (85 g)	8

Curly's

Pulled chicken, barbecue sauce, hickory smoked, ¼ cup	3

Curly's Sauceless

Roasted and seasoned pulled chicken, 2 oz	1

Daily Chef

Chicken breasts with rib meat, 4 oz	1
Pulled pork, 2 oz	4

Del Real

Fried pork, carnitas, 3 oz	5

Dining In

Baby back ribs, 5 oz	11

Earth's Best Kidz

Baked chicken nuggets, 4 pieces (56 g)	3

Eating Right

Chicken methi malai, 1 tray (234 g)	9
Chicken parmesan, 1 tray (257 g)	9
Chicken poblano, 1 tray (255 g)	8
Chicken with basil cream sauce, 1 tray (241 g)	8
Meatloaf, turkey, 1 tray (255 g)	11
Turkey lasagna, 1 tray (319 g)	11

Evol

Chipotle chicken mac & cheese, 1 bowl (227 g)	14

Evol Bowls

Fire grilled steak, 1 bowl (255 g)	12

Evol Lean & Fit

Lemongrass chicken, 1 bowl (241 g)	7

Farm Rich Smokehouse

Pulled pork bbq, ¼ cup	3

Farmland Oven Perfect

Parmesan garlic herb fresh pork loin fillet, 4 oz	2

FarmRich

Meatballs, Italian style, 6 meatballs (85 g)	9
Meatballs, original, 6 meatballs (85 g)	9
Meatballs, turkey, 5 meatballs (88 g)	4

Prepared Foods, Salads & Sides

	SmartPoints™ value
Fast Fixin' Restaurant Style	
Country fried steak with gravy (serves 5), 1 piece (128 g)	10
Country fried steaks, 1 piece (112 g)	8
Foster Farms	
Chicken breast nuggets, 4 nuggets (78.3 g)	4
Chicken patties, value pack, 1 patty (73 g)	5
Grilled chicken strips, 3 oz	1
Honey bbq glazed chicken wings, 3 wings (92 g)	6
Turkey meatballs, homestyle, 3 meatballs (84 g)	4
Turkey meatballs, Italian style, 3 meatballs (84 g)	4
Gardein	
Chick'n scallopini, lightly seasoned, 1 scallopini (71 g)	1
Chick'n sliders, crispy, 1 slider (80 g)	5
Chick'n strips, meat-free, teriyaki, without sauce, 1/3 package (100 g)	2
Turk'y cutlet, lightly breaded (without gravy), 2 cutlets (125 g)	6
Golden Platter	
Chicken nuggets, gluten free, 5 nuggets (85 g)	4
Chicken tenders, gluten free, 2 ½ pieces (85 g)	4
Great Value	
Breaded chicken nuggets, 4 (75 g)	4
Chicken nuggets, fully cooked, 5 nuggets (84 g)	6
Fully cooked homestyle meatballs, 5 meatballs (84 g)	9
Fully cooked Italian style meatballs, 6 meatballs (85 g)	9
Hamburger Helper	
Stroganoff meal kit, 2/3 cup	4
Ultimate beef stroganoff, ½ cup	3

	SmartPoints™ value
Hamburger Helper Classic	
Beef pasta, ½ cup	3
Philly cheesesteak, ½ cup dry	4
Stroganoff, 2/3 cup	4
Hannaford	
Shepherd's pie, beef, 1 cup	9
Healthy Choice	
Honey balsamic chicken, 1 meal (255 g)	6
Healthy Choice Baked	
Chicken and rice cheddar bake, 1 meal (243 g)	6
Roasted chicken and potatoes meal, 1 meal (275 g)	4
Slow roasted turkey bake, 1 meal (255 g)	5
Healthy Choice Cafe Steamers	
Balsamic garlic chicken, 1 entrée (269 g)	7
Beef merlot entrée, 1 entrée (269 g)	5
Chicken and potatoes with peach bbq sauce, 1 meal (276 g)	11
Chicken fettuccini Alfredo, 1 entrée (326 g)	8
Chicken linguini with red pepper Alfredo, 1 meal (227 g)	6
Chicken margherita with balsamic, 1 meal (269 g)	8
Chicken marsala, roasted, 1 meal (295 g)	7
Crustless chicken pot pie, 1 meal (272 g)	8
Crustless chicken pot pie, 1 meal (290 g)	8
General tso's spicy chicken, 1 meal (292 g)	9
Grilled basil chicken, 1 entrée (280 g)	7
Grilled chicken marinara with parmesan, 1 meal (269 g)	8

	SmartPoints™ value
Grilled chicken marsala with mushrooms, 1 entrée (280 g)	7
Honey glazed turkey and potatoes, 1 entrée (269 g)	7
Rosemary chicken and sweet potatoes, 1 entrée (269 g)	7
Simply chicken pasta primavera, 1 entrée (283 g)	6
Simply lemon herb chicken, 1 entrée (283 g)	7
Simply meatball marinara, 1 entrée (283 g)	8
Sweet sesame chicken, 1 meal (276 g)	10
Top chef grilled chicken pesto with vegetables, 1 entrée (280 g)	8
Whiskey steak, 1 meal (269 g)	10
Healthy Choice Complete Meals	
Beef pot roast, 1 meal (312 g)	10
Beef tips portobello, 1 meal (319 g)	9
Chicken parmigiana, 1 meal (329 g)	12
Country fried chicken, 1 meal (326 g)	11
Country herb chicken, 1 meal (322 g)	9
Homestyle salisbury steak, 1 meal (326 g)	10
Meat loaf, classic, 1 meal (340 g)	13
Oven roasted chicken, 1 meal (323 g)	8
Turkey breast, golden roasted, 1 meal (298 g)	8
Healthy Choice Modern Classics	
Beef and broccoli, 1 meal (312 g)	10
Healthy Choice Select Entrées	
Chicken Alfredo florentine, 1 meal (241 g)	6
H-E-B	
Chicken, roasted, rotisserie, lemon pepper, 3 oz	5

	SmartPoints™ value
Herdez	
Bowl, beef barbacoa, 1 bowl (283 g)	8
Bowl, pork chile verde, 1 bowl (283 g)	10
Hillshire Farm	
Polska kielbasa, beef, 2 oz	6
Home Market Foods	
Meatballs, Italian style, 3 pieces (82.5 g)	8
Home Market Foods Cooked Perfect	
Meatballs, turkey, 3 meatballs (88.2 g)	3
HoneySuckle White Italian Style	
Lean turkey meatballs, 3 meatballs (85 g)	4
Hooters	
Chicken wings, hot, 3 oz	7
Hormel	
Apple bourbon pork chops, 5 oz	6
Beef roast, Italian style au jus, 5 oz	6
Meat loaf & tomato sauce, homestyle, 5 oz	8
Slow simmered beef tips & gravy, ½ cup	5
Hormel Compleats	
Beef tips & mashed potatoes, 1 tray (283 g)	8
Chicken & dumplings, 1 tray (283 g)	8
Chicken Alfredo, 1 tray (283 g)	11
Chicken breast & mashed potatoes, with rib meat, 1 tray (283 g)	5
Homestyle beef pot roast, 1 tray (283 g)	6
Roast beef and mashed potatoes, 1 entrée (283 g)	5
Hormel Compleats Homestyle	
Turkey & dressing, 1 tray (283 g)	8
Jack Daniel's	
Pulled beef, ⅓ package (151 g)	8
Pulled chicken, 4 oz	5

SmartPoints™ value

Jack Link's

Turkey strip, original, 1 package (56 g)	4

Jennie-O

Lean turkey & gravy in roasting pan, white, 4 oz	4
Turkey meatballs, homestyle, 3 meatballs (85.1 g)	5
Turkey meatballs, Italian style, 3 meatballs (84 g)	4

Jimmy Dean

Pancakes & sausage on a stick, original, 1 each (71 g)	8
Pancakes & sausage, on a stick, blueberry, 1 piece (71 g)	9

Jimmy Dean Delights

Golden roasted turkey in a creamy herb sauce, 1 bowl (226 g)	6

John Soules Foods

Chicken breast strips with rib meat, grilled, 3 oz	1
Chicken fajitas fully cooked chicken breast strips, 3 oz	1

John Soules Foods Fully Cooked

Certified angus beef steak strips, 3 oz	3

Jones Dairy Farm

Sausage & rice links, light, 3 links (59 g)	4

Kashi

Chicken florentine, 1 entrée (283 g)	8
Lemongrass coconut chicken, 1 entrée (283 g)	9

Kirkland Disney

Whole grain chicken nuggets, 5 pieces (89 g)	6

Kirkland Signature

Meatballs, 5 meatballs (90 g)	9

Kirkwood Snack Time Chicken

Chicken breast nuggets, 5 nuggets (88 g)	5

SmartPoints™ value

Knorr Pasta Sides

Fettuccini, chicken broccoli flavor, ⅔ cup	6

Koch Foods Tender Cravers

Chicken breast, chicken parm, 1 piece (127 g)	7

Kraft

Recipe makers, slow cooker, hickory bbq beef (combined sauces), ¼ cup	5

Kroger

Boneless skinless chicken tenderloins, 2 tenders (136 g)	1
Chicken breasts, 1 piece (202 g)	2
Chicken wing drummettes, 2 pieces (100 g)	5
Chicken wings, 3 pieces (134 g)	7
Fully cooked crispy chicken breast strips, 2 pieces (104 g)	5
Grilled and glazed chicken breast fillets, 1 fillet (98 g)	1
Seasoned lean turkey burgers, 1 burger (151 g)	4

Laura's

Meatloaf, with tomato sauce, 5 oz	8

Lean Cuisine Culinary Collection

Baked chicken, 1 package (244 g)	7
Beef pot roast, 1 package (255 g)	6
Chicken carbonara, 1 package (255 g)	6
Chicken marsala, 1 package (230 g)	7
Chicken parmesan, 1 package (308 g)	10
Chicken pecan, 1 package (255 g)	10
Chicken with almonds, 1 package (240 g)	9
Chicken with basil cream sauce, 1 package (240 g)	6
Chile lime chicken, 1 package (251 g)	7

Prepared Foods, Salads & Sides

	SmartPoints™ value
Glazed chicken, 1 package (240 g)	6
Glazed turkey tenderloins, 1 package (255 g)	10
Grilled chicken Caesar, 1 package (241 g)	7
Herb roasted chicken, 1 package (226 g)	4
Lemon chicken, 1 package (255 g)	9
Meatloaf with mashed potatoes, 1 package (265 g)	7
Ranchero braised beef, 1 package (233 g)	9
Roasted chicken and garden vegetables, 1 package (297 g)	7
Roasted turkey and vegetables, 1 package (226 g)	6
Roasted turkey breast, 1 package (276 g)	10
Salisbury steak with macaroni and cheese, 1 package (269 g)	7
Steak tips portabello, 1 package (212 g)	4

Lean Cuisine Dinnertime Collection

Chicken fettuccini, 1 package (340 g)	8

Lean Cuisine Market Collection

Roasted turkey breast, 1 package (340 g)	9

Lean Cuisine Salad Additions

Asian style chicken, 1 package (205 g)	9
Cranberry and chicken, 1 package (209 g)	10
Southwest style chicken, 1 package (202 g)	7

Lean Cuisine Simple Favorites

Chicken fettuccini, 1 entrée (262 g)	7
Swedish meatballs, 1 package (258 g)	8

Lean Cuisine Spa Collection

Apple cranberry chicken, 1 package (272 g)	12
Grilled chicken primavera, 1 package (265 g)	6

	SmartPoints™ value
Lemongrass chicken, 1 package (265 g)	7
Roasted honey chicken, 1 package (276 g)	10

Lean Cuisine Wrap Additions

Chicken teriyaki, 1 package (209 g)	6
Creamy balsamic chicken, 1 package (212 g)	5

Libby's

Corned beef, 2 oz	3

Little Salad Bar Deli Collection

Cranberry almond chicken salad, ⅓ cup	10

Lloyd's Barbeque Company

Original bbq sauce with seasoned shredded beef, ¼ cup	3

Luvo

Chicken chile verde, with polenta & black beans, 1 pouch (283 g)	9

Mama Lucia

Meatballs, cocktail-size, homestyle, 8 meatballs (90.8 g)	7
Meatballs, cocktail-size, Italian style, 8 meatballs (90 g)	7
Meatballs, Italian style, fully cooked, 8 meatballs (90 g)	7
Turkey meatballs, 4 meatballs (90 g)	6

Mama Mancini's

Turkey meatballs, 2 meatballs (142 g)	3

Marie Callender's

Beef tips in mushroom sauce, 1 meal (385 g)	9
Cheesy chicken & rice, 1 meal (369 g)	13
Chicken pot pie, 1 cup	11
Chicken pot pies, 1 pie (284 g)	22
Country fried pork chop, 1 meal (425 g)	15
Herb roasted chicken, 1 meal (397 g)	13

SmartPoints™ value

	SmartPoints™ value
Honey roasted turkey, 1 meal (369 g)	9
Meat loaf and gravy, 1 meal (397 g)	13
Pot pie, beef, 1 cup	14
Pot pie, chicken, 1 cup	13
Pot pie, turkey, 1 cup	17
Pot pies, white meat chicken, 1 pie (284 g)	22
Salisbury steak, 1 meal (397 g)	11
Slow roasted beef, 1 meal (411 g)	10
Turkey breast with stuffing, 1 meal (397 g)	10
Marie Callender's Comfort Bakes	
Cheesy chicken and rice, 1 cup	10
Mary Kitchen	
Corned beef hash, homestyle, 1 cup	9
Michelina's Lean Gourmet	
Chicken Alfredo florentine, 1 package (227 g)	8
Creamy rigatoni, with broccoli & chicken, 1 package (227 g)	8
Salisbury steak, 1 package (213 g)	5
Michelina's Traditional Recipes	
Beef & peppers, 1 package (227 g)	8
Fettuccine Alfredo, with chicken & broccoli, 1 package (227 g)	10
Salisbury steak, 1 package (227 g)	8
Murry's	
Chicken wings, honey bbq, 3 wings (80 g)	5
Chicken wings, wow, buffalo style, 3 wings (80 g)	5
On-Cor	
4 stuffed green peppers with beef in tomato sauce, 1 each (226.8 g)	7
On-Cor Classics	
Breaded chicken parmagiana patties, with tomato sauce, family size, 1 patty (132 g)	7

	SmartPoints™ value
On-Cor Traditionals	
Gravy & salisbury steaks, family size, 1 patty with gravy (132 g)	4
P.F. Chang's Home Menu	
Beef with broccoli, ½ package (312 g)	12
General Chang's chicken, ½ package (312 g)	14
Orange chicken, ½ package (312 g)	15
Shanghai style beef, ½ package (312 g)	13
Sweet and sour chicken, ½ package (312 g)	14
Pasta Roni	
Linguine, chicken & broccoli flavor, 2 ½ oz	7
Perdue	
Chicken breast cutlets, original, 1 cutlet (85 g)	6
Chicken breast nuggets, 4 pieces (76 g)	5
Chicken breast nuggets, whole grain, 5 pieces (85 g)	7
Chicken breast patties, 1 patty (82 g)	6
Chicken breast, breaded tenders, 3 pieces (99 g)	7
Chicken breast, wholegrain breaded tenders, 3 pieces (90 g)	6
Chicken wings, buffalo style, 3 pieces (85 g)	4
Chicken wings, lightly breaded, buffalo style, 3 wings (80 g)	4
Chicken, bourbon, 3 oz	5
Chicken, breast strips, original, 2 pieces (74 g)	5
Chicken, filets, lightly breaded, 1 fillet (115 g)	4
Chicken, original breast nuggets, 5 nuggets (85 g)	5
Turkey meatballs, Italian style, 4 meatballs (85 g)	5

Prepared Foods, Salads & Sides

Perdue Fun Shapes

Chicken breast nuggets, dinosaur shapes, 4 nuggets (76 g)	5

Perdue Short Cuts

Chicken breast, carved, rotisserie seasoned, ½ cup	1
Curved chicken breast, honey roasted, ½ cup	2

Perdue Simply Smart

Chicken breast cutlets, lightly breaded, 1 piece (90 g)	4
Chicken breast tenders, breaded, gluten free, 3 pieces (87 g)	5
Chicken strips, lightly breaded, 3 oz	3
Chicken strips, original grilled, 3 oz	1

Publix

Beef tips, homestyle, with seasoned gravy, 5 oz	3
Meatloaf, homestyle beef, 5 oz	7

Ready Pac Bistro

Smokehouse bbq style ranch salad, 1 container (220 g)	9

Sabatino's

Smoked mozzarella with artichoke and garlic chicken sausage, 1 link (97 g)	4

Safeway

Chicken tenderloins, young, ice glazed, boneless & skinless, 4 oz	1
Chicken tenders, 2 tenders (94 g)	6

Safeway Kitchens

Meatballs, turkey, 3 meatballs (85 g)	4

Safeway Select

Chicken breast strips, breaded, 2 pieces (90 g)	4

Saffron Road

Bibimbop with beef and brown rice, 10 oz	13

Santiago's

Chile sauce, authentic green, with pork, medium, ½ cup	3

Sea Pak Shrimp & Seafood Co.

Wild Alaskan salmon burgers, 1 burger (113 g)	2

Shelton's

Meat balls, free range turkey, 6 meatballs (71 g)	6

Signature Cafe

Chicken fajita wrap, grilled, 1 fajita (255 g)	16
Chicken tortilla casserole, baked, family size, 1 cup	8

Signature Cafe World Cuisine

Chicken picatta, 1 package (312 g)	9

Simek's

Turkey meatballs, 6 meatballs (85 g)	4

Simply Smart

Lightly breaded chicken tenders, 2 pieces (71 g)	4

Skyline

Chili spaghetti, 2-way, 1 cup	9

So Good

Bbq beef, ½ cup	4

Steak Umm

Sandwich steaks, chicken breast, 1 ½ oz	1

Stouffer's

Chicken & broccoli pasta bake, family size, 1 cup	10
Chicken & vegetable rice bake, grandma's, family size, 1 cup	10
Chicken Alfredo, large, family size, 1 cup	8
Meatloaf, in gravy, family size, 1 loaf & gravy (156 g)	6

Stouffer's Craveable Classics

Creamed chipped beef, ½ cup	5

Prepared Foods, Salads & Sides

SmartPoints™ value

Stouffer's Homestyle Classics

Baked chicken breast, 1 package (251 g)	7
Fried chicken, 1 package (251 g)	10
Meatloaf, 1 package (279 g)	11
Salisbury steak, 1 package (272 g)	11

Stouffer's Large Family

Grandma's chicken & vegetable rice bake, 1 cup	11

Stouffer's Restaurant Classics

Green pepper steak, 1 package (297 g)	7

Stouffer's Satisfying Servings

Grandma's chicken and vegetable rice bake, 1 cup	10

Sycamore Farms

Chicken salad, ⅓ cup	9

Tai Pei

Bourbon street chicken, 1 cup	6
Chicken potstickers with dipping sauce, 5 pieces (162 g)	9
Seasoned chicken for lettuce wraps (with sauce), 2 oz	2

Tandoor Chef

Chicken tikka masala, 1 tray (283 g)	11

Trader Joe's

Applewood smoked peppered uncured turkey bacon, 1 slice (28 g)	1
Bbq marinated beef tri-tip, 4 oz	5
Butter chicken with basmati rice, 1 cup	8
Chicken fried rice, 1 cup	6
Chile lime chicken burgers, 1 burger (114 g)	3
Field fresh chopped salad with chicken (with dressing), ½ package (152 g)	8
Fully cooked grilled chicken burger patties, 1 burger (113 g)	3

SmartPoints™ value

Fully cooked pork belly, 3 oz	8
Fully cooked turkey meatballs, 2 meatballs (71 g)	3
Grilled balsamic vinegar & rosemary chicken, 3 oz	2
Grilled chicken strips, 3 oz	1
Grilled lemon pepper chicken breasts, 3 oz	2
Italian style turkey meatloaf topped with tomato sauce, 5 oz	6
Lemon chicken and arugula salad (with dressing), 1 container (260 g)	10
Mandarin orange chicken, 1 cup	9
Marinated chicken breasts, 3 oz	3
Party size mini meatballs, 6 meatballs (85 g)	7
Pasadena chicken salad (with dressing), ½ salad (188 g)	8
Pulled chicken breast, ⅓ package (151 g)	4
Roasted chicken patties, 1 patty (112 g)	4
Rotisserie style roasted chicken, 3 oz	4
Shepard's pie, 1 cup	4
Sliced roast chicken breast, 3 slices (84 g)	2
Turkey breast roasted and sliced, 3 oz	1
Turkey burgers, 1 burger (112 g)	4

Trader Ming's

Reduced fat Chinese style salad with chicken, 1 container (340 g)	10

Tyson

Beef steak tips, in bourbon sauce, 5 oz	5
Beef tips, in gravy, 5 oz	6
Boneless chicken wings, buffalo style, 3 wings (78 g)	3
Breaded chicken breast tenderloins, 4 oz	5

	SmartPoints™ value
Breast tenders, honey battered, 5 pieces (85 g)	7
Buffalo style hot wings, 2 pieces (77 g)	5
Chicken breast strips, southwestern style, 3 oz	2
Chicken breast tenderloins, southern style, 3 oz	5
Chicken nuggets, 5 pieces (90 g)	8
Chicken strips, buffalo style, 2 pieces (101 g)	6
Chicken strips, honey bbq, 1 piece (75 g)	5
Chicken wings, tequila lime flavored, 3 oz	5
Fully cooked buffalo style boneless chicken wyngz, 3 oz	5
Fully cooked white meat chicken nuggets, 5 pieces (88 g)	7
Hot wings, buffalo style, 3 pieces (100 g)	6
Panko breaded chicken breast tenderloins, 4 oz	5
Rock cornish game hen, premium, without giblets, 4 oz	5

Tyson 100% All Natural

Fun nuggets, 5 pieces (92 g)	8

Tyson Any'tizers

Boneless chicken bites, buffalo style, 3 pieces (84 g)	4
Boneless chicken wyngs, honey bbq, 3 pieces (84 g)	6
Chicken wings, boneless, honey bbq, 3 pieces (80 g)	6
Chicken wyngs, boneless, buffalo style, 3 pieces (84 g)	4
Hot wings, buffalo style, 3 oz	5
Popcorn chicken, 3 oz	4
Wings, honey bbq seasoned, 3 oz	6

Tyson Gluten Free

Fully cooked breaded chicken breast strips, 3 oz	5
Fully cooked chicken nuggets, 4 pieces (79 g)	4

Tyson Grilled & Ready

Diced oven roasted chicken breast, 3 oz	2
Fully cooked pulled chicken breast, 2 oz	1
Sweet Asian flavored chicken thigh fillets, 3 oz	3

Velveeta Cheesy Casseroles

Chicken and broccoli bake dinner kit, 2 oz	6

Velveeta Cheesy Skillets

Cheeseburger mac, ultimate, singles, 1 package (255 g)	10
Dinner kit, chicken and broccoli, 1 serving (84 g)	8
Dinner kit, creamy beef stroganoff (makes 5 servings), 1 serving (70 g)	7

Vienna Beef

Italian style sliced beef and gravy with giardiniera peppers, 2 ¼ oz beef	4

Wegman's Food You Feel Good About

Chicken breast strips, breaded, club pack, 2 strips (84 g)	4

Wegman's Italian Classics

Meatballs, oven-baked, turkey, 3 meatballs (85 g)	3
Meatballs, oven-baked, with romano cheese, 3 meatballs (85 g)	8

WelcomeHomeCafe

Meatloaf, 3 slices (140 g)	5

Wolf

Chili, no beans, 1 cup	12

Yummy Dino Buddies

Chicken breast nuggets, dinosaur-shaped, 5 pieces (93 g)	6

Zatarain's New Orleans Style

Blackened chicken Alfredo, 1 package (297 g)	17
Jambalaya, with sausage, 1 package (340 g)	15

Prepared Foods, Salads & Sides

Meat Substitutes Entrées

Amy's

Gluten free tofu scramble breakfast wrap, 1 wrap (156 g)	9
Tofu scramble, with hash browns & veggies, 1 each (255 g)	9

Amy's Bowls

Country cheddar, 1 entrée (269 g)	13

Amy's Light & Lean

Meatless Swedish meatballs, 1 bowl (227 g)	7

Amy's Whole Meals

Veggie loaf, mashed potatoes & vegetables, 1 entrée (284 g)	9

Boca

All American flamed grilled veggie burger, 1 burger (71 g)	3
Cheeseburger veggie burger, 1 burger (71 g)	2
Grilled vegetable veggie burger, 1 burger (71 g)	1
Original chik'n veggie patty, 1 patty (71 g)	4
Original vegan veggie burger, 1 burger (99 g)	1
Savory mushroom mozzarella veggie patty, 1 patty (71 g)	2
Veggie burgers, original vegan, 1 burger (71 g)	1

Boca Essentials

Chile relleno burger, 1 burger (71 g)	3

Dominex

Vegetarian meatballs, eggplant, 5 balls (85 g)	2

Dr. Praeger's

Veggie burger, 1 patty (113 g)	4
Veggie burgers, tex mex, 1 burger (78 g)	3

Dr. Praeger's Sensible Foods

Black bean burger, 1 burger (71 g)	3
California veggie burgers, 1 burger (78 g)	3
Veggie burgers, Asian, 1 burger (71 g)	4

Gardein

Beefless ground, ½ cup	1
Beefless strips, sizzling szechuan, without sauce, ⅓ package (72 g)	5
Breakfast patties, 1 patty (52 g)	2
Chipotle black bean burger, 1 burger (85 g)	4
Classic meatless meatballs, 2 meatballs (90 g)	3

Gardenburger

Veggie burgers, black bean chipotle, 1 patty (71 g)	3
Veggie burgers, portabella, 1 patty (71 g)	3

Gardenburger Eat Positive

Malibu vegan burger, 1 patty (91 g)	5

Hilary's Eat Well

Burger, veggie, 1 burger (91 g)	7

Kashi

Mayan harvest bake, 1 entrée (283 g)	12

Lightlife

Veggie burgers, backyard grill'n burgers, 1 burger (85 g)	4

Morningstar Farms

Chik patties original veggie patties, 1 patty (71 g)	4
Chik'n parmesan garlic veggie wings, 5 wings (85 g)	5
Chipotle black bean burger (¼ lb), 1 burger (120 g)	5
Chipotle black bean veggie burger, 1 burger (120 g)	5
Grillers vegan burgers, 1 burger (71 g)	2

Sausage patties, veggie, 1 patty (38 g)	2
Tomato and basil pizza veggie burger, 1 burger (67 g)	3
Veggie buffalo wings, 5 wings (85 g)	6
Veggie burgers, garden veggie patties, 1 burger (67 g)	3
Veggie burgers, grillers prime, 1 burger (71 g)	4
Veggie burgers, spicy black bean, 1 burger (67 g)	3
Veggie burgers, spicy black bean, value pack, 1 burger (67 g)	3
Veggie corn dogs, 1 corn dog (71 g)	5
Veggie patties, grillers chik'n, 1 patty (67 g)	2
Veggie riblets, hickory bbq, 1 riblet with sauce (142 g)	8
Veggie sausage pattie, maple flavored, 1 patty (38 g)	2
Veggie sausage patties, hot & spicy, 1 patty (38 g)	1
Veggie sausage patties, original, 1 patty (38 g)	2
Morningstar Farms Breakfast	
Veggie bacon strips, 2 strips (16 g)	2
Morningstar Farms Classics	
Veggie dogs, 1 link (40 g)	1
Morningstar Farms Grillers	
California turk'y veggie burger, 1 burger (64 g)	2
Morningstar Farms Meal Starters	
Veggie crumbles, grillers recipe, ½ cup	2
Veggie meatballs, 5 meatballs (80 g)	3
Nasoya Tofubaked	
Teriyaki marinated baked tofu, 1 piece (57 g)	2

Quorn	
Burgers, gourmet, meatless & soy-free, 1 burger (80 g)	3
Chik'n cutlets, meatless & soy-free, naked, 1 cutlet (69 g)	2
Chik'n cutlets, meatless and soy-free, gruyere, 1 cutlet (110 g)	8
Chik'n patties, meatless and soy-free, 1 patty (75 g)	4
Chik'n tenders, meatless and soy-free, 1 cup	2
Sunshine Burger	
Veggie burgers, organic, garden herb, 1 patty (75 g)	6
Trader Joe's	
Meatless breakfast patties, 1 patty (35 g)	2
Meatless corn dogs, 1 corn dog (71 g)	5
Meatless meatballs, 6 pieces (85 g)	3
Quinoa cowboy veggie burgers with black beans & roasted corn, 1 burger (91 g)	5
Soy chorizo, 2 ½ oz	4
Veggie sausage patties, 1 patty (38 g)	2
Trader Joe's Organic	
Tofu veggie burgers, 1 patty (85 g)	5
Veggie Patch	
Mediterranean spinach and chickpea patties, 1 patty (70 g)	4

Meat, Poultry & Seafood Salads

Acme	
Smoked whitefish salad, 4 Tbsp	5
Bumble Bee	
Chicken salad with crackers, 1 package (99 g)	7
Tuna salad, with crackers, 1 can (82 g)	7
Bumble Bee Snack On The Run!	
Fat-free tuna salad with wheat crackers, 1 can (82 g)	2

SmartPoints™
value

SmartPoints™
value

Prepared Foods, Salads & Sides

GoodFoods

Reduced fat and calorie cranberry almond chicken salad, ½ cup	5

Marketside

Seafood salad with dressing, 1 ½ cups	4

Open Nature

Salad, chopped, kale & chicken, with raspberry balsamic vinaigrette, 1 container (163 g)	7

Ready Pac Bistro

Salad, chicken Caesar, 1 container (177 g)	7
Salad, chicken cranberry walnut, 1 container (142 g)	8

Ready Pac Bistro Bowl

Italian style chopped salad, 1 container (149 g)	7

Safeway Farms

Asian sesame chopped salad kit, 1 ½ cups	4

Signature Cafe

Cobb salad, 1 salad (340 g)	15

StarKist

Tuna salad, chunk light, 1 pouch (85 g)	2

StarKist Charlie's Chunk Light

Lunch kit, tuna salad, tuna in water, 1 kit (126 g)	5

StarKist Lunch To-Go

Tuna salad, chunk light, 1 kit (107 g)	6

StarKist Ready To Eat

Albacore tuna salad, 1 pouch (85 g)	2

Trader Joe's

Citrus salad with chicken (with dressing), 1 container (248 g)	8
Reduced guilt chicken salad (white meat), ½ cup	2

Packaged Lunches

Armour LunchMakers

Ham cracker crunchers with crunch bar, 1 package (73 g)	8
Turkey cracker crunchers with butterfinger bar, 1 package (73 g)	8

Cracker Barrel

Cracker cuts, cheddar, sharp-white, 3 slices (28 g)	4

Hamburger Helper Ultimate

Cheeseburger macaroni, ⅓ cup	5

Healthy Choice Cafe Steamers

Chicken fresca with chardonnay, 1 meal (280 g)	5
Honey balsamic chicken, 1 meal (280 g)	6

Hormel Gatherings

Smoked turkey snack tray with mild cheddar cheese and butter crisp crackers, 1 package (102 g)	8

Kraft Natural

Cracker cuts, cheese, marbled colby & Monterey Jack, 3 slices (28 g)	4
Cracker cuts, mild cheddar cheese, 3 slices (28 g)	5
Cracker cuts, sharp cheddar cheese, 3 slices (28 g)	5

Lunchables

Bologna and American cracker stackers lunch combinations, 1 package (87 g)	12
Extra cheesy pizza lunch combinations, 1 package (119 g)	8
Ham and American cracker stackers lunch combinations, 1 package (87 g)	13
Ham and cheddar cracker stackers lower fat lunch combinations, 1 package (144 g)	13
Ham and cheddar cracker stackers lunch combinations, 1 package (99 g)	13

Pepperoni and mozzarella with crackers, 1 package (63 g)	9
Pizza with pepperoni lunch combinations, 1 package (121 g)	10
Turkey and American cracker stackers lunch combinations, 1 package (82 g)	14
Lunchables Cracker Stackers	
Turkey and American lunch combinations, 1 package (96 g)	13
Old El Paso Stand 'n Stuff	
Taco dinner kit, hard & soft, 2 shells (50 g)	5
Oscar Mayer P3	
Portable protein pack (applewood smoked ham, cheese & cashews), 1 package (56 g)	5
Portable protein pack (chicken breast, Monterey Jack cheese & cashews), 1 package (56 g)	6
Portable protein pack chicken breast, cheddar cheese and dry roasted peanuts, 1 package (56 g)	5
Portable protein pack, smoked ham, sharp cheddar cheese and dry roasted almonds, 1 package (56 g)	4
Portable protein pack, turkey breast, cheddar cheese and dry roasted peanuts, 1 package (56 g)	5
Portable protein pack, turkey breast, marbled colby and Monterey Jack cheeses with dry roasted almonds, 1 package (56 g)	4
Safeway Farms	
Buffalo style chicken tortilla wrap kit, 1 container (163 g)	9
Turkey avocado tortilla wrap kit, 1 container (156 g)	9
StarKist Charlie's Lunch Kit	
Tuna salad, with chunk light tuna in water, 1 kit (130 g)	6

Pasta & Vegetable Salads

Allens	
3-bean salad, ½ cup	4
AzumaGourmet	
Seaweed salad, 2 oz	1
Cedar's	
Chickpea salad, 2 Tbsp	1
Taboule salad, fresh, party size, 2 Tbsp	1
Dole	
Cole slaw, classic, 1 ½ cups	0
Kale Caesar all natural salad kit, 2 cups	7
Salad kit, ceasar, 1 ½ cups	5
Salad kit, light Caesar, 1 ½ cups	3
Salad kit, southwest, 1 ½ cups	5
Salad, mediterranean blend, 2 cup	0
Dole All Natural	
Caesar salad kit, 1 ½ cups	5
Creamy coleslaw kit with dressing, 1 cup	6
Dole Chopped	
Bacon and bleu cheese salad kit, 2 cups	5
Bbq ranch salad kit, 2 cups	6
Chipotle and cheddar salad kit, 2 cups	4
Sesame Asian salad kit, 1 ½ cups	6
Sunflower crunch salad kit, 1 ½ cups	7
Dole Distinctively Dole	
Salad kit, Asian island crunch, 1 ½ cups	5
Salad kit, ultimate Caesar, 1 ½ cups	6
Eat Smart	
Sweet kale vegetable salad kit, 3 oz	6
Fresh Express	
Asian chopped salad kit, 1 ½ cups	5
Baby spinach salad, almond & cranberry, 3 ½ cups	5

Prepared Foods, Salads & Sides

	SmartPoints™ value
Caesarlite salad kit, 2 ½ cups	3
Cole slaw kit, 1 ½ cups	6
Salad, Asian, 2 ½ cups	4
Salad kit, Caesar, 2 ½ cups	5
Salad, broccoli salad, 1 cup	7
Salad, iceberg garden, 1 ½ cups	0
Southwest chopped salad kit, 1 ½ cups	5
Veggie lover's, 2 cups	0
Fresh Express Early Harvest	
Salad, double carrots, 2 cups	0
Salad, green & crisp, 2 cups	0
Fresh Express Kit	
Bacon Caesar salad, 2 ½ cups	5
Giant	
Chef salad, 1 container (283 g)	11
Green Giant	
Three bean salad, ½ cup	4
Hamburger Helper Italian	
Four cheese lasagna, Italian, ½ cup dry	3
Hannaford	
Cole slaw, country, ½ cup	8
Hellmann's	
Cole slaw, 1 serving (106 g)	7
Hidden Valley	
Kit, pasta salad, Southwest ranch, ½ cup	4
Kroger	
Cole slaw, creamy, ½ cup	7
Mustard potato salad, ⅔ cup	6
Sweet cole slaw, ½ cup	7
Marketside	
Asian chopped salad kit with dressing, 1 ½ cups	5
Chef salad with toppings and dressing, 1 package (184 g)	6
Chicken Caesar salad with dressing, 1 cup	6

	SmartPoints™ value
Light Caesar salad, 2 cups	4
Southwest salad with dressing, ½ cup	4
Nature's Promise Organic	
Baby spinach & spring mix, 2 ½ cups	0
O Organics	
Baby kale salad, organic, sweet onion Dijon, 1 container (120 g)	9
Salad, organic, baby spinach & chicken, 1 container (128 g)	9
Salad, organic, cranberry walnut, 1 container (128 g)	10
Open Nature	
Salad, chopped, Greek, with feta vinaigrette, 1 container (198 g)	7
Paisley Farm	
Four bean salad, ½ cup	4
Pita Pal	
Organic balela salad, ½ cup	6
Read	
3 bean salad, ⅓ cup	3
Ready Pac	
Salad, bistro, Italiano, 1 container (163 g)	7
Ready Pac Bistro	
Asian style chicken salad, 1 container (177 g)	6
Organic baby spinach and chicken salad, 1 container (128 g)	9
Organic cranberry walnut salad, 1 container (128 g)	10
Salad, chef, 1 container (220 g)	9
Salad, Santa Fe style Caesar, 1 container (177 g)	6
Salad, spinach Dijon, 1 container (135 g)	10
Ready Pac Bistro Bowl	
Cranberry walnut salad, 1 container (128 g)	8

Ready Pac Bistro Dinner Solutions

Salad, southwestern, 2 ¼ cups	4

Ready Pac Complete Salad

Fancy lettuce blend salad kit, 2 ½ cups	5

Reser's

Cole slaw, ½ cup	8

Safeway

Italian chopped salad kit, 1 ¾ cups	4

Safeway Farms

Bacon and bleu chopped salad kit, 1 ½ cups	4
Bbq ranch chopped salad kit, 2 cups	4
Cafe bowl, apple bleu pecan salad, 1 container (128 g)	9
Cafe bowl, Asian style chicken salad, 1 container (177 g)	6
Cafe bowl, chef salad, 1 container (220 g)	9
Cafe bowl, chicken Caesar salad, 1 container (177 g)	7
Cafe bowl, cranberry walnut salad, 1 container (128 g)	8
Cafe bowl, Italiano, turkey and salami salad, 1 container (163 g)	7
Cafe bowl, Santa Fe style salad, 1 container (177 g)	10
Cafe bowl, spinach Dijon salad, 1 container (135 g)	10
Chopped kale cranberry pecan salad kit, 2 cups	8
Complete salad kit, apple, blue cheese & pecan, 3 cups	6
Mediterranean chopped salad kit, 2 cups	5
Salad kit, baby kale, 2 cups	7
Salad kit, complete, royal parisian, 2 ½ cups	6

Signature Cafe

Apple and walnut with chicken salad, 1 salad (269 g)	16
Asian style salad with chicken, 1 salad (291 g)	16
Bbq style salad with chicken, 1 salad (326 g)	13
Chicken Caesar salad, with dressing, 1 salad (191 g)	8
Greek style salad, 1 salad (262 g)	8
Mediterranean style salad with chicken, 1 salad (248 g)	8
Salad, cobb with chicken, 1 salad (305 g)	14
Southwest style salad with chicken, 1 salad (340 g)	13
Spinach salad with bacon, 1 salad (241 g)	14

Simply Potatoes

Red potato wedges, rosemary & garlic, ½ cup	2
Cole slaw, ½ cup	5
Crisp garden salad, 2 cups	0
Garden salad, crisp, fresh, 2 cups	0

Suddenly Salad

Pasta salad, classic, value size, ½ cup	5
Pasta salad, southwest style ranch, ¾ cup	5
Suddenly pasta salad, Caesar, ⅔ cup	5
Suddenly pasta salad, classic, twin pack, ½ cup	5
Suddenly pasta salad, ranch & bacon, twin pack, ½ cup	5

The Deli Counter

Baked potato salad, loaded, ½ cup	9
Cole slaw, classic, ½ cup	7
Cole slaw, southern style, ½ cup	6

Prepared Foods, Salads & Sides

Prepared Foods, Salads & Sides

	SmartPoints™ value
Trader Joe's	
Balela, ½ cup	3
Broccoli slaw & kale salad with white chicken meat (with dressing), 1 container (263 g)	20
Egg white salad with chives, ½ container (85 g)	1
Honey glazed miso salmon on salad greens with dressing, 1 container (276 g)	10
Salad with bbq flavored chicken with dressing, 1 container (369 g)	18
Wegman's Food You Feel Good About	
Greek pasta with feta salad, 1 cup	9
Salad, fresh garden, 2 cups	0
Yoders	
Cole slaw, ½ cup	5

Pasta Entrées

	SmartPoints™ value
Amy's	
Lasagna, garden vegetable, 1 each (291 g)	9
Macaroni and cheese, 1 cup	13
Amy's Bowls	
Broccoli & cheddar bake, 1 bowl (269 g)	15
Mushroom risotto, 1 bowl (269 g)	8
Pesto tortellini, 1 entrée (269 g)	14
Ravioli, cheese with sauce, 1 each (269 g)	12
Amy's Light & Lean	
Asian noodle, sweet & sour, 1 bowl (227 g)	8
Macaroni and cheese, 1 entrée (227 g)	9
Pasta & veggies, 1 bowl (227 g)	6
Penne marinara, 3 cheese, 1 bowl (227 g)	8
Roasted polenta with Swiss chard, 1 package (227 g)	5

	SmartPoints™ value
Spaghetti Italiano, 1 bowl (227 g)	7
Spinach lasagna, 1 lasagna (227 g)	8
Annie's	
Macaroni & cheese, Bernie's farm, 2 ½ oz	8
Macaroni & cheese, classic, family size, 1 cup	14
Macaroni & cheese, real aged cheddar, 1 package (57 g)	7
Macaroni & cheese, rice pasta & cheddar, 1 package (57 g)	8
Macaroni & cheese, shells & white cheddar, 2 ½ oz dry	9
Macaroni & cheese, white cheddar, 1 package (57 g)	7
Annie's Homegrown	
Aged cheddar macaroni and cheese, 1 container (57 g)	7
Shells and real aged cheddar macaroni and cheese, 2 ½ oz	8
White cheddar macaroni and cheese, 1 container (57 g)	7
Annie's Homegrown Totally Natural	
Macaroni & cheese, rice pasta & cheddar, 2 ½ oz	9
Annie's Organic	
Macaroni & cheese, shells & real aged cheddar, 2 ½ oz	8
Macaroni & cheese, whole wheat shells & white cheddar, 2 ½ oz	8
Annie's Totally Natural	
Classic macaroni and cheese, 2 ½ oz dry	9
Mac & cheese, microwavable, 1 packet (61 g)	7
Mac & cheese, microwavable, gluten free, 1 packet (61 g)	8
Shells and white cheddar macaroni and cheese, 2 ½ oz dry	9

Atkins

Chicken & broccoli Alfredo, 1 tray (255 g)	10
Italian style pasta bake, 1 tray (255 g)	11

Back to Nature

Shells & white cheddar dinner, organic, 1 cup	8

Banquet

Fettuccini Alfredo, 1 meal (198 g)	7
Macaroni & cheese meal, 1 meal (227 g)	8
Spaghetti and meatballs, 1 meal (255 g)	12

Barilla

Tortellini, three cheese, ¾ cup	7

Barilla Collezione Regional Specialties

Tortellini, cheese & spinach, ¾ cup	7

Barilla Italian Entrées

Gemelli, meat sauce, 9 oz	10
Marinara penne, 1 entrée (255 g)	9
Penne, whole grain, tomato and basil, 1 entrée (255 g)	9
Rotini, sausage and tomato, 1 tray (255 g)	10

Bertolli Classic Meal for 2

Chicken Alfredo and penne, ½ package (340 g)	17
Chicken alla vodka and farfalle, ½ package (340 g)	14
Chicken florentine and farfalle, ½ package (340 g)	15
Chicken marsala and roasted redskin potatoes, ½ package (340 g)	11
Chicken parmigiana and penne, ½ package (340 g)	15
Italian sausage and rigatoni, ½ package (340 g)	17
Ricotta & lobster ravioli, ½ package (340 g)	15

Roasted chicken risotto, ½ package (340 g)	11
Shrimp scampi and linguine, ½ package (340 g)	16
Shrimp, asparagus and penne, ½ package (340 g)	14

Bertolli Rustico Bakes

Stuffed shells alla vodka, 1 meal (300 g)	16

Betty Crocker

Mac and cheese, original unprepared, ½ cup	6

Birds Eye Steamfresh

Lightly sauced pasta, penne & vegetables with Alfredo sauce, 1 ⅓ cups	9
Lightly sauced pasta, rotini & broccoli with cheese sauce, 2 cups	7
Rigatoni & vegetables, lightly sauced, with tomato parmesan sauce, 2 cups	7
Rotini & vegetables, lightly sauced, with garlic butter sauce, 2 cups	8

Birds Eye Steamfresh Chef's Favorites

Couscous pasta & spinach, with olive oil & lemon sauce, lightly sauced, ½ bag (142 g)	5

Bob Evans

Macaroni & cheese, special recipe, 1 cup	11

Bob Evans Oven Bake

Macaroni and cheese, 1 cup	9

Bob Evans Special Recipe

Macaroni & cheese, 1 bowl (170 g)	7

Buitoni

Ravioli, spicy beef & sausage, 1 cup	9
Sweet Italian sausage tortelloni, 1 cup	11

Buitoni Riserva

Crab ravioli, 1 cup	10

Prepared Foods, Salads & Sides

	SmartPoints™ value
Campbell's	
Spaghettios, plus calcium, 1 cup	6
Spaghettios, sliced franks, 1 cup	8
Celentano	
Ravioli, cheese, 4 ravioli (123 g)	6
Ravioli, cheese, mini rounds, 12 ravioli (113 g)	6
Stuffed shells, with sauce, 3 shells (284 g)	12
Cheese Club	
Creamy cheese sauce and shell pasta, ⅓ box (112 g)	11
Chef Boyardee	
Beef ravioli in tomato & meat sauce, 1 cup	8
Beefaroni, 1 cup	9
Mini ravioli, 1 cup	8
Ravioli, beef, 1 cup	8
Ravioli, beef, in tomato & meat sauce, 1 cup	8
Spaghetti & meatballs, in tomato sauce, 1 cup	9
Chicken Helper	
Fettuccine pasta & Alfredo sauce mix, fettuccine Alfredo, ½ cup	4
Evol	
Truffle parmesan mac & cheese, 1 bowl (227 g)	17
Evol Bowls	
Teriyaki chicken, 1 bowl (255 g)	7
Evol Meals for 2	
Butternut squash and sage ravioli, ½ bag (225 g)	10
Farm Rich	
Toasted ravioli, 2 pieces (50 g)	5
Frankly Fresh Wholesome Food	
Turkey and spinach lasagna, 1 cup	10
Great Value	
Thick and creamy macaroni and cheese dinner, ⅓ box (70 g)	8

	SmartPoints™ value
Green Giant Just for One	
Macaroni and cheese with broccoli, 1 tray (120 g)	3
Hamburger Helper	
Cheese lover's lasagna, ½ cup	3
Pasta and sauce mix, chili macaroni, ¼ cup	3
Hamburger Helper Classic	
Double cheeseburger macaroni, ¼ cup	3
Pasta & sauce mix, cheddar cheese melt, ½ cup	3
Pasta & sauce mix, three cheese, ¼ cup	3
Ultimate cheeseburger macaroni, 1 ¼ cups as packaged	3
Hamburger Helper Italian	
Lasagna, ⅓ cup	4
Pasta & sauce mix, tomato basil penne, ⅓ cup dry	5
Hamburger Helper Whole Grain	
Cheeseburger macaroni, ¼ cup	3
Healthy Choice Baked	
Alfredo bake fettuccini, 1 meal (249 g)	8
Four cheese ziti marinara, 1 meal (260 g)	10
Italian sausage pasta bake, 1 meal (249 g)	8
Lasagna with meat sauce, 1 meal (269 g)	9
Healthy Choice Cafe Steamers	
100% natural pumpkin squash ravioli, 1 entrée (269 g)	9
100% natural tortellini primavera parmesan, 1 entrée (269 g)	8
Portabella marsala pasta, 1 meal (255 g)	7
Portabella spinach parmesan, 1 meal (277 g)	7
Healthy Choice Complete Meals	
Spaghetti and meatballs, 1 meal (297 g)	9

Healthy Choice Modern Classics

Four cheese tortellini, 1 meal (340 g)	10

Healthy Choice Select Entrées

Ravioli florentine marinara, 1 meal (241 g)	8

Healthy Choice Top Chef Cafe Steamers

Ricotta & spinach ravioli & chicken marinara, 1 meal (283 g)	8

Horizon Organic Mac

Macaroni and mild cheddar cheese, 2 ½ oz	8

Hormel Compleats Homestyle

Spaghetti, meat sauce, 1 tray (283 g)	10

Hormel Simple Ideas

Country crock side dished elbow macaroni & cheese, 1 cup	11

Jimmy Dean Delights

Three cheese pasta, 1 bowl (226 g)	10

Kashi

Pesto pasta primavera, 1 entrée (283 g)	9

Kirkland Signature

Five cheese tortelloni with parmigiano reggiano, 1 cup	9
Italian sausage and beef lasagna, 1 cup	14

Knorr Italian Sides

Four cheese bow tie, ¾ cup	6

Knorr Pasta Sides

Fettuccini, Alfredo, ⅔ cup	7
Fettuccini, Alfredo broccoli, ⅔ cup	7
Fettuccini, butter & herb, ⅔ cup	7
Fettuccini, creamy chicken flavor, ⅔ cup	6
Fettuccini, parmesan, ⅔ cup	7
Fettuccini, smokehouse bacon flavor parmesan, ⅔ cup	6
Rotini pasta, cheesy cheddar, ¾ cup	6

Kraft

Macaroni & cheese dinner cup, extreme cheese, 1 package (57 g)	7
Macaroni & cheese dinner, disney pixar monsters university (unprepared), ½ box as packaged (70 g)	8
Macaroni & cheese dinner, nickelodeon spongebob squarepants (unprepared), ½ box as packaged (70 g)	8
Macaroni & cheese dinner, original flavor (cup), 1 package (58 g)	7
Macaroni & cheese dinner, original flavor (unprepared), ⅓ box (70 g)	8
Macaroni & cheese dinner, phineas & ferb shapes (unprepared), ½ box as packaged (70 g)	8
Macaroni & cheese dinner, spirals (unprepared), ½ box (70 g)	8
Macaroni & cheese dinner, spongebob squarepants shapes (cup), 1 package (55 g)	7
Macaroni & cheese dinner, thick 'n creamy, unprepared, ⅓ box (70 g)	8
Macaroni & cheese dinner, three cheese (unprepared), ⅓ box (70 g)	8
Macaroni & cheese dinner, triple cheese (cup), 1 package (58 g)	7
Macaroni & cheese dinner, whole grain, original flavor (unprepared), ⅓ box as packaged (70 g)	8
Macaroni and cheese dinner (microwave cup), 1 package (58 g)	7
Macaroni and cheese, organic, cheddar, unprepared, 2 ½ oz	8
Original flavor macaroni and cheese dinner, 1 single cup (58 g)	7
Star wars shapes macaroni & cheese dinner, ½ box as packaged (70 g)	8
Velveeta, shells & cheese, original, 5 pack, 4 oz	11

	SmartPoints™ value
Kraft Deluxe	
Macaroni & cheese dinner, made with 2% milk, ¼ box (98 g)	9
Macaroni & cheese dinner, original, cheddar cheese sauce, ¼ box (98 g)	10
Macaroni & cheese dinner, sharp cheddar cheese sauce, ¼ box (98 g)	10
Macaroni and cheese dinner, 2% milk cheese, ¼ box (98 g)	9
Macaroni and cheese dinner, original cheddar, ¼ box (98 g)	10
Kraft Easy Mac	
Macaroni and cheese dinner, animal shapes, 1 pouch (57 g)	7
Macaroni and cheese dinner, extreme cheese flavor, 1 pouch (61 g)	8
Original macaroni and cheese dinner, 1 pouch (61 g)	7
Kraft Homestyle	
Hearty four cheese macaroni and cheese dinner (as packaged), 3 oz	8
Macaroni & cheese dinner, classic cheddar (unprepared), ¼ package (84 g)	8
Kraft Velveeta	
Cheesy skillets dinner kit, chicken Alfredo (unprepared), 1/5 package (70 g)	7
Kroger Meal-Ready Sides	
Vegetables, stir-fry, with noodles, 1 ¼ cups	2
Lean Cuisine Culinary Collection	
Asparagus and cheese ravioli, 1 package (258 g)	9
Mushroom mezzaluna ravioli, 1 package (244 g)	9
Three cheese stuffed rigatoni, 1 package (255 g)	8
Lean Cuisine Dinnertime Collection	
Grilled chicken and penne pasta, 1 package (340 g)	11

	SmartPoints™ value
Lean Cuisine Simple Favorites	
Alfredo pasta with chicken and broccoli, 1 package (283 g)	8
Angel hair pomodoro, 1 package (283 g)	7
Cheese ravioli, 1 package (241 g)	9
Classic five cheese lasagna, 1 package (326 g)	11
Classic macaroni and beef in tomato sauce, 1 package (269 g)	9
Fettuccini Alfredo, 1 package (262 g)	9
Five cheese rigatoni, 1 package (283 g)	11
Four cheese cannelloni, 1 package (258 g)	8
Lasagna with meat sauce, 1 package (297 g)	10
Macaroni and cheese, 1 package (283 g)	10
Pasta romano with bacon, 1 package (283 g)	8
Spaghetti with meat sauce, 1 package (326 g)	9
Spaghetti with meatballs, 1 package (269 g)	8
Lean Cuisine Spa Collection	
Butternut squash ravioli, 1 package (280 g)	9
Marie Callender's	
Lasagna, three meat and four cheese, 1 cup	10
Marie Callender's Comfort Bakes	
Mac and cheese, 1 cup	12
Michael Angelo's	
Lasagna, meat, 1 cup	9
Michelina's Authentico	
Fettuccine Alfredo, 1 package (241 g)	11
Five cheese ziti, 1 package (255 g)	9
Macaroni & cheese, 1 package (227 g)	10
Wheels & cheese, 1 package (227 g)	11

Michelina's Lean Gourmet

Lasagna, five cheese, 1 package (227 g)	9
Ziti marinara, three cheese, 1 package (269 g)	9

Michelina's Traditional Recipes

Cheese manicotti, 1 package (213 g)	8
Tortellini Alfredo, 1 package (213 g)	9

Minute Ready To Serve!

Multi-grain rice medley, 1 cup	6

Monterey Gourmet Foods

Organic fresh spinach and cheese ravioli, 1 cup	7

Newman's Own

Complete skillet meal for two, chicken florentine & farfalle, ½ package (340 g)	10

On-Cor

Vegetable lasagna, with spinach, zucchini, carrots, corn, broccoli and ricotta cheese, 1 cup	7

Panera Bread

Mac and cheese, 1 cup	14

Pasta Prima

Ravioli, spinach and mozzarella, 1 cup	6
Ravioli, wild mushroom, 1 cup	8

Pasta Prima 100% Natural

Ravioli, grilled chicken and mozzarella, 1 cup	7

Pasta Roni

Angel hair pasta, parmesan cheese flavor, 2 oz	6
Angel hair pasta, parmesan cheese flavor, family size, 2 oz	6
Pasta, butter and garlic flavor corkscrew, 1 container (61 g)	7
Pasta, fettuccini Alfredo, 2 ½ oz	8
Pasta, four cheese corkscrew flavor, 2 ½ oz	8

Pasta Roni Nature's Way

Linguine, olive oil & Italian herb, 2 oz	6

Rana

Ravioli, mushroom, 1 cup	9
Ravioli, spinaci e ricotta, 1 cup	9
Tortellini, cheese delicato, family size!, 1 cup	7

Red Baron Pan Pasta

Rotini with meat sauce, 1 cup	8

Rosetto

Ravioli, beef, 9 pieces (124 g)	7
Ravioli, cheese, 9 pieces (141.6 g)	8
Tortellini, cheese, 1 cup	7

Safeway Select

Lasagna, Mexican style, 1 serving (216 g)	12

ShopRite

Spaghetti and meatballs i n meat sauce, 1 cup	10

Simply Nature

Southwestern fresca, 1 package (255 g)	10

SpaghettiOs

Original, 1 can (213 g)	6
Pasta with meatballs in tomato sauce, 1 can (206 g)	6
Spaghetti o's with meatballs, 1 cup	7
Spaghettios, shapes, disney princesses, meatballs, 1 cup	8

Stouffer's

Chicken Alfredo, family size, 1 cup	8
Classic mac and cheese mac cup, 1 (170 g)	8
Lasagna with meat sauce family size, 1 cup	8
Lasagna, five cheese, large family size, 1 cup	10
Lasagna, Italiano, family size, 1 cup	8
Macaroni & cheese, family size, 1 cup	11

	SmartPoints value
Vegetable lasagna, party size, 1 cup	11
White cheddar and bacon mac cup, 1 (170 g)	8
Stouffer's Classics	
Lasagna, Italiano, 1 package (297 g)	12
Lasagna, meat lovers, 1 package (283 g)	13
Stouffer's Craveable Classics	
Macaroni & cheese, large size, 1 cup	11
Macaroni & cheese, 1 cup	11
Stouffer's Easy Express	
Cheesy garlic lasagna with meat & sauce, family size, 1 cup	11
Stouffer's Family	
Rigatoni with chicken and pesto, 1 cup	8
Stouffer's Farmers' Harvest	
Lasagna, vegetable, 1 package (297 g)	13
Lasagna, vegetable, family size, 1 cup	9
Stouffer's Homestyle Classics	
Lasagna, with meat & sauce, 1 package (297 g)	11
Spaghetti with meat sauce, 1 package (340 g)	11
Spaghetti with meatballs, 1 package (357 g)	11
Stouffer's Restaurant Classics	
Rigatoni with roasted white meat chicken, 1 package (237 g)	12
Stouffer's Satisfying Servings	
Lasagna, meat lovers, 1 cup	10
Lasagna, with meat sauce, large, 1 cup	8
Trader Giotto's	
Penne pasta with creamy vodka marinara sauce, 1 package (145 g)	12

	SmartPoints value
Trader Joe's	
Mushroom risotto, 1 cup	5
Pesto pasta salad, 1 cup	10
Reduced guilt mac & cheese, 1 container (198 g)	8
Reduced guilt spinach and cheese stuffed shells with marinara sauce, 1 container (241 g)	8
Tuna Helper Classic	
Cheesy pasta, ½ cup	3
Creamy pasta, ½ cup	3
Tuna Helper Italian	
Fettuccine Alfredo, ½ cup	3
Velveeta	
Rotini & cheese, whole grain, ⅓ box (98 g)	10
Shells & cheese, ½ the fat, ⅓ box (112 g)	10
Shells & cheese, 2% milk cheese, 1 package (62 g)	6
Shells & cheese, original, 1 package (68 g)	7
Velveeta Cheesy Skillets	
Dinner kit, chicken bacon ranch (unprepared), 1/5 package (70 g)	7
Dinner kit, lasagna (makes 5 servings), 1 serving (70 g)	7
Velveeta Cheesy Skillets Singles	
Chicken chili cheese mac, 1 package (255 g)	7

Pizza

	SmartPoints value
American Flatbread	
Pizza, fine artisan, ½ pizza (128 g)	9
Amy's	
Pizza, 4 cheese, ⅓ pizza (113 g)	9
Pizza, cheese, 1 pizza (176 g)	13
Pizza, margherita, ⅓ pizza (123 g)	8
Pizza, mushroom & olive, ⅓ pizza (123 g)	8
Pizza, roasted vegetable, no cheese, ⅓ pizza (113 g)	9
Pizza, spinach, 1 pizza (204 g)	14

Prepared Foods, Salads & Sides

Amy's Light & Lean

Pizza, cheese, 1 pizza (142 g)	8
Pizza, Italian vegetable, 1 pizza (142 g)	8

Archer Farms

Handmade spinach and goat cheese wood fired pizza, ⅓ pizza (157 g)	12

Atkins High Protein

Stone fired cheese pizza, 1 pizza (156 g)	11
Stone fired vegetable pizza, 1 pizza (163 g)	10

Bagel Bites

Mini bagels, cheese & pepperoni, 4 pieces (88 g)	6
Mini bagels, mozzarella cheese, 4 pieces (88 g)	5
Mini bagels, three cheese, 4 pieces (88 g)	6

Bellatoria Ultra Thin Crust

Pizza, garlic chicken Alfredo, ⅓ pizza (151 g)	10
Pizza, ultimate supreme, personal size, ½ pizza (114 g)	8

California Pizza Kitchen

Bbq recipe chicken crispy thin crust pizza, 1 pizza (172 g)	12
Pizza, bbq chicken, 1 serving (132 g)	10
Pizza, crispy thin crust, bbq recipe chicken, ⅓ pizza (139 g)	10
Pizza, crispy thin crust, four cheese, 1 pizza (153 g)	14
Pizza, crispy thin crust, Hawaiian recipe, 1 pizza (175 g)	12
Pizza, crispy thin crust, margherita, ⅓ pizza (146 g)	11
Pizza, crispy thin crust, sicilian recipe, ⅓ pizza (147 g)	12
Pizza, crispy thin crust, signature pepperoni, ⅓ pizza (128 g)	12
Pizza, crispy thin crust, white, ⅓ pizza (127 g)	11

Pizza, margherita, ⅓ pizza (151 g)	14
Sicilian recipe crispy thin crust pizza, 1 pizza (161 g)	13

California Pizza Kitchen For One

Pizza, crispy thin crust, margherita, 1 pizza (172 g)	14

California Pizza Kitchen Limited Edition

Pizza, crispy thin crust, spinach & artichoke, ⅓ pizza (135 g)	10

Celeste Pizza For One

Pizza, deluxe, 1 pizza (167 g)	12
Pizza, original, 1 pizza (158 g)	11
Pizza, original 4 cheese, 1 pizza (148 g)	12
Pizza, pepperoni, 1 pizza (142 g)	12

Culinary Circle

Flatbread pizza, spinach and artichoke, ½ pizza (159 g)	11
Pizza, ultra thin crust, margherita, ⅓ pizza (113 g)	10

DiGiorno

Digiorno original rising crust supreme pizza (serves 6), 1 serving (149 g)	11
Four cheese original rising crust pizza (serves 6), 1 serving (133 g)	10
Pepperoni original rising crust pizza (serves 6), 1 serving (130 g)	10
Pizza, cheese stuffed crust, pepperoni, ½ pizza (120 g)	12
Pizza, cheese stuffed crust, pepperoni (serves 5), 1 serving (150 g)	13
Pizza, cheese stuffed crust, supreme pizza, 1 serving (145 g)	12
Pizza, cheese stuffed crust, three meat (serves 6), 1 serving (136 g)	11
Pizza, classic thin crust, four cheese pizza, 1 serving (130 g)	10
Pizza, classic thin crust, four meat pizza, 1 serving (133 g)	10
Pizza, classic thin crust, pepperoni pizza, 1 serving (125 g)	11

Prepared Foods, Salads & Sides

Prepared Foods, Salads & Sides

	SmartPoints™ value
Pizza, classic thin crust, supreme pizza, 1 serving (141 g)	10
Pizza, rising crust, pepperoni, 1 serving (134 g)	10
Pizza, rising crust, sausage & pepperoni, 1 serving (143 g)	12
Pizza, rising crust, spinach, mushroom & garlic, ⅙ pizza (143 g)	9
Pizza, rising crust, supreme, 1 serving (155 g)	11
Pizza, rising crust, three meat, 1 serving (144 g)	11
Rising crust pizza, four cheese, ⅓ pizza (113 g)	9
Rising crust pizza, pepperoni pizza, ⅓ pizza (120 g)	10
Rising crust three meat pizzas, 1 serving (144 g)	11
DiGiorno For One	
Pizza, thin crispy crust, pepperoni, 1 pizza (238 g)	19
Pizza, traditional crust, four cheese, 1 pizza (260 g)	24
DiGiorno Italian Style Favorites	
Pizza, chicken parmesan, 1 serving (130 g)	9
Pizza, meatball marinara, 1 slice (132 g)	11
DiGiorno Original Rising Crust	
Three meat pizza (serves 6), 1 serving (141 g)	11
DiGiorno Pizzeria!	
Pizza, Italian style meat trio, ¼ pizza (145 g)	12
Pizza, quattro formaggi/four cheese pizza, ¼ pizza (130 g)	11
Pizza, supreme speciale, ¼ pizza (151 g)	12
Pizza, white, ¼ pizza (128 g)	10
Primo pepperoni pizza, ¼ pizza (133 g)	11

	SmartPoints™ value
DiGiorno Thin & Crispy	
Pizza, pepperoni and peppers, ½ pizza (150 g)	13
Pizza, spinach and garlic, ⅓ pizza (112 g)	9
Pizza, tomato mozzarella with pesto, ½ pizza (162 g)	12
Digiorno Thin Crispy Crust	
Four cheese pizza, ½ pizza (113 g)	8
Dr. Oetker	
Pizza, ristorante, mozzarella, ⅓ pizza (108 g)	9
Pizza, ristorante, spinaci, ⅓ pizza (130 g)	10
Ellio's	
Pizza five cheese, 2 slices (115 g)	7
Fit & Active	
Pepperoni pizza lean stuffed sandwich, 1 sandwich (128 g)	7
Freschetta	
Pizza, naturally rising crust, signature pepperoni (serves 6), 1 slice (129 g)	11
Freschetta Brick Oven	
Pizza, 3 meat medley, 1 serving (131 g)	12
Pizza, 5-Italian cheese, ¼ pizza (131 g)	12
Pizza, chicken club, ¼ pizza (155 g)	12
Pizza, pepperoni & Italian style cheese, ¼ pizza (154 g)	14
Pizza, roasted portabella mushrooms & spinach, ¼ pizza (143 g)	11
Freschetta Flat Bread	
Pizza, 5-cheese, ⅓ pizza (121 g)	11
Pizza, pepperoni, ⅓ pizza (119 g)	11
Pizza, roasted garlic & spinach, ⅓ pizza (119 g)	10
Freschetta Gluten Free	
4 cheese medley pizza, ⅓ pizza (152 g)	13

Freschetta Naturally Rising

Pizza, bake to rise crust, 4 cheese medley, 1 serving (140 g)	12
Pizza, Canadian style bacon & pineapple pizza, 1 serving (142 g)	10

Gourmet Parlor Gluten-Free

Pizza, cheese, ½ pizza (141.7 g)	6

Home Run Inn Classic

Pizza, sausage, ¼ pizza (147 g)	11

Home Run Inn Ultra Thin

Pizza, cheese, 1 pizza (113 g)	9
Pizza, sausage, 1 pizza (142 g)	10

Hot Pockets Crispy Crust

Pepperoni pizza sandwich, 1 piece (127 g)	12

Hot Pockets Garlic Buttery

Pepperoni pizza sandwich, 1 piece (127 g)	11

Hot Pockets Pizzeria

Stuffed sandwiches, pepperoni pizza, 1 piece (127 g)	12
Stuffed sandwiches, pepperoni pizza, family value pack, 1 piece (127 g)	12

Jack's

Original thin crust pepperoni pizza, ⅓ pizza (146 g)	12

Jack's Original

Cheese pizza, ⅓ pizza (142 g)	10
Pepperoni pizza, ⅓ pizza (156 g)	13
Pizza, cheese, ⅓ pizza (142 g)	10
Pizza, pepperoni, ⅓ pizza (156 g)	13
Pizza, pepperoni & sausage, ½ pizza (146 g)	12
Pizza, supreme, ¼ pizza (128 g)	10

Kashi

Pizza, margherita, stone-fired thin crust, ⅓ pizza (113 g)	8
Pizza, mediterranean, ⅓ pizza (120 g)	9
Pizza, roasted vegetable, ⅓ pizza (116 g)	8
Pizza, stone-fired thin crust, mushroom trio & spinach, ⅓ pizza (113 g)	8

Kirkland Signature

Cheese pizza, ¼ pizza (120 g)	9

Kirkland Signature Rising Crust

Pepperoni pizza (serves 6), 1 serving (143 g)	12

Lean Cuisine Culinary Collection

Cheese and tomato snack pizza, 1 pizza (91 g)	5
Deep dish spinach and mushroom pizza, 1 Package (173 g)	10
Deep dish three meat pizza, 1 Package (180 g)	11
Pepperoni snack pizza, 1 serving (90 g)	6
Spinach and artichoke snack pizza, 1 pizza (91 g)	5
Traditional deluxe pizza, 1 package (170 g)	10
Traditional four cheese pizza, 1 package (170 g)	10
Traditional pepperoni pizza, 1 package (170 g)	11
Wood fire roasted garlic chicken pizza, 1 pizza (170 g)	10
Wood fire style bbq recipe chicken pizza, 1 package (170 g)	10
Wood fire style margherita pizza, 1 package (170 g)	10

Lean Cuisine Simple Favorites

French bread cheese pizza, 1 pizza (170 g)	10
French bread deluxe pizza, 1 pizza (173 g)	10
French bread pepperoni pizza, 1 package (148 g)	9

Lean Pockets

Reduced fat pepperoni pizza garlic buttery seasoned crust sandwich, 1 piece (127 g)	9

Prepared Foods, Salads & Sides

Prepared Foods, Salads & Sides

	SmartPoints™ value
McCain Ellio's	
Pizza slices, cheese, 27 slices, 1 slice (66.4 g)	6
Pizza, cheese, 2 slices (138 g)	9
Michelina's Authentico	
Snackers, pizza snack rolls, 1 package (142 g)	12
Michelina's Lean Gourmet	
Pepperoni pizza snackers, 11 snacks (85 g)	6
Morningstar Farms	
Veggie pizza, baja black bean, single serve, 1 pizza (160 g)	12
Newman's Own	
All natural thin and crispy buffalo style chicken pizza, ⅓ pizza (132 g)	10
Pizza, thin & crispy, four cheese, ⅓ pizza (126 g)	10
Newman's Own Thin & Crispy	
Pizza, margherita, ⅓ pizza (131 g)	9
Pizza, supreme, ⅓ pizza (139 g)	10
Pizza, uncured pepperoni, ⅓ pizza (125 g)	10
Pizza, white, ⅓ pizza (114 g)	9
Roasted vegetable pizza, ⅓ pizza (133 g)	7
Old City Cafe New York Style	
Pizza, cheese, 9", 1 slice (85 g)	5
Palermo's Hearth Baked Crust	
Roasted vegetable flatbread, ⅓ pizza (145 g)	8
Palermo's Primo Thin	
Pizza, ultra-thin crust, cheese lovers, ⅓ pizza (138 g)	11
Pizza, ultra-thin crust, margherita pizza, ⅓ pizza (140 g)	8
Pizza, ultra-thin crust, pepperoni, ⅓ pizza (139 g)	12

	SmartPoints™ value
Red Baron	
Pizza, classic crust, 4 cheese, ¼ pizza (146 g)	13
Pizza, classic crust, 4-meat pizza, ¼ pizza (149 g)	12
Pizza, classic crust, sausage & pepperoni, ¼ pizza (150 g)	13
Pizza, classic crust, special deluxe, 1 serving (125 g)	10
Pizza, classic crust, supreme pizza, 1 serving (128 g)	11
Pizza, fire baked original crust, pepperoni, ¼ pizza (141 g)	12
Rising crust pepperoni pizza, ¼ pizza (137 g)	11
Red Baron Classic Crust	
Hawaiian style pizza, ¼ pizza (134 g)	10
Mexican style pizza, ¼ pizza (149 g)	13
Pepperoni pizza, ¼ pizza (146 g)	13
Red Baron Fire Baked	
Pizza, thin crust, 5-cheese, ⅓ pizza (139 g)	13
Red Baron Pizza Singles	
Thin crust 4 cheese pizza, 1 pizza (102 g)	10
Red Baron Pizzeria Style	
Pizza, thin & crispy, supreme, ¼ pizza (124 g)	11
Pizza, thin & crispy, tuscan style crust, pepperoni, ⅓ pizza (149 g)	14
Red Baron Rising Crust	
Cheese pizza, ¼ pizza (135 g)	11
Red Baron Singles	
Pizza, deep dish, pepperoni, 1 pizza (159 g)	15
Pizzas, deep dish, 4 cheese, 1 pizza (159 g)	15
Pizzas, deep dish, cheese, 1 pizza (159 g)	14

Pizzas, deep dish, supreme, 1 pizza (163 g) — 15

Pizzas, French bread, 5 cheese & garlic, 1 pizza (125 g) — 14

Pizzas, French bread, pepperoni, 1 pizza (153 g) — 12

Pizzas, French bread, supreme, 1 pizza (164 g) — 12

Red Baron The Big Baron

Pizza, classic style crust, pepperoni, 1 serving (134 g) — 12

Sam's Choice Rising Crust

Four cheese pizza, 1 serving (141 g) — 12

Pepperoni pizza, 1 serving (143 g) — 12

Stouffer's

Pizza, French bread, cheese, 1 piece (147 g) — 12

Pizza, French bread, deluxe, 1 piece (175 g) — 14

Pizza, French bread, extra cheese, 1 piece (167 g) — 13

Pizza, French bread, pepperoni, 1 piece (159 g) — 14

Tombstone

Pizza, original, extra cheese, ¼ pizza (145 g) — 11

Pizza, original, pepperoni, ¼ each (146.5 g) — 13

Pizza, thin crust, three cheese, ¼ pizza (134 g) — 11

Tombstone Original

Pepperoni and sausage pizza (21.4 oz pizza serves 4), ¼ pizza (153 g) — 13

Pizza, 4 meat, 1 serving (130 g) — 10

Pizza, classic sausage, ⅓ pizza (114 g) — 9

Pizza, deluxe, ⅓ pizza (124 g) — 9

Pizza, pepperoni, ¼ pizza (153 g) — 13

Pizza, pepperoni & sausage, ⅓ pizza (118 g) — 10

Pizza, supreme, 1 serving (130 g) — 10

Tony's

Garlic cheese bread, 1 serving (57 g) — 6

Totino's

Pizza rolls, cheese, 6 rolls (85 g) — 6

Pizza rolls, combination, 6 rolls (85 g) — 7

Pizza rolls, triple cheese, 6 rolls (85 g) — 6

Pizza, party, cheese, ½ pizza (139 g) — 11

Pizza, party, classic pepperoni, ½ pizza (139 g) — 11

Pizza, party, combination, ½ pizza (152 g) — 12

Pizza, party, hamburger, ½ pizza (155 g) — 12

Pizza, party, pepperoni, ½ pizza (145 g) — 12

Pizza, party, sausage, ½ pizza (153 g) — 12

Pizza, party, supreme, ½ pizza (155 g) — 12

Pizza, party, triple cheese, ½ pizza (138 g) — 11

Pizza, party, triple meat, ½ pizza (149 g) — 12

Totino's Party Pizza

Pepperoni pizza pack, ½ pizza (145 g) — 12

Triple cheese pizza, ½ pizza (138 g) — 10

Totino's Pizza Rolls

Brand pizza snacks, cheese, 6 rolls (85 g) — 6

Brand pizza snacks, combination, 6 rolls (85 g) — 7

Brand pizza snacks, pepperoni, 6 rolls (85 g) — 7

Combination pizza snacks, 6 rolls (85 g) — 6

Pepperoni pizza snacks, 6 (85 g) — 7

Pizza snacks, combination, 6 rolls (85 g) — 7

Prepared Foods, Salads & Sides

Prepared Foods, Salads & Sides

	SmartPoints™ value
Trader Joe's	
Artisan flatbread pizza, ½ pizza (140 g)	9
Bambino pizza formaggio, 1 pizza (113 g)	8
Roasted vegetable pizza, ⅓ pizza (113 g)	8
Pizza al pollo asado, 1 pizza (284 g)	13
Udi's Gluten Free	
Margherita pizza, ½ pizza (142 g)	10
Pepperoni pizza, ½ pizza (143 g)	12
Three cheese pizza, ½ pizza (142 g)	11
Uno	
Calzone, hearty Italian, 1 serving (125 g)	11
Calzone, Italian, personal size, 1 calzone (227 g)	21
Deep dish pizza, cheese, 1 serving (129 g)	11
Pizza, flatbread, margherita, ½ flatbread (130.5 g)	10
Pizza, margherita flatbread, ⅓ pizza (104 g)	8
VitaPizza	
Cheese and tomato, 1 pizza (152 g)	5
Meatless pepperoni supreme, 1 pizza (151 g)	5

Rice & Grain Sides

	SmartPoints™ value
Alessi	
Risotto, with porcini mushrooms, ¼ package dry (56 g)	6
Amy's	
Rice mac & cheese, 1 entrée (255 g)	14
Amy's Bowls	
Brown rice & vegetables, 1 each (283 g)	8
Brown rice, black-eyed peas and veggies, 1 bowl (255 g)	9

	SmartPoints™ value
Amy's Light & Lean	
Quinoa and black beans with butternut squash and chard, 1 bowl (227 g)	7
Back To Nature	
Granola, vanilla almond agave, ½ cup	7
Birds Eye Steamfresh	
Chicken flavored rice, 1 ½ cups	7
Long grain white rice, ¾ cup	5
Rice, southwestern style, 1 ½ cups frozen	7
Birds Eye Steamfresh Chef's Favorites	
Lightly sauced mushroom and green bean risotto, ½ package (142 g)	5
Birds Eye Steamfresh Selects	
Brown & wild rice with broccoli & carrots, 1 ½ cups frozen	4
Brown & wild rice, with corn, carrots & peas, 1 ½ cups	6
Multi-grain blend with spinach, tomato & onions, 1 ⅔ cups	5
Carolina	
Rice mix, saffron yellow with seasonings, 2 oz	5
Casbah Timeless Cuisine	
Cous cous, roasted garlic & olive oil, ¼ cup	4
CedarLane	
Baked spinach quinoa cake, 1 cake (43 g)	1
Chicken Helper	
Sweet & sour chicken mix, ⅓ cup	8
Chinese Cuisine	
Vegetable fried rice frozen, 1 cup	4
FarmRich	
Mozzarella sticks, breaded, 2 sticks (57 g)	6
Fit & Active	
Rosemary and olive oil quinoa and brown rice blend, ⅓ cup	7

Giant/Stop & Shop 90 Second

Brown rice, 1 cup	3

Green Giant Just for One

Cheesy rice and broccoli, 1 tray (120 g)	2

Green Giant Steamers

Brown rice risotto with carrots, peas, onion & kale, in a parmesan asiago sauce, 2 cups	9
Corn and black beans with brown rice in a southwestern style sauce, 1 ¾ cups frozen	9

Hamburger Helper Mexican

Rice & sauce mix, crunchy taco, ⅓ cup	5

InnovAsian Cuisine

Vegetable fried rice, 1 cup	4

Joseph's Mediterranean Cuisine

Taboule salad, party size, 2 Tbsp	1

Knorr Asian Sides

Teriyaki rice, ½ cup	7

Knorr Fiesta Sides

Spanish rice, ½ cup mix	7
Taco rice, mild, ½ cup	7

Knorr Menu Flavors

Rice sides, steak fajitas, ½ cup	6

Knorr Rice Sides

Cheddar broccoli rice and pasta blend, ½ cup	7
Chicken flavor rice and pasta blend, ½ cup mix	7
Rice & pasta blend, chicken broccoli, ⅔ cup	6
Rice medley, ½ cup	7
Rice pilaf, ½ cup	7
White cheddar queso rice and pasta blend, ½ cup mix	7

Knorr Rice Sides Menu Flavors

Buffalo chicken, ½ cup	6
Rice & pasta blend, creole garlic butter, ½ cup	7

Lean Cuisine Simply Favorites

Santa Fe style rice and beans, 1 package (294 g)	9

Lipton Rice Sides

Rice and orzo blend in a savory mushroom sauce, ½ cup	7

Lundberg Eco-Farmed

Creamy parmesan risotto, ⅓ package (53 g)	6

Lundberg Risotto

Risotto, butternut squash, 2 oz	6

Mahatma

Rice, long grain, saffron yellow seasonings, 2 oz dry rice mix	6

Meijer

Spanish rice, ½ cup	3

Minute

Multi-grain medley, ½ bag (43 g)	4

Minute Ready To Serve!

Brown and wild rice mix, 1 cup	7
Chicken rice mix, 1 container (125 g)	5
Fried rice mix, 1 cup	7

Near East

Broccoli and cheese couscous mix, 2 oz	5
Couscous mix, herbed chicken flavor, 2 oz	5
Couscous mix, mediterranean curry, 2 oz	5
Couscous mix, original plain, ⅓ cup	6
Couscous mix, parmesan, 2 oz	6
Couscous mix, pearled, roasted garlic & olive oil, 2 ½ oz	7
Couscous mix, wild mushroom & herb, 2 oz	5
Garlic and herb rice pilaf mix, 2 oz	5
Long grain & wild rice mix, garlic & herb, 1 cup	5
Rice pilaf mix, 2 oz	5
Rice pilaf mix, chicken, 2 oz	5

	SmartPoints™ value
Rice pilaf mix, original, 2 oz	5
Rice pilaf mix, toasted almond, 2 oz	6
Roasted garlic and olive oil couscous mix, 2 oz	5
Toasted pine nut couscous mix, ⅓ cup	6
Wild mushroom and herb rice pilaf mix, 2 oz dry	6
Near East Whole Grain Blends	
Brown rice pilaf, 2 oz dry	5
Wheat couscous, original plain, ⅓ cup dry	5
Wheat couscous, roasted garlic & olive oil, 2 oz dry	5
Old El Paso	
Rice, Mexican, 1 cup	8
P.F. Chang's Home Menu	
Rice, Chang's signature, 1 cup	5
Rice, steamed white, 1 cup	6
Steamed brown rice, 1 cup	6
Path of Life	
Organic quinoa & kale with garlic, olive oil and sea salt, 1 cup	4
Pictsweet Deluxe Sides	
Garden vegetable medley, with savory seasoning, ½ carton (99 g)	3
Qrunch	
Burger, quinoa, spicy Italian, 1 burger (91 g)	6
Ramona's	
Chile relleno, rice & beans, 1 meal (283 g)	23
Rice A Roni	
Broccoli cheese rice & vermicelli mix, ½ cup	6
Chicken flavor rice, 2 ½ oz	7
Creamy four cheese, 1 container (64 g)	8
Rice & vermicelli, chicken flavor, 2 oz	6

	SmartPoints™ value
Rice meal, creamy four cheese flavor, ¼ cup dry	7
Rice side, Mexican style, 2 oz dry	5
Rice, broccoli au gratin flavor, 2 ½ oz	8
Rice, chicken & broccoli flavor, 2 oz	5
Rice, lower sodium, chicken flavor, 2 ½ oz	6
Rice A Roni Express	
Long grain & wild rice, garlic & herb, 1 cup	8
Rice meal, Mexican, 1 cup	8
Rice A Roni Fast Cook	
Chicken, rice & vermicelli mix with chicken flavored seasoning, ½ cup	6
Rice A Roni Fast Cook	
Spanish rice & vermicelli mix with Spanish style seasonings, ½ cup	6
Rice A Roni Nature's Way	
Rice side, parmesan & romano cheese, 2 oz dry	7
Rice A Roni Whole Grain Blends	
Rice, Spanish, 2 oz dry	6
Rice Select	
Couscous, original, ¼ cup dry	4
Couscous, tri-color, ¼ cup dry	4
Seeds of Change	
Certified organic quinoa & brown rice with garlic, 1 oz	1
Rice, brown, quinoa & whole grain, uyuni, with garlic, 1 cup	7
ShopRite	
Cooked brown rice, ¾ cup	4
Simple Truth Organic	
Red quinoa and brown rice with garlic, olive oil and sea salt, 1 cup	7
Trader Joe's	
Garlic and butter mashed potatoes, ¼ cup dry	3
Israeli couscous, ⅓ cup dry	5
Rice medley, 1 cup	6

Prepared Foods, Salads & Sides

Trader Joe's Duo

Quinoa with vegetable melange, 1 cup cooked	7

Uncle Ben's

Long grain & wild rice, original recipe, ¼ cup dry	6
Long grain and wild rice fast cook recipe, ¼ cup	6

Uncle Ben's Country Inn

Broccoli rice au gratin, 1 cup cooked	6
Chicken and broccoli flavored rice, ¼ cup dry	6
Chicken and wild rice, ⅓ cup dry	6
Chicken flavored rice, ¼ cup dry	6
Rice pilaf, ⅓ cup dry	6

Uncle Ben's Ready Rice

Brown basmati, 1 cup	7
Butter and garlic flavored, 1 cup	7
Chicken flavored whole grain brown rice, 1 cup	6
Creamy four cheese flavored with vermicelli, 1 cup	7
Garden vegetable with peas carrots and corn, 1 cup	6
Long grain and wild rice, 1 cup	5
Rice pilaf with orzo pasta, 1 cup	6
Roasted chicken flavored with carrots and herbs rice, 1 cup	6
Spanish style rice, 1 cup	6
Teriyaki style, 1 cup	6

Uncle Ben's Ready Whole Grain Medley

Brown and wild rice, 1 cup	6
Quinoa and brown rice with garlic rice, 1 cup	6
Santa Fe flavored rice, 1 cup	6

Veetee Dine In

Basmati rice, ½ container (140 g)	5
Thai jasmine rice, ½ container (150 g)	4

Vigo

Black beans & rice, ⅓ cup	5
Mexican rice with corn, 1 cup prepared	5
Red beans & rice, ⅓ cup dry	5
Yellow rice, saffron, ⅓ cup dry	5

Vigo Saffron

Yellow rice, ⅓ cup	5

Zatarain's

Jambalaya mix, new orleans style, mild, 3 Tbsp	4
Spanish rice, new orleans style, ¼ cup dry mix	5
Yellow rice, ⅓ cup	6

Zatarain's New Orleans Style

Black beans & rice, ⅓ cup	6
Dirty rice, 1 cup	8
Dirty rice mix, 3 Tbsp	4
Dirty rice mix, family size, 1 cup	4
Gumbo mix with rice, 1 cup	2
Jambalaya mix, original, 3 Tbsp	4
Jambalaya mix, reduced sodium, 3 Tbsp	4
Jambalaya rice, 1 cup	9
Original jambalaya mix, ¼ cup dry	4
Red beans and rice, family size, 1 cup	5
Red beans and rice, original, ⅓ cup dry	5
Red beans and rice, reduced sodium, 1 cup prepared	5
Rice pilaf, ⅓ cup dry	6

Vegetable Sides

Alexia

Hashed browns, yukon select, ⅔ cup	2
Italian herb corn with sundried tomatoes, ½ cup	3
Onion rings, 6 rings (85 g)	8
Oven crinkles, classic, 13 pieces (85 g)	3

	SmartPoints™ value
Oven fries, olive oil, rosemary & garlic, family size, 8 pieces (85 g)	4
Oven reds, olive oil, parmesan & roasted garlic, 8 pieces (85 g)	3
Potato puffs, crispy seasoned, 14 pieces (84 g)	5
Rib cut bbq sweet potato fries with skin on, twelve 2-3" pieces	7
Southern sweet potato blend, ⅔ cup	3
Sweet potato, crinkle cut, sea salt & pepper, 30 pieces (84 g)	5
Waffle fries, family size, 1 cup	5
Allens Sunshine	
Blackeyed peas, southern style, with pork, ½ cup	3
Amy's Indian	
Paneer, mattar, 1 meal (284 g)	10
Paneer, palak, 1 meal (283 g)	9
Amy's Vegetarian Organic	
Traditional refried beans, ½ cup	4
Archer Farms	
Roasted garlic cauliflower, 1 package (99 g)	3
Aunt Nellie's	
Cabbage, red, sweet & sour, 2 Tbsp	1
B&M	
Baked beans, original, ½ cup	6
Banquet	
Cheesy rice and chicken, 1 meal (198 g)	6
Betty Crocker	
Homestyle sweet potatoes, ⅓ cup	4
Loaded potatoes, ⅓ cup as packaged	2
Mashed potato, savory roasted garlic, ⅓ cup as packaged	2
Mashed potatoes, homestyle, butter and herb potatoes, ⅓ cup dry	2
Mashed potatoes, homestyle, creamy butter, ⅓ cup as packaged	2

	SmartPoints™ value
Mashed potatoes, roasted garlic & cheddar, ⅓ cup dry	2
Potatoes, au gratin, ½ cup as packaged	3
Potatoes, scalloped, ½ cup	3
Potatoes, sour cream and chives, ⅓ cup	2
Potatoes, three cheese, ⅔ cup as packaged	3
Birds Eye	
Broccoli & cheese sauce, ½ cup	4
Green beans & spaetzle, in a bavarian style sauce, 1 cup	5
Vegetables & shells, in garlic butter sauce, 1 package (255 g)	10
Birds Eye Steamfresh	
Broccoli, with cheese sauce, lightly sauced, 1 cup	2
Roasted red potatoes, lightly sauced, with garlic butter sauce, 1 ¼ cups	7
Southwestern corn, specially seasoned, ⅔ cup	3
Super sweet corn, with butter sauce, lightly sauced, ¾ cup	4
Vegetables, lightly sauced, roasted red potatoes, with chive butter sauce, 1 cup	4
Birds Eye Steamfresh Chef's Favorites	
Lightly sauced creamed spinach, 1 ¼ cups	3
Lightly sauced primavera vegetable risotto, ½ package (142 g)	6
Lightly sauced roasted red potatoes and green beans, 1 ⅔ cups	4
Roasted potatoes, with bacon, in a cheese sauce, ⅔ cup	4
Tuscan vegetables, with marinara sauce, lightly sauced, 1 ¼ cups frozen	3
Blue Runner	
Red beans, creole cream style, ½ cup	3

Bob Evans

Diced potatoes, seasoned home fries, 3 oz	2
Mashed potatoes, original, family size, ½ cup	5
Shredded potatoes, seasoned hash browns, 3 oz	2
Sweet potatoes, mashed, ½ cup	6

Bob Evans Flavorful Selections

Loaded mashed potatoes, ½ cup	6

Boston Market

Mashed potatoes, homestyle, ½ cup	6

Bush's Best

Baked beans, barbecue, ½ cup	6
Baked beans, bold & spicy, ½ cup	4
Baked beans, Boston recipe, ½ cup	5
Baked beans, country style, ½ cup	6
Baked beans, homestyle, ½ cup	5
Baked beans, honey, ½ cup	6
Baked beans, maple cured bacon, ½ cup	5
Baked beans, onion, ½ cup	5
Baked beans, vegetarian, ½ cup	5
Country style baked beans, ½ cup	6
Grillin' beans, black bean fiesta, ½ cup	3
Grillin' beans, bourbon and brown sugar, ½ cup	6
Grillin' beans, smokehouse tradition, ½ cup	6
Grillin' beans, southern pit barbecue, ½ cup	7
Grillin' beans, steakhouse recipe, ½ cup	7
Grillin' beans, Texas ranchero, ½ cup	3
Reduced sodium vegetarian baked beans, ½ cup	5
Vegetarian baked beans, ½ cup	5

Bush's Best Chili Beans

Black beans in mild chili sauce, ½ cup	3

Campbell's

Pork & beans, ½ cup	5

Cape Cod Kettle Cooked

Potato chips, waffle cut, seasoned pepper, 1 oz	4

CedarLane

Eggplant parmesan with roasted vegetables and sun dried tomato sauce, 10 oz	10
Roasted chile relleno, 1 entrée (284 g)	12

Cedar's Premium Select

Fresh taboule salad, 2 Tbsp	1

Chef's Cupboard

Homestyle buttery instant mashed potatoes, ⅓ cup	4

Country Crock Side Dishes

Homestyle mashed potatoes, ⅔ cup	6

Crystal Farms Simply Potatoes

Garlic and herb hash browns, ⅔ cup	2

Dole Distictively Dole

Spinach cherry almond bleu kit, 1 cup	7

Dominex

Cutlets, eggplant, 3 oz	3

Dr. Praeger's

Pancakes, broccoli, 1 pancake (57 g)	2
Pancakes, spinach, 1 pancake (57 g)	2

Earthbound Farm Organic

Roasted sweet potato slices, ⅔ cup	7

Essential Everyday

Curly fries, 1 ⅓ cups	6
Hash browns, patties, 1 patty (64 g)	5

	SmartPoints™ value
Mashed potatoes, instant, ⅓ cup flakes	2
Sweet potato fries, 12 pieces (84 g)	5
Flav-R-Pac	
Baja roasted corn blend, ⅓ cup	4
Supreme stir fry, 1 cup	2
Garden Lites	
Soufflé, broccoli, 7 oz	4
Soufflé, butternut squash, 7 oz	7
Soufflé, roasted vegetable, 7 oz	4
Soufflé, spinach, 7 oz	4
Soufflé, zucchini, 7 oz	4
Golden	
Potato pancakes, 1 piece (37.6 g)	2
Vegetable pancakes, 1 piece (37.6 g)	2
Zucchini pancakes, 1 pancake (37 g)	2
Great Value	
Broccoli, with cheese sauce, steamable, 1 ⅓ cup	2
Green Giant	
Creamed spinach, ½ cup	3
Green Giant	
Green beans and butter sauce, 1 cup	2
Green Giant Just for One	
Broccoli and cheese sauce, 1 tray (120 g)	1
Broccoli carrots and Italian seasoning, 1 tray (99 g)	1
Cauliflower and cheese sauce, 1 tray (120 g)	1
Niblets corn and butter sauce, 1 tray (120 g)	3
Peas and corn in a basil butter sauce, 1 tray (120 g)	3
Green Giant Seasoned Steamers	
Mediterranean vegetable blend, ½ cup	3

	SmartPoints™ value
Green Giant Steamers	
Baby brussels sprouts and butter sauce, ⅔ cup frozen	2
Baby brussels sprouts and butter sauce family size, 1 cup frozen	2
Baby sweet peas and butter sauce, ¾ cup	3
Baby vegetable medley seasoned, ¾ cup frozen	2
Backyard grilled potatoes, 1 cup frozen	3
Basil vegetable medley, 1 ⅓ cups frozen	2
Broccoli and cheese sauce, ⅔ cup	2
Broccoli and zesty cheese sauce, ¾ cup	2
Broccoli cauliflower carrots and cheese sauce, ⅔ cup	2
Broccoli spears and butter sauce, 3 spears	2
Cauliflower and cheese sauce, ½ cup	2
Cauliflower broccoli and red peppers with brown rice in a butter sauce, 2 cups	6
Corn and butter sauce, bagged, ¾ cup frozen	3
Cut leaf spinach and butter sauce, ½ cup	1
Green beans and almonds, ¾ cup frozen	1
Healthy vision (mixed vegetables with rosemary butter sauce), 1 cup frozen	2
Healthy weight (mixed vegetables with butter sauce), 1 cup frozen	3
Honey glazed carrots, 1 cup	5
Italian herb vegetable blend with rice, 1 package (226 g)	5
Limited edition teriyaki mixed vegetables and brown rice, 1 package (226 g)	6

Prepared Foods, Salads & Sides

Mixed vegetables with barley and beans in a rosemary butter sauce, 1 package (226 g)	7
Niblets corn and butter sauce, boxed, ⅔ cup	4
Roasted potatoes with garlic and herbs, 1 ¼ cups frozen	6
Roasted red potatoes, green beans & rosemary butter sauce, 1 ¼ cups frozen	3
Shoepeg white corn and butter sauce, boxed, ¾ cup	4

Hannaford

Mashed potatoes, instant, ⅓ cup flakes	2

Heinz

Beans, vegetarian, premium, ½ cup	5
Beans, with tomato sauce, ½ cup	3

Hungry Jack

Mashed potatoes, ⅓ cup flakes	2
Potatoes, cheesy scalloped, ½ cup	3
Potatoes, hashbrown, premium, ⅓ cup dry	2
Potatoes, premium cheesy hashbrown, ½ cup	3

Hungry Jack Easy Mash'd

Mashed potatoes, creamy butter, ¼ cup dry mix	3
Potatoes, mashed, premium homestyle, ¼ cup	3

Ian's

Sweet potato fries, 2 ½ oz	3

Idahoan

Buttery homestyle mashed potatoes, ¼ cup	4
Mashed potatoes, ⅓ cup mix	2
Mashed potatoes, applewood smoked bacon flavor, ¼ cup dry	3
Mashed potatoes, butter & herb, ¼ cup	4
Mashed potatoes, flavored, buttery golden selects, ¼ cup dry mix	4

Mashed potatoes, four cheese, ½ cup mix	4
Mashed potatoes, loaded baked, ¼ cup	4
Potato slices, au gratin, ⅔ cup	3
Red potatoes, premium, steakhouse bacon & ranch, ½ cup dry	4
Red potatoes, premium, steakhouse scalloped, ½ cup dry	4
Roasted garlic mashed potatoes, ¼ cup mix	4

Idahoan Baby Reds

Mashed potatoes, ¼ cup	4

KC Masterpiece Baked Beans

Hickory brown sugar baked beans, ½ cup	6

Kirkland Signature

Artichoke hearts, 2 pieces (28 g)	1

Kroger

Hash brown patties, 1 patty (63 g)	5
Potato nuggets, tater bites, 8 pieces (85 g)	5
Potato nuggets, tater rounds, 11 pieces (85 g)	5
Potatoes, French fried, French fries, 17 fries (85 g)	4
Potatoes, French fried, shoestring fries, 45 fries (85 g)	4
Potatoes, French fried, steak fries, 8 pieces (85 g)	4
Potatoes, French fried, with skins, potato wedges, 9 pieces (85 g)	3
Roasted redskin potatoes, ⅔ cup	3
Sweet potato waffle fries, 1 cup	5

La Costena

Charro beans, ½ cup	2

La Fe

Tostones, 3 oz	5

Larry's

Mashed potatoes, cheddar cheese, 1 tray (142 g)	7

Prepared Foods, Salads & Sides

Prepared Foods, Salads & Sides

	SmartPoints™ value
Lean Cuisine Simple Favorites	
Cheddar potatoes with broccoli, 1 package (290 g)	7
Stuffed cabbage, 1 package (269 g)	7
Lucks	
Blackeye peas, seasoned with pork, ½ cup	3
Marie Callender's	
Scalloped potatoes & ham, in a creamy cheese sauce, 1 cup	11
Marie Callender's Signature Family Meals	
Scalloped potatoes and ham, 1 cup	10
Marketside	
Green beans and red potatoes with roasted garlic butter, ¾ cup	7
McCain	
Baby cakes, homestyle, 4 pieces (76 g)	5
Potatoes, seasoned crinkle cut, 3 oz	5
Smiles, 3 oz	5
McCain Premium	
Oven fries, golden crisp, seasoned, 3 oz	4
McCain Roasters	
Oven roast potatoes, all American, 3 oz	4
Michael Angelo's	
Eggplant parmesan, 1 cup	8
Eggplant parmesan, with tomato sauce & mozzarella cheese, 6 oz	9
Morningstar Farms Meal Starters	
Chipotle black bean crumbles, ½ cup	1
Mr. Dell's	
All natural shredded hash browns, 1 cup	2
Mrs. T's	
Pierogies, potato & 5 cheese blend, 3 pierogies (114 g)	5

	SmartPoints™ value
Nathan's Famous	
French fries, crinkle cut, jumbo, 3 oz	4
Onion rings, battered, thick sliced, 6 pieces (85 g)	6
Omaha Steaks	
Potatoes au gratin, 1 piece (83 g)	6
Stuffed baked potatoes, 1 piece (163 g)	10
Ore-Ida	
Easy breakfast potatoes, extra crispy, ¾ cup	5
Golden crinkles, 12 pieces (84 g)	4
Golden crinkles, extra crispy, 14 pieces (84 g)	5
Golden crinkles, family size, 15 pieces (84 g)	4
Golden crinkles, value size!, 12 pieces (48 g)	4
Golden fries, 14 pieces (84 g)	4
Golden fries, family size, 3 oz	4
Golden twirls, 3 oz	5
Seasoned crinkles, extra crispy, 13 pieces (84 g)	5
Shoestrings, 3 oz	4
Steak fries, 7 pieces (84 g)	3
Steak fries, country style, 8 pieces (84 g)	4
Sweet potato crinkle fries, 31 pieces (90 g)	5
Sweet potato fries, 22 pieces (84 g)	6
Sweet potato steak fries, 8 pieces (90 g)	5
Tater tots, 9 pieces (86 g)	5
Tater tots, abc, 9 pieces (81 g)	5
Tater tots, extra crispy, 12 pieces (86 g)	5
Tater tots, family pack!, 9 pieces (86 g)	5
Tater tots, family size, 9 pieces (86 g)	5
Tater tots, mini, 19 pieces (87 g)	5

	SmartPoints™ value
Tater tots, onion, 9 pieces (90 g)	5
Waffle fries, 8 pieces (84 g)	5
Zesties!, 12 pieces (84 g)	5
Zesty twirls, 1 ¼ cups	5
Ore-Ida Bold & Crispy	
French fried potatoes, seasoned, spicy sriracha fries, 3 oz	6
French fried potatoes, smoky bbq oven chips, 8 pieces (84 g)	6
Steakhouse fries, garlic and pepper, 7 pieces (84 g)	6
Ore-Ida Easy Fries	
Golden crinkles, extra crispy, 22 pieces (84 g)	6
Ore-Ida Extra Crispy	
Easy tater tots crispy crowns, 14 pieces (84 g)	7
Ore-Ida Golden Crinkles	
French fried potatoes, 12 pieces (85 g)	4
Patel's	
Roasted eggplant, baingan bharta, 1 cup	4
Pictsweet	
Stir-fry, Chinese style vegetables, family size, 1 ¼ cups	2
Pictsweet Deluxe Sides	
Brussels sprouts, baby, in butter sauce, ½ carton (99 g)	2
Tuscan vegetable medley, with extra virgin olive oil, ½ carton (99 g)	1
PictSweet Steam'ables	
Asian vegetables, seasoned, 1 cup	1
Spring vegetables, seasoned, ¾ cup	1
Poppers	
Stuffed jalapeños, cream cheese, 3 pieces (98 g)	11
Ranch Style	
Beans, ½ cup	4

	SmartPoints™ value
Ready Pac Ready Snax	
Snack pac, veggie, cheese & pretzel, 1 container (122 g)	6
Snack pac, veggies & cheese with ranch dip, 1 container (116 g)	5
Red Robin	
Onion rings, crispy, 3 rings (94 g)	8
Safeway	
Hash brown patties, 1 patty (64 g)	5
Hash brown potatoes, shredded, 3 oz	2
Hash browns, shredded potatoes, country style, 1 cup	2
San Miguel	
Chilaquiles, red, ¼ package (105 g)	6
Savannah Classics	
Original hushpuppies, 3 pieces (49 g)	4
Season's Choice	
Hash brown potato patties, old fashioned, 1 patty (60 g)	4
ShopRite	
Instant mashed potatoes, ⅓ cup flakes	2
Shur Fine	
Hashbrown patties, 1 piece (63 g)	4
Shurfresh	
Mashed potatoes, instant, butter, ½ cup mix	4
Signature Cafe	
Bbq beef brisket, smoky, 1 cup	9
Signature Cafe World Cuisine	
Roasted root vegetables, 3 oz	3
Simply Potatoes	
Shredded hash browns, ½ cup	2
Stouffer's	
Stuffed peppers, family size, 1 pepper	7

Prepared Foods, Salads & Sides

Prepared Foods, Salads & Sides

	SmartPoints™ value
Stouffer's Craveable Recipes	
Cheddar potato bake, ½ package (142 g)	9
Corn soufflé, ½ cup	5
Spinach soufflé, ½ cup	5
Stouffer's Family Style Recipes	
Side dish, hash brown potato casserole, 1 serving (181 g)	10
Stouffer's Homestyle Classics	
Stuffed pepper, 1 package (283 g)	7
Stouffer's Homestyle Selects	
Stuffed peppers, large size, 1 pepper	6
T.G.I. Friday's	
Cheese and bacon loaded fries, ⅓ tray (85 g)	7
T.J. Farms	
Shredded hashbrowns, 1 cup	2
Tandoor Chef	
Palak (saag) paneer, 5 oz	6
Tasty Bite 1 Step 1 Minute	
Madras lentils, 5 oz	5
The Little Potato Company	
Garlic parsley fresh creamer potatoes, ¼ package (114 g)	2
Savory herb seasoned creamer potatoes, ¼ package (114 g)	2
Tops	
Instant mashed potatoes, Idaho, ⅓ cup	2
Trader Joe's	
Artichoke antipasto, 2 Tbsp	3
Cowboy caviar salsa, 2 Tbsp	1
Eggplant cutlets, 3 oz	5
Handsome cut potato fries, 3 oz	4
Hashbrowns, 1 oz	2
Mashed potatoes, 8 pieces (112 g)	3
Multigrain blend with vegetables, ⅓ package (140 g)	6
Roasted brussels sprouts (ready to eat), ½ cup	2

	SmartPoints™ value
Roasted mashed sweet potatoes, 5 pieces (85 g)	3
Shredded hash browns, 3 oz	2
Steamed lentils (ready to eat warm or cold), ½ cup	4
Sweet potato tots, 3 oz	5
Traditional latkes potato pancakes, 2 pancakes (75 g)	4
Vegetable fried rice, 1 cup	5
Vegetable masala burger, 1 burger (71 g)	4
Zucchini fries, 1 cup	4
Trader Ming's	
Asian vegetables with beijing style soy sauce, ⅓ package (151 g)	3
Van Camps	
Pork and beans, in tomato sauce, ½ cup	4
Van Camps Beanee Weenee	
Beans, original, 1 can (220 g)	8
Veggie Patch	
Falafel chickpea balls, 4 pieces (84 g)	4
Velveeta	
Cheesy au gratin potatoes, ½ cup	6
Cheesy potatoes, hash browns, 1 serving (51 g)	5
Cheesy potatoes, southwest diced, 1 serving (55 g)	5
Wegman's	
Cabbage rolls, 1 piece (198.5 g)	5
Chick pea salad, tri-color, ½ cup	4
Instant mashed potatoes, roasted garlic, ⅓ cup	3
Wegman's Italian Classics	
Eggplant rollatini, 3 ½ oz	6
WelcomeHomeCafe	
Twice baked potatoes, bacon & cheddar, 1 potato (227 g)	9
Zatarain's	
Red beans & rice, 1 cup	7

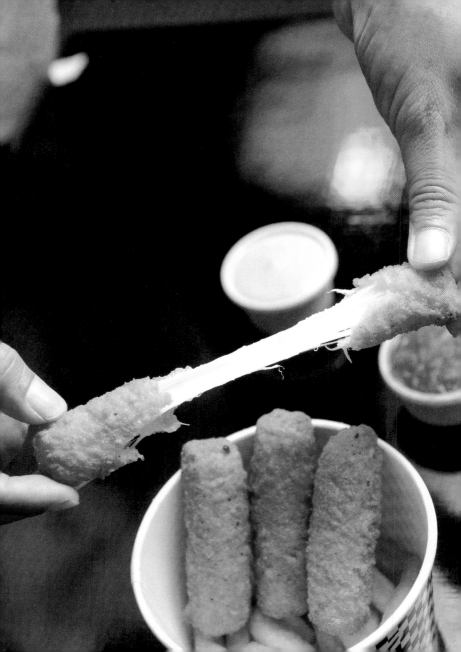

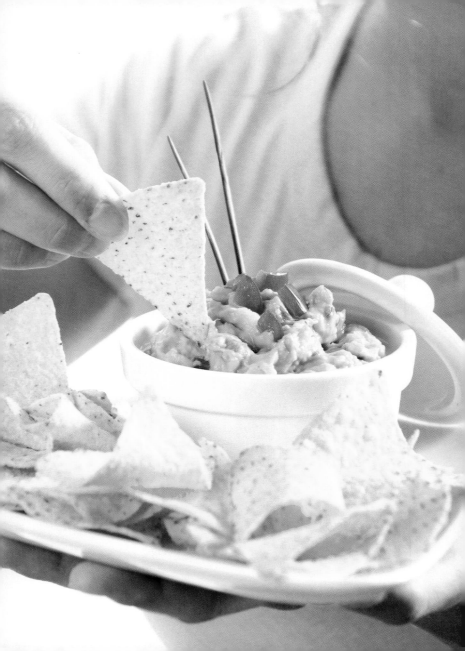

snacks

Snacks

Bagel & Pita Snacks

365
Pita chips, 7 chips (28 g)	3

Athenos
Pita chips, baked, original, 11 chips (28 g)	3
Pita chips, baked, roasted garlic & herb, 11 chips (28 g)	3
Pita chips, baked, whole wheat, 11 chips (28 g)	3

Clancy's Baked
Parmesan garlic and herb pita chips, 11 chips (29 g)	5

Glutino
Bagel chips, bagel chips, original, 7 pieces (30 g)	4

Kangaroo
Pita chips, sea salt, 9 chips (28 g)	3

New York Style
Bagel crisps, original, cinnamon raisin, 6 crisps (28 g)	5
Bagel crisps, original, everything, 6 crisps (28 g)	4
Bagel crisps, original, plain, 6 crisps (28 g)	4
Bagel crisps, original, roasted garlic, 6 crisps (28 g)	4
Bagel crisps, original, sea salt, 6 crisps (28 g)	4
Pita chips, parmesan, garlic & herb, 11 chips (29 g)	5

Open Nature
Pita chips, original, with sea salt, 9 chips (28 g)	3

Stacy's
Cinnamon sugar pita chips, 7 chips (28 g)	5
Fire roasted jalapeño pita chips, 9 chips (28 g)	4
Pita chips, baked, naturally cheddar, 9 chips (28 g)	4

Pita chips, baked, parmesan garlic & herb, 9 chips (28 g)	4
Pita chips, multigrain, 9 chips (28 g)	4
Pita chips, salted caramel, 7 chips (28 g)	4
Pita crisps, c'est la cheese, 11 chips (28 g)	4
Pita crisps, perfectly thymed, 11 chips (28 g)	4
Simply cocoa chips, 7 chips (28 g)	5

Trader Joe's
Multigrain pita chips, 8 chips (28 g)	4
Pita chips, 1 oz	4
Pita chips with cinnamon and sugar, 8 chips (28 g)	4
Pita chips with sea salt, 10 chips (28 g)	4
Reduced guilt multigrain pita chips with sesame seeds, 1 oz	3
Reduced guilt pita chips with sea salt, 1 serving (28 g)	3

Trader Joe's Reduced Guilt
Pita chips with sea salt, 8 chips (28 g)	3

Cereal Bars & Snack Bars

Abbott Perfectly Simple by Zone Perfect
Chocolate peanut butter nutrition bar, 2 bars (50 g)	8
Oatmeal chocolate chip nutrition bar, 1 bar (45 g)	7
Toasted coconut nutrition bars, 1 bar (45 g)	8

Annie's Organic
Chocolate chip chewy granola bar, 1 bar (28 g)	5

Atkins Day Break
Snack bar, chocolate chip crisp, 1 bar (35 g)	4

Atkins Meal

Bar, blueberry Greek yogurt, 1 bar (48 g)	6
Bar, chocolate chip cookie dough, 1 bar (60 g)	8
Bar, chocolate peanut butter, 1 bar (60 g)	8
Bar, chocolate peanut butter pretzel, 1 bar (48 g)	6
Bar, cinnamon bun, 1 bar (48 g)	6
Bar, cookies n' creme, 1 bar (48 g)	6
Bar, mudslide, 1 bar (48 g)	6
Bar, peanut butter granola, 1 bar (48 g)	5
Bar, strawberry almond, 1 bar (48 g)	6

Atkins Snack

Bar, caramel chocolate nut roll, 1 bar (44 g)	6
Bar, caramel double chocolate crunch, 1 bar (44 g)	5
Bar, cashew trail mix, 1 bar (40 g)	6
Bar, coconut almond delight, 1 bar (44 g)	9
Bar, dark chocolate almond coconut crunch, 1 bar (40 g)	7
Bar, triple chocolate, 1 bar (40 g)	5
Daybreak bar, chocolate hazelnut, 1 bar (40 g)	6
Daybreak bar, chocolate oatmeal fiber, 1 bar (40 g)	4
Daybreak bar, cranberry almond, 1 bar (35 g)	5
Daybreak bar, peanut butter fudge crisp, 1 bar (37 g)	5

Atkins Treat

Endulge caramel nut chew bar, 1 bar (34 g)	5
Endulge chocolate caramel mousse bar, 1 bar (34 g)	5
Endulge chocolate coconut bar, 1 bar (40 g)	8

Endulge nutty fudge brownie, 1 bar (40 g)	6
Endulge peanut caramel cluster bar, 1 bar (34 g)	4

Balance Bar

Nutrition energy bar, cookie ough, 1 bar (50 g)	8
Nutrition energy bar, dark chocolate coconut, 1 bar (45 g)	7
Nutrition energy bar, dark chocolate crunch, 1 bar (45 g)	7
Nutrition energy bar, dark chocolate peanut, 1 bar (45 g)	7
Nutrition energy bar, yogurt honey peanut, 1 bar (50 g)	8

Balance Bar Gold

Nutrition energy bar, caramel nut blast, 1 bar (50 g)	8
Nutrition energy bar, chocolate peanut butter, 1 bar (50 g)	8
Nutriton energy bar, chocolate mint cookie crunch, 1 bar (50 g)	8

BelVita Soft Baked

Mixed berry breakfast biscuits, 1 pack (50 g)	7

Betty Crocker

Brownie bar, caramel, 1 bar (48 g)	9

Cascadian Farm

Granola bars, organic, oatmeal raisin, kid-sized, 1 bar (22 g)	3

Cascadian Farm Organic

Granola bar, sweet & salty peanut pretzel, 1 bar (35 g)	7
Granola bars, chewy, dark chocolate almond, 1 bar (35 g)	5
Granola bars, chewy, harvest berry, 1 bar (35 g)	5
Granola bars, chewy, vanilla chip, 1 bar (35 g)	6
Granola bars, chewy. chocolate chip, 1 bar (35 g)	6

Snacks

SmartPoints™ value

Granola bars, crunchy, oats & honey, 2 bars (40 g)	6
Granola bars, crunchy, peanut butter, 2 bars (40 g)	7
Cascadian Farm Sweet & Salty	
Granola bars, chewy, peanut pretzel, 1 bar (35 g)	7
Caveman Foods	
Dark chocolate almond coconut bar, 1 package (40 g)	8
Fruit & nut bar, wild blueberry nut, 1 bar (40 g)	7
Cheerios	
Milk 'n cereal bar, 1 bar (40 g)	7
Cinnamon Toast Crunch	
Milk n cereal bars, 1 bar (45 g)	7
Milk 'n cereal bars, 1 bar (45 g)	8
Treats, cinnamon (24g bar), 1 bar (24 g)	4
Clif	
Energy bar, blueberry crisp, 1 bar (68 g)	9
Energy bar, chocolate almond fudge, 1 bar (68 g)	9
Energy bar, chocolate brownie, 1 bar (68 g)	9
Energy bar, chocolate chip peanut crunch, 1 bar (68 g)	10
Energy bar, cool mint chocolate, 1 bar (68 g)	9
Energy bar, iced gingerbread, 1 bar (68 g)	10
Energy bar, oatmeal raisin walnut, 1 bar (68 g)	9
Energy bar, peanut toffee buzz, 1 bar (68 g)	9
Energy bar, spiced pumpkin pie, 1 bar (68 g)	10
Energy bar, white chocolate macadamia nut, 1 bar (68 g)	9

SmartPoints™ value

Clif Builder's	
Chocolate mint protein bar, 1 bar (68 g)	10
Chocolate peanut butter protein bar, 1 bar (34 g)	5
Protein bar, chocolate, 1 bar (68 g)	10
Protein bar, chocolate mint, 1 bar (68 g)	10
Protein bar, crunchy peanut butter, 1 bar (68 g)	11
Protein bar, peanut butter, 1 bar (68 g)	10
Protein bar, vanilla almond, 1 bar (68 g)	10
Clif Crunch	
Granola bar, chocolate chip, 2 bars (42 g)	7
Granola bar, chocolate peanut butter, 2 bars (42 g)	7
Granola bar, peanut butter, 2 bars (42 g)	7
Granola bar, white chocolate macadamia nut, 2 bars (42 g)	7
Clif Kid	
Chocolate brownie organic z bar, 1 bar (36 g)	5
Chocolate chip organic z bar, 1 bar (36 g)	5
Chocolate chip protein z bar, 1 bar (36 g)	5
Organic iced oatmeal cookie z bar, 1 bar (36 g)	5
Z bar protein peanut butter chocolate flavor whole grain protein snack, 1 bar (36 g)	5
Z bar, organic, honey graham, 1 bar (36 g)	5
Z bar, protein, chocolate mint, 1 bar (36 g)	5
Zbar, organic, chocolate chip, 1 bar (36 g)	5

Snacks

Clif Kid Organic Z Bar

Iced oatmeal cookie energy bar, 1 bar (36 g)	5

CLIF Kid ZBar

Organic chocolate brownie bar, 1 bar (36 g)	5

Clif Mini

Chocolate chip energy bar, 1 bar (28 g)	4

Clif Mojo

Dark chocolate almond sea salt trail mix bar, 1 bar (40 g)	7
Trail mix bar, sweet & salty, chocolate almond coconut, 1 bar (45 g)	8
Trail mix bar, sweet & salty, mountain mix, 1 bar (45 g)	6
Trail mix bar, sweet & salty, peanut butter pretzel, 1 bar (45 g)	7

Clif Mojo Dark Chocolate

Dark chocolate almond sea salt trail mix bar, 1 bar (40 g)	7
Dark chocolate cherry almond trail mix bar, 1 bar (40 g)	7

Corazonas

Chocolate chip mini oatmeal square, 1 square (25 g)	3
Oatmeal square, mini, peanut butter, 1 square (25 g)	3

EAS Lean 15

Nutrition bar, chocolate peanut butter, 1 bar (50 g)	7

Eating Right

Chewy bar, chocolate chip, 1 bar (23 g)	4
Chewy bar, peanut butter, 1 bar (23 g)	4

Elisabeth Hasselbeck's NoGii

Chocolate caramel bliss protein d'lites bar, 1 bar (28 g)	4

Enjoy Life

Snack bars, soft and chewy, cocoa loco, 1 bar (28 g)	5

Essential Everyday

Granola bar, chewy, chocolate chunk, 1 bar (24 g)	4

Fiber One

Blueberry streusel bar, 1 bar (40 g)	6
Chocolate mocha chewy bar, 1 bar (40 g)	6
Chocolate peanut butter meal bar, 1 bar (45 g)	6
Dark chocolate almond meal bar, 1 bar (45 g)	6
Mint fudge brownie, 1 brownie (25 g)	4
Oats and caramel chewy bar, 1 bar (40 g)	6
Oats and chocolate chewy bar, 1 bar (40 g)	6
Oats and strawberries with almonds chewy bar, 1 bar (40 g)	5
Protein peanut butter chewy bars, 1 bar (33 g)	5
Soft baked oatmeal raisin cookie, 1 bar (31 g)	5
Strawberry Greek yogurt meal bar, 1 bar (45 g)	6
Strawberry streusel bar, 1 bar (40 g)	6
Trail mix chewy bar, 1 bar (38 g)	5

Fiber One 90 Calorie

Caramel sea salt soft baked bar, 1 bar (25 g)	4
Chocolate caramel and pretzel chewy bar, 1 bar (23 g)	4
Chocolate chewy bar, 1 bar (23 g)	4
Chocolate peanut butter chewy bar, 1 bar (23 g)	4
Gingerbread bars, 1 bar (25 g)	4
Lemon bar, 1 bar (25 g)	4

Snacks

Snacks

	SmartPoints™ value
Fiber One 90 Calorie Brownie	
Chocolate peanut butter, 1 brownie (25 g)	4
Fiber One Meal Bar	
Sweet and salty nut, 1 bar (45 g)	6
Fiber One Protein	
Caramel nut chewy bar, 1 bar (33 g)	5
Coconut almond chewy bar, 1 bar (33 g)	6
Cookies and creme chewy bar, 1 bar (33 g)	5
Peanut butter chewy bar, 1 bar (33 g)	5
Fiber Plus Antioxidants	
Chewy bar, caramel coconut fudge, 1 bar (36 g)	5
Chewy bar, chocolate chip, 1 bar (36 g)	5
Chewy bar, chocolate chip, 1 bar (36 g)	5
Chewy bar, chocolate chip, value pack, 1 bar (36 g)	5
Chewy bar, dark chocolate almond, 1 bar (36 g)	5
Chewy bar, dark chocolate almond, 1 bar (36 g)	5
Chewy bars, chocolatey peanut butter, 1 bar (36 g)	5
Chewy bars, protein, mixed nut, 1 bar (40 g)	6
Chewy bars, protein, peanut, 1 bar (40 g)	6
Fit & Active	
Caramel nut protein energy bar, 1 bar (50 g)	7
Chocolate peanut butter protein meal bars, 1 bar (45 g)	7
Chocolatey pretzel light & crispy vitality cereal bars, 1 bar (22 g)	4
Cranberry walnut protein meal bars, 1 bar (45 g)	6

	SmartPoints™ value
Strawberry fruit and grain cereal bars, 1 bar (37 g)	6
Wild berry fruit crisps, 3 crisps (44 g)	7
Giant	
Crunchy granola bars, oats and honey, 2 bars (42 g)	7
Granola bars, chewy, chocolate chip, 1 bar (24 g)	4
Glutino	
Breakfast bars, gluten free, strawberry, 1 bar (40 g)	6
Glutino Gluten Free	
Breakfast bars, blueberry, 1 bar (40 g)	5
Gnu Foods FiberLove	
Peanut chocolate chip soft baked fiber bar, 1 bar (45 g)	6
Gnu Foods Flavor & Fiber	
Cinnamon raisin bar, 1 bar (45 g)	5
Great Value	
Cereal bars, 90 calorie, blueberry, 1 bar (23 g)	4
Cereal bars, 90 calorie, strawberry, 1 bar (23 g)	4
Chewy bars, high fiber, oats & chocolate, 1 bar (40 g)	6
Chewy bars, high fiber, oats & peanut butter, 1 bar (40 g)	6
Chewy granola bars, 90 calorie, chocolate chunk, 1 bar (24 g)	4
Fruit & grain bar, low fat, apple cinnamon, 1 bar (37 g)	6
Fruit & grain bars, low fat, blueberry, 1 bar (37 g)	6
Fruit & grain bars, low fat, mixed berry, 1 bar (37 g)	6
Fruit & grain bars, low fat, strawberry, 1 bar (37 g)	6
Granola bars, chewy, sweet salty peanut, 1 bar (35 g)	7

	SmartPoints™ value
Granola bars, chewy, sweet & salty, almond, 1 bar (35 g)	6
Granola bars, crunchy, oats & honey, 2 bars (40 g)	7
Peanut butter and dark chocolate chewy protein bar, 1 bar (40 g)	6
Peanut, almond and dark chocolate chewy protein bar, 1 bar (40 g)	6
Health Warrior	
Chia bar, acai berry, 1 bar (25 g)	3
Chia bar, chocolate peanut butter, 1 bar (25 g)	4
Chia bar, coconut, 1 bar (25 g)	4
H-E-B Multi-Fit Bars	
Bars, raspberry vanilla, 1 bar (20 g)	4
Herbalife	
Protein bars, chocolate peanut, 1 bar (35 g)	5
Protein bars, peanut butter, 1 bar (40 g)	4
Protein bars, vanilla almond, 1 bar (35 g)	5
Hy-Vee	
Granola bars, chewy, low fat chocolate chunk, 1 bar (24 g)	4
Kashi	
Apple cobbler soft n' chewy bars, 1 bar (40 g)	5
Berry lemonade with chia chewy granola bars, 1 bar (35 g)	4
Berry muffin soft n' chewy bars, 1 bar (40 g)	5
Chewy granola bar honey almond flax, 1 bar (35 g)	4
Chewy granola bar peanut peanut butter, 1 bar (35 g)	4
Chewy granola bar trail mix, 1 bar (35 g)	5
Chocolate almond & sea salt with chia chewy granola bars, 1 bar (35 g)	5

	SmartPoints™ value
Chocolate almond and sea salt chewy granola bar with chia, 1 bar (35 g)	5
Chocolate almond and sea salt with chia chewy granola bars, 1 bar (35 g)	5
Chocolate chip chia crunchy granola and seed bars, 2 bars (40 g)	7
Dark mocha almond chewy granola bars, 1 bar (35 g)	4
Granola bars, crunchy, honey toasted 7 grain, 2 bars (40 g)	6
Honey oat flax crunchy granola and seed bars, 2 bars (40 g)	6
Trail mix chewy granola bars, 1 bar (35 g)	5
Kashi Chewy Granola Bar	
Cherry dark chocolate, 1 bar (35 g)	4
Chocolate raspberry, 1 bar (32 g)	4
Dark chocolate coconut, 1 bar (32 g)	5
Kashi TLC	
Cereal bars, soft-baked, blackberry graham, 1 bar (35 g)	4
Cereal bars, soft-baked, cherry vanilla, 1 bar (35 g)	4
Cereal bars, soft-baked, ripe strawberry, 1 bar (35 g)	4
Crunchy granola bar, pumpkin spice flax, 2 bars (40 g)	6
Crunchy granola bars, roasted almond crunch, 2 bars (40 g)	6
Fruit & grain bars, dark chocolate coconut, 1 bar (32 g)	5
Granola bar, chewy, peanut peanut butter, 1 bar (35 g)	4
Granola bar, chewy, trail mix, 1 bar (35 g)	5
Granola bar, honey almond flax, 1 bar (35 g)	4
Granola bars, chewy, cherry dark chocolate, 1 bar (35 g)	4

Snacks

	SmartPoints™ value
Granola bars, chewy, dark mocha almond, 1 bar (35 g)	4
Granola bars, chewy, honey almond flax, 1 bar (35 g)	4
Granola bars, chewy, peanut peanut butter, 1 bar (35 g)	4
Granola bars, crunchy, pumpkin spice flax, 2 bars (40 g)	6
Granola bars, peanutty dark chocolate layered, 1 bar (32 g)	5
Soft baked bar, blackberry graham, 1 bar (35 g)	4
Soft baked bar, ripe strawberry, 1 bar (35 g)	4
Kellogg's	
Cereal bars, cran-vanilla crunch, 1 bar (28 g)	5
Cranberry walnut protein meal bar, 1 bar (45 g)	7
Kellogg's Fiber Plus Antioxidants	
Chewy bar, chocolatey peanut butter, 1 bar (36 g)	5
Kellogg's Nutri-Grain	
Cereal bar, apple cinnamon, 1 bar (37 g)	5
Cereal bar, blueberry, 1 bar (37 g)	5
Cereal bar, raspberry, 1 bar (37 g)	5
Cereal bar, strawberry, 1 bar (37 g)	5
Cereal bars with wheat, whole-grain oats and fruit, strawberry, 1 bar (37 g)	6
Cereal bars, 16 apple cinnamon, 32 strawberry, 1 bar (37 g)	6
Cereal bars, apple cinnamon, 1 bar (37 g)	5
Cereal bars, apple cinnamon, value pack, 1 bar (37 g)	5
Cereal bars, assorted, 1 bar (37 g)	5
Cereal bars, blackberry, 1 bar (37 g)	5
Cereal bars, blueberry, 1 bar (37 g)	5

	SmartPoints™ value
Cereal bars, cherry, 1 bar (37 g)	5
Cereal bars, mixed berry, 1 bar (37 g)	5
Cereal bars, raspberry, 1 bar (37 g)	5
Cereal bars, strawberry, 1 bar (37 g)	5
Cereal bars, strawberry, value pack, 1 bar (37 g)	5
Granola bars, fruit crunch, apple cobbler, 2 bars (42 g)	8
Yogurt bars, strawberry, 1 bar (37 g)	5
Kellogg's Nutri-Grain Crunch	
Chocolatey chip granola bars, 2 bars (42 g)	8
Chocolatey toffee granola bars, 2 bars (42 g)	8
Kellogg's Nutri-Grain Fruit & Oat Harvest	
Blueberry bliss hearty fruit and oat bar, 1 bar (50 g)	7
Kellogg's Nutri-Grain Fruit Crunch	
Granola bars, strawberry parfait, 2 bars (42 g)	8
Kellogg's Rice Krispies Treats	
Blasted chocolatey chip marshmallow crispy squares, 1 bar (22 g)	4
Blasted double chocolatey chunk crispy squares, 1 bar (22 g)	5
Blasted s'mores crispy marshmallow squares, 1 bar (22 g)	4
Original crispy marshmallow squares monsters treats sheet (20 servings), 1 serving (45 g)	8
Kellogg's Special K	
Bars, cranberry apple, 1 bar (23 g)	4
Berry medley snack bar (variety pack), 1 bar (25 g)	4
Blueberry bliss snack bar, 1 bar (25 g)	4

Snacks

Caramel peanut protein meal bar, 1 bar (45 g)	7
Cereal bar, blueberry, 1 bar (23 g)	4
Cereal bar, chocolatey drizzle, 1 bar (22 g)	4
Cereal bar, chocolatey pretzel, 1 bar (22 g)	4
Cereal bar, honey nut, 1 bar (22 g)	3
Cereal bar, raspberry cheesecake, 1 bar (22 g)	4
Chocolate caramel protein bar, 1 bar (45 g)	7
Granola bars, protein & fiber, chocolatey peanut butter, 1 bar (27 g)	4
Protein meal bar, double chocolate, 1 bar (45 g)	7
Protein snack bar, chocolate delight, 1 bar (26 g)	5
Red berries cereal bar, 1 bar (23 g)	4
Salted caramel chocolate snack bars, 1 bar (25 g)	4
Salted pretzel chocolate snack bars, 1 bar (25 g)	4
Strawberry cereal bar, 1 bar (23 g)	4
Vanilla crisp cereal bar, 1 bar (22 g)	4

Kellogg's Special K Bliss

Cereal bars, raspberry, 1 bar (22 g)	4

Kellogg's Special K Cereal Bars

Chocolatey strawberry, 1 bar (23 g)	4

Kellogg's Special K Moments

Caramel pretzel bliss indulgent snack bites, 1 pouch (16 g)	3
Dreamy coconut indulgent snack bites, 1 pouch (16 g)	3

Kellogg's Special K Nourish

Cranberry almond bars, 1 bar (45 g)	6

Kellogg's Special K Pastry Crisps

Strawberry flavor bars (variety pack), 2 crisps (25 g)	4

Kellogg's Special K Protein

Chocolate peanut butter meal bar, 1 bar (45 g)	7
Chocolatey peanut butter granola snack bar, 1 bar (27 g)	4
Greek yogurt and fruit granola snack bar, 1 bar (27 g)	4
Meal bar, chocolate peanut butter, 1 bar (45 g)	7
Meal bar, strawberry, 1 bar (45 g)	7
Snack bars, almond honey oat granola, 1 bar (27 g)	4

Kellogg's Special K Protein Granola Bars

Dark chocolate granola, 1 bar (27 g)	4
Almond honey nut, 1 bar (27 g)	4

Kidz Zone Perfect

Yellow cupcake nutrition bar, 1 bar (36 g)	6

Kind

Almond and coconut fruit and nut bar, 1 bar (40 g)	8
Caramel almond and sea salt nuts and spices bar, 1 bar (40 g)	7
Dark chocolate chili almond nuts and spices bar, 1 bar (40 g)	7
Dark chocolate nuts and sea salt nut and spice bar, 1 bar (40 g)	7
Fruit & nut bar, almond & apricot, 1 bar (40 g)	8
Fruit & nut bar, almonds & apricots in yogurt, 1 bar (45 g)	10
Fruit & nut bar, in yogurt, 1 bar (45 g)	9
Fruit & nut bar, nut delight, 1 bar (40 g)	7
Fruit & nut bars, cranberry almond plus antioxidants, 1 bar (40 g)	7
Fruit & nut bars, minis, variety 12-pack, 1 bar (24 g)	4

Snacks

	SmartPoints™ value
Fruit & nut, peanut butter & strawberry, 1 bar (40 g)	7
Maple glazed pecan and sea salt nuts ans spices bar, 1 bar (40 g)	7
Nuts & spices bar, dark chocolate nuts & sea salt, 1 bar (40 g)	7
Nuts & spices bars, dark chocolate cinnamon pecan, 1 bar (40 g)	7
Nuts & spices bars, dark chocolate nuts & sea salt, 1 bar (40 g)	7

Kind Fruit & Nut

Almond & coconut bar, 1 bar (40 g)	9
Blueberry vanilla cashew bar, 1 bar (40 g)	7

Kind Healthy Grains

Dark chocolate chunk bar, 1 bar (35 g)	6
Gluten free dark chocolate chunk granola bars, 1 bar (35 g)	6
Maple pumpkin seeds granola bars, 1 bar (35 g)	5
Maple pumpkin seeds with sea salt bar, 1 bar (35 g)	5
Oats and honey with toasted coconut bar, 1 bar (35 g)	6
Peanut butter dark chocolate gluten free granola bar, 1 bar (35 g)	5
Vanilla blueberry bars, 1 bar (35 g)	5
Vanilla blueberry granola bar, 1 bar (35 g)	5

Kind Healthy Snacks Fruit & Nut

Almond & coconut, 1 bar (40 g)	9

Kind Nuts & Spices

Caramel almond and sea salt bar, 1 bar (40 g)	7
Cashew and ginger spice bar, 1 bar (40 g)	7
Dark chocolate mocha almond bar, 1 bar (40 g)	7
Madagascar vanilla almond bar, 1 bar (40 g)	7

Kind Plus

	SmartPoints™ value
Blueberry pecan and fiber bar, 1 bar (40 g)	7
Cranberry almond plus antioxidants fruit and nut bar, 1 bar (40 g)	7
Dark chocolate cherry cashew and antioxidant bar, 1 bar (40 g)	7
Fruit & nut bars, dark chocolate & cherry cashew, 1 bar (40 g)	7
Fruit & nut bars, almond walnut macadamia plus protein, 1 bar (40 g)	6
Fruit & nut bars, peanut butter dark chocolate, 1 bar (40 g)	8
Fruit & nut bars, pomegranate blue berry pistachio plus antioxidants, 1 bar (40 g)	7
Fruit & nut bars, almond & cashew, 1 bar (40 g)	6
Fruit & nut bars, protein, almond, walnut & macadamia, 1 bar (40 g)	7
Peanut butter dark chocolate and protein bars, 1 bar (40 g)	7
Protein bars, peanut butter dark chocolate, 1 bar (40 g)	8

Kind Snack Bars Nuts & Spices

Dark chocolate nuts and sea salt bar, 1 bar (40 g)	7

Kirkland Signature

Soft and chewy granola bars, 1 bar (24 g)	4

Kroger

Cereal bars, fruit and grain, blueberry, 1 bar (37 g)	6
Cereal bars, fruit and grain, mixed berry, 1 bar (37 g)	6
Cereal bars, fruit and grain, strawberry, 1 bar (37 g)	6
Crunchy granola bars, oats & honey, 2 bars (42 g)	7
Granola bars, chewy sweet & salty, almond, 1 bar (35 g)	7

Snacks

	SmartPoints™ value
Granola bars, chewy, chocolate chip, 1 bar (24 g)	4
Granola bars, chewy, peanut butter chocolate chip, 1 bar (24 g)	4
Granola bars, crunchy, variety pack, 2 bars (42 g)	7
High fiber oats and chocolate chewy bars, 1 bar (40 g)	6
Peanut butter and dark chocolate chewy protein bar, 1 bar (40 g)	6
Sweet and salty pretzel bars, 1 bar (35 g)	7
Trail mix bars, chewy, fruit & nut, 1 bar (35 g)	6

Kroger Fruit & Grain

Apple cinnamon low fat cereal bar, 1 bar (37 g)	6

Kroger Sweet & Salty

Granola bars, chewy, peanut dipped in peanut butter coating, 1 bar (34.8 g)	7

Kudos

Granola bars, milk chocolate, with m&m's brand mini's milk chocolate candies, 1 bar (24 g)	4

Larabar

Apple pie fruit and nut bar, 1 bar (45 g)	8
Blueberry muffin bar, 1 bar (45 g)	8
Carrot cake flavored fruit and nut bar, 1 bar (45 g)	9
Cashew cookie fruit and nut bar, 1 bar (48 g)	9
Cherry pie fruit and nut bar, 1 bar (48 g)	9
Chocolate chip brownie food bar, 1 bar (45 g)	9
Chocolate chip cherry torte fruit and nut bar, 1 bar (45 g)	9
Chocolate chip cookie dough fruit and nut bar, 1 bar (45 g)	9

	SmartPoints™ value
Chocolate coconut chew fruit and nut bar, 1 bar (51 g)	10
Coconut cream pie fruit and nut bar, 1 bar (48 g)	11
Lemon bar fruit and nut bar, 1 bar (51 g)	9
Peanut butter and jelly fruit and nut bar, 1 bar (48 g)	8
Peanut butter chocolate chip fruit and nut bar, 1 bar (45 g)	9
Peanut butter cookie flavored fruit and nut bar, 1 bar (48 g)	9
Peanut butter cookie fruit and nut bar, 1 bar (55 g)	9
Pecan pie fruit and nut bar, 1 bar (45 g)	9

Larabar Alt

Chocolate peanut butter fruit and nut bar, 1 bar (60 g)	11
Lemon pound cake fruit and nut bar, 1 bar (50 g)	7
Peanut butter cookie fruit and nut bar, 1 bar (55 g)	9

Larabar Mini Bars

Apple pie fruit and nut bar, 1 bar (22 g)	4

Larabar Über

Coconut macaroon sweet and salty fruit and nut bar, 1 bar (40 g)	8
Coconut macroon sweet and salty fruit nut bar, 1 bar (40 g)	8
Fruit & nut bar, sweet & salty, dark chocolate peanut, 1 bar (40 g)	8
Fruit & nut bar, sweet & salty, dark chocolate turtle, 1 bar (40 g)	8
Fruit & nut bar, sweet and salty, cherry cobbler, 1 bar (40 g)	7
Roasted nut roll sweet and salty fruit and nut bar, 1 bar (40 g)	8

Life

Nutrition bars, for adults, banana walnut bread, 1 bar (42 g)	5

Snacks

	SmartPoints™ value
Lucky Charms	
Treats, marshmallow, 1 bar (24 g)	4
Luna	
Caramel nut brownie whole nutrition bar for women, 1 bar (48 g)	7
Chocolate peppermint stick nutrition bar for women, 1 bar (48 g)	7
Nutrition bar, berry almond, 1 bar (48 g)	6
Nutrition bar, blueberry bliss, 1 bar (48 g)	7
Nutrition bar, chocolate cupcake, gluten free, 1 bar (48 g)	7
Nutrition bar, chocolate dipped coconut, 1 bar (48 g)	7
Nutrition bar, for women, chocolate dipped coconut, 1 bar (48 g)	7
Nutrition bar, for women, nutz over chocolate, 1 bar (48 g)	6
Nutrition bar, for women, peanut butter cookie, 1 bar (48 g)	7
Nutrition bar, for women, peanut honey pretzel, 1 bar (48 g)	7
Nutrition bar, for women, vanilla almond, 1 bar (48 g)	7
Nutrition bar, for women, white chocolate macadamia, 1 bar (48 g)	7
Nutrition bar, iced oatmeal raisin, 1 bar (48 g)	7
Nutrition bar, lemon zest, 1 bar (48 g)	7
Nutrition bar, nutz over chocolate, 1 bar (44 g)	7
Nutrition bar, vanilla almond, 1 bar (48 g)	7
Nutrition bars, for women, minis, assorted, 1 bar (20 g)	3
Peanut caramel cluster whole nutrition bar for women, 1 bar (48 g)	7
Protein bar, chocolate, 1 bar (45 g)	7

	SmartPoints™ value
Protein bar, chocolate cherry almond, 1 bar (45 g)	7
Protein bar, chocolate peanut butter, 1 bar (45 g)	7
Protein bar, cookie dough, 1 bar (45 g)	7
Protein bar, mint chocolate chip, 1 bar (45 g)	7
S'mores whole nutrition bar for women, 1 bar (48 g)	7
Luna Minis	
Chocolate peppermint stick snack bar, 1 bar (23 g)	3
Nutrition bar, assorted, 1 bar (20 g)	3
Luna Protein	
Chocolate salted caramel high protein bar, 1 bar (45 g)	7
High protein bar, chocolate coconut almond, 1 bar (45 g)	7
High protein bar, lemon vanilla, 1 bar (45 g)	7
Lemon vanilla flavored bar, 1 bar (45 g)	7
Marathon	
Energy bar, chewy chocolate peanut, 1 bar (55 g)	8
Market Pantry	
Chocolate chunk chewy granola bars, 1 bar (24 g)	3
Granola bars, chewy, s'mores, 1 bar (24 g)	4
Market Pantry 90 Calories	
Fiber and chocolate chewy bars, 1 bar (23 g)	4
Meta Health Bar	
Cinnamon oatmeal raisin, 1 bar (40 g)	6
Cinnamon oatmeal raisin 3 in 1 multihealth fiber! bars, 1 bar (40 g)	6
Cranberry lemon drizzle 3 in 1 multihealth fiber! bars, 1 bar (40 g)	6

Snacks

MET-Rx

Meal replacement bar, big 100, chocolate chip cookie dough, 1 bar (100 g)	12

MET-Rx Big 100 Colossal

Meal replacement bar, super cookie crunch, 1 bar (100 g)	15

MET-Rx Protein Plus

Protein bar, peanut butter cup, 1 bar (85 g)	8

Millville

Chocolate coconut chewy bar, 1 bar (40 g)	7
Granola bars, chewy, chocolate chip, 1 bar (24 g)	4
Granola bars, chewy, peanut butter chocolate chip, 1 bar (24 g)	4
Granola bars, sweet & salty nut, with almonds, 1 bar (35 g)	7
Granola bars, sweet & salty nut, with peanuts, 1 bar (35 g)	7
Peanut butter crunchy granola bars, 2 bars (42 g)	7

Millville Chewy

Chocolate chunk granola bars, 1 bar (24 g)	4
Oatmeal raisin granola bar, 1 bar (24 g)	3
Trail mix fruit and nut bars, 1 bar (35 g)	5

Millville Crispy Rice Treats

Original crispy marshmallow squares, 1 bar (22 g)	4

Millville Fiber Now

90 calorie chocolate chunk and peanut chewy bar, 1 bar (23 g)	4
Oats and peanut butter chewy bar, 1 bar (40 g)	6

Nature Valley

Almond crunch roasted nut crunch bars (gluten free), 1 bar (35 g)	7
Almond dark chocolate nut crisps bar, 1 bar (25 g)	5
Chew bars, protein, peanut, almond & dark chocolate, 1 bar (40 g)	6
Chewy trail mix bars, mixed berry, 1 bar (35 g)	6
Crispy squares, dark chocolate, 1 pouch (17 g)	3
Crunchy coconut granola bar, 2 bars (42 g)	7
Dark chocolate granola thins, 1 pouch (17 g)	3
Granola bars, chewy, trail mix, dark chocolate cherry, 1 bar (35 g)	6
Granola bars, crunchy, apple crisp, 2 bars (42 g)	6
Granola bars, crunchy, cinnamon, 2 bars (42 g)	7
Granola bars, crunchy, dark chocolate peanut butter, 2 bars (42 g)	7
Granola bars, crunchy, maple brown sugar, 2 bars (42 g)	7
Granola bars, crunchy, oats 'n dark chocolate, 2 bars (42 g)	7
Granola bars, crunchy, roasted almond, 2 bars (42 g)	7
Granola bars, crunchy, variety pack, 2 bars (42 g)	7
Granola bars, sweet & salty nut, roasted mixed nut, 1 bar (35 g)	7
Granola thins, crispy squares, dark chocolate peanut butter, 1 pouch (17 g)	3
Granola thins, peanut butter, 1 pouch (17 g)	4
Mixed berry and Greek yogurt protein bar, 1 bar (40 g)	7

Snacks

	SmartPoints™ value
Mixed berry Greek yogurt protein bar, 1 bar (40 g)	7
Nut crunch bar, roasted, almond crunch, 1 bar (35 g)	6
Nut crunch bars, roasted, peanut crunch, 1 bar (35 g)	6
Roasted nut crunch, almond crunch, 1 bar (35 g)	6
Salted caramel peanut nut crisp bar, 1 bar (25 g)	5
Salted caramel peanut nut crisp bars, 1 bar (25 g)	5
Soft baked blueberry oatmeal squares, 1 bar (35 g)	6
Sweet and salty dark chocolate peanut and almonds bar, 1 bar (35 g)	7
Sweet and salty nut granola bars, cashew, 1 bar (35 g)	7
Trail mix bar, chewy, cranberry & pomegranate, 1 bar (32 g)	5
Trail mix bars, chewy, cranberry & pomegranate, 1 bar (32 g)	5
Trail mix bars, chewy, fruit & nut, 1 bar (35 g)	6
Trail mix bars, chewy, variety pack, value size, 1 bar (35 g)	6

Nature Valley Chewy

Dark chocolate and nut trail mix bar, 1 bar (35 g)	6

Nature Valley Crunchy

Granola bars, peanut butter, 2 bars (42 g)	7
Oats 'n honey granola bars, 2 bars (42 g)	7
Pecan crunch granola bars, 2 bars (42 g)	7

Nature Valley Fruteria

Mango strawberry chewy granola bar, 1 bar (26 g)	4
Strawberry apple chewy granola bar, 1 bar (26 g)	4

	SmartPoints™ value
Nature Valley Greek Yogurt Protein	
Chewy bar, mixed berry, 1 bar (40 g)	7
Chewy bar, strawberry, 1 bar (40 g)	7
Nature Valley Protein	
Coconut almond chewy bar, 1 bar (40 g)	7
Peanut butter dark chocolate chewy bars, 1 bar (40 g)	6
Salted caramel nut chewy bar, 1 bar (40 g)	6
Nature Valley Soft Baked	
Blueberry flavored oatmeal squares, 1 bar (35 g)	6
Cinnamon brown sugar oatmeal squares, 1 bar (35 g)	6
Peanut butter oatmeal squares, 1 bar (35 g)	6
Nature Valley Sweet & Salty Nut	
Dark chocolate peanut and almond granola bar, 1 bar (35 g)	7
Granola bars, almond, 1 bar (35 g)	7
Granola bars, cashew, 1 bar (35 g)	7
Granola bars, peanut, 1 bar (35 g)	7
Granola bars, roasted mixed nut, 1 bar (35 g)	7
Chocolate pretzel nut granola bars, 1 bar (35 g)	6
Nature Valley Yogurt	
Chewy granola bar, vanilla yogurt, 1 bar (35 g)	6
Chewy granola bars, strawberry yogurt, 1 bar (35 g)	6
Nature's Bakery	
Apple cinnamon fig bar, ½ package (28 g)	4
Fig bar, stone ground whole wheat, 1 oz	4
Fig bar, whole wheat apple cinnamon, 1 oz	4

Snacks

	SmartPoints™ value
Fig bar, whole wheat blueberry, 1 oz	4
Fig bar, whole wheat raspberry, 1 oz	4
Raspberry fig bar, ½ package (28 g)	4
Stone ground whole wheat fig bar, 1 bar (28 g)	4
Whole wheat blueberry fig bar, ½ bar (28 g)	4
Nature's Path Organic	
Granola bars, chewy, chococonut, 1 bar (35 g)	6
Nature's Path Organic Flax Plus	
Granola bars, chewy, trail mix, flax plus, pumpkin-n-spice, 1 bar (40 g)	6
Nature's Path Organic Gluten Free Selections	
Granola bars, chewy, chunky chocolate peanut, 1 bar (35 g)	5
Granola bars, chewy, dark chocolate chip, 1 bar (35 g)	6
Granola bars, chewy, trail mixer, 1 bar (35 g)	5
NuGo	
Chocolate bar, 1 bar (50 g)	6
Peanut butter chocolate bar, 1 bar (50 g)	6
Vanilla yogurt bar, 1 bar (50 g)	6
NuGo Dark	
Bars, mint chocolate chip, 1 bar (50 g)	8
Chocolate chocolate chip bar, 1 bar (50 g)	8
Mint chocolate chip bar, 1 bar (50 g)	8
Mocha chocolate bar, 1 bar (50 g)	8
NuGo Slim	
Crunchy peanut butter bar, 1 bar (45 g)	5

	SmartPoints™ value
Odwalla	
Nourishing food bar, original bar, berries gomega, 1 bar (56 g)	8
Nourishing food bar, original bar, chocolate chip peanut, 1 bar (56 g)	8
Nourishing food bar, original, super food, blueberry swirl, 1 bar (56 g)	8
Nourishing food bar, protein, chocolate peanut butter, 1 bar (56 g)	8
Odwalla Original Bar	
Nourishing food bar, banana nut, 1 bar (56 g)	8
Nourishing food bar, super protein, 1 bar (56 g)	7
Oh Yeah	
Brownie, almond fudge, 1 bar (45 g)	6
Energy bar, chocolate & caramel, 1 bar (45 g)	6
Perfect Bar	
Almond butter, 1 bar (64 g)	11
Peanut butter, 1 bar (71 g)	10
Perfect Bar Lite	
Cranberry crunch, 1 bar (45 g)	7
Perfectly Simple	
Nutrition bar, peanut crunch, 1 bar (45 g)	7
Pop-Tarts Go-Tarts!	
Snack bars, frosted brown sugar cinnamon, 1 bar (35 g)	6
Snack bars, frosted strawberry, 1 bar (35 g)	6
Power Crunch	
Protein energy bar, original peanut butter creme, 1 bar (40 g)	7
Protein energy bar, peanut butter fudge, 1 bar (40 g)	7

SmartPoints™ value

Power Crunch Original

Chocolate mint protein energy bar, 1 bar (40 g)	7
French vanilla creme protein energy bar, 1 bar (40 g)	7

PowerBar

Energy bar, chocolate flavor, 1 bar (65 g)	10
Energy bites, chocolate, 4 pieces (38 g)	6

PowerBar Harvest

Energy bar, whole grain, double chocolate crisp, 1 bar (65 g)	10
Energy bar, whole grain, toffee chocolate chip, 1 bar (65 g)	10

PowerBar Performance

Energy bar, peanut butter, 1 bar (65 g)	10

PowerBar Performance Energy

Wafer bar, chocolate peanut butter, 1 pack (40 g)	7

PowerBar Protein Plus

Bar, chocolate peanut butter bar, 1 bar (60 g)	7
Bar, vanilla, 1 bar (60 g)	7
High protein bars, reduced sugar, chocolate peanut butter flavor, 1 bar (70 g)	7

PowerBar Triple Threat

Energy bar, long lasting energy, caramel peanut fusion flavor, 1 bar (55 g)	9

Premier Protein

Bar, yogurt peanut crunch, 1 bar (72 g)	8

Premier Protein Crisp

Crunchy chocolate mint protein bar, 1 bar (52 g)	6
Crunchy peanut butter caramel protein bar, 1 bar (52 g)	7

SmartPoints™ value

Pure

Bar, organic ancient grains peanut butter chocolate, 1 bar (35 g)	6

Pure Organic

Nut bar, chocolate chunk, 1 bar (35 g)	6
Triple berry nut bar, 1 bar (35 g)	6

Pure Protein

Bar, chewy chocolate chip (gluten free), 1 bar (50 g)	5
Bar, chocolate deluxe (gluten free), 1 bar (50 g)	5
Bar, chocolate peanut butter (gluten free), 1 bar (50 g)	5
Bar, chocolate peanut caramel (gluten free), 1 bar (50 g)	5
bar, chocolate salted caramel (gluten free), 1 bar (50 g)	6
Bar, dark chocolate coconut (gluten free), 1 bar (50 g)	5

Pure Protein High Protein Bar

Blueberry with Greek yogurt style coating, 1 bar (50 g)	5
Chocolate deluxe, 1 bar (50 g)	5
Peanut butter caramel surprise, 1 bar (57 g)	6

Pure Protein Soft Baked Protein Bar

Double chocolate peanut butter crunch, 1 bar (45 g)	6

Quaker

Bars, granola, yogurt, fruit & nut quinoa, 1 bar (35 g)	6

Quaker Big Chewy

Chocolate chip granola bar, 1 bar (42 g)	8
Granola bar, sweet & salty, caramel popcorn crunch, 1 bar (40 g)	7
Peanut butter chocolate chip granola bar, 1 bar (42 g)	7

Sweet and salty caramel popcorn granola bar, 1 bar (40 g) — 7

Sweet and salty chocolate and salted caramel granola bar, 1 bar (40 g) — 7

Quaker Breakfast Cookies

Oatmeal chocolate chip, 1 cookie (48 g) — 7

Quaker Chewy

25% less sugar chocolate chip granola bar, 1 bar (24 g) — 4

Caramel apple granola bar, 1 bar (24 g) — 4

Chocolate chip cookie dough granola bar, 1 bar (24 g) — 3

Chocolate chip granola bar, 1 bar (24 g) — 4

Chocolate strawberries flavor granola bar, 1 bar (24 g) — 4

Chocolate strawberries granola bar, 1 bar (24 g) — 4

Low fat oatmeal raisin granola bar, 1 bar (24 g) — 3

Peanut butter chocolate chip granola bar, 1 bar (24 g) — 4

S'mores granola bar, 1 bar (24 g) — 4

Quaker Chewy 25% Less Sugar

Peanut butter chocolate chip granola bar, 1 bar (24 g) — 4

Quaker Chewy 90 Calories

Low fat chocolate chunk granola bar, 1 bar (24 g) — 4

Peanut butter granola bar, 1 bar (24 g) — 3

Quaker Chewy Dipps

Chocolatey covered caramel nut granola bar, 1 bar (31 g) — 7

Chocolatey covered chocolate chip granola bar, 1 bar (31 g) — 7

Chocolatey covered peanut butter granola bar, 1 bar (30 g) — 7

Dark chocolatey covered granola bar, 1 bar (31 g) — 7

Quaker Chewy Yogurt

Blueberry granola bar, 1 bar (35 g) — 6

Strawberry granola bar, 1 bar (35 g) — 6

Quaker Harvest

Chocolate nut medley quinoa granola bars, 1 bar (35 g) — 6

Quaker Oatmeal To Go

Apples and cinnamon breakfast bar, 1 bar (60 g) — 9

Brown sugar cinnamon breakfast bar, 1 bar (60 g) — 8

Oatmeal raisin breakfast bar, 1 bar (60 g) — 9

Quaker Protein

Oatmeal raisin nut flavor baked bar, 1 bar (47 g) — 7

Peanut butter chocolate baked bar, 1 bar (47 g) — 7

Quaker Real Medleys

Apple nut harvest multigrain fruit and nut bar, 1 bar (38 g) — 7

Cherry pistachio multigrain fruit and nut bar, 1 bar (38 g) — 6

Dark chocolate chunk almond coconut multigrain bar, 1 bar (38 g) — 8

Peach almond multigrain fruit and nut bar, 1 bar (38 g) — 6

Quaker Soft Baked

Cinnamon pecan bar, 1 bar (42 g) — 5

Quest Bar

Bar, protein, peanut butter supreme, 1 bar (60 g) — 5

Protein bars, apple pie, 1 bar (60 g) — 4

Protein bars, banana nut muffin flavor, 1 bar (60 g) — 3

Protein bars, chocolate brownie, 1 bar (60 g) — 4

Protein bars, chocolate chip cookie dough, 1 bar (60 g) — 5

Snacks

Snacks

	SmartPoints™ value
Protein bars, chocolate peanut butter, 1 bar (60 g)	3
Protein bars, cinnamon roll, 1 bar (60 g)	3
Protein bars, coconut cashew, 1 bar (60 g)	4
Protein bars, cookies and cream flavored, 1 bar (60 g)	4
Protein bars, double chocolate chunk, 1 bar (60 g)	4
Protein bars, mixed berry bliss, 1 bar (60 g)	5
Protein bars, strawberry cheesecake, 1 bar (60 g)	3
Protein bars, vanilla almond crunch, 1 bar (60 g)	4
Protein bars, white chocolate raspberry, 1 bar (60 g)	5
Quest Bar Protein Bar	
Peanut butter and jelly bar, 1 bar (60 g)	5
Reese's Puffs Treats	
Cereal bars, peanut butter and cocoa, 1 bar (24 g)	4
Rice Krispies Treats	
Crispy marshmallow squares, assorted, 1 bar (22 g)	4
Crispy marshmallow squares, holiday color, 1 bar (22 g)	4
Crispy marshmallow squares, with colored rice cereal, 1 bar (22 g)	4
Marshmallow squares, crispy, the original, 1 bar (22 g)	4
The original crispy marshmallow squares, 1 bar (22 g)	4
Rice Krispies Treats Mini Squares	
The original crispy marshmallow treat, 4 bars (44 g)	7
Rice Krispies Treats Scotcheroos	
Crispy marshmallow squares, chocolate and butterscotch, 1 piece (25 g)	5

	SmartPoints™ value
Rice Krispies Treats The Original	
Crisp rice cereal and marshmallow square, 1 bar (22 g)	4
Simple Truth	
Double chocolate protein bar, 1 bar (50 g)	6
Peanut butter extreme protein bar, 1 bar (50 g)	6
Skinny Cow Blissful Truffle	
Milk chocolate candy bar, 1 bar (22 g)	7
Skinny Girl	
Banana oatmeal dark chocolate tasty nutrition bar, 1 bar (39 g)	5
Chocolate peanut butter with sea salt tasty nutrition bar, 1 bar (41 g)	7
Dark chocolate pretzel tasty nutrition bar, 1 bar (39 g)	6
Slim Fast	
Chocolate cookie dough protein meal bar, 1 bar (52 g)	7
Protein meal bars, vanilla, 1 bar (45 g)	7
Slim Fast 3-2-1 Plan	
Meal bars, chocolate fudge brownie, 1 bar (52 g)	8
Snack bar, peanut butter crunch time, 1 bar (23 g)	5
Snack bars, chocolate mint, 1 bar (23 g)	4
South Beach Diet	
Cereal bar, high, protein, peanut butter, 1 bar (35 g)	5
Chocolate caramel nut snack bars, 1 bar (28 g)	4
Coconut crunch phase 1 snack bars, 1 bar (28 g)	4
Fiber bars, good to go, extra fiber, fudge graham flavored, 1 bar (35 g)	4
Good to go bars, cinnamon raisin, 1 bar (35 g)	5

Good to go bars, extra fiber, dark chocolate flavored, 1 bar (35 g) — 4

Good to go bars, peanut butter, 1 bar (35 g) — 5

Meal bars, chocolate chunk, 1 bar (50 g) — 6

Meal bars, chocolate peanut butter flavored, 1 bar (50 g) — 6

Snack bars, fudgy chocolate mint flavored, 1 bar (28 g) — 4

Snack bars, toffee nut flavored, 1 bar (28 g) — 4

Snack bars, whipped chocolate almond flavored, 1 bar (28 g) — 4

Snack bars, whipped peanut butter, 1 bar (28 g) — 4

South Beach Diet Good to Go Bars

Cereal bars, gluten-free, dark chocolate raspberry flavored, 1 bar (34 g) — 5

Chocolate brownie soft baked bars, 1 bar (37 g) — 5

South Beach Diet Protein Fit

Cereal bars, chocolate, 1 bar (35 g) — 5

Vanilla caramel nutrition bars, 1 bar (53 g) — 7

Southern Grove 100 Calorie Packs

Natural almond and walnut mix, 1 package (16 g) — 3

Special K

Berry medley snack bar, 1 bar (25 g) — 4

Strong & Kind

Hickory smoked almond protein bar, 1 bar (45 g) — 7

Honey mustard almond protein bar, 1 bar (45 g) — 7

Honey smoked bbq almond protein bar, 1 bar (45 g) — 7

Honey smoked bbq almond protein bar, 1 bar (45 g) — 7

Roasted jalapeño almond protein bar, 1 bar (45 g) — 7

Roasted jalapeño almond protein bar, 1 bar (45 g) — 7

Thai sweet chili almond protein bar, 1 bar (45 g) — 7

Sunbelt

Chewy granola bars, chocolate chip, 1 bar (35 g) — 6

Chewy granola bars, oats & honey, 1 bar (28.4 g) — 6

Fruit and grain bars, apple cinnamon, 1 bar (39 g) — 6

Fruit and grain bars, strawberry, pre-priced, 1 bar (39 g) — 6

Sunbelt Bakery

Banana harvest chewy granola bar, 1 bar (25 g) — 5

Chewy chocolate chip granola bars, 1 bar (30 g) — 6

Chewy oats and honey granola bars, 1 bar (27 g) — 5

Chocolate chip chewy granola bars, 1 bar (30 g) — 6

Fudge dipped chocolate chip granola bars, 1 bar (30 g) — 7

Fudge dipped coconut chewy granola bar, 1 bar (29 g) — 7

Golden almond chewy granola bars, 1 bar (28 g) — 5

Sunbelt Bakery Sweet & Salty

Almond chewy granola bar, 1 bar (30 g) — 6

Sunbelt Chewy Granola Bars

Oatmeal raisin low fat, 1 bar (30 g) — 5

Peanut butter chip, 1 bar (31 g) — 6

Sunrise

Energy bars with omega-3, 1 bar (28 g) — 6

Taste of Nature

Fruit and nut bar, organic, California almond valley, 1 bar (40 g) — 7

Snacks

SmartPoints™ value

SmartPoints™ value

Think Thin

Chocolate peanut butter toffee fiber bar, 1 bar (50 g)	5
Fiber bar, chocolate almond coconut, 1 bar (50 g)	5
Fiber bar, milk chocolate toffee almond, 1 bar (50 g)	5
High protein bar, chocolate fudge, 1 bar (60 g)	6
Lean protein & fiber bar, dark chocolate peppermint, 1 bar (40 g)	5
Lean protein & fiber bars, pumpkin spice, 1 bar (40 g)	5
Meal alternative nutrition bar, chunky peanut butter, 1 bar (60 g)	6
Protein bar, brownie crunch, 1 bar (60 g)	6
Protein bar, chocolate fudge, 1 bar (60 g)	6
Protein bar, white chocolate chip, 1 bar (60 g)	6

Think Thin Crunch

Bar, caramel chocolate dipped mixed nuts, 1 bar (40 g)	6
Bar, coconut chocolate mixed nuts, 1 bar (40 g)	6
Protein bar, nut and soy, mixed nuts & chocolate, 1 bar (40 g)	5

Think Thin High Protein Bar

Brownie crunch, 1 bar (60 g)	6
Caramel fudge, 1 bar (60 g)	6
Chunky peanut butter, 1 bar (60 g)	6
Chunky peanut butter chocolate, 1 bar (60 g)	6
Creamy peanut butter, 1 bar (60 g)	6
Creamy peanut butter chocolate, 1 bar (60 g)	6

Think Thin Lean Protein & Fiber

Chocolate almond brownie protein bar, 1 bar (40 g)	5
Chunky chocolate peanut protein bar, 1 bar (40 g)	5

Cinnamon bun white chocolate protein bar, 1 bar (40 g)	5
Honey drizzle peanut protein bar, 1 bar (40 g)	5
Salted caramel protein bar, 1 bar (40 g)	5

Tiger's Milk

Nutrition bar, protein rich, 1 bar (35 g)	6
Apple and coconut fruit bar, 1 bar (30 g)	5
Apple and strawberry fruit bar, 1 oz	4
Apple mango fruit bar, 1 bar (30 g)	5
Chocolate chip brownie & oat bars, 1 bar (35 g)	5
Chocolate chip chewy coated granola bar, 1 bar (35 g)	7
Peanut butter & oat bars, 1 bar (35 g)	6
Rolled oats & chocolate chips fiberful granola bars, 1 bar (35 g)	4
Rolled oats & peanut butter fiberful granola bars, 1 bar (35 g)	5
This "apple walks into a bar..." cereal bars, 1 bar (37 g)	6
This "blueberry walks into a bar..." cereal bars, 1 bar (37 g)	6
This "cranberry walks into a bar" cereal bars, 1 bar (37 g)	6
This "fig walks into a bar..." cereal bars, 1 bar (37 g)	5
This "strawberry walks into a bar..." cereal bars, 1 bar (37 g)	6

Trader Joe's Fiberful

Rolled oats and chocolate chips granola bars, 1 bar (35 g)	4

Twix

Milk chocolate coated cookie bars with caramel, 1 cookie (16 g)	4

Tyson Grilled & Ready

Chicken breast chunks, 3 oz	2

Udi's

Granola bars, chocolate chip,
1 bar (35 g) — 5

V8

Chocolate peanut butter
protein bar, 1 bar (49 g) — 8

Oatmeal raisin protein bar,
1 bar (50 g) — 7

Van's

Sandwich bars, pb&j blueberry
and peanut butter, 1 bar (40 g) — 6

Sandwich bars, pb&j strawberry
and peanut butter, 1 bar (40 g) — 7

Snack bars, chewy baked whole
grain, chocolate chip, 1 bar (35 g) — 6

Snack bars, chewy baked
whole grain, cranberry almond,
1 bar (35 g) — 6

Whole Foods 365 Everyday Value

Mixed berry flavored cereal bars,
1 bar (37 g) — 6

Woats

Peanut butter graham slam oat
snack, ¼ cup — 5

World Gourmet Sensible Portions

100 calorie bar, cinna-swirl,
1 each (30 g) — 4

Zone Perfect

Nutrition bar, all-natural, chocolate
almond raisin, 1 bar (50 g) — 8

Nutrition bar, all-natural,
cinnamon roll, 1 bar (50 g) — 8

Nutrition bar, all-natural, classic,
fudge graham, 1 bar (50 g) — 8

Nutrition bar, all-natural,
strawberry yogurt, 1 bar (50 g) — 8

Nutrition bar, Greek yogurt
chocolate, 1 bar (45 g) — 7

Nutrition bars, all-natural,
chocolate mint, 1 bar (50 g) — 8

Nutrition bars, all-natural,
dark chocolate caramel pecan,
1 bar (45 g) — 7

Nutrition bars, all-natural, double
dark chocolate, 1 bar (45 g) — 8

Nutrition bars, chocolate chip
cookie dough, 1 bar (44 g) — 7

Nutrition bars, chocolate peanut
butter, 1 bar (50 g) — 8

Nutrition bars, sweet & salty,
cashew pretzel, 1 bar (45 g) — 7

Zone Perfect Classic

Nutrition bar, all-natural, chocolate
caramel cluster, 1 bar (50 g) — 8

Nutrition bars, all-natural, chocolate
peanut butter, 1 bar (50 g) — 8

Nutrition bars, chocolate peanut
butter, 1 bar (50 g) — 8

Nutrition bars, fudge graham,
1 bar (50 g) — 8

Zone Perfect Dark

Nutrition bar, dark chocolate
almond, 1 bar (45 g) — 7

Nutrition bars, dark chocolate
almond, 1 bar (45 g) — 7

Nutrition bars, double dark
chocolate, 1 bar (45 g) — 8

Zone Perfect Fruitified

Nutrition bars, strawberry yogurt,
1 bar (50 g) — 8

Cheese Snacks

Bachman Jax

Puffed curls, real cheddar cheese,
23 pieces (28 g) — 5

Cheetos

Cheese flavored snacks,
baked, puffs, reduced fat,
1 package (20 g) — 3

Cheese snacks, crunchy,
xxtra flamin' hot flavored,
21 pieces (28 g) — 5

Snacks

Snacks

SmartPoints™ value

Flamin' hot flavored oven baked snack, 34 pieces (28 g)	4
Flamin' hot limon flavored crunchy cheese snacks, 21 pieces (28 g)	5
Cheetos Baked!	
Crunchy cheese flavored snacks, 34 pieces (28 g)	4
Cheetos Crunchy	
Cheddar jalapeño cheese flavored snack, 21 pieces (28 g)	5
Cheese flavored snack (treat size), 1 bag (18.4 g)	3
Cheese flavored snacks, 21 pieces (28 g)	5
Flamin hot cheese flavored snacks, 21 pieces (28 g)	5
Xxtra flamin' hot cheese flavored snacks, 21 pieces (28 g)	5
Cheetos Mix-Ups	
Xtra cheezy flavored snack mix, 1 cup	5
Cheetos Oven Baked	
Crunchy cheese flavored snacks, 1 single bag (21.25 g)	3
Cheetos Puffs	
Cheese flavored snacks, 13 pieces (28 g)	5
Flamin' hot cheese flavored snacks, 13 pieces (28 g)	5
Cheetos Simply Natural	
White cheddar puffed corn snacks, 32 pieces (28 g)	5
Cheetos Simply Puffs	
White cheddar cheese flavored snacks, 1 package (28 g)	5
Cheez-It	
Baked cheese snacks, crisps, cheddar crunch, 36 crackers (32 g)	5
Original baked snack crackers, 1 package (28 g)	4

SmartPoints™ value

Cheez-It Crisps	
Baked cheese snacks, white cheddar, 36 crackers (30 g)	5
Cheez-It Crunch'd	
Cheddar cheese baked cheese snack, 34 pieces (28 g)	5
Chester's	
Flamin hot flavor fries, 33 pieces (28 g)	5
Puffcorn, cheese, 3 cups	5
Combos	
Baked snacks, 7 layer dip, tortilla, ⅓ cup	5
Earth Balance	
Vegan aged white cheddar flavor puffs, 1 ¼ cups	4
Eating Right For Calorie Counting	
Popped crisps, cheddar, 22 (28 g)	3
Golden Flake	
Puff corn, cheddar cheese, 3 cups	6
Goldfish	
Cheddar goldfish crackers (variety pack), 1 package (28 g)	4
Xtra cheddar flavor blasted goldfish crackers, 1 package (26 g)	4
Handi Snacks Ritz	
Crackers 'n cheese dip, 1 pack (27 g)	3
Herr's	
Cheese curls, baked, 15 curls (28 g)	5
Hi I'm Skinny	
Skinny sticks, multi-grain cheddar, 34 sticks (28 g)	4
Hy-Vee	
Rice crisps, cheddar cheese, 9 chips (15 g)	2
LesserEvil Super 4	
White bean bites, cheesy nacho, 46 pieces (28 g)	3

Nabisco Ritz

Cheese cracker sandwich packs, 1 pack (38 g)	7

Pepperidge Farm Goldfish

Crackers, bold blasted, extra cheddar baked snacks, 51 pieces (30 g)	4

Pepperidge Farm Goldfish Puffs

Crackers, cheddar bacon flavored baked snacks, 41 pieces (30 g)	4
Crackers, mega cheese flavored baked snacks, 41 pieces (30 g)	4

Pirate's Booty

Aged white cheddar baked rice and corn puffs, 1 oz	4

PopCorners

White cheddar, popped corn chips, 1 oz	4

Pringles Stix

Cheese flavored baked snack sticks, 1 pack (17 g)	3
Pizza flavored baked snack sticks, 1 pack (17 g)	3

Quest

Chips, protein, cheddar & sour cream flavor, 1 bag (32 g)	2

Ritz

Toasted chips, cheddar, 1 oz	4
Toasted chips, dairyland cheddar, 14 chips (28 g)	4

Sage Valley

Puffs, white cheddar, 65 puffs (28 g)	4

Saputo Frigo Cheese Heads

100% natural cheese snack sticks, 1 piece (24 g)	3

Smart Puffs

Cheese puffs, baked, real Wisconsin cheddar, 1 oz	4
Snacks, real Wisconsin cheddar, 1 oz	4

Snikiddy

Baked grilled cheese corn puffs, 70 puffs (28 g)	4
Baked, mac n' cheese puffs, 60 pieces (28 g)	4

Snyder's Naturals

Cheese puffs, multigrain, white cheddar cheese, 1 ½ cups	4

Sunshine Cheez-It 100 Calorie Right Bites

Extra cheddar party mix, 1 pouch (21 g)	3

Trader Joe's

Baked cheese crunchies, 33 pieces (28 g)	4
Reduced fat cheese puffs, 1 serving (28.35 g)	4

Utz

Cheese balls, 32 balls (28 g)	4
Cheese curls, 1 package (28 g)	5

Wise

Cheez doodles, crunchy, 1 bag (28 g)	5

Wise Cheez Doodles

Cheese flavored corn snacks, puffed, 23 pieces (28 g)	5

Corn Chips & Snacks

Barcel

Takis, fuego, 14 pieces (28 g)	5

Bugles

Baked crispy corn snacks, original flavor, 1 ½ cups	4
Corn snacks, crispy, nacho cheese flavor, 1 ⅓ cup	7
Corn snacks, crispy, original flavor, 1 ⅓ cups	7

Cheetos Sweetos

Cinnamon sugar puffs, 25 pieces (28 g)	6

Snacks

	SmartPoints™ value
Chester's	
Puffcorn, butter, 1 oz	5
Chex Mix Muddy Buddies	
Snickerdoodle corn snacks, ⅓ cup	5
Corn Nuts	
Corn kernels, crunchy, ranch flavored, 1 pack (28 g)	4
Corn snack, crunchy, original, ⅓ cup	4
Cosmos Creations	
Salted caramel premium puffed corn, 1 oz	6
Eating Right For Calorie Counting	
Popped crisps, barbeque, 21 crisps (28 g)	4
Popped crisps, sea salt, 23 crisps (28 g)	4
Frito Lay	
Chili cheese flavored corn chips, 31 pieces (28 g)	5
Scoops!® corn chips, 10 chips (28 g)	5
The original corn chips, 32 chips (28 g)	5
Frito Lay Flavor Twists	
Honey bbq flavored corn snacks, 23 chips (28 g)	5
Fritos	
Bar-b-q corn chips, 29 chips (28 g)	5
Corn chips, chili cheese flavored, 31 chips (28 g)	5
Lightly salted corn chips, 34 chips (28 g)	5
Original corn chips, 1 oz	3
Fritos Flavor Twists	
Honey bbq corn snacks, 1 package (28 g)	5
Fritos Scoops	
Lightly salted corn chips, 1 oz	5

	SmartPoints™ value
Garden of Eatin'	
Blue corn chips, 1 oz	4
Kellogg's	
Baked popcorn chips butter flavored snacks, 1 pouch (22 g)	3
Baked popcorn chips sweet and salty flavored snacks, 1 pouch (22 g)	3
Kellogg's Special K	
Butter-flavored popcorn chips, 28 chips (28 g)	4
Cocoa with fudge drizzle popped delights, 1 pouch (11.76 g)	3
White cheddar flavored popcorn chips, 25 chips (28 g)	4
White cheddar popcorn chips, 25 chips (28 g)	4
O-Ke-Doke	
Corn puffs, 2 ½ cups	5
PopCorners	
Butter, popped corn chips, 1 serving (32 g)	4
Cheesy jalapeño, popped corn chips, 1 serving (32 g)	5
Kettle, popped corn chips, 1 package (32 g)	4
Sea salt, popped corn chips, 1 oz	4
The Better Chip	
Corn chips, jalapeño, with sea salt, 10 chips (28 g)	4
Corn chips, spinach & kale, 10 chips (28 g)	4
Corn chips, spinach & kale with sea salt, 10 chips (28 g)	4
Tom's	
Bugles, original flavor, 37 bugles (28 g)	6
Tostitos Scoops!	
Fajita corn chips, 10 chips (28 g)	4

Snacks

Trader Joe's

Kettle popped sweet & salty whole grain popcorn chips, 1 oz	3
Organic corn chip dippers, 10 chips (28 g)	5

Wise Original

Dipsy doodles, 1 bag (24 g)	5

Xochitl

Corn chips, blue, organic, Mexican style, 1 oz	4
Corn chips, Mexican style, 1 oz	4
Corn chips, stone-ground, 1 oz	4
Corn chips, stone-ground, organic, white, 1 oz	4
Corn chips, stone-ground, salted, 1 oz	4

Crackers

34 Degrees

Crispbread, cracked pepper, 19 crackers (30 g)	3
Crispbread, natural, 19 crackers (30 g)	4
Crispbread, rosemary, 19 crackers (30 g)	4
Crispbread, sesame, 19 crackers (30 g)	4
Crispbread, whole grain, 9 crackers (15 g)	1

Ak-Mak

Sesame crackers, 5 crackers (28 g)	3

Annie's

Cheddar bunnies, 51 crackers (30 g)	4
Cheddar squares, 27 crackers (30 g)	4
Snack crackers, baked, cheddar bunnies, 1 packet (28 g)	4

Annie's Organic

Bunnies, cheddar, 50 crackers (30 g)	5

Annie's Totally Natural

White cheddar bunny crackers, 44 crackers (30 g)	5

Archer Farms

Sesame water crackers, 4 crackers (15.6 g)	2

Asian Gourmet

Rice crackers, wasabi, 18 pieces (33 g)	4
Sea salt and lime rice crackers, 18 pieces (30 g)	4

Austin

Cheese crackers with cheddar cheese, 1 package (39 g)	7
Cheese crackers with peanut butter, 1 package (26 g)	4
Cheese crackers, with cheddar cheese, 1 package (26 g)	5
Crackers, peanut butter, 1 package (26 g)	4
Toasty crackers with peanut butter, 1 each (39 g)	7
Toasty crackers, with peanut butter, 1 package (26 g)	4

Back To Nature

Crackers, classic round, 5 crackers (15 g)	2
Crackers, crispy, cheddar, 24 crackers (30 g)	4
Crackers, flatbread, seeded, multigrain flax, 3 pieces (26 g)	4
Crackers, gluten free, multi-seed, 15 crackers (30 g)	4
Crackers, gluten free, white cheddar rice, 18 crackers (30 g)	4
Crackers, harvest whole wheat, 6 crackers (28 g)	3
Crackers, organic, stoneground wheat, 5 crackers (16 g)	2
Crackers, spinach & roasted garlic, 20 crackers (30 g)	4

Snacks

	SmartPoints™ value
Barnum's Animals	
Crackers, Lilly Pulitzer special edition, 8 crackers (28 g)	5
Barnum's Animals Snak-Saks	
Crackers, 17 crackers (31 g)	5
Bauducco	
Whole wheat toast, 3 crackers (28 g)	3
Better Cheddar	
Baked snack crackers, 20 crackers (30 g)	5
Bisca	
Water crackers, cracked pepper, 4 crackers (14 g)	2
Water crackers, original, 4 crackers (14 g)	2
Blue Diamond Artisan Nut-Thins	
Cracker snacks, almonds, 13 crackers (30 g)	4
Cracker snacks, almonds, asiago cheese with poppy & sunflower seeds, 13 crackers (30 g)	4
Cracker snacks, natural, flax seeds, 13 crackers (30 g)	4
Cracker snacks, natural, multi-seeds, 13 crackers (30 g)	4
Cracker snacks, natural, sesame seeds, 13 crackers (30 g)	4
Blue Diamond Honey Nut-Thins	
Honey cinnamon cracker snacks, 17 crackers (30 g)	4
Honey mustard cracker snacks, 17 crackers (30 g)	4
Blue Diamond Natural Nut-Thins	
Cracker snacks, nut & rice, almond, hint of sea salt, 17 crackers (30 g)	4
Cracker snacks, nut & rice, almond, smokehouse, 16 crackers (30 g)	4

	SmartPoints™ value
Blue Diamond Nut-Thins	
Cracker snacks, country ranch, 16 pieces (30 g)	4
Cracker snacks, nut & rice, barbeque, 17 crackers (30 g)	4
Cracker snacks, nut & rice, cheddar cheese, 16 crackers (30 g)	4
Nut & rice cracker snacks, almond, 16 crackers (30 g)	4
Nut & rice cracker snacks, pecan, 16 crackers (30 g)	4
Cambridge Fit & Active	
Reduced fat wheat crackers, 18 crackers (29 g)	4
Carr's	
Crackers, rosemary, 4 crackers (16 g)	2
Crackers, whole wheat, 2 pieces (17 g)	3
Table water crackers with roasted garlic & herbs, 4 crackers (14 g)	1
Table water crackers, baked with toasted sesame seeds, 5 pieces (17 g)	2
Table water crackers, with cracked pepper, 5 crackers (17 g)	2
Cheese Nips	
Baked cheddar snack cracker, 23 crackers (28 g)	4
Baked snack crackers, cheddar, 29 crackers (30 g)	5
Cheddar baked snack crackers, 29 crackers (30 g)	4
Crackers, snack, cheddar baked, nickelodeon, spongebob square pants, 27 crackers (31 g)	4
Reduced fat cheddar baked snack crackers, 31 crackers (30 g)	4
Cheese Nips Mini	
Despicable me baked cheddar snack cackers, 1 pack (28 g)	4

Snacks

Cheez-It

Baked snack crackers, 27 crackers (30 g)	5
Baked snack crackers, big, 14 crackers (30 g)	5
Baked snack crackers, cheddar Jack, 25 crackers (30 g)	4
Baked snack crackers, colby, 25 crackers (30 g)	5
Baked snack crackers, creamy & mild mozzarella, 25 crackers (30 g)	5
Baked snack crackers, hot & spicy, 25 crackers (30 g)	5
Baked snack crackers, Italian four cheese, 25 crackers (30 g)	5
Baked snack crackers, pepper Jack, 25 crackers (30 g)	5
Baked snack crackers, reduced fat, 29 crackers (30 g)	4
Baked snack crackers, reduced fat, white cheddar, 25 crackers (30 g)	4
Baked snack crackers, white cheddar, 25 crackers (30 g)	5
Reduced fat baked snack crackers, 1 package (28 g)	4
Snack crackers, baked, grab bags, 27 crackers (30 g)	5
Snack crackers, baked, Italian four cheese, 25 crackers (30 g)	5
Snack mix, double cheese, ¾ cup	4

Cheez-It Duoz

Baked snack crackers, sharp cheddar, parmesan, 25 crackers (30 g)	5

Cheez-It Gripz

Mighty tiny baked snack crackers, 1 package (25 g)	4

Cheez-It Grooves

Crispy cracker chips, sharp white cheddar, 18 cracker chips (29 g)	4
Crispy cracker chips, zesty cheddar ranch, 18 cracker chips (29 g)	4

Cheez-It Reduced Fat

Baked snack crackers, 29 crackers (30 g)	4

Cheez-It Zingz

Chipotle cheddar baked snack crackers, 18 crackers (29 g)	5
Queso fundido baked snack crackers, 18 crackers (29 g)	5

Chicken in a Biskit

Baked snack crackers, original, 12 crackers (31 g)	5

Chicken in a Biskit

Crackers, baked snack, original, 12 crackers (31 g)	5

Clover Valley

Saltine crackers, 5 crackers (14 g)	2

Club

Crackers, minis, original, 17 crackers (15 g)	2
Crackers, multi-grain, 4 crackers (14 g)	2
Crackers, original, 4 (14 g)	2
Crackers, original, 4 crackers (14 g)	2
Crackers, reduced fat, 5 (16 g)	2
Original crackers, 4 crackers (14 g)	2
Reduced fat crackers, 5 crackers (16 g)	2
Sandwich crackers, club & cheddar, 1 package (39 g)	7

Combos

Baked snacks, cheddar cheese cracker, ⅓ cup	5
Baked snacks, pepperoni pizza cracker, ⅓ cup	5

Crunchmaster

Crackers, multi-grain, five seed, 15 crackers (30 g)	4
Crackers, multi-grain, white cheddar, 15 crackers (30 g)	4
Crackers, multi-seed, original, 15 crackers (30 g)	4

SmartPoints™ value

Crackers, multi-seed, roasted garlic, 14 crackers (30 g)	4
Crackers, multi-seed, roasted vegetable flavor, 15 crackers (30 g)	4
Crackers, multi-seed, rosemary & olive oil, 14 crackers (30 g)	4
Crackers, multi-seed, sea salt, 16 crackers (30 g)	4
Crackers, rice, artisan four cheese, 15 crackers (30 g)	4
Rice crackers, toasted sesame, 15 crackers (30 g)	4
Snack crackers, multi-grain crisps, sea salt, 28 crackers (30 g)	4

Crunchmaster Crisps

Original multi grain snack crackers, 30 crackers (30 g)	4

Crunchmaster Healthy Gatherings

Multigrain crackers, 15 crackers (30 g)	4

Dare Breton

Crackers, crisp & buttery, cabaret, 3 crackers (14 g)	2
Crackers, herb and garlic, 4 crackers (18 g)	3
Crackers, multigrain, 3 crackers (16 g)	3
Crackers, original, 4 crackers (18 g)	3
Crackers, original with flax, 4 crackers (18 g)	3
Crackers, sesame, 3 crackers (14 g)	3

Dare Grainsfirst

Whole grain crackers, 4 crackers (18 g)	2

Devonsheer

Melba rounds, garlic, 5 pieces (16 g)	2
Melba rounds, plain, 5 pieces (16 g)	1

SmartPoints™ value

Diamond Bakery

Crackers, soda, 4 crackers (15 g)	2
Soda crackers, 3 crackers (18 g)	2

Doctor Kracker

Asiago cheese culinary crisps, 10 crackers (28 g)	4
Flatbreads, klassic 3 seed, 1 flatbread (25 g)	3
Flatbreads, pumpkin seed cheddar, 1 flatbread (25 g)	3
Flatbreads, seedlander, 1 flatbread (25 g)	3

Doctor Kracker Culinary Crisps

Apple oat crunch crisps, 10 crackers (28 g)	4

Eat Smart Naturals 100 Calorie Pack

Crisps, garden veggie, potato, tomato & spinach, 1 package (21 g)	3

Edward & Sons

Brown rice snaps, vegetable, 8 crackers (15 g)	2

Essential Everyday

Cheddar cheese rice snacks, 9 chips (15 g)	2

Excelsior

Water crackers, 5 crackers (33 g)	3

Finn Crisp

Rye crispbread, 3 pieces (18 g)	2
Rye crispbread, caraway, 3 pieces (18 g)	2
Thin crispbread, multigrain, 2 each (13 g)	1

Finn Crisp Plus 5 Wholegrains

Thin crispbread with sourdough rye, 2 slices (15 g)	2

Fit & Active

Zesty tomato cracker crisps, 1 oz	4

Fit & Active 100 Calorie

Baked cheese crackers, 1 package (22 g)	3

Snacks

Food Should Taste Good

Sea salt brown rice crackers, 10 crackers (28 g)	4

Frito Lay Munchies

Peanut butter on golden toast crackers, 1 package (40 g)	8
Peanut butter sandwich crackers, 1 package (40 g)	7

Gamesa Saladitas

Crackers, saltine, 15 cookies (29 g)	4

Gardetto's Special Request

Rye chips, roasted garlic, ½ cup	5

Giant

Crackers, soup & oyster, 35 crackers (15 g)	2
Saltines, original, 5 crackers (14 g)	2

Glutino

Crackers, gluten free, multigrain, 8 crackers (30 g)	5
Crackers, original, 8 crackers (30 g)	5
Crackers, table, gluten free, 3 crackers (33 g)	6

Glutino Gluten Free

Crackers, 4 crackers (15 g)	2

Goldfish

Baked snack crackers, American cheese, 55 pieces (30 g)	4
Baked snack crackers, cheddar, 55 pieces (30 g)	4
Baked snack crackers, cheddar, colors, 55 pieces (31 g)	4
Baked snack crackers, cheddar, finn smile pack, 55 pieces (30 g)	4
Baked snack crackers, made with whole grain, cheddar, 55 pieces (30 g)	4
Baked snack crackers, original, 55 pieces (30 g)	4
Baked snack crackers, original, soup crackers, 55 pieces (28 g)	5

Baked snack crackers, pizza, 55 pieces (29 g)	5
Baked snack crackers, saltine original, 55 pieces (30 g)	4
Cheddar baked snack crackers, 55 pieces (30 g)	4
Crackers, baked snack, cheddar, finn smile pack, 55 pieces (30 g)	4
Crackers, baked snack, pizza, 55 pieces (30 g)	4
Graham snacks, vanilla cupcake, 1 package (34 g)	6
Parmesan baked snack crackers, 60 pieces (30 g)	4
Snack crackers, baked pretzel, 41 pieces (31 g)	4
Snack crackers, baked, cheddar, 55 pieces (30 g)	4
Snack crackers, baked, whole grain, cheddar, 55 pieces (30 g)	4
Team goldfish baked snack crackers, American cheese, 55 pieces (28 g)	4
Team goldfish baked snack crackers, fun baseball shapes, American cheese, 55 pieces (28 g)	4

Goldfish 100 Calorie Flavor Blasted

Crackers, baked snack, xtra cheddar, 1 pouch (21 g)	3

Goldfish 100 Calorie Pouches Colors

Snack crackers, baked, 1 pouch (21 g)	3

Goldfish Colors

Snack crackers, baked, cheddar, 55 pieces (30 g)	4

Goldfish Flavor Blasted

Baked snack crackers, slammin' sour cream & onion, 57 pieces (30 g)	4
Baked snack crackers, wild white cheddar, 51 pieces (30 g)	4
Baked snack crackers, xtra cheddar, 51 pieces (30 g)	4

Snacks

	SmartPoints™ value
Crackers, baked snack, xplosive pizza, 51 pieces (30 g)	4
Crackers, baked snack, xtra cheddar, 51 pieces (30 g)	4
Snack crackers, baked, xtra cheddar, 1 pouch (26 g)	4
Goldfish Grahams	
Cinnamon baked graham snacks, 41 pieces (30 g)	5
Goldfish Mix-Up Adventures	
Crackers, baked snack, pretzel & flavor blasted xtra cheddar, 43 pieces (30 g)	4
Goldfish Princess	
Baked snack crackers, cheddar, 55 pieces (30 g)	4
Goya	
Soda crackers, ½ oz	2
Great Value	
Cheese crackers, 28 crackers (30 g)	5
Crackers, buttery smooth, 4 crackers (14 g)	2
Crackers, saltine, 5 crackers (15 g)	2
Crackers, soup & oyster, 36 crackers (15 g)	2
Crackers, unsalted tops, 5 crackers (15 g)	2
Crackers, wheat, 16 crackers (31 g)	5
Crackers, wheat, reduced fat, 16 crackers (28 g)	4
Multigrain crackers, 4 crackers (14 g)	2
Multigrain saltine crackers, 5 crackers (15 g)	2
Hannaford	
Crackers, oyster, 35 crackers (15 g)	2
Health Valley GG	
Crispbread, bran, Scandinavian, 2 crackers (20 g)	1

	SmartPoints™ value
Honey Maid	
Grahamfuls, banana vanilla creme filled, 1 package (25 g)	5
Horizon Organic	
Crackers, sandwich, cheddar, 12 sandwiches (30 g)	5
Peanut butter sandwich crackers, 12 sandwiches (30 g)	5
Hy-Vee	
Saltine crackers, 5 crackers (15 g)	2
Jacob's	
Crackers, cream, 2 crackers (15 g)	2
Jacobsen's	
Snack toast, cinnamon, 1 slice (10 g)	1
Snack toast, cinnamon raisin, 1 slice (10 g)	1
KA-ME	
Rice crunch crackers, plain, 19 crackers (33 g)	3
Rice crunch crackers, sesame, 19 crackers (33 g)	3
Rice crunch crackers, wasabi, 17 crackers (33 g)	3
Kashi	
Garlic pesto pita chips, 11 crisps (31 g)	4
Kashi Crackers	
Tlc crackers original 7 grain, 15 crackers (30 g)	4
Kashi TLC	
Crackers, fire roasted vegetable, 15 crackers (30 g)	4
Pita crisps, original 7 grain, with sea salt, 11 crisps (30 g)	4
Snack crackers, original 7 grain, 15 crackers (30 g)	4
Kavli	
Crispbread, 5 grain, 2 pieces (17 g)	2
Crispbread, crispy thin, 3 pieces (15 g)	2

Keebler

Cheese and peanut butter sandwich crackers, 1 package (39 g)	6
Crackers, export sodas, 3 crackers (14 g)	2
Light buttery crackers, wheat, 5 crackers (28 g)	3
Sandwich crackers, cheese & cheddar, 1 package (52 g)	9
Sandwich crackers, cheese & peanut butter, snack pack, 1 package (51 g)	8
Sandwich crackers, club & cheddar, snack pack, 1 package (51 g)	9
Sandwich crackers, pb 'n j, 1 package (39 g)	7
Sandwich crackers, toast & peanut butter, snack pack, 1 package (51 g)	8
Toast and peanut butter sandwich crackers, 1 package (39 g)	7

Keebler Club

Crackers, buttery garlic, 4 crackers (14 g)	2
Crackers, minis, multi-grain, 17 crackers (15 g)	2
Jalapeño cornbread cracker bites, 8 crackers (30 g)	5
Multi-grain crackers, 4 crackers (14 g)	2
Original crackers, 4 crackers (14 g)	2
Reduced fat crackers, 5 crackers (16 g)	2

Keebler Gripz

Cheez-it (variety pack), 1 package (25 g)	4

Keebler Town House

Cinnamon sugar pita oven baked crackers, 6 crackers (15 g)	2
Original light buttery crackers, 5 crackers (16 g)	3

Keebler Town House Pita

Mediterranean herb oven baked crackers, 6 crackers (16 g)	2
Sea salt oven baked crackers, 6 crackers (15 g)	2

Kellogg's Special K

Cracker chips, baked snacks, sea salt, 30 chips (30 g)	3
Cracker chips, cheddar, 1 package (25 g)	3
Cracker chips, chili lime, 27 chips (30 g)	3
Cracker chips, honey barbecue, 27 chips (30 g)	3
Cracker chips, sour cream & onion, 27 chips (30 g)	3
Cracker chips, southwest ranch, 27 chips (30 g)	3
Crackers, Italian tomato & herb, 24 crackers (30 g)	4
Crackers, savory herb, 24 crackers (30 g)	4
Salt and vinegar cracker chips, 25 chips (30 g)	4
Sea salt cracker chips, 1 package (25 g)	3
Sour cream and onion cracker chips, 1 package (25 g)	3

Kellogg's Special K 90 Calories

Sea salt cracker chips, 1 package (25 g)	3

Kellogg's Special K Cracker Chips

Sour cream and onion baked snack, 1 pack (25 g)	27

Kirkland Signature

Crackers, 3 crackers (18 g)	3
Organic animal crackers, 11 crackers (28 g)	4
Rice crackers with nuts, ¼ cup	5

Krispy

Original saltine crackers, 5 crackers (15 g)	2

Snacks

	SmartPoints™ value
Kroger	
Baked original flavour oyster crackers, 19 crackers (15 g)	2
Cheese bits, baked, reduced fat, 36 crackers (30 g)	4
Crackers, cheese peanut butter, 6 crackers (39 g)	7
Crackers, country club, multi-grain, 4 crackers (30 g)	5
Crackers, country club, original, 4 crackers (30 g)	5
Crackers, oyster, 19 crackers (15 g)	2
Crackers, oyster, baked, reduced sodium, 19 crackers (15 g)	2
Crackers, toasty peanut butter, 6 crackers (35 g)	6
Saltines, low fat, 5 crackers (14 g)	1
Saltines, original, 5 crackers (14 g)	2
Saltines, unsalted top, 5 crackers (14 g)	2
Snack crackers, 100% whole wheat crisps, baked, 17 crackers (31 g)	5
Snack crackers, multigrain crisps, baked, 17 crackers (31 g)	4
Snack crackers, wheat, 5 crackers (15 g)	2
Thin and crispy wheat saltines, 5 crackers (14 g)	2
Wheat crisps, original, reduced fat, 17 crackers (31 g)	4
La Panzanella	
Croccantini, mini, original, 1 oz	3
Croccantini, mini, rosemary, 1 oz	3
Rosemary croccantini, 1 oz	3
Lance	
Captain's wafers, 4 crackers (13 g)	2
Captain's wafers, grilled cheese, 1 package (39 g)	7
Crackers, captain's wafers, four cheese, 6 crackers (39 g)	7

	SmartPoints™ value
Crackers, toast chee, 1 package (28 g)	5
Crackers, wheat, peanut butter, 1 package (39 g)	7
Cream cheese and chive sandwich crackers, 1 package (39 g)	7
Real peanut butter malt crackers, 6 crackers (36 g)	6
Real peanut butter toasty crackers, 6 crackers (36.5 g)	6
Toast chee, 1 package (43 g)	7
Toastchee, rich 'n creamy peanut butter, reduced fat, 1 package (39 g)	6
Whole grain cracker sandwiches with real peanut butter, 1 package (43 g)	7
Lance Captain's Wafers	
Crackers, cream cheese & chives, 1 package (39 g)	1
Crackers, grilled cheese, 1 package (39 g)	7
Crackers, peanut butter & honey, 6 crackers (39 g)	7
Cream cheese and chives filled crackers, 1 package (39 g)	7
Jalapeño cheddar filled crackers, 1 package (39 g)	8
Peanut butter and honey filled crackers, 1 package (39 g)	7
Lance Nip Chee	
Real cheddar cheese filled crackers, 6 crackers (39 g)	7
Lance Toast Chee	
Real peanut butter crackers, 6 crackers (43 g)	7
Lance Toasty	
Crackers, peanut butter, 1 package (35 g)	6
Real peanut butter filled crackers, 6 crackers (36 g)	6

Lance Whole Grain

Cheddar cheese filled crackers, 1 package (42 g) — 8

Peanut butter cracker packs, 6 crackers (42.5 g) — 7

Sharp cheddar cheese filled crackers, 1 package (42 g) — 8

Le Pain Des Fleurs

Crispbread, 100% organic, quinoa, 4 crispbreads (16 g) — 2

Lesley Stowe

Cranberry and hazelnut raincoast crisps, 6 crackers (30 g) — 4

LiveGfree

Gluten free sea salt multiseed snack crackers, 13 crackers (28 g) — 4

Rosemary and olive oil gluten free multiseed crackers, 11 crackers (28 g) — 4

M.Y. San SkyFlakes

Crackers, saltine, 3 crackers (25 g) — 5

Market Pantry

Saltine crackers, 5 crackers (15 g) — 2

Sandwich crackers, peanut butter, 6 crackers (39 g) — 7

Soup and oyster crackers, 36 crackers (15 g) — 2

Mary's Gone Crackers

Crackers, organic, black pepper, 13 crackers (30 g) — 4

Crackers, organic, caraway, 13 crackers (30 g) — 4

Crackers, organic, herb, 13 crackers (30 g) — 4

Crackers, organic, hot 'n spicy jalapeño, 13 crackers (30 g) — 4

Crackers, organic, onion, 13 crackers (30 g) — 4

Crackers, organic, original, 13 crackers (30 g) — 4

Crackers, organic, super seed, 13 crackers (30 g) — 5

Mediterranean Snack Food

Crackers, lentil, sea salt, 18 crackers (28 g) — 3

Meijer Select

Crackers, saltine, 5 crackers (14 g) — 2

Crackers, saltine, wheat, 5 crackers (15 g) — 2

Crackers, soup & chili, 35 crackers (15 g) — 2

Milton's

Crackers, baked, original multi-grain, 2 crackers (16 g) — 2

Crackers, multi-grain, everything, 2 crackers (16 g) — 2

Multi-grain crackers, whole wheat sesame, 2 crackers (16 g) — 2

Milton's Craft Bakers

Gluten free crispy sea salt baked crackers, 14 crackers (30 g) — 4

Milton's Gluten Free

Crackers, baked, crispy sea salt, 14 crackers (30 g) — 4

Everything baked crackers, 14 crackers (30 g) — 4

Multi-grain baked crackers, 14 crackers (30 g) — 4

Munchies

Sandwich crackers, cheddar cheese, 1 package (39 g) — 8

Sandwich crackers, jalapeño cheddar, 1 package (39 g) — 7

My Essentials

Original saltines, 5 crackers (14 g) — 2

Nabisco 100 Calorie Packs

Thin crisps, cheese nips, 1 package (21 g) — 3

Snacks

Snacks

Nabisco Barnum's Animals

Chewy cookies, fig, whole grain, 1 package (28 g)	5

Nabisco Premium

Crackers, saltine, original, minis, 17 crackers (15 g)	2

Nabisco Premium Rounds

Rosemary and olive oil saltine crackers, 6 crackers (15 g)	2

Nabisco Rice Thins

Gluten free sweet barbecue brown rice snacks, 13 pieces (30 g)	4

Nabisco Ritz

Crackers, 5 crackers (16 g)	3

Nabisco Sociables

Crackers, baked savory, 5 crackers (14 g)	2

Nabisco Wheat Thins

Dill pickle flavored snacks, 14 crackers (29 g)	5
Zesty salsa snack crackers, 15 crackers (31 g)	5

Natural Nectar

Cracklebred, original, 3 crackers (14 g)	2

Nonni's THINaddictives

Cranberry almond thins, 1 package (23 g)	4
Mango coconut almond thins, 1 package (21 g)	4

Old London

Ancient grains melba toast, 3 pieces (15 g)	2
Melba snacks, roasted garlic, 4 pieces (15 g)	1
Melba snacks, sea salt, 4 pieces (15 g)	1
Melba snacks, sesame, 4 pieces (15 g)	2

Melba snacks, whole grain, 4 pieces (15 g)	1
Melba toast, classic, 3 pieces (17 g)	2
Melba toast, rye, 3 pieces (17 g)	2
Melba toast, sesame, 3 pieces (17 g)	2
Melba toast, sourdough, 3 pieces (17 g)	2
Melba toast, unsalted, whole grain, 3 pieces (18 g)	2
Melba toast, wheat, 3 pieces (18 g)	2
Melba toast, whole grain, 3 pieces (18 g)	2

Olde Cape Cod

Oyster crackers, soup & chowder, 1 package (14 g)	2

Osem

Matzah ball & soup mix, 3 balls (27 g)	4

P$$t...

Oyster crackers, 38 crackers (15 g)	2
Saltines, 5 crackers (14 g)	2

Pepperidge Farm

Cracker trio, 3 crackers (13 g)	2
Crackers, distinctive, golden butter, 4 crackers (15 g)	2
Crackers, distinctive, harvest wheat, 3 crackers (16 g)	3

Pepperidge Farm 100 Calorie Pouches

Baked snack crackers, goldfish pretzel, 1 pouch (23 g)	3

Pepperidge Farm Baked Naturals

Cracker chips, cheddar & sour cream potato, 25 pieces (30 g)	4
Cracker chips, simply cheddar, 27 pieces (30 g)	4

Pepperidge Farm Cracker Chips

Classic bbq flavored snacks, 26 pieces (30 g)	4
Zesty chili and lime snacks, 24 pieces (30 g)	4

Pepperidge Farm Goldfish

Crackers, baby baked cheddar snacks, 89 pieces (30 g)	4
Crackers, cheddar baked snacks, 55 pieces (30 g)	4
Crackers, flavor blasted kick it up a nacho baked snacks, 50 crackers (30 g)	4
Crackers, flavor blasted queso fiesta baked snacks, 54 crackers (30 g)	4
Crackers, mega size cheddar baked snacks, 55 pieces (30 g)	4
Crackers, pretzel baked snacks, 43 pieces (30 g)	4

Pepperidge Farm Goldfish Colors

Crackers, cheddar baked snacks, 55 pieces (30 g)	4

Pepperidge Farm Goldfish Grahams

Crackers, cookies & cream flavor baked snacks, 35 pieces (30 g)	6
Crackers, French toast flavor baked snacks, 34 pieces (30 g)	5
Crackers, holiday vanilla cupcake flavor baked snacks, 35 pieces (30 g)	5

Pepperidge Farm On The Go!

Goldfish, cheddar, baked snack crackers, 55 pieces (28 g)	4

Pepperidge Farm Slime Blasted Goldfish

Crackers, xtra cheddar, 51 pieces (31 g)	4

Premium

Crackers, saltine, unsalted tops, 5 crackers (16 g)	2
Crackers, saltines, hint of salt, 5 crackers (15 g)	2
Crackers, saltines, original, 5 crackers (16 g)	2
Crackers, saltines, with whole grain, topped with sea salt, 2 full sheets (31 g)	3
Crackers, soup & oyster, 22 crackers (15 g)	2
Crackers, soup & oyster, 22 crackers (15 g)	2
Saltine crackers, with whole grain, topped with sea salt, 5 crackers (14 g)	2

Premium Rounds

Saltine crackers with whole grain topped with sea salt, 6 crackers (15 g)	2

Private Selection

Crisps, classic water, 4 crackers (15 g)	2

Publix

Soup and oyster crackers, 1 serving (15 g)	2

Quaker Multigrain Fiber Crisps

Blackberry pomegranate flavor baked snack, 13 pieces (28 g)	4
Wild blueberry flavor baked snacks, 13 pieces (28 g)	4

Red Oval Farms

Crackers, mini stoned wheat thins, original, 19 pieces (31 g)	4
Crackers, wheat, stoned wheat thins, 2 crackers (14 g)	2

Red Oval Farms Stoned Wheat Thins

Crackers, wheat, lower sodium, 2 crackers (14 g)	2
Snack crackers, mini, 19 crackers (30 g)	4

Rice Thins Gluten Free

Original thin rice snacks, 18 pieces (31 g)	4
Sea salt and pepper thin rice snacks, 13 pieces (30 g)	4
White cheddar thin rice snacks, 13 pieces (30 g)	4

Snacks

	SmartPoints™ value
Ritz	
Cracker sandwiches, cheese, 1 package (38 g)	7
Cracker sandwiches, peanut butter, 1 pack (39 g)	7
Crackers, 5 crackers (16 g)	3
Crackers, bacon flavor, 5 crackers (16 g)	3
Crackers, baked with whole wheat, fresh stacks, 5 crackers (15 g)	2
Crackers, everything, fresh stacks, 5 crackers (16 g)	3
Crackers, fudge covered, 4 crackers (33 g)	8
Crackers, hint of salt, 5 crackers (16 g)	3
Crackers, honey wheat, 5 crackers (16 g)	3
Crackers, reduced fat, 5 crackers (15 g)	2
Crackers, roasted vegetable, 5 crackers (16 g)	3
Crackers, snowflakes, 5 crackers (16 g)	3
Crackers, whole wheat, 5 crackers (15 g)	2
Crackers, whole wheat, 5 crackers (15 g)	2
Roasted vegetable crackers, 5 crackers (16 g)	3
Toasted chips, main street original, 16 chips (28 g)	4
Toasted chips, original, 13 chips (28 g)	4
Toasted chips, sour cream and onion, 1 oz	4
Toasted chips, sweet home sour cream & onion, 14 chips (28 g)	4
Ritz 100 Calorie Packs	
Ritz chips, minis, original, 1 package (22 g)	3

	SmartPoints™ value
Ritz Bits	
Cracker sandwiches, cheese, 1 package (28 g)	6
Cracker sandwiches, cheese, 13 crackers (31 g)	6
Cracker sandwiches, cheese, big bag, 13 sandwiches (28 g)	6
Cracker sandwiches, peanut butter, 12 crackers (30 g)	5
Cracker sandwiches, ritz bits with cheese, 13 sandwiches (30 g)	6
Ritz Chips	
Toasted southwest chili flavored snacks, 12 chips (28 g)	4
Ritz Crackerfuls	
Filled crackers, bold buffalo & ranch, 1 pack (28 g)	5
Filled crackers, classic cheddar, 1 package (28 g)	5
Filled crackers, four cheese, 1 package (28 g)	5
Filled crackers, peanut butter, 1 pack (28 g)	5
Peanut butter and chocolate filled crackers, 1 pack (28 g)	5
Ritz Crisps	
Crispy baked snack crackers, 24 crisps (28 g)	5
Ritz Fresh Stacks	
Crackers, 5 crackers (16 g)	3
Original crackers, 5 crackers (16 g)	3
Ritz Handi-Snacks	
Crackers 'n cheese dip, 1 pack (27 g)	3
Ritz Mini	
Bite size crackers, 1 pack (28 g)	5
Chips, toasted original flavor, 1 pack (21 g)	3
Cracker sandwiches, peanut butter, 14 pieces (31 g)	5

Ritz Mini Toasted

Sour cream and onion chips, 1 package (21 g)	3

Ry Krisp

Crackers, light rye, 2 crackers (14 g)	1
Crackers, seasoned, 2 crackers (14 g)	2
Crackers, sesame, 2 crackers (14 g)	1

Ryvita

Crispbread, wholegrain rye, fruit & seed crunch, 2 slices (30 g)	4
Whole grain rye crispbread, dark rye, 1 slice (10 g)	1
Whole grain rye crispbread, sesame rye, 1 (10 g)	1

Safeway

Crackers, oyster & soup, 25 crackers (15 g)	3
Saltine crackers, 5 crackers (14 g)	2

Safeway Select

Crackers, rice, sesame, 16 crackers (30 g)	4

Savoritz

Crackers, cheese baked, 28 crackers (30 g)	5
Crackers, garlic and chive pita, 9 crackers (28 g)	3
Crackers, Original wheat, 3 crackers (15 g)	2
Crackers, wheat round, 5 crackers (15 g)	2

Sensible Portions Pita Bites

Pita crackers, naturally baked, black olive feta, 9 crackers (28 g)	3
Pita crackers, naturally baked, original sea salt, 9 crackers (28 g)	3

Sesmark

Rice thins, savory, original, 16 crackers (30 g)	4

Sesmark Ancient Grains

Snack crackers, all natural, sea salt, 17 crackers (33 g)	4

Sesmark Rice Thins

Crackers, rice, brown rice, 17 crackers (30 g)	3
Crackers, rice, sesame, 16 crackers (30 g)	4

ShopRite

Oyster crackers, soup and chili, 35 crackers (15 g)	2
Saltines, 5 crackers (14 g)	2

Simple Truth

Multigrain rice crackers with sea salt, 16 crackers (30 g)	4

Simply Balanced

Crackers, brown rice, gluten free, multigrain with flax, 18 crackers (30 g)	4
Crackers, brown rice, gluten free, multi-seed, 18 crackers (30 g)	4
Crackers, brown rice, gluten free, sesame, 18 crackers (30 g)	4
Multigrain pita crackers with quinoa and flax, 10 crackers (28 g)	3
Sea salt pita crackers, 10 crackers (28 g)	4

Snack Factory Pretzel Crisps

Original pretzel crackers, 11 crackers (28 g)	3

Stauffer's

Baked snack crackers, whales, 33 crackers (30 g)	4

Stauffer's Whales

Crackers, baked snack, with real cheddar cheese, 33 crackers (30 g)	4

Stonefire

Everything naan crisps, 13 crisps (28 g)	4

Sultana

Soda crackers, ½ oz	2

Snacks

	SmartPoints™ value
Sunshine	
Crackers, soup & oyster, 16 crackers (15 g)	2
Saltine crackers, wheat, 5 crackers (15 g)	2
Sunshine Cheez-It	
Baked snack crackers (disney pixar monsters university), 29 crackers (30 g)	4
Suzie's	
Spelt and flax seeds thin whole grain cakes, 3 cakes (14 g)	1
Suzie's Kamut	
Flat breads, sesame topping, 3 flatbreads (25 g)	3
Suzie's Thin Cakes	
Crackers, puffed, corn, quinoa & sesame, 3 cakes (13 g)	1
Crackers, puffed, lightly salted corn, 3 cakes (13 g)	1
Toasted's	
Buttercrisp lightly toasted crackers, 5 crackers (16 g)	3
Crackers, onion, 5 crackers (16 g)	3
Crackers, sesame, 5 crackers (16 g)	3
Harvest wheat lightly toasted crackers, 5 crackers (16 g)	2
Tops	
Thin wheats, reduced fat, 16 crackers (29 g)	4
Town House	
Crackers, light buttery, original, 5 crackers (16 g)	3
Crackers, original, light buttery flavor, 5 crackers (16 g)	3
Light buttery crackers, reduced fat, 6 crackers (15 g)	2
Light buttery wheat crackers, 5 crackers (16 g)	2
Original light and buttery crackers, 5 crackers (16 g)	3

	SmartPoints™ value
Town House Flatbread Crisps	
Italian herb crackers, 8 crackers (15 g)	2
Roasted garlic crackers, 8 crackers (15 g)	2
Sea salt and olive oil crackers, 8 crackers (15 g)	2
Town House Flip Sides	
Original pretzel crackers, 5 crackers (15 g)	2
Town House Reduced Fat	
Light buttery crackers, 15 crackers (15 g)	2
Trader Joe's	
12 grain mini snack crackers, 22 crackers (30 g)	4
Bit size everything crackers, 14 crackers (30 g)	4
Cheddar rocket crackers, 46 crackers (30 g)	4
Classic original water crackers, 4 crackers (15 g)	2
Fig & olive crisps, 11 crackers (30 g)	3
Golden rounds crackers, 9 crackers (30 g)	4
Honey graham crackers, 2 sheets (31 g)	5
Multigrain and flaxseed water creackers, 4 crackers (15 g)	2
Multigrain pita bite crackers, 8 crackers (28 g)	3
Multiseed with soy sauce savory thin mini rice crackers, 1 oz	3
Organic mini cheese sandwich crackers, 12 crackers (28 g)	5
Organic mini peanut butter sandwich crackers, 12 crackers (28 g)	5
Oriental rice crackers, ½ cup	3
Original savory thin mini crackers, 1 oz	3

Pita bite crackers with sea salt, 9 crackers (28 g)	3
Raisin rosemary crisps, 10 pieces (30 g)	3
Roasted gorgonzola flavored oven crisp crackers, 31 crackers (30 g)	4
Savory thin mini edamame crackers, 38 chips (28 g)	3
Sesame sticks, 28 pieces (30 g)	5
Social snackers, 8 crackers (28 g)	4
Soup & oyster crackers, 14 crackers (15 g)	2

Trader Joe's Reduced Guilt

Wheat crisps, 14 crackers (30 g)	4
Woven wheats wafers, 8 crackers (32 g)	3

Triscuit

Balsamic vinegar & basil crackers, 6 crackers (28 g)	4
Brown rice and wheat sweet potato and sea salt crackers, 6 crackers (30 g)	4
Crackers, baked, fire roasted tomato & olive oil, 6 crackers (28 g)	4
Crackers, baked, wheat, garden herb, 6 crackers (28 g)	4
Crackers, baked, wheat, hint of salt, 6 crackers (28 g)	4
Crackers, baked, wheat, original, 6 crackers (28 g)	4
Crackers, baked, wheat, roasted garlic, 6 crackers (28 g)	4
Crackers, baked, wheat, rye, with caraway seeds, 6 crackers (28 g)	4
Crackers, cracked pepper & olive oil, 6 crackers (28 g)	3
Crackers, fire roasted tomato & olive oil, 6 crackers (28 g)	3
Crackers, garden herb, 6 crackers (28 g)	3

Crackers, hint of salt, 6 crackers (28 g)	3
Crackers, original, 6 crackers (28 g)	3
Crackers, reduced fat, with sea salt, 7 crackers (30 g)	3
Crackers, roasted garlic, 6 crackers (28 g)	3
Crackers, rosemary & olive oil, 6 crackers (28 g)	3
Crackers, rye with caraway seeds, 6 crackers (28 g)	3
Crackers, wheat, baked whole grain, reduced fat, 7 crackers (29 g)	3
Dill sea salt and olive oil crackers, 6 crackers (28 g)	3
Limited edition cranberry and sage crackers, 6 crackers (28 g)	4
Reduced fat crackers made with whole wheat, 7 crackers (30 g)	3
Tomato and sweet basil brown rice and wheat cracker, 6 crackers (29 g)	4

Triscuit Brown Rice

Crackers, sea salt & black pepper, 6 crackers (29 g)	4
Roasted red pepper crackers, 9 crackers (29 g)	4
Roasted sweet onion crackers, 6 crackers (29 g)	4
Savory red bean crackers, 6 crackers (29 g)	4

Triscuit Thin Crisps

Brown rice wasabi and soy sauce crackers, 10 crackers (30 g)	4
Crackers, baked, original, 15 crackers (30 g)	4
Crackers, baked, wheat, parmesan garlic, 15 crackers (31 g)	4
Crackers, brown rice & wheat, sour cream & chive, 10 crackers (30 g)	4
Crackers, brown rice & wheat, wasabi & soy sauce, 10 crackers (30 g)	4

	SmartPoints™ value
Crackers, original, 15 crackers (30 g)	4
Crackers, parmesan garlic, 14 crackers (29 g)	4
Twistos	
Asiago flavoured baked snack bites, 24 pieces (28 g)	4
Van's	
Baked crackers, crispy whole grain, lots of everything!, 30 crackers (30 g)	4
Baked crackers, crispy whole grain, multigrain, 30 crackers (30 g)	4
Crackers, baked, fire-roasted veggie, 12 crackers (30 g)	4
Crackers, baked, the perfect 10, 12 crackers (30 g)	4
Vegetable Thins	
Crackers, baked snack, 21 crackers (28 g)	5
Wasa	
Crispbread, fiber, 1 slice (10 g)	1
Crispbread, flax seed, 2 slices (19 g)	2
Crispbread, hearty, 1 slice (14 g)	1
Crispbread, light rye, 2 slices (17 g)	2
Crispbread, sesame, 1 slice (17 g)	2
Crispbread, sourdough, 1 slice (11 g)	1
Crispbread, whole grain, 1 slice (12 g)	1
Crispbread, whole wheat, 1 slice (14 g)	1
Multi grain crispbread, 1 slice (15 g)	2
Wasa Crisp'n Light	
7 grains crackerbread, 3 slices (18 g)	2
Crackerbread, mild rye, 3 slices (18 g)	2
Crackerbread, wholesome wheat, 3 slices (18 g)	2

	SmartPoints™ value
Wegman's	
Crackers, wheat, thin & crispy, reduced fat, 16 crackers (28 g)	4
Westminster Bakers Co.	
Oyster crackers, 1 package (14 g)	2
Wheat Thins	
Baked snack crackers, 16 crackers (32 g)	4
Baked snack crackers, harvest garden vegetable, 15 crackers (30 g)	4
Crackers, 100% whole grain, 16 crackers (31 g)	5
Crackers, flatbread, garlic & parsley, 2 crackers (15 g)	2
Crackers, hint of salt, 16 crackers (31 g)	5
Crackers, lime, 14 pieces (30 g)	5
Crackers, multigrain, 15 crackers (30 g)	5
Crackers, original whole grain, 16 crackers (31 g)	5
Crackers, oven baked, toasted pita, garlic herb, 14 crackers (30 g)	4
Crackers, oven baked, toasted pita, original, 15 crackers (30 g)	4
Crackers, reduced fat, 16 crackers (29 g)	4
Crackers, reduced fat whole grain, 16 crackers (29 g)	4
Crackers, sundried tomato & basil, 15 pieces (30 g)	5
Flatbread, tuscan herb, 2 crackers (15 g)	2
Garden valley veggie toasted chips, 13 chips (28 g)	4
Original baked snack, 16 pieces (31 g)	5
Snacks, chili cheese, 15 pieces (30 g)	5
Snacks, honey mustard, 15 pieces (30 g)	5

Snacks, multigrain, 14 pieces (31 g)	4
Snacks, ranch, 15 pieces (30 g)	5
Snacks, reduced fat, 16 pieces (29 g)	4
Snacks, spicy buffalo, 14 pieces (29 g)	5
Snacks, sundried tomato & basil, 15 pieces (30 g)	5
Snacks, whole grain, hint of salt, 16 pieces (31 g)	5
Snacks, zesty salsa, 15 pieces (31 g)	5
Spicy buffalo grain snacks, 14 pieces (29 g)	5
Sundried tomato and basil snacks, 1 pack (28 g)	5
Sweet onion whole grain snacks, 14 pieces (29 g)	5
Toasted chips, little Italy roasted garlic, 12 chips (28 g)	4
Toasted chips, veggie, 1 pack (47 g)	7
Wheat thins, original, 16 pieces (31 g)	5

Wheat Thins 100 Calorie Packs

Toasted chips, wheat thins, multi-grain, minis, 1 package (22 g)	3
Wheat thins, minis, 1 package (21 g)	3

Wheat Thins Big

Whole grain crackers, 11 crackers (31 g)	5

Wheat Thins Crispy Thins

Baked snack crackers, seasoned original, 24 crackers (30 g)	4

Wheat Thins Fiber Selects

Garden vegetable whole grain snacks, 15 pieces (30 g)	4
Snacks, garden vegetable, 15 pieces (30 g)	4

Wheat Thins Holiday

Whole grain snacks, 16 pieces (31 g)	5

Wheat Thins Popped

Chips, popped, barbecue, 24 chips (30 g)	4
Chips, sour cream & onion, 1 package (22 g)	3
Popped chips, spicy cheddar, 26 chips (30 g)	4
Sour cream and onion popped chips, 26 chips (30 g)	4

Wheatsworth

Wheat crackers, stone ground, 5 crackers (16 g)	3

Zesta

Crackers, unsalted tops, 5 crackers (15 g)	2
Saltine crackers, original, 5 crackers (16 g)	2
Saltine crackers, whole wheat, 5 crackers (15 g)	2
Soup & oyster crackers, 45 each (16 g)	2

Fruit & Nut Mixes

Aurora Natural

Salad fixins', original, ¼ cup	5

Daily Chef Gourmet Foods

Tropical fruit and nutblend, ¼ cup	6

Fresh Gourmet

Cranberries & glazed walnuts, ½ Tbsp	1

Kirkland Signature Sahale Snacks

Pecan-cashew nut crisp, ¼ cup	6

Kroger

Salad toppers, dried cranberries & honey roasted pecans, 1 Tbsp	1

Marzetti Salad Accents

Salad toppings, Asian sesame, 1 Tbsp	1
Salad toppings, bac'n almond crunch, 1 Tbsp	1

Snacks

SmartPoints™ value

McCormick

Crunchy and flavorful salad toppins, 1 ⅓ Tbsp	1

Nut Harvest

Nut and fruit mix, ¼ cup	5

Ocean Spray Craisins

Cranberry almond fruit clusters, 1 oz	5

Orchard Valley Harvest

Cranberry almond cashew trail mix, 1 package (28 g)	5

Planters NUT-rition

Blueberry nut sustaining energy mix, 1 pack (51 g)	9

Safeway Kitchens

Salad toppers, gourmet, cranberry and roasted almonds, 1 Tbsp	1

Salad Pizazz

Cherry cranberry pecano, 1 Tbsp	1
Orange cranberry almondine, 1 Tbsp	1
Pomecranate honey walnut fusion, 1 Tbsp	1
Raspberry cranberry walnut frisco, 1 Tbsp	1

Second Nature

Simplicity medley, ¼ cup	5
Wholesome medley fruit, nut and chocolate mix, 3 Tbsp	5

Trader Joe's

Just a handful of oh my! omega trek mix, 1 bag (34 g)	6
More than a mouthful trek mix, ¼ cup	8

Whole Foods 365 Everyday Value

Cranberry and nut trail mix, ⅓ cup	5

Wonderful

Almond accents, honey roasted with cranberries, 1 Tbsp	1

SmartPoints™ value

Nuts

Archer Farms

Almonds, raw, unsalted, ¼ cup	5
Mixed nuts, raw, unsalted, ¼ cup	5
Unsalted raw mixed nuts, ¼ cup	5

Aurora Natural

Cashews, raw, ¼ cup	6

Bachman

Honey roasted peanuts, 3 Tbsp	5

Blue Diamond

Almonds, 1 oz	5
Almonds, bold, jalapeño smokehouse, 1 package (43 g)	8
Almonds, bold, wasabi & soy sauce, 1 package (43 g)	8
Almonds, honey roasted, 28 nuts (28 g)	5
Almonds, lightly salted, 28 nuts (28 g)	5
Almonds, oven roasted, blueberry flavor, 24 nuts (28 g)	5
Almonds, oven roasted, butter toffee flavor, 1 oz	5
Almonds, roasted salted, 28 nuts (28 g)	5
Almonds, salted caramel flavored, 28 nuts (28 g)	5
Almonds, smokehouse, 28 nuts (28 g)	5
Almonds, strawberry flavored, 24 nuts (28 g)	5
Almonds, toasted coconut, 1 oz	5
Almonds, whole natural, 24 nuts (28 g)	5
Almonds, whole natural, value pack, 24 nuts (28 g)	5
Honey roasted cinnamon almonds, 28 pieces (28 g)	5
Nut thins, almond, pepper Jack cheese, 16 crackers (30 g)	4

Snacks

Blue Diamond Bold

Almonds, habanero bbq, 28 nuts (28 g)	5
Almonds, honey Dijon, 28 nuts (28 g)	5
Almonds, lime 'n chili, 1 package (43 g)	8
Almonds, salt 'n vinegar, 28 nuts (28 g)	5
Almonds, wasabi & soy sauce, 28 nuts (28 g)	5

Blue Diamond Low Sodium

Lightly salted sea salt almonds, 1 oz	5

Blue Diamond Natural

Almonds, oven roasted, 24 nuts (28 g)	5
Almonds, oven roasted, cinnamon brown sugar, 24 nuts (28 g)	5
Almonds, oven roasted, dark chocolate flavor, 24 nuts (28 g)	5

Blue Diamond Smokehouse

Almonds, 1 package (43 g)	6

CVS

Peanuts, dry roast, honey roasted, 1 oz	5
Peanuts, dry roast, lightly salted, 40 pieces (28 g)	5
Peanuts, dry roasted, 1 oz	5

Diamond of California Nut Toppings

Almonds, sliced, ¼ cup	5
Pecans, glazed, ¼ cup	6
Walnuts, finely diced, ¼ cup	6
Walnuts, glazed, ¼ cup	6

Emerald

100 calorie packs dry roasted almonds, 1 package (17.5 g)	3
Almonds, cinnamon roast, cinnamon flavor, ¼ cup	5
Almonds, cocoa roast, dark chocolate, ¼ cup	5
Almonds, cocoa roast, dark chocolate flavor, ¼ cup	4
Almonds, dry roasted, ¼ cup	5
Almonds, smoked, ¼ cup	5
Cocoa roast almonds, ¼ cup	5
Honey roasted peanuts, old fashioned, 1 oz	5
Mixed nuts, sweet & salty, original, ¼ cup	5
Vanilla bean flavoured roast almonds, ¼ cup	4
Walnuts, glazed, original, 1 oz	5
Whole jumbo cashews, ¼ cup	5

Emerald 100 Calorie Pack

Cocoa roast almonds, 1 package (18 g)	3
Halves and pieces cashew, 1 package (18 g)	3
Natural walnuts and almonds, 1 package (16 g)	3
Natural walnuts and almonds, 1 package (16 g)	3
Smoked almonds, 1 pack (16 g)	3
Vanilla roast almonds, 1 package (18 g)	3

Emerald Breakfast On The Go!

Nut & granola mix, berry nut blend, 1 pouch (42.5 g)	8

Emerald Cocoa Roast

Dark chocolate almonds, ¼ cup	4

Emerald Simply

Natural almonds, ¼ cup	5

Finest

Boiled peanuts, large, green, ¼ cup	3

Fisher

Nut topping, mixed nut variety, 2 Tbsp	3

Fisher Chef's Naturals

Walnut halves and pieces, ¼ cup	6

Snacks

	SmartPoints™ value
Fresh Gourmet	
Almonds, sliced, toasted, 1 Tbsp	1
Pecan pieces, honey roasted, 2 tsp	1
Walnut pieces, glazed, 2 tsp	1
Frito Lay	
Almonds, roasted, salted, 1 oz	6
Deluxe mixed nuts, ¼ cup	5
Pistachios in shell, 1 package (25 g)	4
Whole salted cashews, 3 Tbsp	6
Gefen	
Chestnuts, whole, roasted & peeled, ¼ cup	3
Good Sense	
Sunflower nuts, roasted & salted, ¼ cup	6
Sunflower nuts, roasted/ no salt, ¼ cup	6
Great Value	
Cashew cranberry and almond trail mix, ¼ cup	6
Roasted salted almonds, ¼ cup	5
Hershey's	
Candy bar, milk chocolate with almonds, snack size, 3 pieces (38 g)	10
Hoody's	
Roasted in-shell peanuts, ½ cup	5
Hy-Vee	
Almonds, raw, ¼ cup	5
Peanuts, salted in the shell, 1 oz	5
Kirkland Signature	
Almonds, ¼ cup	5
Cashew clusters with almonds and pumpkin seeds, 1 oz	5
Dry roasted sea salt almonds, ¼ cup	5
Extra fancy mixed nuts, ¼ cup	6
Extra fancy unsalted mixed nuts, 1 oz	5

	SmartPoints™ value
Marcona almonds, 1 oz	5
Pecan halves, ¼ cup	6
Super extra-large peanuts, 3 Tbsp	5
Walnuts, 1 oz	6
Whole fancy indian cashews, 1 oz	6
Whole fancy unsalted cashews, 16 pieces (28 g)	5
Kirkland Signature Everybody's Nuts!	
California pistachios, ½ cup	5
Kroger	
Almonds, ¼ cup	5
Peanuts, dry roasted, salted, 40 pieces (28 g)	5
Peanuts, honey roasted, ¼ cup	5
Peanuts, light salted, ¼ cup	5
Peanuts, unsalted, ¼ cup	5
Unsalted dry roasted almonds, 1 oz	5
Lance Fresh	
Peanuts, salted, 1 package (39 g)	7
Mareblu Naturals	
Cashew crunch, ¼ cup	6
Mariani	
Sliced almonds, ¼ cup	5
Sliced premium almonds, ¼ cup	5
Meijer	
Peanuts, dry roasted, ¼ cup	5
Munchies	
Peanuts, flamin' hot, 1 package (46 g)	9
Peanuts, honey roasted, 1 package (39 g)	8
Peanuts, salted, 1 package (46 g)	8
Nice!	
Pistachios, in shells, 35 nuts (23 g)	4
Nutclub	
Pistacios, ¼ cup	6
Our Family Recipe	
Sliced almonds salad toppings, 1 Tbsp	1

Planters

Almonds, pumpkin spice, 25 pieces (28 g)	5
Almonds, roasted, 27 pieces (28 g)	5
Cashews, halves & pieces, lightly salted, 50 pieces (28 g)	5
Cashews, honey roasted, 25 pieces (28 g)	6
Cashews, whole, deluxe, 1 oz	5
Deluxe mixed nuts, 21 pieces (28 g)	5
Deluxe mixed nuts, lightly salted, 1 oz	5
Dry roasted peanuts, 1 oz	5
Dry roasted peanuts, honey roasted, value pack, 1 oz	5
Dry roasted peanuts, lightly salted, 1 oz	5
Fancy whole cashews with sea salt, 18 pieces (28 g)	5
Mixed nuts, 30 pieces (28 g)	5
Mixed nuts, deluxe, made with sea salt, 19 pieces (28 g)	5
Mixed nuts, honey roasted, 28 pieces (28 g)	5
Mixed nuts, lightly salted, less than 50% peanuts, 29 pieces (28 g)	5
Mixed nuts, unsalted, 30 pieces (28 g)	5
Peanuts, chipotle, 39 pieces (28 g)	5
Peanuts, classic, 35 pieces (28 g)	5
Peanuts, cocktail, 35 pieces (28 g)	5
Peanuts, cocktail, 35 pieces (28 g)	5
Peanuts, cocktail, lightly salted, 35 pieces (28 g)	5
Peanuts, cocoa, 39 pieces (28 g)	5
Peanuts, dry roasted honey roasted, 39 pieces (28 g)	5
Peanuts, honey roasted, 1 package (28 g)	5
Peanuts, honey roasted, 1 package (56 g)	10

Peanuts, lightly salted, 1 package (56 g)	10
Peanuts, salted, 1 package (28 g)	5
Peanuts, sweet 'n crunchy, 40 pieces (28 g)	6
Pistachio blend, 28 pieces (28 g)	5
Pistachios, dry roasted, ½ cup	5
Pistachios, sea salt and black pepper, 1 oz	5
Smoked peanuts, 39 pieces (28 g)	5
Spanish peanuts, redskin, 1 oz	6
Stadium peanuts, roasted in-shell salted, 19 pieces (28 g)	5

Planters Deluxe

Cashews, whole, honey roasted, 25 pieces (28 g)	5
Cashews, whole, lightly salted, 23 pieces (28 g)	5
Mixed nuts, lightly salted, with California pistachios, 20 pieces (28 g)	5
Pistachio mix, 35 pieces (28 g)	5

Planters Limited Edition

Winter spice mix, 3 Tbsp	5

Planters NUT-rition

Heart healthy mix, 1 pack (42 g)	8
Nut mix, wholesome, 1 pack (35 g)	7
Sustaining energy mix, honey nut, 1 pack (47 g)	8
Wholesome nut mix, 18 pieces (28 g)	5

Roland

Almonds, oven roasted, sea salt, 1 oz	5

Safeway Kitchens

Sliced almond no salt oven roasted salad toppers, 1 Tbsp	1

Sahale Snack Better

Almonds, glazed, ¼ cup	5

Second Nature

California medley, ¼ cup	5

Snacks

SmartPoints™ value

Simple Truth

Raw almonds, ¼ cup	5

Snak Club

Almonds, raw, 22 pieces (30 g)	5

Southern Grove Simply Nature's Best

Dry roasted peanuts, 40 pieces (28 g)	5

Southern Style Nuts Hunter Mix

Gourmet mixed nuts, ¼ cup	5

Sunkist Almond Accents

Flavored sliced almonds, honey roasted, 1 Tbsp	1

Trader Joe's

Candied pecans, 1 oz	7
Candied walnuts, ¼ cup	7
Coconut cashews, ¼ cup	6
Just a handful of dry roasted unsalted almonds, 1 bag (35 g)	6
Mesquite smoked seasoned almonds, ¼ cup	5
Organic raw almonds, ¼ cup	5
Organic raw almonds, ¼ cup	5
Raw fancy mixed nuts, ¼ cup	5
Raw pistachios (with shells), ½ cup	5
Sliced honey roasted almonds, ¼ cup	6

Trader Joe's Nuts

Dry roasted unsalted almonds, 1 package (35 g)	6
In shell pumpkin seeds, ¼ cup	6
Raw cashew pieces, ¼ cup	5
Reduced salt almonds, ¼ cup	5

True North

Almond pecan cashew clusters, 5 clusters (28 g)	6

Walgreen's

Almonds, natural raw, ¼ cup	5
Pistachios, in shells, 28 pieces (18 g)	3

SmartPoints™ value

Wonderful

Almond accents, honey roasted, 1 Tbsp	1
Almond accents, original oven roasted, 1 Tbsp	1
Almond accents, oven roasted no salt, 1 Tbsp	1
Almond accents, sea salt & cracked pepper, 1 Tbsp	1
Almonds, natural raw, ¼ cup	5
Almonds, roasted & salted, ¼ cup	5
Almonds, roasted, no salt, ¼ cup	5
Pistachios, roasted & salted, 1 package (43 g)	4
Pistachios, roasted lightly salted, ½ cup with shells	5
Pistachios, roasted, no salt, ½ cup	5
Pistachios, salt & pepper, ½ cup	5
Pistachios, sweet chili, ½ cup	5
Roasted & salted pistachios (without shells), 1 oz	5
Roasted and salted pistachios (with shells), ½ cup	5

Young Pecan

Golden sweet pecan halves, ¼ cup	7

Popcorn

479°

Popcorn, artisan, asiago parmesan and cheddar, 3 cups	4
Popcorn, artisan, sea salt, 4 cups	4
Popcorn, artisan, toasted coconut caramel, 1 cup	5

Act II

Micorwave popcorn, butter, light, 3 Tbsp unpopped	4
Microwave popcorn, butter flavored, 2 Tbsp unpopped	4
Microwave popcorn, butter flavored, 94% fat free, 3 Tbsp unpopped	4

Snacks

Microwave popcorn, butter lovers, 2 Tbsp unpopped	5
Microwave popcorn, extreme butter, 1 bag (100 g)	7
Microwave popcorn, movie theatre butter, 2 Tbsp unpopped	5

Act II Mini Bags

Microwave popcorn, butter flavored, bags, 1 bag (45 g)	6

American Farmer

Kettle popped corn, 2 ½ cups	5

American Farmer Skinny N'Light

Kettle popped corn, 2 ½ cups	4

Angie's Boom Chicka Pop

Caramel and cheddar popcorn mix, 1 ¼ cups	5
Lightly sweet popcorn, 3 ¼ cups	4
Popcorn, sea salt, 4 cups	4
Salted caramel popcorn, 1 ¾ cups	5
Sea salt popcorn, 1 package (6 g)	1
Sweet and salty kettle corn, 2 cups	5
Sweet and spicy popcorn, 2 cups	5
White cheddar popcorn, 2 ½ cups	5

Angie's Delightfully Different

Sweet and salty classic kettle corn, 2 cups	5

Bachman

Popcorn, air popped, 2 ¾ cups	5

Better Made Signature

Popcorn, gourmet, movie theater butter, 3 cups	5

Cape Cod

Lightly sweet kettle corn popcorn, 3 ¾ cups	4
Sea salt popcorn, 4 cups	4
White cheddar popcorn, 2 ¼ cups	5

Chester's

Cheddar cheese flavored popcorn, 3 cups	5
Popcorn, cheddar cheese, 3 cups	5

Clancy's

Extra butter microwave popcorn, 2 Tbsp unpopped	4

Cosmos Creations

Baked corn creations, salted caramel, 1 ¼ cups	6

Cracker Jack

Butter toffee flavored popcorn, ½ cup	5
Caramel coated popcorn & peanuts, the original, ½ cup	5
Caramel coated popcorn & peanuts, the original, 3 pack, 1 package (28 g)	5

Earth Balance

Vegan aged white cheddar flavor popcorn, 2 ¾ cups	5
Vegan buttery flavor popcorn, 3 ½ cups	4

Fit & Active

Butter flavor microwave popcorn, 3 Tbsp unpopped	4
Butter microwave popcorn unpopped, 1 bag (35 g)	4

From the Kitchen of Cooking Light Magazine

Simply sea salt popcorn gluten free, 4 cups	4

G.H. Cretors

Chicago mix popcorn, 1 ¼ cups	6
Popped corn, just the cheese, 2 cups	6

Gaslamp Popcorn

Popcorn, kettle corn, sweet and salty, 2 ¼ cups	5

Good Health

Popcorn, half naked, with a hint of olive oil, 4 cups	4
Popcorn, organic, with a hint of sea salt, 3 ½ cups	4

Snacks

Great Value

Popping corn, yellow, 3 Tbsp unpopped	4

Herr's

Popcorn, original, 3 cups	5

Jay's

Caramel corn, 1 oz	5

Jenny's

Carmel corn ditto's, ¾ cup	6

Jensen's Finest

Caramel corn, old fashioned, ¾ cup	5

Jiffy Pop

Microwave popcorn, light butter, 2 Tbsp	3
Popcorn, butter flavored, 2 Tbsp	4

Jolly Time

100 calorie kettle corn, 94% fat free, 5 cups	3
100% organic yellow popcorn (unpopped), 2 Tbsp	3
Microwave pop corn, better butter flavor, 2 Tbsp	5
Pop corn, yellow, 2 Tbsp	3
White cheddar delicious white popcorn, 3 ⅔ cups	4

Jolly Time 100 Calorie Healthy Pop

94% fat free kettle corn mini bags, 2 Tbsp unpopped	3
94% fat free pop corn mini bags, 2 Tbsp unpopped	3
Low sodium butter flavor microwave popcorn, 1 bag unpopped (34 g)	3
Microwave pop corn, butter flavor, 2 Tbsp unpopped	2

Jolly Time American's Best

94% fat free butter flavor microwave popcorn (3 pack), 2 Tbsp	3

Jolly Time Blast O Butter

Ultimate theatre style microwave pop corn, 2 Tbsp unpopped	6

Jolly Time Healthy Pop

94% fat free butter popcorn, 2 Tbsp unpopped	3
94% fat free kettle corn microwave popcorn, 2 Tbsp unpopped	3
Butter flavor microwave popcorn (12 pack), 2 Tbsp unpopped	3
Butter microwave popcorn, 2 Tbsp unpopped	3
Crispy n white microwave popcorn, 2 Tbsp unpopped	3
Jolly time healthy pop caramel apple, 94% fat free, 5 cups	3
Jolly time healthy pop low sodium, 94% fat free, 5 cups	3
Kettle corn 100 calorie microwave popcorn, 1 bag unpopped (34 g)	3
Microwave popcorn, kettle corn, 2 Tbsp unpopped	3

Jolly Time Light

Crispy n white microwave popcorn, 2 Tbsp unpopped	4

Jolly Time Ready to Eat

Kettle corn, 3 ½ cups	4
Sea salted, 4 ½ cups	4
White cheddar, 3 ⅔ cups	4

Kellogg's Special K

Popcorn chips, butter, 1 pouch (22 g)	3
Popcorn chips, sweet and salty, 1 pouch (22 g)	3

Kirkland Signature

Microwave popcorn, unpopped, 2 Tbsp	7

Kroger

94% fat free butter flavoured popcorn mini bag, 1 bag (34 g)	4
94% fat free microwave popcorn, 2 Tbsp	3
Microwave popcorn, movie theater butter, 2 Tbsp	5

Popcorn, butter, 2 ½ cups	5
Popcorn, white, 3 Tbsp	4
Popcorn, white cheddar, 2 ½ cups	5
Popcorn, yellow, 3 Tbsp	4

Lance

Popcorn, movie theater butter, 1 oz	5
Popcorn, white cheddar cheese, 2 ⅛ cups	6

LesserEvil

Chia pop, aged white cheddar, 2 ½ cups	3
Chia pop, sea salt and cracked pepper, 2 ½ cups	3

LesserEvil Buddha Bowl

Himalayan sweetness organic popcorn, 2 cups	5

LesserEvil Kettle Corn

Classic, 1 cup	5

Market Pantry

Microwave popcorn with 94% fat free butter, 3 Tbsp unpopped	4
Single serve microwave popcorn, 1 bag unpopped (31 g)	3
Yellow kernel popping corn, 3 Tbsp unpopped	4

Martin's

Popcorn, butter flavored, value size, 3 ½ cups	5

Nature's Promise Naturals

Kettle corn, 2 cups	5

Newman's Own

Microwave popcorn, 94% fat free butter, 3 ½ cups	3
Microwave popcorn, natural, 3 ½ cups	4

Newman's Own All Natural

Popcorn, light butter flavor, 1 oz	4

Newman's Own Organic Pop's Corn

Microwave popcorn, organic, light butter, 1 serving (28 g)	4

O-Ke-Doke

Popcorn, cheese flavored, 1 oz	5
Popcorn, chicago mix, 2 cups	5

Orville Redenbacher

Butter flavored gourmet popping corn, 2 Tbsp	7
Gourmet popcorn, kettle korn, classic, 2 ½ cups	5
Gourmet popping corn, movie theater butter, mini bags, 5 cups	7
Gourmet popping corn, white corn, 3 Tbsp	3
Movie theater butter gourmet popping corn, 2 Tbsp	6
Original gourmet popping corn, 3 Tbsp	3
Popcorn, natural light, 1 oz	3
Popcorn, original, ½ cup	7
Popping corn, gourmet, light butter, 2 Tbsp	4
Popping corn, gourmet, microwave, butter, single serve bags, 1 bag unpopped (42.5 g)	8
Popping corn, gourmet, mini bags, movie theater butter, 1 bag (43 g)	8
Popping corn, gourmet, simply salted, 2 Tbsp	6
Smartpop butter gourmet popping corn, 3 Tbsp	3

Orville Redenbacher Gourmet

Movie theater butter popping corn, 2 Tbsp unpopped	7

Orville Redenbacher Gourmet Naturals

Popping corn, gourmet, classic butter & sea salt, 2 Tbsp	4
Popping corn, gourmet, classic butter & sea salt, 2 Tbsp unpopped	4
Popping corn, gourmet, garlic butter & sea salt, 2 Tbsp unpopped	4
Popping corn, gourmet, simply salted, 2 Tbsp unpopped	4

Snacks

Snacks

	SmartPoints™ value
Orville Redenbacher Mini	
Movie theater butter gourmet popping corn, 1 bag unpopped (42 g)	7
Orville Redenbacher Pop Up Bowl	
Butter flavor gourmet popping corn, 4 cups popped	7
Butter flavored gourmet microwave popping corn, 2 Tbsp	7
Classic recipe microwave popcorn, 2 Tbsp unpopped	7
Gourmet popping corn, butter, smart pop, microwave, 3 Tbsp	3
Gourmet popping corn, kettle korn, 2 Tbsp	6
Gourmet popping corn, movie theater butter, 2 Tbsp	7
Gourmet popping corn, movie theater butter, microwave, 2 Tbsp unpopped	7
Gourmet white popping corn, 2 Tbsp unpopped	6
Light butter popping corn, 5 ½ cups popped	4
Popping corn, gourmet, kettle korn, 2 Tbsp	6
Popping corn, gourmet, tender white, 2 Tbsp	6
Popping corn, gourmet, ultimate butter, 2 Tbsp unpopped	7
Orville Redenbacher Popping & Topping	
Popcorn oil, butter flavor, 1 Tbsp	4
Orville Redenbacher Smart Pop!	
Butter flavored popped corn, 1 bag (33 g)	3
Gourmet popping corn, butter, 3 Tbsp	3
Gourmet popping corn, butter, single serve bags, 1 bag (33 g)	3
Gourmet popping corn, kettle korn, 3 Tbsp	4
Gourmet popping corn, kettle korn, single serve bags, 1 bag (33 g)	3

	SmartPoints™ value
Kettle korn, pop up bowl, 3 Tbsp unpopped	4
Popping corn, gourmet, 94% fat free, mini bags, butter, 1 bag (35 g)	3
Popping corn, gourmet, kettle korn, 1 bag (35 g)	3
Popping corn, gourmet, microwave, butter, 3 Tbsp	3
Single serve butter flavored popping corn, 1 bag (33 g)	3
Sweet and salty kettle corn, 94% fat free, 1 bag (33 g)	3
Orville Redenbacher Smart Pop! Pop Up Bowl	
Gourmet popping corn, kettle korn, 3 Tbsp	4
Popping corn, gourmet, butter, 3 Tbsp	3
Our Family	
Popcorn, movie theater butter, mini bags, 1 bag (43 g)	8
Pop Weaver	
Popcorn, microwave butter flavored, 1 bag unpopped (61 g)	9
Popcorn, microwave, extra butter, 1 bag unpopped (65 g)	10
Popcorn, microwave, light butter, 1 bag unpopped (61 g)	7
Popcorn, Indiana	
Dark fudge sea salt caramel drizzlecorn, ½ cup	6
Kettlecorn, all natural, 2 cups	5
Kettlecorn, chocolate peanut butter, 1 ½ cups	6
Kettlecorn, dark fudge chocolate chip, 1 ½ cups	7
Kettlecorn, drizzled black & white, 1 ½ cups	7
Popcorn, Indiana Chip'ins	
Popcorn chips, sea salt, all natural, 20 chips (28 g)	3
Popcorn chips, white cheddar, all natural, 18 chips (28 g)	4

Popcorn, Indiana Fit

Extra virgin oil popcorn, 3 ¾ cups	4
Parmesan and herb popcorn, 3 ¾ cups	4
Popcorn, extra virgin olive oil, 3 ¼ cups	4
Popcorn, parmesan & herb, 3 ¼ cups	4
Popcorn, real butter, 4 cups	3
Sea salt popcorn, 3 ½ cups	4

Popcorn, Indiana Original

Movie theater popcorn, 2 cups	5

PopCorners

Sweet chili, popped corn chips gluten free, 1 oz	4

Pop-Secret

Popcorn, homestyle butter, 3 cups	5
Popcorn, kettle corn, 3 cups	5
Popcorn, microwave, homestyle, 2 Tbsp unpopped	1
Popcorn, microwave, old fashion kettle corn, sweet and salty, 3 Tbsp unpopped	6
Popcorn, premium, butter, 94% fat free, 3 Tbsp	5
Popcorn, premium, extra butter, 3 Tbsp	6
Popcorn, premium, movie theater butter flavor, 2 Tbsp	6
Popcorn, sweet 'n crunchy microwave kettlecorn, 2 Tbsp unpopped	7
Popcorn, white cheddar, 3 cups	5

Pop-Secret 100 Calorie Pop

Microwave popcorn, premium, butter, snack size, 1 bag (35 g)	4
Microwave popcorn, premium, kettle corn, 1 bag (35 g)	4
Popcorn, premium, butter, kettle corn, 3 Tbsp	3
Premium butter popcorn snack bag prepared, 1 Tbsp	3

Premium kettle corn snack bag prepared, 1 bag (31 g)	3
Premium popcorn, homestyle, 3 Tbsp	3

Pop-Secret Jumbo

Microwave popcorn, premium, movie-theater butter, 3 Tbsp	6
Popcorn, premium, butter, 3 Tbsp	7
Popping corn, 3 Tbsp unpopped	3

Pop-Secret Snack Size

Premium popcorn, kettle corn, 94% fat free, 3 Tbsp unpopped	4

Popz

Popcorn, microwave, movie butter, ⅓ tub (39 g)	8

Quinn

Popcorn, kale and sea salt, 4 cups	5

Rocky Mountain Popcorn Company Just Honest

White cheddar popcorn, 2 cups	4

Safeway The Snack Artist

Popcorn, microwave, butter 94% fat free, 2 Tbsp	3

Sage Valley

Popcorn, lite organic, 1 oz	3

Simple Truth

Kettle popcorn, 2 cups	5

Simple Truth Organic

Low sodium popcorn, 3 ½ cups	4

Simply Balanced

Popcorn, whole grain, lightly salted, 3 cups	4

Skinny Girl

Butter and sea salt popcorn, 6 cups	5
Lime and salt microwave popcorn, 6 cups	5

Skinny Girl Snacks

Kettle corn popcorn, 1 cup	5
Olive oil and pink himalayan salt flavored popcorn, 3 ½ cups	4
White cheddar chipotle popcorn, 3 cups	4

Snacks

Snacks

SmartPoints™ value

SkinnyPop

Black pepper popcorn, 4 cups	5
Original flavor popcorn, 4 cups	5
Popcorn, 3 ¾ cups	5
Popcorn 100 calorie bag, 1 package (18 g)	3
Popcorn, skinny pack, 1 package (18 g)	3
Popcorn, ultra lite, 3 ½ cups	5
Popcorn, ultra lite, white cheddar flavor, 3 ½ cups	5
Popcorn, xl skinny, 3 ¾ cups	5
Skinnypack popcorn, 1 package (18 g)	3
Ultra lite white cheddar popcorn, 1 oz	5
Microwave popcorn, deluxe, light butter, 2 Tbsp unpopped	4

Smart Balance

Microwave popcorn, deluxe, smart n' healthy, 3 Tbsp unpopped	3
Popcorn, deluxe microwave light butter flavor, 3 Tbsp unpopped	5

Smart Sense

Popcorn, cheese flavored, 3 cups	5

Smartfood

Kettle corn flavored popcorn, 1 ¼ cups	6
Popcorn, movie theater butter flavored, 1 package (57 g)	9
White cheddar cheese flavored popcorn, 1 ¾ cups	1
White cheddar popcorn, 1 package (18 g)	3

Smartfood 100 Calorie

Popcorn, white cheddar, 1 package (18 g)	3

Smartfood Delight

Sea salt, air popped popcorn, 1 oz	4
White cheddar popcorn, 3 ½ cups	4

SnackWell's 130 Calorie Packs

Popcorn, caramel, fudge drizzled, 1 pack (30 g)	7

SmartPoints™ value

SnackWell's 130 Calorie Packs

Popcorn, caramel, white fudge drizzled, 1 pack (30 g)	7

Snak King

Popcorn, carmel, ¾ cup	5

The Popcorn Factory

Popcorn ball, 1 popcorn ball (31 g)	6

Trader Joe's

94% fat free microwave popcorn, 1 bag (40 g)	4
Caramel popcorn, ¾ cup	6
Kettle corn, 2 ¼ cups	5
Lite kettle corn, 1 oz	4
Lite popcorn, 2 ½ cups	4
Movie theater buttery popcorn, 2 cups	5
Organic popcorn with olive oil, 2 cups	4
Partially popped popcorn, ⅓ cup	4
Popcorn with herbs and spices, 2 cups	4
Reduced guilt air-popped popcorn, 2 ½ cups	3
White cheddar popcorn, 2 cups	6
World's puffiest white cheddar corn puffs, 2 ½ cups	4

Potato Chips

Kettle

Backyard barbeque potato chips, 13 chips (28 g)	5
Chips, lightly salted, 1 oz	5
Maple bacon potato chips, 13 chips (28 g)	5
Olive oil real sliced potatoes baked potato chips, 20 chips (28 g)	4
Potato chips, 40% reduced fat, salt & fresh ground pepper, 13 chips (28 g)	4
Potato chips, 40% reduced fat, sea salt, 13 chips (28 g)	4
Potato chips, baked, hickory honey barbeque, 20 chips (28 g)	4

	SmartPoints™ value
Potato chips, baked, lightly salted, 1 bag (23 g)	3
Potato chips, baked, sea salt & vinegar, 23 chips (28 g)	4
Potato chips, jalapeño, 13 chips (28 g)	5
Potato chips, jalapeño, hot, 13 chips (28 g)	5
Potato chips, krinkle cut, 40% reduced fat, sea salt & vinegar, 9 chips (28 g)	4
Potato chips, krinkle cut, salt & fresh ground pepper, 9 chips (28 g)	5
Potato chips, krinkle cut, salt & fresh ground pepper, sharing size, 9 chips (28 g)	5
Potato chips, krinkle cut, sea salt, party size, 9 chips (28 g)	5
Potato chips, lightly salted, 13 chips (28 g)	5
Potato chips, sea salt, 13 chips (28 g)	5

Kirkland Kettle

Lightly salted krinkle cut chips, 1 oz	5

Kitchen Cooked

Potato chips, classic, 18 chips (28 g)	5

Kroger

Potato chips, bar-b-q flavored, 15 chips (28 g)	5
Potato chips, classic, 15 chips (28 g)	5
Potato chips, sour cream & onion, 15 chips (28 g)	6
Potato chips, wavy, 15 chips (28 g)	5

Kroger Kettle Cooked

Reduced fat original potato chips, 18 chips (28 g)	4

Lay's

Baked potato crisps (variety pack), 1 package (31.8 g)	4
Cheddar bacon mac and cheese flavored potato chips, 15 chips (28 g)	5

	SmartPoints™ value
Cheesy garlic bread flavored potato chips, 17 chips (28 g)	5
Classic potato chips, 15 chips (28 g)	5
Dill pickle potato chips, 17 chips (28 g)	5
Flamin' hot flavored potato chips, 17 chips (28 g)	5
Honey barbeque flavored potato chips, 15 chips (28 g)	5
Lightly salted potato chips, 1 oz	5
Limon potato chips, 15 chips (28 g)	5
Original deli style potato chips, 17 chips (28 g)	5
Potato chips, barbecue flavored, 1 package (28 g)	5
Potato chips, cheddar & sour cream, 15 chips (28 g)	5
Potato chips, classic, 1 package (28 g)	5
Salt and vinegar potato chips, 17 chips (28 g)	5
Sour cream & onion potato chips, 17 chips (28 g)	5
Sweet southern heat barbecue flavored potato chips, 15 chips (28 g)	5

Lay's Air Pops

Barbeque flavored crisps, 20 crisps (28 g)	4
Original potato crisps, 24 crisps (28 g)	4
Sour cream and onion flavored crisps, 19 crisps (28 g)	4

Lay's Baked!

Cheddar & sour cream potato crisps, 1 package (32 g)	5

Lay's Kettle Cooked

40% less fat applewood smoked bbq potato chips, 16 chips (28 g)	4
40% less fat original potato chips, 18 chips (28 g)	4

Snacks

Snacks

	SmartPoints™ value
40% less fat sea salt & vinegar flavored potato chips, 1 package (39 g)	6
40% less fat sea salt and vinegar potato chips, 16 chips (28 g)	4
Jalapeño flavored potato chips, 15 chips (28 g)	5
Mesquite bbq flavored potato chips, 18 chips (28 g)	5
Original potato chips, 1 single bag (39 g)	6
Original potato chips, 16 chips (28 g)	5
Potato chips, jalapeño cheddar flavored, 40% less fat, 16 chips (28 g)	4
Roasted garlic and sea salt lattice cut potato chips, 13 chips (28 g)	5
Sea salt & cracked pepper potato chips, 18 chips (28 g)	5
Sea salt & vinegar flavored potato chips, 18 chips (28 g)	5
Wasabi ginger flavored potato chips, 18 chips (28 g)	5

Lay's Kettle Cooked Lattice Cut

Aged cheddar and black pepper lattice cut potato chips, 13 chips (28 g)	5

Lay's Oven Baked

Barbecue potato crisps, 1 package (32 g)	5
Original potato crisps, 1 package (32 g)	4
Sour cream and onion potato crisps, 1 package (32 g)	4

Lay's Simply

Sea salted thick cut potato chips, 15 chips (28 g)	5

Lay's Stax

Bacon & cheddar potato skins flavored potato crisps, 12 crisps (28 g)	5
Cheddar flavored potato crisps, 12 crisps (28 g)	5

	SmartPoints™ value
Mesquite barbecue flavored potato crisps, 12 crisps (28 g)	5
Original potato crisps, 12 crisps (28 g)	5
Salt & vinegar potato crisps, 12 crisps (28 g)	5
Sour cream & onion potato crisps, 12 crisps (28 g)	5

Lay's Wavy

Hickory bbq potato chips, 13 chips (28 g)	5
Lightly salted potato chips, 11 chips (28 g)	5
Milk chocolate covered potato chips, 3 chips (28 g)	7
Original potato chips, 11 chips (28 g)	5
Ranch flavored potato chips, 12 chips (28 g)	5
Roasted garlic & sea salt potato chips, 12 chips (28 g)	5

Martin's

Potato chips, kettle-cook'd, 19 chips (28 g)	5

Miss Vickie's

Jalapeño kettle cooked potato chips, 1 mini bag (39 g)	7
Potato chips, jalapeño flavored, 1 oz	5
Potato chips, kettle cooked, sea salt & vinegar, 1 package (38.9 g)	7
Potato chips, simply sea salt, original recipe, 1 package (39 g)	7
Potato chips, smokehouse bbq, 1 package (39 g)	7

Munchos

Light tasting potato crisps, 16 crisps (28 g)	5
Potato chips, 16 crisps (28 g)	1
Potato crisps, big grab, 1 package (37 g)	7

Pik-Nik Original

Shoe string potatoes, ⅔ cup	6

Popchips

Barbeque potato popped chip snacks, 20 chips (28 g)	4
Cheddar & sour cream potato popped chip snacks, 22 chips (28 g)	4
Cheddar potato popped chip snacks, 1 bag (23 g)	3
Cheddar potato popped chip snacks, 22 chips (28 g)	4
Original potato popped chip snack, 1 bag (23 g)	3
Salt & pepper potato popped chip snacks, 22 chips (28 g)	4
Sea salt & vinegar potato popped chip snacks, 22 chips (28 g)	4
Sea salt potato popped chip snacks, 23 chips (28 g)	4
Sour cream & onion potato popped chip snacks, 22 chips (28 g)	4
Sweet potato popped chip snacks, 23 chips (28 g)	4

Pringles

Potao crisps, multigrain farmhouse cheddar, 15 crisps (28 g)	5
Potato crisps, bacon flavor, 15 crisps (28 g)	5
Potato crisps, bbq flavor, 15 crisps (28 g)	5
Potato crisps, cheddar cheese flavored, 15 crisps (28 g)	5
Potato crisps, fat free, original flavor, 15 crisps (28 g)	2
Potato crisps, French onion dip, 16 crisps (28 g)	5
Potato crisps, honey mustard, 15 crisps (28 g)	5
Potato crisps, jalapeño flavored, 15 crisps (28 g)	5
Potato crisps, lightly salted flavored, 16 crisps (28 g)	5
Potato crisps, Loaded baked flavored, 15 crisps (28 g)	5
Potato crisps, original flavor, 16 crisps (28 g)	5

Potato crisps, original flavored, 1 oz	6
Potato crisps, pizza flavored, 15 crisps (28 g)	5
Potato crisps, ranch flavored, 15 crisps (28 g)	5
Potato crisps, reduced fat, original flavor, 16 crisps (28 g)	5
Potato crisps, reduced fat, sour cream & onion flavor, 16 crisps (28 g)	5
Potato crisps, salt and vinegar flavor, 1 oz	5
Potato crisps, sour cream and onion fat free, 15 crisps (28 g)	2
Potato crisps, sour cream and onion flavor, 15 crisps (28 g)	5
Potato crisps, sour cream and onion multigrain, 15 crisps (28 g)	5

Pringles 100 Calorie Packs

Original reduced fat potato crisps, 1 oz	5
Potato crisps, sour cream & onion, 1 tub (18 g)	3
Reduced fat potato crisps, 1 tub (18 g)	3

Pringles Cheez Ummms

Potato crisps, 4 cheese, 15 crisps (28 g)	5
Potato crisps, cheddar & sour cream, 15 crisps (28 g)	5

Pringles Grab and Go! Stack

Potato crisps, the original, 16 crisps (28 g)	5
Sour cream and onion flavored potato crisps, 15 crisps (28 g)	5

Pringles Light

Potato crisps, fat free, original, 1 oz	2
Potato crisps, fat free, sour cream & onion, 1 oz	2
Potato crisps, original, 15 crisps (28 g)	2
Potato crisps, sour cream & onion, 14 crisps (28 g)	2

Snacks

	SmartPoints™ value
Pringles Original	
Potato crisps, 1 tub (18 g)	3
Pringles Reduced Fat	
Potato crisps, original, 1 oz	5
Pringles Rewind Edition	
Original potato crisps, 16 pieces (28 g)	5
Pringles Snack Stacks!	
Potato crisps, original, 1 tub (21 g)	4
Potato crisps, sour cream & onion, 1 tub (21 g)	4
Sour cream and onion flavored crisps, 1 tub (21 g)	4
Pringles Stix	
Honey butter flavored baked snack sticks, 1 pack (17 g)	3
Quest	
Chips, protein, salt & vinegar flavor, 1 bag (32 g)	2
Ruffles	
Potato chips, 1 oz	4
Potato chips, cheddar and sour cream oven baked chips, 11 chips (28 g)	4
Potato chips, cheddar and sour cream potato chips, 11 chips (28 g)	5
Potato chips, original, 12 chips (28 g)	5
Potato chips, reduced fat, 13 chips (28 g)	4
Ruffles Baked!	
Cheddar and sour cream potato chips, 1 package (32 g)	4
Cheddar and sour cream potato crisps, 1 package (32 g)	4
Cheddar and sour cream potato crisps, 10 chips (28 g)	4
Naturally baked potato crisps, cheddar & sour cream, 1 oz	4
Original potato crisp, 9 crisps (28 g)	4

	SmartPoints™ value
Original potato crisps, 1 package (25 g)	3
Potato crisps, original, 9 chips (28 g)	4
Ruffles Flavor-Rush	
Potato chips, zesty sour cream & onion, 1 oz	6
Ruffles Light	
Potato chips, original, 15 chips (28 g)	2
Ruffles Natural	
Potato chips, reduced fat, sea salted, 15 chips (28 g)	4
Potato chips, sea salted, reduced fat, 15 chips (28 g)	4
Ruffles Ready To Go Snacks	
Oven baked cheddar and sour cream flavored potato crisps, 1 package (32 g)	4
Sensible Portions Garden Veggie Chips	
Bbq flavored potato crisps, 14 pieces (28 g)	5
Cheddar cheese flavored potato crisps, 14 pieces (28 g)	5
Sea salt flavored potato crisps, 14 pieces (28 g)	5
Sour cream & onion flavored potato crisps, 14 pieces (28 g)	5
Sensible Portions Onion Straws	
Southwestern vegetable and potato snack, 38 pieces (28 g)	4
Starbucks	
Smoky sweet barbecue kettle potato chips, 1 package (43 g)	6
Sun Chips	
French onion multigrain snacks, 15 chips (28 g)	5
T.G.I. Friday's	
Snack chips, potato skins cheddar & bacon, 16 chips (28 g)	5
Terra Blues	
Potato chips, 1 oz	4

Snacks

Terra Sweets Medley

Sweet potatoes chips seasoned with sea salt, 15 chips (28 g)	5

Trader Joe's

Barbecue popped potato chips, 20 chips (28 g)	4
Kettle cooked potato chips with sea salt, 1 bag (28 g)	5
Popped potato chips, 22 chips (28 g)	4

Trader Joe's Reduced Guilt

Lightly salted kettle cooked potato chips, 12 chips (28 g)	4

Twistos

Parmesan and garlic flavored baked snack bites, 27 pieces (28 g)	4

Utz

Potato chips, 20 chips (28 g)	5
Potato chips, bar-b-q, 1 package (28 g)	5
Potato chips, family size, 20 chips (28 g)	5
Potato chips, honey bbq, 20 chips (28 g)	5
Potato chips, no salt added, 20 chips (28 g)	5
Potato chips, reduced fat, family size, 20 chips (28 g)	4
Potato chips, ripple cut, sour cream and onion flavored, 20 chips (28 g)	6
Potato chips, ripples, 20 chips (28 g)	5
Potato chips, salt 'n vinegar, 20 chips (28 g)	5
Potato chips, sour cream and onion flavored, 1 package (28 g)	6

Utz Classic Russets

Potato chips, gourmet dark, 20 chips (28 g)	5

Utz Kettle Classics

Potato chips, crunchy, 20 chips (28 g)	5
Potato chips, crunchy, reduced fat, 20 chips (28 g)	4
Potato chips, crunchy, salt and malt vinegar, 20 chips (28 g)	5
Potato chips, crunchy, smokin' sweet, bbq flavored, 20 chips (28 g)	5
Potato chips, gourmet sweet potato, 18 chips (28 g)	5

Utz Natural

Potato chips, kettle cooked, gourmet medley, 20 chips (28 g)	5

Wheat Thins

Sea salt popped chips, 27 chips (30 g)	4

Wise

Potato chips, 16 chips (28 g)	5
Potato chips, honey bbq, 14 chips (28 g)	5

Wise Kettle

Salt and vinegar potato chips, 13 chips (28 g)	5

Wise Ridgies

Potato chips, ridged, 15 chips (28 g)	5

Pretzels

Bachman

Mini baked pretzels, bite size, 1 oz	3
Pretzel twists, 1 oz	3
Pretzels, baked rods, 2 pretzels (28 g)	3
Pretzels, pretzel stix, 1 oz	3
Pretzels, thins, 11 pretzels (28 g)	3

Clancy's

Old fashioned pretzel minis, 17 pieces (28 g)	3
Pretzel sticks, old fashioned, 32 pieces (28 g)	3

Snacks

Snacks

	SmartPoints™ value
Clover Valley	
Pretzel sticks, 42 sticks (30 g)	3
Combos	
Baked snacks, buffalo blue cheese pretzel, ⅓ cup	5
Baked snacks, pizzeria pretzel, ⅓ cup	5
Pretzel, cheddar cheese flavored filling, ⅓ cup	5
Combos Sweet & Salty	
Vanilla frosting pretzel, ⅓ cup	5
Dream Pretzels Pressels	
Everything pretzel chips, 20 pieces (28 g)	4
Original pretzel chips, 22 (28 g)	4
Essential Everyday	
Pretzel, sticks, 42 (30 g)	3
Pretzels, honey wheat, braids, 9 (30 g)	4
Pretzels, mini, 18 (30 g)	3
Fit & Active	
100 calorie dipped prezels, 1 pack (22 g)	5
Flipz	
Chocolate covered pretzels, milk chocolate covered, 8 pieces (28 g)	6
Chocolate covered pretzels, white fudge covered, 7 pieces (28 g)	7
Food Club	
Pretzels, mini twists, classic style, 22 pretzels (30 g)	3
Giant Eagle	
Peanut butter filled pretzels, 10 pretzels (30 g)	5
Giant/Stop & Shop	
Pretzels minis, 18 pretzels (28 g)	3
Glutino	
Pretzel sticks, gluten free, family pack, 33 pretzels (30 g)	5
Pretzel twists, gluten free, family pack, 24 pretzels (30 g)	5

	SmartPoints™ value
Pretzels twists, 24 pretzels (30 g)	5
Pretzels, chips, gluten free, 11 pretzels (30 g)	4
Glutino Gluten Free	
Pretzel sticks, 33 pretzels (30 g)	5
Pretzel twists, 24 pretzels (30 g)	5
H.K. Anderson	
Nuggets, filled, peanut butter, original, 10 nuggets (30 g)	4
Pretzels, braided twists, honey wheat, 10 twists (30 g)	4
Pretzels, old fashioned stick, 7 sticks (29 g)	3
Pretzels, peanut butter filled, 10 pretzels (30 g)	5
Pretzels, rod, 2 ½ rods (28 g)	3
Pretzels, stick, 51 sticks (30 g)	3
Pretzels, ultra thin, salty stix, 88 sticks (30 g)	3
Handi Snacks	
Pretzels 'n cheese dip, mister salty, 1 package (26 g)	3
Herr's	
Pretzel rods, 3 rods (33 g)	3
Pretzel sticks, whole grain, honey wheat, 7 pretzels (28 g)	3
Pretzels, extra thin, 9 pretzels (28 g)	3
Pretzels, hard, sourdough, bite size, 11 pretzels (30 g)	3
Pretzels, low fat, sourdough specials, 4 pretzels (28 g)	3
Pretzels, peanut butter filled, 10 pretzels (28 g)	4
Pretzels, stix, 30 pretzels (28 g)	3
Hill Country Fare	
Pretzels, twists, mini, 21 pieces (28 g)	3
Keebler	
Pretzel thins, 6 crackers (15.6 g)	2
Pretzel thins, parmesan herb, 6 crackers (15.6 g)	2

Keebler 100 Calorie Right Bites Fudge Shoppe

Pretzels, fudge dipped, 1 pouch (21 g)	5

Kellogg's Special K

Fudge dipped pretzels, 1 pouch (21 g)	5
White fudge dipped pretzels, 1 pouch (21 g)	5
White fudge dipped pretzels, 1 pouch (21 g)	5

Kellogg's Special K Moments

Caramel pretzel bliss snack bites, 1 pouch (16 g)	3

Kroger

Braided twist honey wheat pretzels, 9 (28 g)	4
Original pretzel thins, 10 pieces (28 g)	3
Pretzel rods, 3 rods (28 g)	3
Pretzel sticks, 48 pretzels (28 g)	3
Pretzel twists, 1 oz	3
Pretzel waffles, 17 pretzels (28 g)	3
Pretzels, peanut butter filled, 10 pretzels (30 g)	4
Sourdough pretzel nuggets, 12 pieces (31 g)	3
Tiny pretzel twists, 21 pretzels (28 g)	3
Twisted mini pretzels, 50 pieces (42 g)	5

Lean Cuisine Culinary Collection

Monterey Jack jalapeño stuffed pretzels, 4 pieces (99 g)	6

M&M's

Chocolate candies, pretzel, fun size, 3 packs (41 g)	9

Market Pantry

Peanut butter filled pretzels, 10 pretzel bites (30 g)	4

Mary's Gone Crackers

Sticks & twigs, organic, sea salt, 15 pieces (28 g)	4

Mayfair

Pretzel sticks, fat free, 37 pretzels (30 g)	3
Pretzels, fat free, mini, 19 pretzels (30 g)	3

Meijer

Pretzels, butter braids, 10 pretzels (30 g)	3
Pretzels, honey wheat braids, 7 pieces (28 g)	4
Pretzels, low fat, waffle style, 16 pieces (28 g)	3
Pretzels, rings, 19 pretzels (28 g)	3
Pretzels, rods, 3 rods (28 g)	3
Pretzels, stix, 51 pretzels (30 g)	3
Pretzels, tiny twists, 19 pretzels (30 g)	3

Nabisco Snackwell's

Pretzels, yogurt flavored, 100 calorie packs, 1 pack (22 g)	5
Yogurt flavored pretzels single serve pack, 1 pack (22 g)	5

Newman's Own Organic

Pretzels, spelt, 20 pretzels (28 g)	3

Nice!

Pretzels, mini twist, 17 pretzels (28 g)	3

Old Dutch

Mini fat free pretzel thins, 17 pretzels (28 g)	3
Mini pretzels, fat free thins, 17 each (28 g)	3
Pretzel rods, 3 pieces (28 g)	3

Pennysticks

Braided pretzels, honey wheat, 18 pretzels (28 g)	3

Pepperidge Farm Baked Naturals

Pretzel thins, everything & more, 11 crisps (28 g)	4
Simply pretzel thins, 12 pieces (29 g)	3

Snacks

Snacks

	SmartPoints™ value
Pocket Pretzels	
Pocket pretzels, peanut butter filled, 11 pretzels (28 g)	5
Pretzel Crisps	
Buffalo wing, 10 crisps (28 g)	3
Dark chocolate crunch, 5 crackers (28 g)	6
Everything, 11 crackers (28 g)	3
Garlic parmesan, 10 crackers (28 g)	3
Honey mustard and onion, 10 crackers (28 g)	3
Jalapeño Jack, 1 package (43 g)	5
Original deli style, 11 crackers (28 g)	3
Sea salt and cracked pepper, 10 crackers (28 g)	3
Pretzel Crisps Deli Style	
Buffalo wing flavored deli style thin and crunchy pretzel crackers, 1 package (43 g)	5
Pretzel crackers, thin, crunchy, original, 1 package (43 g)	5
Pretzel Crisps Minis	
Cheddar, 35 crackers (28 g)	3
Original, 42 crackers (28 g)	3
Publix	
Pretzel sticks, baked, 35 (28 g)	3
Publix MiniTwist	
Pretzels, 19 (30 g)	3
Rold Gold	
Pretzel thins, garlic parmesan, 13 (28 g)	4
Pretzel thins, original, 14 (28 g)	3
Pretzel thins, three cheese, 13 (28 g)	4
Pretzels thins, classic style, 9 pretzels (28 g)	3
Pretzels, braided twists, 8 pretzels (28 g)	3
Pretzels, dark dipped bavarian twists, 2 pretzels (28 g)	7

	SmartPoints™ value
Pretzels, heartzels, 1 package (20 g)	2
Pretzels, honey mustard, 1 oz	3
Pretzels, honey wheat braided twists, 8 pretzels (28 g)	3
Pretzels, rods, 3 pretzels (28 g)	3
Pretzels, sourdough, 1 pretzel (24 g)	3
Pretzels, sticks, 53 pretzels (28 g)	3
Pretzels, sticks, classic style, 1 oz	3
Pretzels, tiny twists, 18 pretzels (28 g)	3
Pretzels, tiny twists, cheddar flavored, 20 pretzels (28 g)	3
Pretzels, tiny twists, fat free, 18 pretzels (28 g)	3
Pretzels, tiny twists, honey mustard, 20 pretzels (28 g)	3
Pretzels, tiny twists, lightly salted, 18 pretzels (28 g)	3
Rold Gold Go Snacks	
Mini pretzels, classic style twists, 28 pretzels (27 g)	3
Sabra	
Red roasted pepper hummus with rold gold pretzels, 1 snack cup (129 g)	11
Safeway	
Pretzel nuggets, peanut butter filled, 10 pretzels (28 g)	4
Pretzel, sticks, 39 pretzels (30 g)	3
ShopRite	
Pretzels, Amish, fat free, 1 pretzel (21 g)	2
Pretzels, braided twists, honey wheat, 10 pretzels (30 g)	4
Pretzels, gem, 12 pretzels (31 g)	3
Pretzels, log, fat free, 6 pretzels (28 g)	3
Pretzels, mini, 19 pretzels (30 g)	3
Pretzels, mini, fat free, 19 pretzels (30 g)	3

	SmartPoints™ value
Pretzels, mini, no surface salt, 19 pretzels (30 g)	3
Pretzels, stick, fat free, 37 pretzels (30 g)	3
Pretzels, waffle, 16 pretzels (30 g)	3
Shultz	
Mini pretzels, 19 pretzels (30 g)	3
Mini pretzels, deli pack, 18 pretzels (28 g)	3
Pretzels, honey wheat braided twist, 10 pretzels (28 g)	4
Pretzels, mini, 19 pretzels (30 g)	3
Pretzels, sour dough hard, ¾ oz	0
Pretzels, stick, 51 pretzels (30 g)	3
Skinny Girl Snacks	
Cucumber dill baked pretzel thins, 10 pretzels (28 g)	4
Snack Factory	
Classic pretzel crisps, 11 crackers (28 g)	6
Pretzel crackers, Buffalo wing, 10 crackers (28 g)	3
Pretzel crackers, deli style, original, 11 crackers (28 g)	3
Pretzel crisps, deli style, buffalo wing, 10 crackers (28 g)	3
Pretzel snacks, thin crunchy, original, 23 crisps (28 g)	3
Snack Factory Deli Style	
Chipotle cheddar flavor pretzel crisps, 10 crackers (28 g)	3
Jalapeño Jack flavor pretzel crisps, 10 crackers (28 g)	3
Snack Factory Pretzel Crisps	
Buffalo wing pretzel crackers, 10 crackers (28 g)	3
Cheddar horseradish chips, 10 crisps (28 g)	3
Dark chocolate crunch pretzel snacks, 5 (28 g)	6
Garlic parmesan pretzel crackers, 10 crackers (28 g)	3

	SmartPoints™ value
Pretzel crackers, deli style, everything, 11 crisps (28 g)	3
Pretzel crackers, deli style, garlic parmesan, 10 crisps (28 g)	3
Pretzel crackers, deli style, original, 11 crisps (28 g)	3
Pretzel crackers, deli style, sesame, 11 crisps (28 g)	3
Sea salt & cracked pepper pretzel crackers, 10 crackers (28 g)	3
SnackWell's 100 Calorie Packs	
Pretzels, fudge, 1 pack (22 g)	5
Pretzels, yogurt, 1 pack (22 g)	5
Snappers	
Gourmet caramel & pretzel treats with dark chocolate and sea salt caramel, 3 pieces (40 g)	7
Snyder's	
Bacon cheddar pretzel pieces, ⅓ cup	5
Jalapeño pretzel pieces, ⅓ cup	5
Mini pretzels, 20 pretzels (30 g)	3
Nibblers, honey mustard & onion, 1 package (43 g)	5
Pretzel chips, original, 14 chips (30 g)	3
Pretzel dips, dipped in Hershey's milk chocolate, 7 pretzels (28 g)	6
Pretzel dips, dipped in Hershey's special dark mildly sweet chocolate, 8 pretzels (30 g)	6
Pretzel pieces, buttermilk ranch, ⅓ cup	5
Pretzel rings, 20 pretzels (30 g)	3
Pretzel rods, old fashioned, 3 pretzels (30 g)	3
Pretzel sandwiches, cheddar cheese, 9 sandwiches (28 g)	6
Pretzel sandwiches, peanut butter, 9 sandwiches (28 g)	5
Pretzels, hard, sourdough, the pounder, 1 pretzel (28 g)	3
Pretzels, mini, 25 pretzels (30 g)	4

Snacks

	SmartPoints™ value
Pretzels, mini, hungry size, 20 minis (32 g)	3
Pretzels, old tyme, the pounder, 3 pretzels (30 g)	3
Pretzels, sourdough specials, 5 pretzels (28 g)	3
Pretzels, sticks, gluten free, honey mustard & onion, 30 sticks (30 g)	5
Pretzels, thin, 11 (30 g)	3
Snyder's 100 Calorie Pack	
Mini pretzels, 1 mini bag (26 g)	3
Pretzel sticks, 1 serving (26 g)	3
Pretzels, snaps, 1 package (26 g)	3
Snyder's Gluten Free	
Pretzel sticks, 40 sticks (30 g)	4
Snyder's of Hanover	
Bacon cheddar pretzel pieces, 1 oz	5
Butter snap pretzels, 24 pretzels (30 g)	3
Homestyle pretzels, 4 pretzels (31 g)	3
Honey mustard and onion pretzel pieces, 1 oz	5
Honey wheat braided twists, 7 twists (30 g)	4
Hot buffalo wing pretzel pieces, 1 oz	5
Mini pretzel halloween snack sack, 1 pack (14 g)	1
Multigrain braided twists, 8 twists (30 g)	4
Nibblers, sourdough, the pounder, 16 nibblers (30 g)	3
Old fashioned dipping sticks, 14 sticks (30 g)	3
Pretzel dips, Hersheys, milk chocolate, 7 pretzels (28 g)	6
Pretzel packs, 100 calorie, pretzel sticks, gluten-free, 1 bag (26 g)	3
Pretzel pieces, cheddar cheese, ⅓ cup	5
Pretzel pieces, hot buffalo wing, ⅓ cup	5

	SmartPoints™ value
Pretzel poppers, original, 21 pretzels (30 g)	3
Pretzel rods, 3 pretzels (30 g)	3
Pretzel snaps, 24 pretzels (30 g)	3
Pretzels, braided twists, honey wheat, 8 twists (30 g)	4
Pretzels, braided twists, multigrain, 9 twists (30 g)	4
Pretzels, butter snaps, 24 pretzels (30 g)	3
Pretzels, mini, the pounder, 20 minis (30 g)	3
Pretzels, mini, unsalted, 20 minis (30 g)	3
Pretzels, old fashioned dipping sticks, 14 sticks (30 g)	3
Pretzels, olde tyme, 3 pretzels (30 g)	3
Pretzels, sticks, 28 sticks (32 g)	3
Pretzels, thins, 10 pretzels (28 g)	3
Pumpernickel and onion braided twists, 8 twists (30 g)	3
Sourdough hard pretzels, fat free, 1 each (28 g)	3
Unsalted mini pretzels, 20 minis (30 g)	3
Snyder's of Hanover Gluten Free	
Hot buffalo wing pretzel sticks, 29 (30 g)	4
Snyder's Of Hanover Nibblers	
Honey mustard and onion pretzels, 13 nibblers (30 g)	4
Pretzels, honey mustard & onion, 13 nibblers (30 g)	4
Snyder's of Hanover Pretzel Poppers	
Cinnamon sugar pretzel shells, 20 pieces (30 g)	4
Snyder's of Hanover Snack Sack	
Bags of peanut butter pretzel sandwiches, 1 package (14 g)	2
Snyder's of Hanover Spoonz	
Spoon shaped dipping pretzels, 15 pieces (30 g)	3

Snacks

Snyder's Of Hanover Sweet and Salty

Cinnamon sugar pretzel pieces, ⅓ cup	5
Salted caramel pretzel pieces, ⅓ cup	5

Snyder's The Pounder

Pretzels, sticks, 28 sticks (30 g)	3

Stacy's Simply Naked

Pretzel thins, 13 pieces (28 g)	3

Super Pretzel

Baked soft pretzels, 1 pretzel (71.4 g)	5
King size soft pretzel without toppings, 1 pretzel (71 g)	5
Pretzel bites, baked, soft, 5 bites	4
Soft pretzels, baked, 1 pretzel (64 g)	4

Super Pretzel Bavarian Restaurant Style

Soft pretzel stick, 1 stick (43 g)	3

Super Pretzel Soft Stix

Soft pretzel sticks, cheese filled, cheddar, 2 soft stix (50 g)	4

Super Pretzel Sweet Cinnamon

Soft pretzel with cinnamon sugar topping, 1 pretzel (61 g)	6

The Snack Factory Pretzel Crisps Minis

Cheddar flavored pretzel crackers, 35 pieces (28 g)	3
Original pretzel crackers, 42 pieces (28 g)	3

Tom Sturgis

Pretzels, little ones, 17 pretzels (28 g)	3

Town House Flip Sides

Pretzel crackers, original, 5 crackers (15 g)	2
Pretzel crackers, reduced fat, 5 crackers (14 g)	2

Trader Joe's

Dark chocolate covered pretzel slims, 7 pieces (40 g)	8
Honey wheat pretzel sticks, 10 drumsticks (30 g)	4
Multi-grain pretzel nuggets with sesame seeds, 22 pretzels (28 g)	3
Peanut butter filled pretzels, 11 pieces (30 g)	5
Pretzel slims, 23 (28 g)	3
Pretzel slims, 23 pretzels (28 g)	3
Pretzel slims everything, 23 pieces (28 g)	3
Pumpernickel pretzel sticks, 8 (28 g)	3

Unique Pretzels

Pretzels, multi grain, splits, 3 pretzels (28 g)	3
Pretzels, splits, 1 oz	3

Unique Pretzels Splits

Pretzels, 3 pretzels (28 g)	3
Pretzels, extra dark, 3 pretzels (28 g)	3

Utz

Chocolate covered pretzels, 2 pretzels (25 g)	6
Country store pretzel stix, 5 pieces (28 g)	3
Pretzel rods, old fashioned, 3 pretzels (30 g)	3
Pretzel treats, 1 package (14.2 g)	2
Pretzels, butter waffles, 20 pretzels (28 g)	3
Pretzels, chocolate, 2 pretzels (25 g)	5
Pretzels, extra dark specials, 5 pretzels (28 g)	3
Pretzels, extra thin, 10 pretzels (28 g)	3
Pretzels, hard, sourdough, 1 pretzel (23 g)	3

Snacks

	SmartPoints™ value
Pretzels, multigrain specials, family size!, 3 pretzels (28 g)	3
Pretzels, nuggets, sourdough, 10 pretzels (28 g)	3
Pretzels, sourdough hard, old fashioned, 1 pretzel (23 g)	3
Pretzels, sourdough nuggets, 10 pretzels (28 g)	3
Pretzels, sourdough specials, 5 pretzels (28 g)	3
Pretzels, wheels, the pounder, 20 pretzels (28 g)	3
Utz 100 Calorie	
Brick oven pretzel stix, 1 tray (28 g)	3
Utz Organic	
Pretzel sticks, seven whole grains, 7 pretzels (28 g)	3
Utz Select	
Pretzel chips, thinly baked, 15 pretzels (28 g)	3
Pretzels, braided twists, honey wheat, 7 pretzels (28 g)	4
Utz Specials	
Extra dark pretzels, 5 pretzels (28 g)	3
Pretzels, extra dark, the pounder, 5 pretzels (28 g)	3
Pretzels, sourdough, the pounder, 5 pretzels (28 g)	3
Pretzels, sourdough, unsalted, the pounder, 5 pretzels (28 g)	3
Wegman's Food You Feel Good About	
Filled pretzel nuggets, peanut butter filled, 10 pretzels (30 g)	4
Whole Foods 365 Everyday Value	
Crunchy pretzels, 1 oz	3

Rice & Corn Cakes

	SmartPoints™ value
America's Choice	
Rice cakes, caramel corn, 1 cake (13 g)	2
Rice cakes, white cheddar flavor, 1 cake (11 g)	1
Bamboo Lane	
Crunchy rice roller, 1 (12.5 g)	2
Clancy's Fit & Active	
Rice snacks, 15 chips (15 g)	2
Coco Pop Cakes Lite	
Multigrain, 1 piece (5 g)	0
Multigrain, 6 pieces (30 g)	3
Multigrain, blueberry cinnamon, 1 piece (5 g)	0
Multigrain, maui onion, 1 piece (5 g)	0
Essential Everyday	
Apple cinnamon rice cake, 1 cake (13 g)	2
Caramel corn flavor fat free rice cake, 1 cake (13 g)	2
Caramel flavor fat free rice snacks, 7 chips (15 g)	2
Ranch flavor rice snacks, 10 chips (16 g)	2
White cheddar flavor low fat rice cake, 1 cake (11 g)	1
Fit & Active	
Chocolate rice snacks, 7 chips (15 g)	2
Rice snacks, 8 mini cakes (15 g)	2
Food Club	
Rice cakes, caramel corn, 1 cake (13 g)	2
Giant	
Corn cakes, fat free, caramel flavor, 1 cake (13 g)	2
Corn cakes, white cheddar, 1 cake (11 g)	1
Rice cakes, apple cinnamon, 1 cake (12 g)	2

Snacks

	SmartPoints™ value
Rice cakes, fat free, unsalted, multigrain, 1 cake (10 g)	1
Rice cakes, lightly salted, plain, 1 cake (10 g)	1
Rice chips, crunchy minis, cheddar, 9 chips (15 g)	2
Rice chips, crunchy minis, fat free, caramel, 8 chips (15 g)	2
Rice chips, crunchy minis, sour cream & onion, 10 chips (16 g)	2
H-E-B	
Rice cakes, caramel, 1 cake (13 g)	2
Hy-Vee	
Rice cakes, whole grain, caramel corn, 1 cake (13 g)	2
Rice cakes, whole grain, lightly salted, 1 cake (10 g)	1
Rice cakes, whole grain, white cheddar, 1 cake (11 g)	1
Kameda Crisps	
Baked frosted rice crackers, 1 package (12 g)	2
Kellogg's Crackle Snaps	
Caramel drizzle puffed rice snacks, 1 pouch (12 g)	3
Fudge drizzle puffed rice snacks, 1 pouch (12 g)	3
Kellogg's Special K Popped Delights	
Strawberry with fudge drizzle popped snacks, 1 pouch (12 g)	3
Kim's Magic Pop All Natural	
Multigrain cakes, 1 piece (5 g)	0
Kroger	
Cheddar flavored mini rice cakes, 9 mini cakes (16 g)	2
Rice cakes, low sodium, 1 cake (9 g)	1
Rice cakes, mini, apple cinnamon flavored, 7 mini cakes (16 g)	2
Rice cakes, white cheddar flavored, 1 cake (11 g)	1

	SmartPoints™ value
Lundberg	
Lightly salted organic rice cake, 1 cake (19 g)	2
Rice cakes, brown rice, salt-free, 1 cake (19 g)	2
Rice cakes, cinnamon toast, 1 cake (21 g)	3
Lundberg Eco-Farmed	
Rice cakes, brown rice, lightly salted, 1 cake (19 g)	2
Rice cakes, brown rice, salt-free, 1 cake (19 g)	2
Rice cakes, honey nut, 1 cake (21 g)	2
Lundberg Organic	
Rice cakes, kettle corn, 1 cake (23 g)	3
Rice cakes, organic, caramel corn, 1 cake (21 g)	3
Rice cakes, tamari with seaweed, 1 cake (19 g)	2
Rice cakes, wild rice, lightly salted, 1 cake (19 g)	2
Meijer Organics	
Rice cakes, lightly salted, 1 cake (10 g)	1
Mother's	
Rice & popped corn cakes, caramel, 1 cake (13 g)	2
Rice cakes, plain, salted, 1 cake (9 g)	1
Paskesz	
Rice cake squares, ultra-thin, plain, 3 cakes (16 g)	2
Pirate's Booty Disney Pirates of the Caribbean	
Aged white cheddar rice and corn puffs, 1 oz	4
Popped	
Rice snacks, apple cinnamon, 1 bag (26 g)	4
Rice snacks, caramel corn, 13 mini cakes (30 g)	4

Snacks

SmartPoints™ value

Rice snacks, cheddar cheese, 18 mini cakes (30 g)	4
Rice snacks, chocolate, 1 bag (26 g)	4
Rice snacks, ranch, 1 bag (19 g)	2
Rice snacks, sea salt & cracked black pepper, 16 mini cakes (30 g)	4

Quaker

Rice cake, butter popped corn, 1 cake (9 g)	1
Rice cake, caramel corn, 1 cake (13 g)	2
Rice cake, chocolate crunch, 1 cake (15 g)	2
Rice cakes, apple cinnamon, 1 cake (13 g)	2
Rice cakes, lightly salted, 1 cake (9 g)	1
Rice cakes, salt free, 1 cake (9 g)	1
Rice cakes, white cheddar, 1 cake (11 g)	1

Quaker Popped

Bbq flavor rice snacks, 1 mini bag (19 g)	2
Buttered popcorn flavored rice snacks, 18 mini cakes (30 g)	4
Caramel corn flavor rice snacks, 13 mini cakes (30 g)	4
Cheddar cheese flavor rice snacks, 1 mini bag (19 g)	3
Chocolate flavor rice snacks, 13 mini cakes (30 g)	4
Kettle corn rice snacks, 15 mini cakes (30 g)	4
Ranch flavor rice snacks, 17 mini cakes (30 g)	4
Sour cream and onion rice snacks, 18 mini cakes (30 g)	4
Sweet chili flavor rice snacks, 18 mini cakes (30 g)	4

Real Foods

Corn thins, multigrain, 2 slices (12 g)	1
Corn thins, organic, flax & soy, 2 slices (12 g)	1

SmartPoints™ value

Corn thins, organic, original, 2 slices (12 g)	1
Corn thins, sesame, 2 slices (14 g)	1

ShopRite

Rice cakes, fat free, whole grain, apple cinnamon, 1 cake (12 g)	2
Rice cakes, fat free, whole grain, lightly salted, 1 cake (10 g)	1
Rice cakes, fat free, whole grain, multigrain, 1 cake (10 g)	1
Rice cakes, fat free, whole grain, popped corn, caramel, 1 cake (13 g)	2
Rice cakes, fat free, whole grain, popped corn, white cheddar, 1 cake (11 g)	1
Rice cakes, fat-free, whole grain, salt-free, 1 cake (10 g)	1

Stop & Shop

Chocolate mini rice cakes, 7 chips (15 g)	2

Suzie's

Thin cakes, brown rice, 4 cakes (17 g)	2

Suzie's Whole Grain

Thin cakes, puffed multigrain, 3 cakes (16 g)	2
Thin cakes, puffed rice, 3 cakes (16 g)	2

Snack & Trail Mixes

Archer Farms

Caramel cashew trail mix, ¼ cup	8
Monster trail mix, ¼ cup	8
Sweet Cajun trail mix, ¼ cup	6
Tex Mex trail mix, ¼ cup	4

Cheez-It

Baked snack assortment, party mix, ½ cup	4
Snack mix, ½ cup	4
Snack mix baked snack assortment, ½ cup	4

Cheez-It 100 Calorie Right Bites

Snack mix, 1 pouch (21 g)	3

Chex Mix

Snack mix, bold party blend, ½ cup	4
Snack mix, cheddar, ½ cup	4
Snack mix, chocolate, turtle, ½ cup	5
Snack mix, Italian herb & parmesan, ½ cup	4
Snack mix, peanut lovers', ½ cup	4
Snack mix, sweet 'n salty, caramel crunch, ½ cup	4
Snack mix, sweet 'n salty, honey nut, ½ cup	4
Trail mix, sweet 'n salty, ½ cup	6

Chex Mix Muddy Buddies

Brownie supreme snack mix, ⅓ cup	5
Snack mix, cookies & cream, ½ cup	7
Snack mix, peanut butter & chocolate, ⅓ cup	6

Chex Mix Popped

Sweet and salty snack mix, ¾ cup	5
White cheddar snack mix, ¾ cup	4

Chex Mix The Original

Traditional snack mix, ½ cup	4

Cracker Jack'D Hearty Mix

Pb and chocolate flavored snack mix, 1 oz	6

Daily Chef

Mountain trail mix, 3 Tbsp	7

Emerald Breakfast On The Go!

Caramel macchiato nut and granola mix, 1 pouch (42 g)	8
S'mores nut blend, 1 pouch (43 g)	8
Trail mix, breakfast nut blend, 1 pouch (43 g)	8

Gardetto's

Original recipe snack mix, 1 bag (49 g)	7
Snack mix, original recipe, 1 bag (47 g)	7
Snack mix, reduced fat, original recipe, ½ cup	4

General Mills Chex Mix

Mega-size traditional snack mix, ½ cup	4
Traditional snack mix (1.75 oz pouch), 1 pouch (49 g)	7

Great Value

Cajun trail mix, ¼ cup	5
Mountain trail mix, ¼ cup	7
Peanut butter trail mix, ¼ cup	6

Kar's

Sweet and salty mix, 1 package (57 g)	12
Sweet 'n salty mix, 3 Tbsp	6
Sweet 'n salty mix (single serve package), 1 package (35 g)	7

Kimberley's Bakeshoppe

Granola, ⅓ cup	8

Kind

Clusters, with chia & quinoa, maple walnut, ⅓ cup	4

Kind Healthy Grains

Cinnamon oat clusters with flax seeds, ⅓ cup	4
Oats & honey clusters with toasted coconut, ⅓ cup	5
Peanut butter whole grain clusters, ⅓ cup	4
Vanilla blueberry clusters with flax seeds, ⅓ cup	4

Kirkland Signature

Fruit and nut medley, ¼ cup	6
Trail mix, 3 Tbsp	6
Trail mix snack packs, 3 Tbsp	6
Trek mix, ¼ cup	6

Kroger

Trail mix, cranberry delight, ¼ cup	5

Mareblu Naturals

Trail mix crunch, blueberry pomegranate, ¼ cup	6

Munchies

Snack mix, cheese fix, 1 package (49.6 g)	8
Snack mix, cheese fix flavored, ¾ cup	4

Snacks

Snacks

	SmartPoints™ value
Snack mix, flavored, cheese fix, ¾ cup	4
Ultimate cheddar flavored snack mix, ¾ cup	4
Munchies Cheese Fix	
Snack mix, ¾ cup	4
Snack mix, cheetos, doritos, rold gold, sun chips, ¾ cup	4
Nabisco 100 Calorie Packs	
Baked snacks, ritz snack mix, 1 package (22 g)	3
Orchard Valley Harvest	
Trail mix, cranberry almond cashew, ¼ cup	6
Planters	
Nut-rition heart healthy mix, 1 pack (42 g)	8
Nut-rition men's health mix, 1 pack (35 g)	6
Trail mix, nut & chocolate, 1 pack (56 g)	12
Trail mix, nuts, seeds & raisins, 3 Tbsp	6
Planters NUT-rition	
Chocolate nut sustaining energy mix, 1 pack (49 g)	9
Digestive health mix, ¼ cup	6
Energy mix, sustaining, chocolate nut, 1 pack (49 g)	9
Energy mix, sustaining, honey nut, 1 pack (47 g)	8
Post Great Grains The Bar Undone	
Cranberry nuts and seeds granola snack mix, 1 pouch (40 g)	6
Dark chocolate nut granola snack mix, 1 pouch (40 g)	7
Quaker Popped	
Sweet mix variety pack rice snacks assorted flavors, 1 bag (26 g)	4
Ready Pac Ready Snax	
Carrots, grapes & cheese with pretzels, 1 container (122 g)	6

	SmartPoints™ value
Sargento Balanced Breaks	
Natural sharp cheddar cheese, sea salted cashews & cherry juice infused dried cranberries, 1 tray (43 g)	7
Natural sharp white cheddar cheese, sea salted cashews & golden raisin medley, 1 tray (43 g)	7
Natural white cheddar cheese, sea salted roasted almonds & dried cranberries, 1 tray (42 g)	7
Pepper Jack natural cheese, honey roasted peanuts & raisins, 1 tray (43 g)	7
Snack Sensations	
Fruit & cheese bites, 1 container (156 g)	8
Sunshine Cheez-It 100 Calorie Right Bites	
Party mix, 1 pouch (21 g)	3
Trader Joe's	
Chicago style popcorn mix, 1 cup	7
Handfuls of breakfast trek mix, 1 bag (42.5 g)	9
Peanuts, berries and almonds snack mix, ¼ cup	6
Rainbow's end trail mix, ¼ cup	6
Simply almonds, cashews & chocolate trek mix, ¼ cup	7
Simply almonds, cashews and cranberries trek mix, 1 bag (43 g)	7
Trader Joe's Nuts	
Roasted unsalted mixed nut with peanuts, ¼ cup	5
Sweet and spicy pecans, ¼ cup	7
Trader Joe's Wasabi Wow!	
Snack mix, ¼ cup	5
Utz	
Party mix, 1 oz	5
Utz Select	
Pub mix, ½ cup	4

WildRoots

Forest berry trail mix, ¼ cup	6

Woats

Cookies 'n' dreams oatsnack, ¼ cup	5

Tortilla Chips

Archer Farms

Southwestern-style tortilla strips salad topper, 2 Tbsp	1

Bachman

Tortilla chips, restaurant style, black bean, 1 oz	4

Barcel

Takis hot chili pepper and lime tortilla chips, 13 pieces (30 g)	5

Boston Market

Home style meals, hicken broccoli and cheese casserole, 1 tray (397 g)	14

Calidad

Tortilla chips, 12 chips (28 g)	5
White corn tortilla chips, 8 chips (28 g)	5

Casa Sanchez

Tortilla chips, thin & light, 10 chips (28 g)	4

Chef's Finest

Tortilla strips, tri-color, 2 Tbsp	1

Chi-Chi's Authentic

Original white corn tortilla chips, 13 chips (30 g)	5

Clancy's

Big dipper tortilla chips, 10 pieces (28 g)	4

Donkey

Tortilla chips, authentic, salted, 8 chips (28 g)	4

Doritos

Cool ranch flavored tortilla chips, 12 chips (28 g)	5
Cool ranch tortilla chips, 1 package (33 g)	5
Flavored tortilla chips, blazin buffalo & ranch, 12 chips (28 g)	4
Nacho cheese flavored tortilla chips, 11 chips (28 g)	4
Salsa verde flavored tortilla chips, 12 chips (28 g)	4
Spicy nacho tortilla chips, 12 chips (28 g)	4
Spicy sweet chili flavored tortilla chips, 1 package (32 g)	5
Taco flavor tortilla chips, 10 chips (28 g)	4
Toasted corn tortilla chips, 13 chips (28 g)	4
Tortilla chips, blazin' buffalo & ranch, 12 chips (28 g)	5
Tortilla chips, cool ranch, 12 chips (28 g)	5
Tortilla chips, nacho cheese, 11 chips (28 g)	4
Tortilla chips, reduced fat, cool ranch, 1 package (28.3 g)	4
Tortilla chips, reduced fat, nacho cheese, 1 package (28 g)	4
Tortilla chips, spicy nacho flavored, 12 chips (28 g)	4
Tortilla chips, taco flavor, 10 chips (28 g)	4
Tortilla chips, toasted corn, 13 chips (28 g)	4

Doritos Baked!

Nacho cheese tortilla chips, 15 chips (28 g)	4

Doritos Dinamita

Chile limon flavored tortilla chips, 15 pieces (28 g)	5

Doritos Jacked

Jalapeño pepper Jack flavored tortilla snacks, 13 pieces (28 g)	5
Ranch dipped hot wings flavored tortilla chips, 6 chips (28 g)	4
Spicy street taco tortilla chips, 6 chips (28 g)	4

Snacks

	SmartPoints™ value
Doritos Locos Tacos	
Nacho cheese and crunchy taco flavored tortilla chips, 11 chips (28 g)	4
Doritos Party Size!	
Spicy nacho tortilla chips, 12 chips (28 g)	4
Doritos Spicy Sweet Chili	
Spicy sweet chili tortilla chips, 11 chips (28 g)	4
El Milagro	
Tortilla chips, Mexican kitchen style, 10 chips (32 g)	4
Tortilla chips, Mexican kitchen style, salted, 1 oz	4
Tostadas, corn, 2 pieces (33 g)	5
El Ranchero	
Tortilla chips, with salt, 12 pieces (39 g)	4
Food Should Taste Good	
Blue corn tortilla chips, 10 chips (28 g)	4
Multigrain tortilla chips, 10 chips (28 g)	4
Olive tortilla chips (5.5 oz bag), 10 chips (28 g)	4
Sweet potato tortilla chips, 12 chips (28 g)	5
Tortilla chips, guacamole, 10 chips (28 g)	4
Tortilla chips, sweet potato, 12 chips (28 g)	4
Fresh Gourmet	
Sante Fe style tortilla strips, 2 Tbsp	1
Tortilla strips, lightly salted, 2 Tbsp	1
Tortilla strips, tri-color, 2 Tbsp	1
Frontera	
Tortilla chips, lime & sea salt, 1 oz	4
Tortilla chips, thin & crispy, 1 oz	4

	SmartPoints™ value
Garden of Eatin'	
All natural tortilla chips, blue chips, 22 chips (42 g)	7
Blue chips, party size, 15 chips (28 g)	4
Blue corn tortilla chips, 11 chips (28 g)	4
Chia seed corn tortilla chips, 11 chips (28 g)	4
Multi-grain tortilla chips, sea salt with flax seeds, 16 chips (28 g)	4
Sweet potato corn tortilla chips, 9 chips (28 g)	4
Tortilla chips, all natural, yellow chips, 13 chips (28 g)	4
Tortilla chips, blue corn, 1 oz	4
Tortilla chips, blue corn, no salt added, 1 oz	4
Tortilla chips, blue, party size, 1 oz	4
Tortilla chips, corn, sweet potato, 9 chips (28 g)	4
Tortilla chips, red hot blues, 15 chips (28 g)	4
Tortilla chips, restaurant style, blue corn, 7 chips (28 g)	4
Tortilla chips, restaurant style, white corn, 7 chips (28 g)	4
Great Value	
Bite size tortilla chips, 22 chips (28 g)	5
Tortilla chips, white, 8 chips (28 g)	4
Great Value Bowlz	
Tortilla chip dippers, 11 chips (28 g)	4
Green Mountain Gringo	
Tortilla strips, 1 oz	4
Herr's Bite Size	
Tortilla chips, dippers, 16 chips (28 g)	4
Juanita's	
Tortilla chips, 13 tortillas (28 g)	5
Tortilla chips, fiesta bag, 13 chips (28 g)	5

Kirkland Signature

Organic tortilla chips, 11 chips (28 g)	4
Tortilla strips, 9 chips (28 g)	5

Kroger

Tortilla chips, restaurant style, 7 chips (29 g)	5
Tortilla chips, traditional, 12 chips (28 g)	5
Tortilla chips, traditional gold, 11 chips (28 g)	5
Tortilla strips, original, ¼ cup	1
Tortilla strips, Santa Fe style, ¼ cup	1

La Favorita

Tortilla chips, yellow corn, 10 chips (28 g)	2
White corn tortilla chips lightly salted, 10 chips (28 g)	2

Late July Organic

Chia and quinoa restaurant style tortilla chips, 10 chips (28 g)	4
Sea salt by the seashore multigrain tortilla chips, 9 chips (28 g)	4
Sea salt restaurant style tortilla chips, 10 chips (28 g)	4

Margaritaville

Sea salt tortilla chips, 11 chips (28 g)	4

Meijer

Tortilla chips, restaurant style, 7 chips (28 g)	5
Tortilla chips, white round, bite-sized, 13 chips (28 g)	5
Tortilla chips, whole grain, multigrain, 10 chips (28 g)	4

Mission

Restaurant style tortilla strips, 12 chips (28 g)	4
Tortilla chip rounds, 10 chips (28 g)	4
Tortilla chip triangles, 10 chips (28 g)	4
Tortilla chips, super thin, triangles, 12 chips (28 g)	5

Tortilla rounds, 10 chips (28 g)	5
Tortilla rounds, restaurant style, 10 chips (28 g)	5
Tortilla strips, 12 chips (28 g)	5
Tortilla strips, restaurant style, 12 chips (28 g)	4
Tortilla triangles, restaurant style, 10 chips (28 g)	5

Mystic Harvest

Purple corn tortilla chips with golden flax, red & black quinoa, 15 chips (28 g)	4

Nature's Promise Naturals

Tortilla chips, natural blue corn, restaurant style, 14 chips (28 g)	4

New York Texas Toast

Tortilla strips, chili lime flavored, 11 strips (7 g)	1
Tortilla strips, chipotle cheddar flavored, 11 strips (7 g)	1

Nuevo Leon

Nacho chips, totopos, restaurant style, 9 chips (28 g)	4

Old Dutch

Restaurante style bite size premium tortilla chips, 20 chips (29 g)	5

On The Border

Tortilla chips, 7 chips (28 g)	5
Tortilla chips, cafe style, 7 chips (29 g)	4
Tortilla chips, cantina thins, 14 chips (28 g)	4

On The Border Mexican Grill & Cantina

Cafe style tortilla chips, 7 chips (28 g)	5
Cantina thins tortilla chips, 14 chips (28 g)	4

Padrino's

Tortilla chips, reduced fat, 9 chips (28 g)	4

Party 'tizers Dippin' Chips

Kale carrot and spinach tortilla, 10 chips (28 g)	4

Snacks

SmartPoints™ value

Pringles

Tortilla crisps, southwestern ranch flavored, 14 crisps (28 g)	5
Tortilla crisps, truly original flavor, 15 crisps (28 g)	5

Pringles Tortillas

Tortilla crisps, zesty salsa flavored, 14 crisps (28 g)	5

Quaker Popped

Cheesy nacho tortilla style chips, 15 chips (28 g)	4
Tangy ranch tortilla style chips, 15 chips (28 g)	4

RW Garcia Dippers

3 seed veggie dipping chips, 10 strips (28 g)	4

RW Garcia MixtBag

Tortilla chips, classic, yellow & blue, family value pack, 15 chips (28 g)	4

Santitas

Grande lightly seasoned tortilla chips, 9 chips (28 g)	4
Tortilla chips, 9 chips (28 g)	4
Tortilla chips, triangles, white corn blend, 9 chips (28 g)	4
Tortilla chips, triangles, yellow corn blend, 9 chips (28 g)	4
Tortilla chips, yellow corn blend, pounder, 9 chips (28 g)	4
White corn blend tortilla chips, 9 chips (28 g)	4

Simply Balanced

Tortilla chips, organic, blue corn, 11 chips (28 g)	4
Tortilla chips, organic, blue corn with flax seed, 9 chips (28 g)	4
Tortilla chips, organic, white corn, 1 oz	4
Tortilla chips, organic, yellow corn, 1 oz	4

Snyder's

Tortilla chips, restaurant style, 8 chips (28 g)	4
Tortilla chips, yellow corn, the pounder, 13 chips (28 g)	4

SmartPoints™ value

Snyder's Naturals

Tortilla chips, multigrain, sea salt, 9 chips (28 g)	4

Snyder's of Hanover

Whole grain tortilla chips, 10 crackers (28 g)	4

Snyder's of Hanover Dippin' Strips

Reduced fat tortilla strips, 10 strips (28 g)	4

Snyder's of Hanover Reduced Fat

Twist of lime tortilla chips, 13 chips (28 g)	4

Snyder's The Pounder

White corn reduced fat tortilla chips, 13 chips (28 g)	4

Tia Rosa

Megathin tortilla chips, 8 ½ chips (28 g)	4

Tostitos

Baked scoops, 16 chips (28 g)	4
Bite size tortilla chips, 24 chips (28 g)	4
Blue corn, 7 chips (28 g)	4
Crispy rounds tortilla chips, white corn, 13 chips (27 g)	4
Crispy rounds, 100% white corn, 1 oz	4
Hint of lime tortilla chips, 6 Chips (28 g)	5
Original restaurant style tortilla chips, 7 chips (28 g)	4
Tortilla chips, crispy rounds, 13 chips (28 g)	4
Tortilla chips, hint of lime flavored, 6 chips (28 g)	5
Tortilla chips, multigrain, 8 chips (28 g)	5
Tortilla chips, restaurant style, 7 chips (28 g)	4
Tortilla chips, restaurant style, 100% white corn, 7 chips (28 g)	4
Tortilla chips, scoops, 1 oz	4

Snacks

Tostitos Artisan Recipes

Red pepper and tomato salsa flavored tortilla chips, 8 chips (28 g)	5
Roasted garlic and black bean flavored tortilla chips, 8 chips (28 g)	4

Tostitos Baked!

Tortilla chips, scoops, 1 oz	4
Tortilla chips, scoops!, 14 chips (28 g)	4
Tortilla crisps, scoops!, 1 package (25 g)	3

Tostitos Cantina

Thin and crispy tortilla chips, 15 chips (28 g)	5
Traditional tortilla chips, 7 chips (28 g)	5

Tostitos Natural

Restaurant style tortilla chips, yellow corn, 6 chips (28 g)	4
Tortilla chips, restaurant style, yellow corn, 6 chips (28 g)	4

Tostitos Rolls

Rolled tortilla chips, 15 chips (28 g)	5

Tostitos Scoops!

Tortilla chips, 12 chips (28 g)	4
Tortilla chips, 13 chips (28 g)	4
Tortilla chips, 100% white corn, 12 chips (28 g)	4
Tortilla chips, family size, 13 chips (28 g)	4
Tortilla chips, multigrain, 12 chips (28 g)	4

Tostitos Simply

Tortilla chips, blue corn, 6 chips (28 g)	4

Trader Joe's

Organic blue corn tortilla chips, 14 chips (28 g)	4
Organic white corn tortilla chips, 14 chips (28 g)	4
Quinoa & black bean infused tortilla chips, 8 chips (28 g)	4
Soy and flaxseed tortilla chips, 15 chips (28 g)	4

Sweet potato tortilla chip rounds, 11 chips (28 g)	5
Veggie and flaxseed tortilla chips, 7 chips (28 g)	4

Trader Joe's Organic

Blue corn tortilla chips, 12 chips (28 g)	4
Yellow corn tortilla chip rounds, 9 chips (28 g)	4

Trader Joe's Reduced Guilt

Organic white corn tortilla chips, 14 chips (28 g)	3

Tuscan Garden

Tri-color tortilla strips, 2 Tbsp	1

Utz

Tortilla, white corn, 12 chips (28 g)	5
Tortillas, multigrain, 9 chips (28 g)	5

Utz Baked

Tortillas, bite size, 14 chips (28 g)	3
White corn tortilla chips, baked tortillas, 1 oz	3

Utz Organic

Tortilla chips, blue corn, 1 oz	4

Wegman's

Tortilla chips, multi-grain, round, 14 chips (28 g)	4

Wegman's Food You Feel Good About

Get dippin blue corn tortilla chips, 1 oz	4
Get dippin multigrain tortilla chips, 1 oz	4
Tortilla chips, blue corn, 1 oz	4

Whole Foods 365 Everyday Value

Tortilla chips, 9 chips (28 g)	4
Lightly salted black bean tortilla chips, 11 chips (28 g)	4

Wild Roots Wild Chips

Premium tortilla chips with red quinoa and chia, 7 chips (28 g)	4

Xochitl Organic

Mexican style white corn chips, 1 oz	4

Snacks

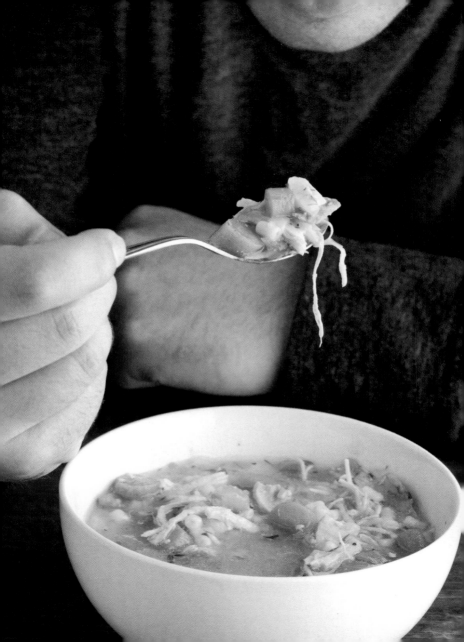

soups
Stews & Chili

Beef Soup

Annie Chun's

Soup bowl, Vietnamese pho, 1 bowl (170 g)	8

Bear Creek

Soup mix, vegetable beef, ¼ cup dry	3

Campbell's

Condensed beef with vegetables and barley soup, ½ cup	3
Condensed vegetable beef soup, ½ cup	3
Soup, vegetable beef, 1 cup	2

Campbell's Chunky

Beef with country vegetables soup, 1 cup	4
Hearty beef barley soup, 1 cup	4
Roasted beef tips with vegetables soup, 1 cup	3
Sirloin burger with country vegetables soup, 1 cup	5
Sirloin burger with country vegetables soup (microwaveable individual size), 1 cup	4
Slow roasted beef with mushrooms soup, 1 cup	4
Soup, beef with country vegetables, family size!, 1 cup	4
Soup, beer-n-cheese with beef & bacon, 1 cup	6
Soup, hearty beef noodle, 1 cup	3
Soup, hearty cheeseburger, 1 cup	7
Soup, philly-style cheesesteak, 1 cup	5
Soup, savory pot roast, 1 cup	4
Soup, vegetable beef, old fashioned, 1 cup	3
Steak and potato soup, 1 cup	3

Campbell's Chunky Healthy Request

Soup, beef with country vegetables, 1 cup	3
Soup, old fashioned vegetable beef, 1 cup	4
Soup, sirloin burger with country vegetables, 1 cup	4

Campbell's Home Style

Soup, Italian-style wedding, light, 1 cup	2

Healthy Choice

Soup, vegetable beef, 1 cup	4

Maruchan Instant Lunch

Beef flavor, 1 container (64 g)	10

Maruchan Ramen

Beef flavor, ½ block (43 g)	6
Beef flavor, ½ block (43 g)	6
Ramen noodle soup, ½ package (43 g)	6

Nissin Cup Noodles

Soup, ramen noodle, beef flavor, 1 container (64 g)	11

Nissin Top Ramen

Ramen noodle soup, beef flavor, 1 ½ oz	6

Progresso

Soup, high fiber, three-bean chili with beef, 1 cup	5

Progresso Light

Beef pot roast soup, 1 cup	2
Savory beef barley vegetable soup, 1 cup	2

Progresso Rich & Hearty

Beef pot roast with country vegetables soup, 1 cup	3
Savory beef barley vegetable soup, 1 cup	3
Sirloin steak and vegetables soup, 1 cup	4

	SmartPoints™ value
Slow cooked vegetable beef soup, 1 cup	4
Steak and homestyle noodles soup, 1 cup	3
Steak burger and country vegetables soup, 1 cup	5
Progresso Traditional	
99% fat free beef barley soup, 1 cup	3
Beef barley soup, 1 cup	4
Raley's	
Soup, beef barley, 1 cup	4
Signature Cafe	
Soup, stuffed pepper with beef, 1 cup	4
Top Ramen	
Soup, ramen noodle, 6-pack, beef flavor, ½ dry block (42 g)	6

Chicken Soup

	SmartPoints™ value
Amy's Soups	
Low fat, no chicken noodle, 1 cup	3
Bear Creek	
Soup mix, chicken noodle, chicken flavored, ¼ cup dry	4
Better Than Bouillon	
Chicken base, 1 tsp	0
Campbell's	
Chicken noodle soup, ½ cup	2
Condensed chicken noodle soup, ½ cup	2
Condensed chicken noodle soup, ½ cup	2
Condensed cream of chicken and mushroom soup, ½ cup	4
Condensed cream of chicken soup, ½ cup	4
Condensed homestyle chicken noodle soup, ½ cup	2

	SmartPoints™ value
Condensed soup, chicken won ton, ½ cup	2
Soup, chicken & quinoa with poblano chilies, 1 cup	4
Soup, condensed, chicken noodle o's, ½ cup	3
Soup, condensed, chicken with rice, family size, ½ cup	2
Soup, homestyle chicken noodle, 1 cup	2
Soup, ready to serve, low sodium, chicken with noodles, 1 container (305 g)	4
Campbell's 100% Natural	
Soup, creamy gouda bisque with chicken, 1 cup	5
Campbell's Chunky	
Chicken pot pie pub style soup, 1 cup	6
Classic chicken noodle soup, 1 cup	3
Creamy chicken and dumplings soup, 1 cup	5
Fajita chicken with rice and beans soup, 1 cup	4
Pub style chicken pot pie soup, 1 cup	6
Savory chicken with white and wild rice soup, 1 cup	3
Soup, chipotle chicken & corn chowder, 1 cup	5
Soup, grilled chicken & sausage gumbo, 1 cup	5
Soup, hearty chicken with vegetables, 1 cup	3
Soup, jammin' jerk chicken with rice & beans, 1 cup	4
Soup, kickin' buffalo-style chicken, 1 cup	4
Soup, roasted chicken with country vegetables, 1 cup	3
Soup, spicy chicken quesadilla, 1 cup	6

Soups, Stews & Chili

	SmartPoints™ value
Campbell's Chunky Healthy Request	
Gumbo, grilled chicken & sausage, 1 cup	4
Soup, chicken corn chowder, 1 cup	5
Soup, chicken noodle, 1 cup	3
Soup, classic chicken noodle, 1 cup	3
Soup, grilled chicken & sausage gumbo, 1 cup	4
Campbell's Classic Recipe	
Chicken noodle soup, ½ cup	2
Condensed chicken and stars soup, ½ cup	2
Condensed double noodle soup, ½ cup	3
Campbell's Go	
Soup, coconut curry with chicken & shiitake mushrooms, 1 cup	5
Soup, creamy Thai style chicken with rice, 1 cup	9
Soup, Moroccan style chicken with chickpeas, 1 cup	5
Soup, spicy chorizo & pulled chicken with black beans, 1 cup	6
Campbell's Healthy Request	
Condensed cream of chicken soup, ½ cup condensed	2
Condensed soup, chicken noodle, ½ cup	2
Soup, chicken noodle, 1 cup	2
Soup, condensed, chicken with rice, ½ cup	2
Soup, condensed, Mexican-style chicken tortilla, ½ cup condensed	4
Campbell's Homestyle	
Light chicken & dumplings soup, 1 fl oz	0
Light chicken corn chowder, 1 fl oz	0
Light savory chicken with vegetables soup, 1 cup	3

	SmartPoints™ value
Mexican-style chicken tortilla soup, 1 cup	4
Soup, chicken noodle, light, 1 cup	2
Soup, creamy chicken & herb dumplings, 1 cup	5
Soup, Mexican-style chicken tortilla, 1 cup	4
Campbell's Kitchen Classics	
Soup, chicken noodle, 1 cup	2
Campbell's Light	
Condensed chicken with white and wild rice soup, ½ cup	2
Soup, condensed, light, chicken gumbo, ½ cup	2
Campbell's Select Harvest	
Chicken with egg noodles soup, 1 cup	3
Mexican style chicken tortilla soup, 1 cup	3
Soup, chicken with whole grain pasta, 1 cup	3
Soup, ready to serve, southwest-style white chicken chili, 1 cup	4
Soup, savory chicken and long grain rice, 1 cup	3
Soup, savory chicken with long grain rice, 1 cup	3
Campbell's Select Harvest Healthy Request	
Soup, savory chicken and brown rice, 1 cup	3
Campbell's Slow Kettle Style	
Creamy broccoli cheddar bisque, 1 cup	7
Roasted chicken noodle soup, 1 cup	3
Tuscan style chicken and white bean soup, 1 cup	4
Campbell's Soup at Hand	
Soup, chicken with mini noodles, 1 container (301 g)	2
Soup, creamy chicken, 1 container (305 g)	4

Campbell's Soup on the Go

Cheesy chicken tortilla, 1 container (310 g)	3
Chicken and star shaped pasta soup, 1 container (305 g)	2

Chunky

Kickin' buffalo-style chicken soup, 1 cup	4

Cuginos

Soup mix, chicken enchilada!, mild, 1 cup prepared	2

Fit & Active

Chicken noodle chunky style soup, 1 cup	3

Gluten Free Cafe

Soup, chicken noodle, 1 cup	2

Healthy Choice

Soup, chicken & dumplings, 1 cup	4
Soup, hearty chicken, 1 cup	4
Soup, mediterranean style chicken with orzo, 1 container (226 g)	2
Soup, old fashioned, chicken noodle, 1 cup	2
Soup, variety pack, 1 cup	2
Soup, zesty gumbo with chicken & sausage, 1 cup	3

Juanita's

Caldo de pollo, 1 cup	2

Kirkland Signature

Chicken tortilla soup, 1 cup	4

Lipton

Cup-a-soup, chicken noodle flavor, 1 envelope (23 g)	3
Noodle soup with real chicken broth, 2 Tbsp	2

Lipton Cup-a-Soup

Instant soup, chicken noodle with white meat, 1 envelope (13 g)	1
Instant soup, cream of chicken flavor, 1 envelope (17 g)	2

Instant soup, hearty chicken noodle, 1 envelope (16.1 g)	2
Soup mix, instant, chicken noodle, with white meat, office pack, 1 envelope (13 g)	1

Lipton Soup Secrets

Ring -o-noodle, with real chicken broth, 2 Tbsp	2
Soup, chicken noodle, with diced white chicken meat, 3 Tbsp	2
Soup, noodle, 2 Tbsp	2

Manischewitz

Soup, chicken matzo ball, 1 cup	5

Marie Callender's

Chicken dumplings soup, 1 cup	5
Soup, chicken & dumplings, 1 cup	5
Soup, chicken pot pie style, 1 cup	5

Maruchan

Chicken flavor instant lunch, 1 container (64 g)	10
Chicken flavor ramen noodle soup, ½ package (43 g)	6
Chicken flavor ramen noodles with vegetables in bowl, 1 bowl (47 g)	7

Maruchan Instant Lunch

Hot & spicy chicken flavor, 1 container (64 g)	10
Roast chicken flavor, 1 container (64 g)	10

Maruchan Ramen

Creamy chicken flavor, ½ block (43 g)	6

Mrs. Grass

Soup mix, extra noodles, ⅓ carton (29 g)	3
Soup mix, noodle soup, ¼ carton (18 g)	2

Nissin Big Cup Noodles

Ramen noodle soup, chicken flavor, ½ container (40 g)	6

Soups, Stews & Chili

SmartPoints™ value

Nissin Top Ramen

Ramen noodle soup, chicken flavor, 1 ½ oz	6

Pacific Natural Foods

Soup, organic, chicken & white rice, 1 cup	3
Soup, organic, chicken noodle, 1 cup	2
Soup, organic, Santa Fe style chicken, 1 cup	4

Panera Bread

Soup, chicken, kale & sweet potato (gluten free), 1 cup	3
Soup, low fat chicken tortilla, 1 cup	3
Soup, low fat, chicken noodle, 1 cup	3
Soup, low fat, chicken tortilla, gluten free, 1 cup	3

Progresso

Soup, light chicken and vegetables with rosemary, 1 cup	2
Soup, light creamy roasted chicken with herb dumplings, 1 cup	3

Progresso Heart Healthy

Chicken and wild rice reduced sodium soup, 1 cup	2
Chicken noodle reduced sodium soup, 1 cup	2
Reduced sodium chicken gumbo soup, 1 cup	3

Progresso Light

Chicken and cheese enchilada flavor soup, 1 cup	3
Chicken and dumpling soup, 1 cup	2
Chicken corn chowder soup, 1 cup	3
Chicken noodle soup, 1 cup	2
Chicken pot pie style soup, 1 cup	3
Chicken vegetable rotini soup, 1 cup	2
Creamy chicken Alfredo with pasta, 1 cup	3

SmartPoints™ value

Roasted chicken and vegetable soup, 1 cup	2
Santa Fe style chicken soup, 1 cup	2

Progresso Rich & Hearty

Chicken and homestyle noodles soup, 1 cup	3
Chicken corn chowder soup, 1 cup	7
Chicken pot pie style soup, 1 cup	4
Creamy Alfredo with penne and chicken soup, 1 cup	6
Creamy roasted chicken wild rice soup, 1 cup	4

Progresso Traditional

99% fat free chicken noodle soup, 1 cup	3
Chicken and herb dumplings soup, 1 cup	3
Chicken and orzo with lemon soup, 1 cup	2
Chicken and sausage gumbo soup, 1 cup	4
Chicken and wild rice soup, 1 cup	3
Chicken barley soup, 1 cup	2
Chicken noodle soup, 1 cup	3
Chicken rice with vegetables soup, 1 cup	3
Chicken tortilla soup, 1 cup	3
Creamy roasted chicken with herb dumplings soup, 1 cup	5
Hearty chicken and rotini soup, 1 cup	3
Homestyle chicken soup with vegetables and pearl pasta, 1 cup	3
Roasted chicken primavera soup, 1 cup	3
Roasted chicken rotini soup, 1 cup	2
Roasted garlic chicken with vegetables and penne soup, 1 cup	3
Southwestern style chicken soup, 1 cup	3

Soups, Stews & Chili

Raley's

Soup, chicken tortilla soup, 1 cup	4

Signature Cafe

Soup, fiesta chicken tortilla, 1 cup	4

Trader Joe's

Chicken, barley and vegetable soup, 1 cup	3

Wegman's

Soup, chicken noodle, 1 cup	3
Soup, chunky chicken noodle, 1 cup	3

Whole Foods 365 Organic

Chicken noodle soup, 1 cup	2

Wolfgang Puck

Soup, organic, chicken with egg noodles, 1 cup	3
Soup, organic, chicken with white & wild rice, 1 cup	4

Chili

Amy's

Organic, chili medium black bean, 1 cup	5
Organic, chili medium with vegetables, 1 cup	7
Organic, medium chili, 1 cup	8
Organic, spicy chili, 1 cup	8

Bear Creek

Chili mix, darn good, ⅓ cup dry	2

Bush's Best Chili Beans

Kidney beans in mild chili sauce, ½ cup	3
Red beans in medium chili sauce, ½ cup	3

Campbell's Chunky

Beef and bean roadhouse chili, 1 cup	8
Roadhouse beef and bean chili, 1 cup	7

Campbell's Home Style Healthy Request

Chili, spicy vegetable, 1 cup	5

Campbell's Slow Kettle Style

Southwest style chicken with beans chili, 1 cup	5

Castleberry's American Originals

Chili sauce, hot dog, 1 Tbsp	0

Dennison's

Chili con carne with beans, original, 1 cup	11
Chili with beans, turkey, 1 cup	6

Eating Right

Turkey chili with beans, 1 cup	7

Great Value

Hot dog chili sauce, 1 Tbsp	0

Hormel

Chili, chunky with beans, 1 cup	8
Chili, chunky, no beans, 1 cup	6
Chili, hot with beans, 1 cup	8
Chili, no beans, 1 cup	7
Chili, vegetarian with beans, 1 cup	5
Chili, with beans, 1 cup	8
Turkey chili with beans, 1 cup	6
Turkey chili with no beans, 1 cup	4

Hormel Chili Master

Chili, white chicken, 1 cup	7
Chili, with beans, made with beef, 1 cup	7

Marie Callender's

White chicken chili with beans, 1 cup	7

Mark Schlereth's

Green chili sauce with pork, stinkin' good, medium, ¼ cup	2

Nalley

Chili con carne, with beans, turkey, 1 cup	6
Original chili con carne with beans, 1 cup	8

	SmartPoints™ value
Nalley 99% Fat Free	
Original vegetarian chili with beans, 1 cup	5
Panera Bread	
Organic vegetarian chili, 1 cup	4
Progresso	
Chili, Southwest style white chicken with beans, 1 cup	6
Ray's	
Chilli with beans, reduced fat, 1 cup	6
Skyline	
Chili & spaghetti, 1 cup	8
Chili, original, 1 cup	9
Stagg	
Chili, four-bean, vegetable garden, 1 cup	6
Trader Joe's	
Chicken chili with beans, 1 cup	8
Turkey chili with beans, 1 cup	7
Wegman's	
Chili, turkey & bean, 1 cup	4
Wolf	
Chili, homestyle with beans, 1 cup	10
Chili, turkey with beans, 1 cup	6
Chili, with beans, 1 cup	11

Seafood Soup

	SmartPoints™ value
Authentic Asia	
Shrimp wonton soup, with noodles, Chinese-style, 6 oz	7
Campbell's	
Kickin' crab and sweet corn chowder, 1 cup	7
Campbell's Chunky	
New England clam chowder soup, 1 cup	6
Soup, Manhattan clam chowder, 1 cup	4

	SmartPoints™ value
Campbell's Chunky Healthy Request	
Soup, New England clam chowder, 1 cup	4
Campbell's Home Style	
New England clam chowder soup, 1 cup	5
Giant	
Maryland crab soup, 1 cup	3
Maruchan Instant Lunch	
Shrimp flavor, 1 container (64 g)	10
Maruchan Ramen	
Shrimp flavor, ½ block (43 g)	6
Phillips Seafood Restaurants	
Soup, Crab, Maryland style, 1 cup	4
Soup, Cream of crab, 1 cup	15
Progresso Light	
New England clam chowder soup, 1 cup	3
Progresso Rich & Hearty	
New England clam chowder, 1 cup	6
Progresso Traditional	
99% fat free New England clam chowder, 1 cup	3
Manhattan clam chowder soup, 1 cup	3
New England clam chowder soup, 1 cup	6
Wegman's	
Soup, shrimp bisque, 1 cup	7

Stew

	SmartPoints™ value
Dinty Moore	
Beef stew, 1 cup	7
Mrs. Fearnow's	
Brunswick stew, with chicken, 1 cup	5
Our Family	
Beef stew, thick & hearty, 1 cup	7
Stoke's	
Green chile stew, with pork, medium, 1 cup	5

Vegetable & Other Soup

Alessi

Sicilian lentil soup, lenticchie, ⅓ cup dry	4
Tuscan white bean soup, zuppa toscana, ⅓ cup dry mix	5

Amy's

Organic, fire roasted southwestern vegetable, 1 cup	4

Amy's Light in Sodium

Organic chunky tomato bisque soup, 1 cup	6
Organic lentil vegetable soup, 1 cup	5
Organic soup, cream of tomato, low fat, 1 cup	5
Soup, organic, lentil, 1 cup	4
Soup, organic, low fat, split pea, 1 cup	3

Amy's Soups

Organic, alphabet, fat free, 1 cup	3
Organic, black bean vegetable, 1 cup	5
Organic, chunky vegetable, 1 cup	2
Organic, hearty, Spanish rice & red bean, ½ can (208 g)	4
Organic, lentil, 1 cup	5
Organic, lentil vegetable, 1 cup	5
Organic, low fat cream of tomato, 1 cup	5
Organic, ready to serve, chunky tomato bisque, 1 cup	6
Organic, ready to serve, low fat, minestrone, 1 cup	3
Organic, ready to serve, low fat, vegetable barley, 1 cup	3
Organic, split pea, 1 cup	3
Ready to serve, minestrone, 1 cup	3
Ready to serve, mushroom bisque, with porcini, 1 cup	4
Thai coconut, tom kha phak, ½ can (200 g)	10

Andersen's Creamy Soup

Split pea, 1 cup	3

Annie Chun's

Miso soup bowl, 1 bowl (169 g)	7
Udon soup bowl, 1 bowl (168 g)	7

Bear Creek

Soup mix, creamy potato, ¼ dry cup (39 g)	5
Soup mix, creamy wild rice, ¼ cup dry	4
Soup mix, gumbo, ¼ cup dry	4
Soup mix, minestrone, ⅓ cup dry	3
Soup mix, navy bean, ¼ cup dry	4
Soup mix, tortilla, ¼ cup dry	3

Campbell's

Condensed bean with bacon soup, ½ cup	5
Condensed broccoli cheese soup, ½ cup	4
Condensed cream of broccoli soup, ½ cup	3
Condensed cream of celery soup, ½ cup	3
Condensed cream of mushroom with roasted garlic soup, ½ cup	2
Condensed cream of potato soup, ½ cup	3
Condensed French onion soup, ½ cup	2
Condensed golden mushroom soup, ½ cup	3
Condensed minestrone soup, ½ cup	3
Condensed soup, cream of mushroom, ½ cup	3
Condensed soup, tomato bisque, ½ cup	6
Condensed split pea with ham soup, ½ cup	5
Condensed tomato soup, ½ cup	4
Condensed tomato soup, ½ cup	4
Condensed vegetable soup, ½ cup	3

Soups, Stews & Chili

Soups, Stews & Chili

	SmartPoints™ value
Condensed vegetarian vegetable soup, ½ cup	3
Cream of mushroom condensed soup, ½ cup	3
Soup, condensed, bean with bacon, ½ cup	5
Soup, condensed, cheddar cheese, less sodium, ½ cup	4
Soup, condensed, cream of mushroom, ½ cup	3
Soup, condensed, old fashioned vegetable, ½ cup	3
Soup, condensed, tomato, ½ cup	4
Soup, creamy tomato, 1 cup	7
Soup, tomato, 1 cup	5
Soup, vegetable, 1 cup	4
Tomato soup, 1 cup	5
Campbell's 100% Natural	
Soup, butternut squash bisque, 1 cup	5
Campbell's Chunky	
Baked potato soup, 1 cup	7
Baked potato with cheddar and bacon bits soup, 1 cup	7
Chicken broccoli cheese with potato soup, 1 cup	6
Chowder, chicken corn, 1 cup	6
Hearty bean and ham with natural smoke flavor soup, 1 cup	5
Jazzy jambalaya soup, 1 cup	4
Mushroom Swiss burger soup, 1 cup	5
Sausage and pepper rigatoni soup, 1 cup	7
Soup, baked potato with steak & cheese, 1 cup	6
Soup, hearty tomato with pasta, 1 cup	6
Soup, old fashioned potato ham chowder, 1 cup	6
Soup, savory vegetable, 1 cup	4
Split pea and ham soup, 1 cup	5

	SmartPoints™ value
Campbell's Chunky Healthy Request	
Hearty Italian style wedding soup, 1 cup	4
Soup, savory vegetable, 1 cup	4
Soup, split pea & ham, 1 cup	5
Campbell's Classics	
Condensed old fashioned tomato rice soup, ½ cup	5
Campbell's Go	
Soup, creamy red pepper with smoked gouda, 1 cup	10
Campbell's Gourmet Bisques	
Bisque, golden butternut squash, 1 cup	5
Campbell's Healthy Request	
Soup, condensed, cheddar cheese, ½ cup condensed	3
Soup, condensed, golden mushroom, ½ cup	2
Soup, condensed, tuscan-style lentil, ½ cup	4
Soup, Italian-style wedding, 1 cup	3
Soup, tomato, 1 cup	5
Southwest style bean and barley condensed soup, ½ cup	3
Campbell's Home Style	
Italian style wedding soup, 1 cup	3
Campbell's Organic	
Garden vegetable soup with herbs, 1 cup	4
Campbell's Select Harvest	
Bisque, zesty tomato, 1 cup	5
Healthy request Italian style wedding soup, 1 cup	3
Soup, harvest tomato, with basil, 1 cup	5
Soup, ready to serve, light, southwestern-style vegetable, 1 cup	2
Soup, whole grain pasta fagioli, 1 cup	3

Campbell's Select Harvest Garden Recipes

Soup, vegetable medley, 1 cup	3

Campbell's Slow Cooker Sauces

Moroccan spiced stew, ¼ cup	1

Campbell's Soup at Hand

Soup, classic tomato, 1 each (301 g)	5
Soup, cream of broccoli, 1 each (305 g)	5
Soup, creamy tomato parmesan bisque, 1 container (305 g)	9
Soup, vegetable beef, 1 container (305 g)	2

Campbell's Soup on the Go

Cheesy potato with bacon soup, 1 container (310 g)	5
Classic tomato soup, 1 container (305 g)	6
Creamy tomato soup, 1 container (305 g)	8

CedarLane

Chopped tomato and vegetable soup with quinoa, 1 cup	3

Cuginos Ridiculously Delicious!

Soup! mix, lemon chicken & rice flavored, ⅛ package (25 g)	3

Dole Garden Soup

Roasted garlic tomato basil soup, 1 cup	4
Soup, carrot ginger, 1 cup	4
Southwestern black bean and corn soup, 1 cup	3
Sweet corn soup, 1 cup	4

Dr. McDougall's

Ramen, vegan, miso, 1 oz	2

Dr. McDougall's Fresh Flavor

Soup, pad Thai noodle, 1 oz	3
Soup, vegan, black bean & lime, 1 ⅔ oz	4

Essential Everyday

Soup, condensed, cream of mushroom, 98% fat free, ½ cup	2

Fit & Active

Vegetable beef homestyle soup, 1 cup	4

Goya

Soup, black bean, 1 cup	6

Harry's

Soup, vegetable minestrone, organic, 1 cup	4

Harry's Fresh Foods Organic

Soup, creamy tomato, 1 cup	8

Health Valley

Soup, vegetable barley, 1 cup	3

Healthy Choice

Cheese tortellini soup, 1 cup	3
Soup, bean & ham, 1 cup	5
Soup, chicken tortilla, 1 cup	4
Soup, garden vegetable, 1 cup	4
Soup, hearty vegetable barley, 1 cup	5
Soup, split pea and ham, 1 cup	4

Hursts HamBeens

15 bean soup, 1 oz dry	3
15 bean soup, Cajun, ½ cup	3

Imagine

Creamy broccoli soup, 1 cup	2
Creamy potato leek soup, 8 oz	3

Imagine Natural Creations Organic

Soup, creamy sweet pea, 1 cup	3

Imagine Organic

Light in sodium creamy butternut squash soup, 1 cup	4
Soup, creamy garden tomato, light in sodium, 1 cup	2
Soup, creamy, butternut squash, 1 cup	4
Soup, creamy, tomato, 1 cup	3

Soups, Stews & Chili

	SmartPoints™ value
Kikkoman	
Instant soup, soybean paste with tofu, tofu miso, 1 packet (10 g)	1
Kirkland Signature	
Roasted corn chowder, 1 cup	5
Lipton Cup-a-Soup	
Instant soup, spring vegetable, 1 envelope (13 g)	1
Lipton Recipe Secrets	
Onion recipe soup and dip mix, 1 Tbsp	1
Extra noodle soup mix, 3 Tbsp	2
Manischewitz	
Matzo ball & soup mix, 1 Tbsp	2
Matzo ball soup, 1 cup	4
Maruchan Ramen	
Oriental flavor, ½ block (43 g)	6
Mrs. Grass	
Soup mix, hearty, homestyle chicken noodle, 1 cup prepared	2
Nong Shim	
Bowl noodle soup, hot & spicy flavor, picante, ½ bowl (43 g)	6
Omaha Steaks	
Classic French onion soup, 8 oz	7
Our Family	
Soup, chunky, beef vegetable, 1 cup	4
Pacific Natural Foods	
Bisque, organic, hearty tomato, 1 cup	7
Bisque, organic, roasted red pepper & tomato, 1 cup	7
Chowder, poblano pepper and corn, 1 cup	7
Soup, Thai sweet potato, 1 cup	6
Soup, vegetable lentil & roasted red pepper, 1 cup	4
Pacific Natural Foods - Organic	
All natural soup, creamy butternut squash, 1 cup	3

	SmartPoints™ value
Pacific Organic	
Creamy tomato soup, 1 container (240 ml)	4
Soup, all natural, light sodium, creamy tomato, 1 cup	4
Soup, cashew carrot ginger, 1 cup	5
Soup, creamy butternut squash, 1 cup	3
Soup, creamy tomato, 1 cup	4
Soup, curried red lentil, 1 cup	6
Soup, light sodium, roasted red pepper and tomato, 1 cup	5
Soup, roasted red pepper & tomato, 1 cup	5
Soup, spicy black bean & kale, 1 cup	4
Soup, vegetable lentil & roasted red pepper, reduced sodium, 1 cup	4
Soup, vegetable quinoa, 1 cup	3
Panera Bread	
Autumn squash soup (gluten free & vegetarian), 1 cup	11
Baked potato soup, 1 cup	9
Broccoli cheddar soup, 1 cup	11
Loaded baked potato soup, 1 cup	9
Organic lentil soup (gluten free & vegetarian), 1 cup	5
Organic tomato bisque, 1 cup	5
Soup, creamy tomato, gluten free, 1 cup	9
Plats Du Chef	
French onion soup (serves 6), 1 soup (285 g)	8
Progresso Artisan	
Creamy tomato with roasted red pepper soup, 1 cup	6
Masala curry butternut squash soup, 1 cup	7
Rustic tomato with chicken and dumplings soup, 1 cup	5

Soups, Stews & Chili

Progresso Heart Healthy

	SmartPoints value
Creamy tomato basil soup, 1 cup	5
Italian style wedding with meatballs reduced sodium soup, 1 cup	2
Reduced sodium garden vegetable soup, 1 cup	3
Reduced sodium minestrone soup, 1 cup	4
Reduced sodium tomato parmesan soup, 1 cup	3
Southwest style black bean and vegetable soup, 1 cup	3

Progresso High Fiber

Creamy tomato basil soup, 1 cup	6
Hearty vegetable and noodles soup, 1 cup	3

Progresso Light

Creamy potato with bacon and cheese soup, 1 cup	3
Homestyle vegetable and rice soup, 1 cup	2
Italian style meatball soup, 1 cup	3
Italian style vegetable soup, 1 cup	2
Savory vegetable barley soup, 1 cup	2
Vegetable soup, 1 cup	2
Zesty southwestern style vegetable soup, 1 cup	2

Progresso Rich & Hearty

Lentil and andouille sausage soup, 1 cup	7
Loaded potato with bacon soup, 1 cup	6
Steak and roasted russet potato soup, 1 cup	4
Tomato florentine with Italian sausage soup, 1 cup	6

Progresso Traditional

Albondigas meatball and rice, 1 cup	4
Beef and vegetable soup, 1 cup	4
Chickarina soup (chicken soup with meatballs), 1 cup	4

	SmartPoints value
Chicken tuscany soup, 1 cup	3
Creamy tomato with bacon and cheese soup, 1 cup	6
Italian style wedding soup, 1 cup	3
Potato broccoli and cheese chowder soup, 1 cup	7
Split pea with ham soup, 1 cup	4
Turkey noodle soup, 1 cup	2

Progresso Vegetable Classics

99% fat free lentil soup, 1 cup	4
99% fat free minestrone soup, 1 cup	3
Creamy mushroom soup, 1 cup	5
French onion soup, 1 cup	2
Garden vegetable soup, 1 cup	3
Hearty black bean soup, 1 cup	4
Hearty tomato soup, 1 cup	5
Hearty tomato soup, 1 cup	5
Lentil soup, 1 cup	4
Macaroni and bean soup, 1 cup	5
Minestrone soup, 1 cup	3
Southwestern style corn with potatoes and peppers soup, 1 cup	4
Tomato basil soup, 1 cup	6
Tomato basil soup, 1 cup	6
Tomato rotini soup, 1 cup	6
Vegetable Italiano soup, 1 cup	4
Vegetable soup, 1 cup	2
Vegetarian vegetable with barley soup, 1 cup	3

Raley's

Soup, butternut squash, 1 cup	5

Shore Lunch

Soup mix, creamy wild rice, 1 cup	5

Signature Cafe

Jambalaya, Cajun-style, with sausage, chicken & ham, 1 cup	7

Signature Cafe Savory

Vegetable barley soup, 1 cup	4

Soups, Stews & Chili

	SmartPoints™ value
Simply Balanced	
Soup, butternut squash, 1 cup	2
Soup, organic, rustic bean & vegetable, 1 cup	3
Soup, organic, tomato basil, 1 cup	4
Sushi Chef	
Clear soup, traditional Japanese style, 1 package (9 g)	1
Tabatchnick	
Cabbage soup, 1 pouch (213 g)	4
Thai Kitchen	
Tom kha soup, coconut ginger, 7 oz	10
Tom yum soup, hot & sour, 7 oz	2
Trader Joe's	
Beef pho soup with rice noodles and vegetables, ½ package (85 g)	3
Butternut squash soup, 1 cup	3
Carrot ginger soup, 1 cup	3
Garden patch veggie soup, 1 cup	2
Latin style black bean soup, 1 cup	2
Organic butternut squash soup - low sodium, 1 cup	3
Organic creamy tomato soup, 1 cup	4
Organic creamy tomato soup - low sodium, 1 cup	4
Organic pea soup, 1 container (567 g)	8
Organic split pea soup, 1 cup	3
Organic tomato & roasted red pepper soup - low sodium, 1 cup	4
Organic tomato and roasted red pepper soup, 1 cup	4
Organic vegetable soup with quinoa & kale, 1 container (567 g)	8
Pumpkin soup, 1 cup	5

	SmartPoints™ value
Trader Ming's	
Chicken and vegetable wonton soup, 1 bowl (305 g)	6
Wegman's	
Soup, Italian style wedding with meatballs & chicken, 1 cup	4
Wegman's Food You Feel Good About	
Soup, tomato basil with orzo, 1 cup	5
Wild Veggie	
Soup, simply carrot, 1 cup	2
Wolfgang Puck	
Soup, organic, thick hearty vegetable, 1 cup	5
Zooop!	
Cream of chicken and rice soup, 1 cup	10

Soups, Stews & Chili

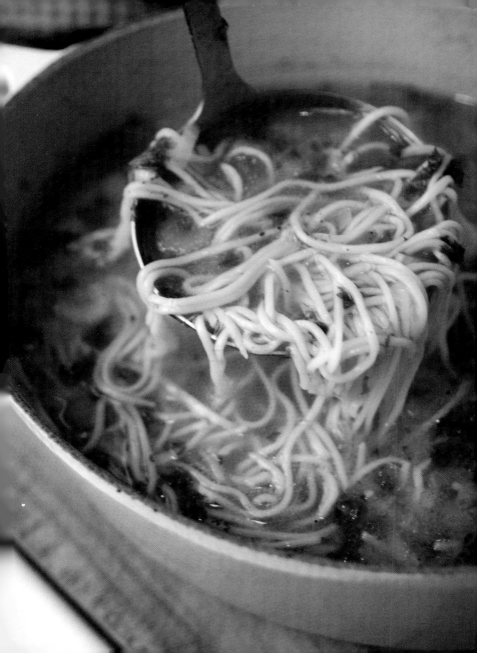

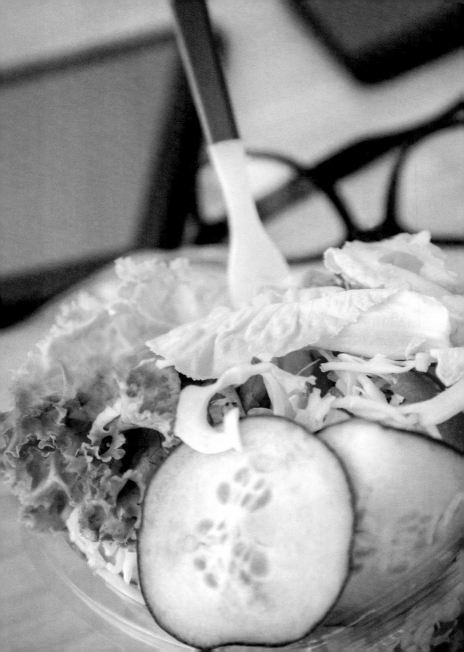

vegetables

Artichokes

Bellino

Artichoke hearts, quartered & marinated, 2 pieces (28 g)	1

Beans, Dried

Amy's Vegetarian Organic

Refried beans, black beans, ½ cup	4

Bush's Best

Black beans, ½ cup	3
Black beans, reduced sodium, ½ cup	3
Black beans, seasoned recipe, ½ cup	3
Butter beans, large, ½ cup	2
Butter beans, speckled, ½ cup	2
Cannellini beans, ½ cup	2
Garbanzos, ½ cup	3
Garbanzos, reduced sodium, ½ cup	3
Great northern beans, ½ cup	2
Kidney beans, dark red, ½ cup	3
Kidney beans, dark red, reduced sodium, ½ cup	3
Kidney beans, light red, ½ cup	3
Pinto beans, ½ cup	2
Pinto beans, reduced sodium, ½ cup	2
Refried beans, fat free, ½ cup	3

Bush's Best Chili Beans

Pinto beans in mild chili sauce, ½ cup	3

Del Monte Fresh Cut Specialties

Green lima beans, ½ cup	3

Glory Foods

Blackeye peas, seasoned, southern style, ½ cup	3

Goya

Beans, black, ½ cup	2
Beans, pinto, premium, ½ cup	2
Beans, red kidney, ½ cup	2
Beans, small red, premium, ½ cup	2
Black beans, low sodium, ½ cup	2
Blacks beans, premium, ½ cup	2
Cannellini, premium, ½ cup	2
Kidney beans, red, ½ cup	2
Pink beans in sauce, ½ cup	3
Red kidney beans, ½ cup	2
Small white beans, ½ cup	2

Goya Prime Premium

Chick peas, garbanzos, ½ cup	2
Red kidney beans, ½ cup	3

Great Value

Black beans, ½ cup	3
Chick peas, garbanzos, ½ cup	3
Kidney beans, dark red, ½ cup	3

Green Giant Steamers

Baby lima beans, ½ cup frozen	2

King's

Black-eyed pea mix, with seasonings, ¼ cup	3

Kroger

Black beans, ½ cup	3
Kidney beans, dark red, ½ cup	3
Pinto beans, ½ cup	3
Red beans, ½ cup	3
Refried beans, fat free, ½ cup	3
Refried beans, vegetarian, ½ cup	3
Seasoned black beans, ½ cup	3

La Preferida

Black beans, refried, ½ cup	3
Refried beans, ½ cup	4
Refried beans, authentic flavor, fat free, ½ cup	2

Meijer

Refried beans, fat free, ½ cup	3

Old El Paso

Refined beans, traditional, ½ cup	3
Refried beans, ½ cup	3
Refried beans, fat free, ½ cup	2

	SmartPoints™ value
Refried beans, fat free, spicy, ½ cup	3
Refried beans, traditional, ½ cup	3
Refried beans, vegetarian, ½ cup	3
Refried beans, with green chiles, ½ cup	2
Refried black beans, ½ cup	4
Ortega	
Refried beans, ½ cup	4
Refried beans, fat free, ½ cup	3
Pictsweet	
Butter beans, ½ cup	3
Lima beans, fordhook, ½ cup	3
Progresso	
Beans, black, ½ cup	2
Beans, kidney, cannellini white, ½ cup	3
Chick peas, ½ cup	3
Publix	
Beans, black, reduced sodium, ½ cup	3
Ranch Style	
Black beans, ½ cup	3
Pinto beans, with jalapeño peppers, ½ cup	3
Red Gold	
Red beans, ½ cup	3
Rosarita	
Black beans, whole, premium seasoned, ½ cup	3
Refried beans, green chile & lime, ½ cup	2
Refried beans, low fat, black, ½ cup	3
Refried beans, no fat, zesty salsa, ½ cup	2
Refried beans, spicy jalapeño, ½ cup	3
Refried beans, traditional, ½ cup	3
Refried beans, vegetarian, ½ cup	3

	SmartPoints™ value
S&W	
Black beans, ½ cup	3
Black beans, 50% less sodium, ½ cup	3
Black beans, organic, ½ cup	3
Seapoint Farms	
Edamame, dry roasted, spicy wasabi, 1 container (22.5 g)	2
ShopRite	
Chick peas, garbanzos, ½ cup	3
Simple Truth Organic	
Tri-bean blend, ½ cup	2
Black beans, ½ cup	3
Sun Vista	
Pinto beans, ½ cup	3
Taco Bell	
Refried beans, fat free, ½ cup	3
Refried beans, original, ½ cup	3
Trader Joe's	
Fat free traditional style refried beans, ½ cup	3
Trader Joe's Organic	
Baked beans, ½ cup	5
Allens	
Italian cut green beans, ½ cup	0
Italian cut green beans, seasoned southern style, ½ cup	1

Beans, Other

	SmartPoints™ value
Birds Eye Steamfresh	
Green beans, cut, ⅔ cup	0
Birds Eye Steamfresh Premium Selects	
Green beans, whole, 1 cup	0
Bush's Grillin' Beans	
Sweet mesquite flavor baked beans, ½ cup	6
Butter Kernel	
Green beans, cut, ½ cup	0

Vegetables

Vegetables

	SmartPoints™ value
Del Monte	
Cut green beans, blue lake, ½ cup	0
Low sodium cut green beans, ½ cup	0
Del Monte Fresh Cut	
Blue lake cut green beans, ½ cup	0
Blue lake French style green beans, ½ cup	0
Cut green beans and potatoes, ½ cup	1
French style green beans, ½ cup	0
Green beans, cut, blue lake, no salt added, ½ cup	0
Green beans, cut, no salt added, ½ cup	0
Green beans, French style, blue lake, no salt added, ½ cup	0
Del Monte Fresh Cut Specialties	
Whole green beans, ½ cup	0
Del Monte Seasoned Vegetables	
French style green beans with roasted garlic, ½ cup	1
Freshlike	
Green beans, French style, ½ cup	0
Giant Steam Ready	
Green beans, extra fine, ¾ cup	0
Glory Foods Seasoned Country Style	
String beans, ½ cup	1
Glory Foods Sensibly Seasoned	
String beans, lower sodium, ½ cup	1
Great Value	
French style green beans, ½ cup	0
Refried beans, fat free, ½ cup	3
Green Giant	
Cut green beans, ½ cup	0
Cut green beans 50% less sodium, ½ cup	0
French style green beans, ½ cup	0

	SmartPoints™ value
Green Giant Fresh	
Green beans, ¾ cup	0
Green Giant Steamers	
Whole green beans, 1 cup frozen	0
GreenLine Quick & Easy	
Green beans, fresh, 1 cup	0
Happy Harvest	
Green beans, cut, ½ cup	0
Kroger	
Green beans, cut, ½ cup	0
Green beans, cut, no salt added, ½ cup	0
Green beans, French style, sliced, ½ cup	0
Libby's	
Cut green beans, ½ cup	0
French style green beans, ½ cup	0
Lucks	
Pinto beans seasoned with pork, ½ cup	3
Margaret Holmes	
Seasoned Italian green beans, ½ cup	1
Pictsweet Deluxe Sides	
Edamame, with sea salt, 1 carton (170 g)	3
Rosarita	
Refried beans, traditional, no fat, ½ cup	3
Seapoint Farms	
Edamame, shelled soybeans, ½ cup	2
Simple Truth Organic	
Garbanzo beans, ½ cup	3
Simply Nature Organic	
Black beans, ½ cup	3

Trader Joe's

Extra fine French green beans, 3 oz	0
Garbanzo beans, ½ cup	3
White kidney beans, ½ cup	3

Beets

Aunt Nellie's

Beets, pickled, sliced, 4 slices (29 g)	1
Harvard beets, ruby red, sweet & sour, ⅓ cup	3

Kroger

Beets, pickled, sliced, 2 slices (30 g)	1

Love Beets

Beets, 3 ½ oz	0

Safie's

Pickled beets, home style sweet, ⅓ cup	5

Trader Joe's

Cut beets in vinaigrette, ⅓ cup	2
Steamed and peeled baby beets, 2 baby beets	0

Brussels Sprouts

Green Giant Steamers

Brussels sprouts with sea salt and cracked pepper, ¾ cup frozen	2

Pictsweet Steam'ables

Lightly sauced baby brussels sprouts, 6 brussels sprouts	2

Cabbage

Full Circle Organic

Kale, baby, 2 cups	0

King's Kimchi

Korean marinated cabbage, spicy, 2 oz	0

Margaret Holmes

Cabbage, seasoned, ½ cup	1

Corn

Birds Eye

Baby gold & white corn, 1 cup	3
Corn on the cob, sweet mini, 1 ear (85 g)	3
Sweet kernel corn, ⅔ cup	3

Birds Eye Steamfresh

Corn, super sweet, ⅔ cup	3
Gold & white corn, premium selects, ⅔ cup	3
Super sweet corn, ⅔ cup	3
Super sweet corn, singles, 1 bag (92 g)	3

Del Monte

Fire roasted corn blend, ½ cup	2
Low sodium whole kernel corn, ½ cup	2
Whole kernel corn, ½ cup	2

Del Monte Fresh Cut

Corn, whole kernel, golden sweet, no salt added, ½ cup	2
Corn, whole kernel, no salt added, ½ cup	2
Golden sweet whole kernel corn, ½ cup	2
Sweet corn cream style, golden, ½ cup	3

Del Monte Fresh Cut Specialties

Whole kernel gold and white super sweet corn, ½ cup	2

Del Monte Summer Crisp

Whole kernel golden sweet corn, ½ cup	3

Freshlike

Sweet corn, whole kernel, ½ cup	5

Green Giant Niblets

Extra sweet whole kernel sweet corn, ½ cup	2

Vegetables

Vegetables

	SmartPoints™ value
Green Giant Steam Crisp	
Mexicorn, ½ cup	3
Mexicorn, canned, ½ cup	3
Niblets whole kernel sweet corn, canned, ½ cup	4
Southwestern style corn, canned, ½ cup	2
White shoepeg whole kernel corn, canned, ½ cup	3
Whole kernel corn super sweet yellow and white, canned, ½ cup	3
Green Giant Steamers	
Cream-style corn, ½ cup	3
Niblets corn, boxed, ⅔ cup frozen	2
White shoepeg corn, boxed, ⅔ cup frozen	3
Hannaford	
Whole kernal corn, frozen fresh, ⅔ cup	3
Happy Harvest	
Sweet corn, whole kernel, ½ cup	2
Kirkland Signature	
Golden sweet corn, ½ cup	2
Kroger	
Corn, golden sweet, ⅔ cup	3
Corn, sweet golden, whole kernel, ½ cup	3
Libby's	
Sweet corn, whole kernel, ½ cup	3
Sweet corn, whole kernel, jumbo-can, ½ cup	3
Whole kernel sweet corn, ½ cup	2
Pictsweet All Natural Steam'ables	
Sweet corn, ¾ cup	3
Trader Joe's	
Roasted corn, ⅔ cup	4

Edamame

	SmartPoints™ value
Birds Eye Steamfresh Premium Selects	
Edamame, in the pod, ⅔ cup	1
Pictsweet Deluxe Steam'ables	
Soybeans, shelled, edamame, ½ cup	3
PictSweet Steam'ables	
Edamame soybeans, in the pod, ½ cup	3
Edamame, seasoned, with sea salt, ½ cup	3
Roland Feng Shui	
Edamame, lightly salted, ¼ cup	3
Seapoint Farms	
Edamame, dry roasted, wasabi, ¼ cup	3
Edamame, lightly salted, ½ cup	2
Soybeans, in pods, edamame, steam bags, ½ cup	2
Sensible Foods	
Crunch dried snacks, roasted edamame, 1 bag (21 g)	2

Giardiniera

	SmartPoints™ value
Tiffes	
Okra, Louisiana, mild pickled, 2 pods (28 g)	0

Hominy

	SmartPoints™ value
Bush's Best	
Hominy, golden, ½ cup	2

Lentils

	SmartPoints™ value
Tasty Bite	
Madras lentils indian cuisine, ½ pack (143 g)	5
Trader Joe's	
Red split lentils, ¼ cup dry	3

Mixed Vegetables

Birds Eye

Baby corn bean and pea mix frozen, ¾ cup	2
Mixed vegetables, classic, 3 cups	2
Stir-fry vegetables, broccoli, 3 cups	0
Stir-fry vegetables, green bean, 3 cups	3
Stir-fry vegetables, pepper, 3 cups	0

Birds Eye C&W

The ultimate southwest blend, ⅔ cup	3

Birds Eye Recipe Ready

Broccoli stir fry, 1 cup	0
Grilling blend mix of zucchini yellow squash red onions and red bell peppers, ¾ cup	0
Southwest blend, ⅔ cup	3
Tri color pepper and onion blend, ¾ cup	0

Birds Eye Steamfresh

Baby potato blend, ¾ cup	1
Broccoli & cauliflower, 3 cups	0
Broccoli, carrots, sugar snap peas & water chestnuts, ¾ cup	0
Broccoli, cauliflower, & carrots, 3 cups	0
Lightly seasoned Asian medley, 1 cup	2
Vegetables, fresh frozen, baby broccoli blend, 1 cup	2
Vegetables, fresh frozen, Italian blend, 3 cups	1
Vegetables, lightly sauced, ¾ cup	2

Birds Eye Steamfresh Chef's Favorites

Italian green beans lightly sauced, 1 ¼ cups	2

Daily Chef

Normandy blend, steamable, 1 cup	0
Steamable mixed vegetables, ⅔ cup	2

Del Monte Fresh Cut Specialties

Seasoned green beans with onions, red peppers and garlic, ½ cup	0

Del Monte Specialties

Peas & carrots, ½ cup	2

Del Monte Whole Kernel

Southwest corn with poblano and red peppers, ½ cup	2

Dole

American blend, 1 ½ cups	0
Classic iceberg, 1 ½ cups	0
Greener selection, 1 ½ cups	0
Lettuce, classic iceberg, 1 ½ cups	0
Very veggie blend, 1 ½ cups	0

Dole Chopped

Asian blend salad, 1 ½ cups	0
Summer garden blend salad, 1 ½ cups	0

Dole Fresh Discoveries

Field greens, 3 oz	0

Dole Fresh Favorites

Classic iceberg, 3 oz	0

Eat Smart

Broccoli carrots and cauliflower, ¼ packet (85 g)	0

Essential Everyday

Steamy vegetables, broccoli, cauliflower & carrots, ⅔ cup	0

Flav-R-Pac

Nantucket vegetable blend with cranberries, 1 cup	2
Northwest vegetable blend, 1 cup	0

Food Club

Mixed vegetables, freshly frozen, ¾ cup	2

Fresh Express

Fancy greens, 2 ½ cups	0
Iceberg garden salad, 1 ½ cups	0
Iceberg lettuce, red cabbage & carrots, 1 ½ cups	0

Vegetables

	SmartPoints™ value
Fresh Express Veggie Medleys	
Farmers garden salad, 2 cups	0
Freshlike	
California blend, family pack, 1 cup	0
Giant	
Onions & peppers, chopped, 1 cup	0
Giant Steam Ready	
Broccoli & cauliflower, ¾ cup	0
Great Value	
Broccoli & cauliflower, steamable, 1 cup	0
Mixed vegetables, ⅔ cup	2
Mixed vegetables, steamable, 3 cups	0
Steamable grilled vegetables, ¾ cup	2
Vegetable blend, ½ cup	2
Green Giant Fresh	
Broccoli slaw, ¾ cup	0
Vegetable medley broccoli, carrots and snow peas, ¾ cup	0
Green Giant Steamers	
Garden vegetable medley, 1 cup frozen	2
Teriyaki vegetables, 1 ¼ cups	2
Green Giant Valley Fresh Steamers	
Valley blend (colorful blend of vegetables lightly tossed in a butter sauce), 1 ¼ cups frozen	1
Hannaford	
Broccoli, cauliflower & carrots, 1 cup	0
Hy-Vee Grand Selections	
Gourmet vegetables, fresh frozen, normandy blend, 1 cup	0
Hy-Vee Steam Quick	
Mixed vegetables, ⅔ cup	2

	SmartPoints™ value
Kirkland Signature	
Normandy style vegetable blend, 1 cup	0
Organic normandy vegetables, 1 cup	0
Premium stir fry vegetables, 3 oz	1
Kroger	
Mixed vegetables, ½ cup	2
Peas & carrots, ⅔ cup	2
Kroger Meal-Ready Sides	
Vegetables, California style, ¾ cup	0
Vegetables, Mexican style, ¾ cup	2
Vegetables, stir-fry, 1 cup	0
Kroger Value Recipe Beginnings	
3 pepper and onion blend, 1 cup	0
Mann's	
Broccoli cole slaw, 3 oz	0
Rainbow salad, 3 oz	0
Margaret Holmes	
Hoppin' john, with blackeye peas, tomatoes, onions & jalapeños, ½ cup	3
Succotash, triple, ½ cup	2
Tomatoes okra and corn, ½ cup	2
Meijer	
California blend, steamable, ¾ cup	0
Frozen mixed vegetables, ⅔ cup	2
Ore-Ida	
Potatoes o'brien with onions and peppers, ¾ cup	2
Peas of Mind Veggie Wedgies	
Cauliflower fries, baked, 14 pieces (85 g)	2
Pictsweet	
Mixed vegetables, family size, ⅔ cup	2

Pictsweet Steam'ables

Broccoli florets, cauliflower and carrots, 1 cup	0
Green and yellow whole beans and baby carrots, 1 cup	0
Harvest vegetables, seasoned, 1 cup	2

Private Selection

Broccoli and carrots, fresh, 3 oz	0
Broccoli and cauliflower, fresh, 3 oz	0
Broccoli slaw, fresh, 3 oz	0
Vegetable medley, broccoli, cauliflower, carrots, fresh, 3 oz	0

Publix

Vegetables, mixed, steam in bag, ⅔ cup	2
Safeway Farms	
Broccoli & cauliflower, steam in bag, 1 cup	0
Vegetable medley, steam in bag, 1 cup	0

ShopRite

Stir-fry, Asian, steam in bag!, ⅔ cup	0
Vegetables, California style, 1 cup	0
Winter mix vegetables, 1 cup	0

Trader Joe's

Cruciferous crunch collection mixed greens, 3 cups	0
Dolmas, 4 dolmas (110 g)	4
Fire roasted bell peppers and onions, ¾ cup	0
Healthy 8 chopped veggie mix, ¾ cup	0
Stir fry vegetables, ½ cup	1

Trader Joe's Fresh Cut and Ready

Veggie stir fry, 1 cup	0

Veg All Steam Supreme

Broccoli florets, cauliflower, whole baby carrots, 3 cups	0
Mixed vegetables, original, 3 cups	2
Winter blend, broccoli florets and cauliflower, 3 cups	0

Onions

French's

French fried onions, cheddar, 2 Tbsp	2
French fried onions, original, 2 Tbsp	2
Original French fried onions, 2 Tbsp	2

Fresh Gourmet

Lightly salted crispy onions, 1 ½ Tbsp	1
Onions, crispy, garlic pepper, 1 ½ Tbsp	1

Kroger

Onions, crispy fried, 2 Tbsp	2

Loeb's

Onion crunch, 2 Tbsp	2

New York Texas Toast

Lightly salted crispy onions, 2 Tbsp	2

Trader Joe's

Gourmet fried onion pieces, 2 Tbsp	2

Peas, Dried

Allens

Blackeyed peas, with bacon, ½ cup	3

Bush's Best

Blackeye peas, with snaps, ½ cup	2
Crowder peas, ½ cup	2
Field peas with snaps, ½ cup	2
Peas, blackeye, ½ cup	2
Purple hull peas, ½ cup	2

Vegetables

Vegetables

	SmartPoints™ value
Eden Organic	
Black eyed peas, ½ cup	2
Goya	
Blackeye peas, premium, ½ cup	2
Chick peas, premium, ½ cup	3
Hanover	
Peas, blackeye, ½ cup	2
Kroger	
Peas, blackeye, ½ cup	3
Margaret Holmes	
Peas & snaps, field, seasoned, ½ cup	3
Pictsweet	
Blackeye peas, ½ cup	3
Pictsweet Premium	
Field peas with snaps, ½ cup	3
Swad	
Toor dal, ¼ cup	3
Trappey's	
Black eye peas, ½ cup	3

Peas, Other

	SmartPoints™ value
Allens	
Blackeyed peas with snaps, ½ cup	3
Field peas and snaps, seasoned, ½ cup	3
Purple hull peas, ½ cup	3
Birds Eye	
Baby sweet peas, ⅔ cup	2
Sweet garden peas, ⅔ cup	2
Birds Eye Steamfresh	
Sweet peas, family size, ⅔ cup	2
Sweet peas, singles, 1 single (91 g)	2
Calbee Harvest Snaps	
Caesar snapea crisps, 22 pieces (28 g)	3
Del Monte	
Low sodium sweet peas, ½ cup	3

	SmartPoints™ value
Del Monte Fresh Cut	
Sweet peas, ½ cup	2
Sweet peas, no salt added, ½ cup	2
Giant Steam Ready	
Green peas, ⅔ cup	2
Great Value	
Sweet peas, ⅔ cup	0
Green Giant	
Sweet peas, ½ cup	2
Green Giant Steamers	
Sweet peas, ⅔ cup	2
Hapi	
Peas, wasabi, hot, 55 pieces (28 g)	4
Kroger	
Peas, green, ⅔ cup	2
Le Sueur	
Early peas, very young small, ½ cup	2
Very young small sweet peas, ½ cup	2
Libby's	
Sweet peas, ½ cup	2
Mann's	
Stringless sugar snap peas, 1 cup	0
Pictsweet	
Purple hull peas, ½ cup	3
Trader Joe's	
English peas, ⅔ cup	3

Potatoes

	SmartPoints™ value
Alexia	
Fries, house cut, with sea salt, 3 oz	4
Hashed browns, ⅔ cup	2
Julienne fries, sweet potato, family size, 12 pieces (84 g)	5
Julienne fries, with chipotle seasoning, spicy sweet potato, 30 pieces (84 g)	6

	SmartPoints™ value
Julienne fries, yukon gold, with sea salt, 24 pieces (85 g)	4
Seasoned fries, sweet potato, waffle cut, 1 cup	4
Sweet potato, crispy bite-sized puffs, ⅔ cup	5
Sweet potato, julienne fries, 12 pieces (84 g)	5
Alexia Smart Classics	
Fries, crinkle cut, roasted, with sea salt, 12 pieces (84 g)	3
Fries, straight cut, roasted, with sea salt, 12 pieces (84 g)	3
Potatoes, tri-cut, roasted, with sea salt, ¾ cup	3
Bob Evans	
Mashed potatoes, cheddar, ½ cup	6
Mashed potatoes, garlic, ½ cup	5
Mashed potatoes, original, 1 bowl (170 g)	7
Mashed potatoes, original, twin pack, ½ cup	5
Mashed potatoes, sour cream & chives, ½ cup	5
Bob Evans Top Bake	
Hash brown casserole, ⅔ cup	8
Boulder Canyon Natural Foods	
Sweet potato fries, baked, lightly salted, 20 fries (28 g)	4
Cascadian Farm	
Fries, shoe string, 30 pieces (85 g)	3
Country Crock Simple Ideas	
Garlic mashed potatoes (serves 5), 1 serving (142 g)	5
Crystal Farms	
O'brien hash browns, ⅔ cup	2
Steakhouse seasoned diced potatoes, ⅔ cup	2

	SmartPoints™ value
Del Monte Fresh Cut	
Diced new potatoes, ½ cup	2
Sliced new potatoes, ⅔ cup	2
Whole new potatoes, 2 potatoes (158 g)	2
Express Bake PotatOH!	
Russet potato, small, 1 (170 g)	4
Golden Grill Russet	
Premium hashbrown potatoes, ⅓ cup	2
Great Value	
French fried potatoes, crinkle cut, 15 pieces (84 g)	4
Fries, seasoned, 22 pieces (84 g)	5
Hash brown patties, 1 patty (64 g)	5
Potato wedges, deli style, seasoned, 8 pieces (84 g)	4
Steak fries, 3 oz	4
Taters, 10 pieces (84 g)	5
Hannaford	
Curly fries, 20 pieces (85 g)	6
Hashbrowns, country style, 3 oz	2
Hormel Country Crock Side Dishes	
Mashed potatoes, loaded, ⅔ cup	7
Hy-Vee	
Potatoes, hash brown, country style, shredded, 1 cup	2
Idaho Spuds	
Classic flakes mashed potatoes, ½ cup dry	2
Idahoan	
Mashed potatoes, bacon & cheddar chipotle, ¼ cup dry	4
Mashed potatoes, microwaveable, buttery homestyle, ¼ cup dry	4
Idahoan Microwavable	
Roasted garlic mashed potatoes, ¼ cup dry	4

Vegetables

Vegetables

	SmartPoints™ value
Idahoan Premium Steakhouse	
Cheesy hashbrown potatoes, ½ cup dry	5
Joy of Cooking	
Red potato halves, roasted, ¾ cup	3
Klondike Goldust Express	
Baby potatoes, ⅓ package (148 g)	3
Klondike Rose Express	
Baby Idaho potatoes, ⅓ package (148 g)	3
Kroger	
Crinkle cut sweet potato fries, 16 pieces (85 g)	6
Crinkle fries, 18 pieces (85 g)	4
Crispy fries, 18 pieces (85 g)	4
Extra crispy crinkle cut fries, 18 pieces (85 g)	5
Hash browns, country style, 3 oz	2
Potatoes, diced, hash browns, southern style, 3 oz	2
Potatoes, diced, with onions & peppers, potatoes o'brien, 3 oz	2
Kroger Meals Made Simple	
Mashed potatoes, homestyle, ½ cup	6
McCain	
Cross trax, seasoned, 3 oz	5
French fried potatoes, classic cut, 3 oz	3
French fried potatoes, crinkle cut, 18 pieces (82 g)	4
Fries, 5 minute, 3 oz	4
Fries, crinkle cut, sweet potato, 3 oz	5
McCain Purely Potatoes	
Potatoes, premium yellow, whole baby, skin on, 3 oz	3
Omaha Steaks	
Sweet potato steak fries, 3 oz	5

	SmartPoints™ value
Ore-Ida	
Cottage fries, 12 pieces (84 g)	4
Country style hash browns, 1 cup	2
Crispers!, 20 pieces (84 g)	7
Crispy crowns!, 11 pieces (84 g)	6
Crispy crunchies!, 3 oz	5
Extra crispy fast food fries, 27 pieces (84 g)	5
French fried potatoes, extra crispy, fast food fries, family size!, 27 pieces (84 g)	5
French fries, country style, 3 oz	4
Hash browns, ⅔ cup	2
Ore-Ida Easy Fries	
French fried potatoes, extra crispy, golden fries, 36 pieces (84 g)	6
Ore-Ida Simply	
Country style French fries, 13 pieces (84 g)	4
Cracked black pepper and sea salt French fries, 13 pieces (84 g)	4
Homestyle potato wedges, 7 pieces (84 g)	4
Roasted garlic and herbs potato wedges, 7 pieces (84 g)	4
Ore-Ida Steam n' Mash	
Potatoes, cut russet, ¾ cup	2
Parade	
Potatoes, white, small whole, ⅔ cup	3
Red Robin	
Fries, steak, seasoned, 10 pieces (84 g)	4
Reser's Fine Foods Main St. Bistro	
Scalloped potatoes, baked, ⅔ cup	8
S&W	
Potatoes, new, small, whole, 2 potatoes (158 g)	2
Safeway	
Potatoes, russet, 1 potato (148 g)	3
Potatoes, russet, jumbo, 12 oz	8

Season's Choice

French fried potatoes, crinkle cut,
16 pieces (85 g) — 3

ShopRite

Frozen potato patties, hashbrowns,
1 patty (60 g) — 4

Hashbrowns, ⅔ cup — 2

Simply Potatoes

Diced potatoes, with onion, ⅔ cup — 2

Mashed potatoes, ⅔ cup — 6

Mashed potatoes, country style,
½ cup — 4

Mashed potatoes, garlic, ½ cup — 5

New potato wedges, ½ cup — 2

Sliced home fries, ⅔ cup — 3

Sour cream and chive mashed
potatoes, ½ cup — 5

Southwest style hash browns,
⅔ cup — 2

Simply Potatoes Diner's Choice

Mashed potatoes, traditional,
family size, ½ cup — 5

Simply Spuds Steamables

Petite sweet potato, 1 potato (130 g) — 4

Spartan

Potatoes, cubed, hash brown
potatoes, southern style, 3 oz — 2

Potatoes, shredded hashbrowns,
3 oz — 2

Wegman's

Fries, sweet potato,
18 pieces (85 g) — 5

Wegman's Food You Feel Good About

Potato medley, fingerling,
1 ⅓ cups chopped — 4

Potatoes, baby Dutch yellow,
¾ cup diced — 2

Pumpkin

Libbys

100% pure pumpkin, ½ cup — 0

Sauerkraut

Claussen

Sauerkraut, premium crisp, ¼ cup — 0

Glory Foods Seasoned Southern Style

Cabbage, country, ½ cup — 1

Silver Floss Krrrrisp Kraut

Sauerkraut, barrel cured, 2 Tbsp — 0

Vlasic

Sauerkraut, old fashioned, ¼ cup — 0

Seaweed

Kirkland Signature

Roasted seasoned seaweed
(serves 5), 1 serving (3.4 g) — 0

Spinach

Birds Eye

Creamed spinach, ½ cup — 3

Seabrook

Creamed spinach, ½ cup — 4

Tasty Bite

Kashmir spinach, ½ pack (143 g) — 4

Squash & Zucchini

Del Monte Fresh Cut Specialties

Zucchini, ½ cup — 1

Margaret Holmes

Squash, with vidalia onions, ½ cup — 1

McKenzie's Southland

Butternut squash, microwavable,
½ cup — 3

Sugar Snap Peas

Green Giant Fresh

Sugar snap peas, 1 ⅓ cups — 0

Green Giant Steamers

Sugar snap peas, ¾ cup frozen — 2

Vegetables

Vegetables

Tomato Paste & Puree

Contadina

Tomato paste, 2 Tbsp	1

Hunt's

Basil garlic and oregano tomato sauce, ¼ cup	0
Sauce, tomatoes, ¼ cup	0
Tomato paste, 2 Tbsp	1
Tomato sauce, ¼ cup	0
Tomato sauce, roasted garlic flavor, ¼ cup	1

Tomatoes

Bella Sun

Tomatoes, sun dried, julienne-cut, ½ oz	0

California Sun Dry

Smoked sun dried tomatoes, julienne cut, ½ oz	0
Sun dried tomatoes, halves, ½ oz	0
Sun dried tomatoes, julienne cut, ½ oz	0
Sun-dried julienne cut tomatoes, with herbs, 2 Tbsp	1

Cherubs

Heavenly salad tomatoes, ½ package (149 g)	0

Del Monte

Tomatoes, stewed, original recipe, ½ cup	1

Giant/Stop & Shop

Grape tomatoes, 1 cup	0

Hunt's

Fire roasted diced tomatoes with garlic, ½ cup	0
Tomato sauce no salt added, ¼ cup	0
Tomatoes, diced, ½ cup	0
Tomatoes, diced, basil, garlic & oregano, ½ cup	2
Tomatoes, diced, no salt added, ½ cup	0
Tomatoes, petite diced, ½ cup	0

Hunt's No Salt Added

Basil garlic and oregano diced tomatoes, ½ cup	0

Margaret Holmes

Tomatoes and okra, southern style blend, ½ cup	1

NatureSweet Glorys

Perfect ingredient tomatoes, 1 (62 g)	0

NatureSweet Sunbursts

Sweet golden tomatoes, 1 tomato	0

Regal

Sundried tomato, 1 Tbsp	0

Ro-Tel

Diced tomatoes & green chilies, mild, ½ cup	0
Diced tomatoes & green chilies, original, ½ cup	0
Diced tomatoes, with habaneros, hot, ½ cup	0
Diced, tomatoes, Mexican lime & cilantro, ½ cup	0

Sunset Zima

Sweet orange tomatoes, 1 tomato	0

Yuca

Goya

Yuca, 2 pieces (199 g)	3

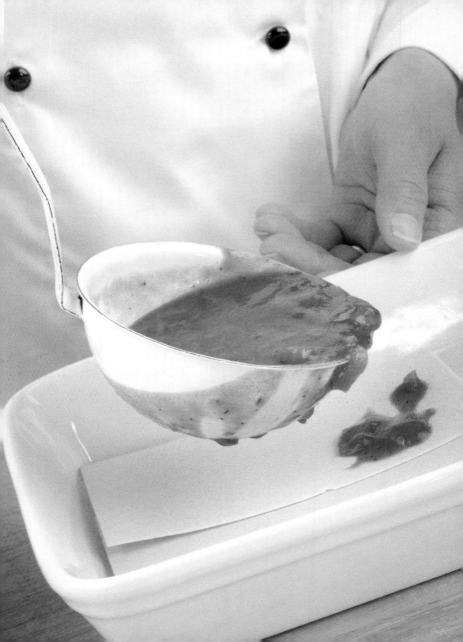

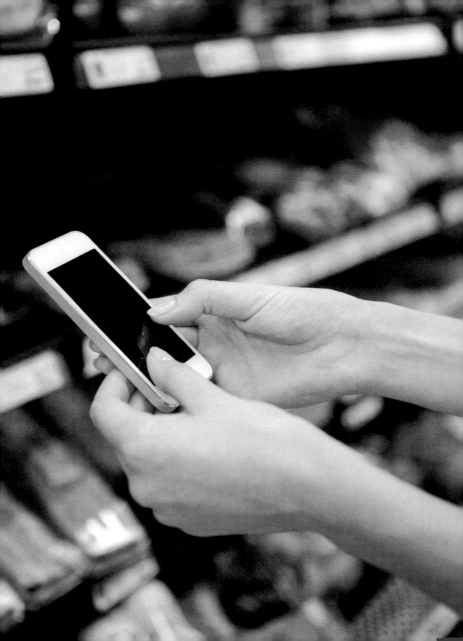

weightwatchers
Food Products

Weight Watchers Food Products

Frozen Entrées

Weight Watchers Smart Ones Classic Favorites

Angel hair marinara, 1 entrée	7
Broccoli and cheddar roasted potatoes, 1 entrée	7
Chicken enchiladas Suiza, 1 entrée	9
Chicken oriental, 1 entrée	7
Creamy pasta Romano with spinach, 1 entrée	7
Creamy rigatoni with broccoli and chicken, 1 entrée	7
Fettuccini Alfredo, 1 entrée	7
Lasagna bake with meat sauce, 1 entrée	7
Lasagna Florentine, 1 entrée	11
Lemon herb chicken piccata, 1 entrée	5
Macaroni and cheese, 1 entrée	8
Mini rigatoni with vodka cream sauce, 1 entrée	8
Pasta primavera, 1 entrée	7
Pasta with ricotta and spinach, 1 entrée	9
Ravioli Florentine, 1 entrée	9
Santa Fe style rice and beans, 1 entrée	9
Sesame noodles with vegetables, 1 entrée	8
Spaghetti with meat sauce, 1 entrée	8
Spicy Szechuan style vegetables, 1 entrée	8
Swedish meatballs, 1 entrée	9
Three cheese macaroni, 1 entrée	9
Three cheese ziti marinara, 1 entrée	9
Traditional lasagna with meat sauce, 1 entrée	10
Tuna noodle gratin, 1 entrée	7
Vegetable fried rice, 1 entrée	9

Weight Watchers Smart Ones Smart Creations

Bacon macaroni & cheese, 1 entrée	9
Chicken carbonara, 1 entrée	8
Chicken fajitas, 1 entrée	7
Chicken fettuccini, 1 entrée	8
Chicken mesquite, 1 entrée	7
Chicken parmesan, 1 entrée	7
Chicken Santa Fe, 1 entrée	4
Chicken strips and fries, 1 entrée	9
Chicken strips with sweet potato fries, 1 entrée	8
Chipotle lime chicken, 1 entrée	4
Creamy basil chicken with broccoli, 1 entrée	5
Crustless chicken pot pie, 1 entrée	5
Fish and chips, 1 entrée	9
Home style beef pot roast, 1 entrée	4
Homestyle turkey breast with stuffing, 1 entrée	7
Meatloaf, 1 entrée	8
Orange sesame chicken, 1 entrée	8
Pulled pork & black beans, 1 entrée	7
Roast beef in gravy, 1 entrée	6
Roasted chicken with herb gravy, 1 entrée	4
Salisbury steak, 1 entrée	7
Slow roasted turkey breast, 1 entrée	5
Spicy chicken strips with salt & pepper fries, 1 entrée	9
Steak fajitas, 1 entrée	8
Teriyaki chicken and vegetables, 1 entrée	8
Thai style chicken and rice noodles, 1 entrée	8
Three cheese ziti marinara with meatballs, 1 entrée	10
Tomato basil chicken with spinach, 1 entrée	4

Frozen Pizzas

Weight Watchers Smart Ones Classic Favorites

Thin crust cheese pizza, 1 pizza	9
Thin crust pepperoni pizza, 1 pizza	10

Weight Watchers Smart Ones Smart Anytime

Brick oven style pizza pepperoni, 1 pizza	12
Cheese mini pizza, 4 pieces	8
Pepperoni mini pizzas, 1 tray	9

Frozen Burgers/Sliders

Weight Watchers Smart Ones Smart Anytime

Chicken slider, 1 sandwich	6
Mini cheeseburger, 1 burger	6
Spicy chicken slider, 1 sandwich	6

Frozen Chicken

Weight Watchers

Chicken breasts, 1 breast	1
Chicken burger, 1 burger	2
Chicken tenders, 1 tender	1

Frozen Quesadilla/Wraps

Weight Watchers Smart Ones Smart Anytime

Chicken quesadilla, 1 piece	5
Chicken ranchero mini wraps, 2 wraps	7

Frozen Soups

Weight Watchers Smart Ones Classic Favorites

Loaded potato soup, 1 bowl	5
Southwest style vegetable soup, 1 bowl	4

Frozen Breakfasts

Weight Watchers Smart Ones Smart Beginnings

Apple and cinnamon oatmeal, 1 cup	7
Breakfast quesadilla, 1 item	7
Cheesy scramble with hashbrowns, 1 entrée	6
English muffin sandwich Canadian style turkey bacon, 1 sandwich	6
English muffin sandwich egg whites and cheese, 1 sandwich	6
English muffin sandwich with turkey sausage, 1 sandwich	7
English muffin turkey sausage sandwich, 1 sandwich	7
French toast with turkey sausage, 1 entrée	10
Maple and brown sugar oatmeal, 1 cup	7
Pancakes with turkey sausage, 1 entrée	10
Peaches and cream oatmeal, 1 cup	6
Smart morning wrap, egg, sausage and cheese, 2 pieces	7
Three cheese omelet, 1 entrée	6

Frozen Desserts

Weight Watchers Smart Ones Smart Delights

Chocolate chip cookie dough sundae, 1 dessert	6
Peanut butter cup sundae, 1 dessert	6
Strawberry shortcake, 1 dessert	5

Frozen Novelties

Weight Watchers

Dark chocolate mint bars, 1 bar	3
Dark chocolate raspberry bars, 1 bar	3
Giant chocolate fudge bars, 1 bar	4
Snack size chocolate fudge bars, 1 bar	2

Weight Watchers Food Products

Weight Watchers Food Products

	SmartPoints™ value
Snack size cookies & cream bars, 1 bar	4
Snack size divine triple chocolate bars, 1 bar	4
Snack size double caramel swirl cones, 1 cone	4
Snack size English toffee crunch bars, 1 bar	4
Snack size mocha latte bars, 1 bar	2
Snack size peanut butter caramel candy bars, 1 bar	4
Snack size salted caramel bars, 1 bar	4
Snack size vanilla fudge swirl cones, 1 cone	4

Frozen Smoothies

Weight Watchers Smart Ones Smart Delights

Mixed berry smoothie, 1 cup	5
Strawberry banana smoothie, 1 cup	5
Tropical fruit smoothie, 1 cup	5

Cheese

Weight Watchers Cheese Shreds

Reduced fat Mexican style blend, ⅓ cup	3
Reduced fat shredded mozzarella cheese, ⅓ cup	2

Weight Watchers Cheese Singles

Reduced fat cheese singles, 1 slice	2
Reduced fat pepper jack singles, 1 slice	1

Weight Watchers Cheese Snacks

Light jalapeño string cheese, 1 stick	1
Natural light mozzarella string cheese, 1 stick	1
Natural light smoked mozzarella string cheese, 1 stick	1
Natural reduced fat colby jack cheese stick, 1 stick	2
Reduced fat mild cheddar cheese sticks, 1 stick	2

	SmartPoints™ value
Weight Watchers Cheese Wedge	
Garlic and herb cheese wedge, 1 wedge	1
Jalapeño pepper cheese wedge, 1 wedge	1
Original Swiss cheese wedge, 1 wedge	1
Weight Watchers Cream Cheese	
Reduced fat cream cheese spread, 1 portion cup	3
Reduced fat soft chive and onion cream cheese spread, 2 Tbsp	5
Reduced fat soft strawberry cream cheese spread, 2 Tbsp	5
Reduced fat whipped cream cheese spread, 2 Tbsp	3

Bread

Weight Watchers

100% whole wheat bread, 2 slices	2
Multi-grain bread, 2 slices	2
Seedless rye bread, 2 slices	2

Cereal

Weight Watchers

Blueberry pomegranate crunch cereal, ¾ cup	4
Chocolate frosted shredded wheat cereal, 1 cup	8
Frosted shredded wheat with protein cereal, 1 cup	7
Oat clusters with almonds cereal, ¾ cup	4
Oat clusters with cherries and almonds cereal, ¾ cup	4
Whole grain honey nut toasted oats cereal, 1 cup	4

Sweet Baked Goods

Weight Watchers

Carrot crème cake, 1 cake	4
Chocolate brownie, 1 brownie	6
Chocolate chip cookie, 1 cookie	4

Chocolate crème cake, 1 cake	4
Coffee cake, 1 cake	5
Lemon crème cake, 1 cake	4
Mint chocolate brownie bliss, 1 brownie	4
Oatmeal raisin cookie, 1 cookie	4
Peanut butter brownie bliss, 1 brownie	4
Red velvet crème cake, 1 cake	4
Salted caramel brownie bliss, 1 brownie	5
Triple chocolate brownie bliss, 1 brownie	4

Chocolate Candy

Weight Watchers by Whitman's

Bite size dark chocolates, 1 pouch	5
Bite size red velvet chocolates, 1 pouch	5
Caramel bite size covered in milk chocolate, 1 pouch	6
Caramel chocolates, 3 pieces	8
Caramel with crispies chocolates, 3 pieces	7
Chocolate mousse dark chocolates, 3 pieces	6
Coconut chocolates, 3 pieces	7
English toffee chocolate candies, 3 pieces	6
Mint patties dark chocolate candies, 3 pieces	6
Pecan crown bite size chocolates, 1 pouch	6
Pecan crowns chocolates, 3 pieces	7

In-Meeting Products

Weight Watchers Café Creations

Mucho mocha, 1 packet	0
Vanilla bean, 1 packet	0

Weight Watchers Candies

Blackberry sugar free candies, 8 candies	1
Citrus drops sugar free candies, 11 candies	1
Strawberry sugar free candies, 8 candies	1

Weight Watchers Crunchy Snacks

Cheddar twists, 1 pouch	2
Garlic parmesan sticks, 1 pouch	2
Original mini pretzel thins, 1 pouch	2
Popped barbeque potato crisps, 1 pouch	2
Popped salt & vinegar potato crisps, 1 pouch	2
Popped sea salt hummus chips, 1 pouch	2

Weight Watchers Snack Bars

Sweet & salty toffee twist, 1 bar	4

Weight Watchers Mini Bars

Chocolate caramel, 1 bar	2
Chocolate pretzel blast, 1 bar	2
Mint cookie crisp, 1 bar	2
Peanut butter cookie explosion, 1 bar	3
So-good salted caramel, 1 bar	3

Weight Watchers Oatmeal

Blueberry vanilla, 1 container	3
Maple brown sugar, 1 container	3

Weight Watchers Smoothies

Creamy chocolate, 1 slim pack	2
French vanilla, 1 slim pack	2

Weight Watchers Water Enhancers

Berry pomegranate, 2 ml	0
Southern sweet tea, 2 ml	0

Weight Watchers Food Products

NOTE: The Weight Watchers line of food products is continuously being revised to meet your needs and help you follow the Weight Watchers program. So although the information for the products listed here was current at the time this guide was compiled, you might find that things are different once a product is purchased. Always check product packaging for the latest information, including SmartPoints values, when you purchase one of these products.

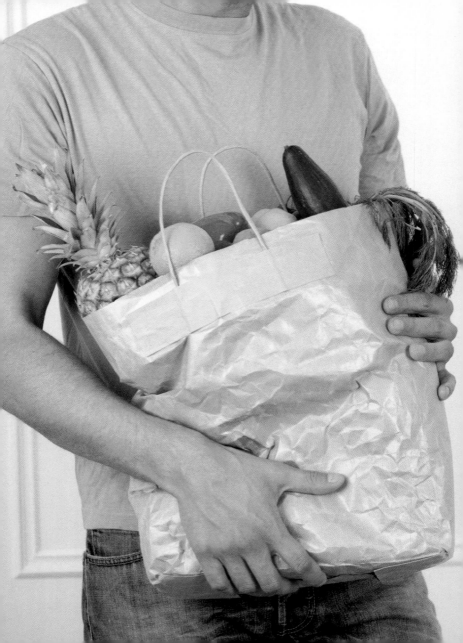

index

Index

Index

Index